THE
DOCTORS' BOOK OF
H⬤ME
REMEDIES

THE
DOCTORS' BOOK OF
H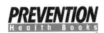ME
REMEDIES

Simple, doctor-approved

self-care solutions for over

140 common health conditions

General Editor: Dr Stephen Amiel

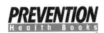
PREVENTION
Health Books

RODALE

This edition first published in the UK in 2004 by
Rodale Ltd
7-10 Chandos Place
London W1G 9AD
www.rodale.co.uk

Printed and bound in the UK by CPI Bath using acid-free paper from sustainable
sources
1 3 5 7 9 8 6 4 2

UK consultants: Dr Stephen Amiel, Sue Livingston and Douglas Schar
Edited by Helen Spence
Designed by Christina Gaugler and Emma Ashby
Index by Hilary Bird

A CIP record for this book is available from the British Library
ISBN 1–4050–4182–X

This paperback edition distributed to the book trade by Pan Macmillan Ltd

Notice
This book is intended as a reference volume only, not as a medical manual. The
information given here is designed to help you make informed decisions about your
health in collaboration with your doctor. It is not intended as a substitute for any
treatment that may have been prescribed by your doctor. If you suspect that you have
a medical problem, we urge you to seek competent medical help.

Beginning on page 570, you will find safe use guidelines for the supplements
recommended in this book that will help you to use these remedies safely and wisely.

Mention of specific companies, organizations or authorities does not imply endorsement by the publisher or contributors, nor does mention of specific companies,
organizations or authorities imply that they endorse this book. Mention of specific
drugs by brand name does not imply endorsement of those particular products.

Internet addresses and phone numbers were accurate at the time of going to press.

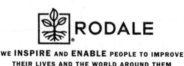

RODALE
WE **INSPIRE** AND **ENABLE** PEOPLE TO IMPROVE
THEIR LIVES AND THE WORLD AROUND THEM

About *Prevention* Health Books

The editors of *Prevention* Health Books are dedicated to providing you with authoritative, trustworthy and innovative advice for a healthy, active lifestyle. In all of our books, our goal is to keep you thoroughly informed about the latest breakthroughs in natural healing, medical research, alternative health, herbs, nutrition, fitness and weight loss. We cut through the confusion of today's conflicting health reports to deliver clear, concise health information that you can trust. And we explain in practical terms what each new breakthrough means to you, so you can take immediate, practical steps to improve your health and well-being.

Every recommendation in *Prevention* Health Books is based upon reliable sources, including interviews with qualified health professionals. In addition, we retain top-level health practitioners who serve on our board of advisors. *Prevention* Health Books are thoroughly fact-checked for accuracy, and we make every effort to verify recommendations, dosages and cautions.

The advice in this book will help to keep you well-informed about your personal choices in healthcare – to help you lead a happier, healthier and longer life.

CONTENTS

G

H

I

J, K

L

M

N

O, P

R

S

T

U, V

W

FOREWORD

It's a great job, being a GP, but it can also be a frustrating one. There's often so much to discuss, and so little time! And if it's frustrating for us GPs, what must it be like for you, our patients?

It can be hard to get an appointment, and then it can often feel like a rush. You may not feel there's enough time for you to ask all the questions you want to about what's wrong with you, and why. Or you don't feel you can bother the doctor with a worry that might sound trivial. Or you want to discuss the latest health scare or wonder drug, but can't. Or maybe you want to know how to help yourself, so that next time you don't have to come to the doctor at all.

That's why *The Doctors' Book of Home Remedies* is such a godsend, both to people who don't want to become patients, and to their doctors. Thousands of nuggets of common sense and good advice have been brought together by eminent doctors, herbalists and pharmacists about 140 of the ailments and worries that can afflict us and our families at any time. The knowledge, wisdom and experience of medical and complementary medicine specialists are combined with folklore remedies proven to work, tried-and-trusted grandmothers' tips and simple kitchen cures.

For this first-ever UK edition (of a book that has already sold 16 million copies worldwide in its original US edition), every tip has been given the once-over, and many completely new ones have been added by our team of British experts. Everything's been updated, checked against the best available evidence for its effectiveness and safety, and where necessary adapted in line with our healthcare system and UK guidelines.

This book is about helping people to help themselves. It won't stop you from getting ill, although there is plenty of good advice in it about how to stay healthy.

Did you know, for example:

- that stopping smoking (apart from quite possibly saving your life) will improve bad breath, irritable bowel syndrome, snoring, ear infections, angina, varicose veins and a host of other problems;

- that you shouldn't take aspirin if you have a black eye – aspirin is an anticoagulant, which means it delays blood clotting;

- that if you are bitten or stung by an insect, you can ease swelling and pain if you moisten the area and rub it with an aspirin tablet;

- that stretch receptors in your jaw send messages to your brain's appetite centre: chew your food more, and your brain tells you you're full sooner – chew more, eat less, lose weight!

- that you can help your PMS (premenstrual syndrome) by cutting down on coffee and alcohol, taking the herbal remedies chasteberry and black cohosh, or making love?

From minor but irritating problems to major and life-threatening illnesses, *The Doctors' Book of Home Remedies* offers reassuring and easy-to-follow advice on what you can do to prevent illness, how to help yourself when you are unwell, and – most importantly – tells you when you really do need to see a doctor.

So I don't expect I'll be put out of a job by this book. If it does its job properly, it will even occasionally alert you to come to the doctor sooner. That's good: I love my work, and I love seeing people who need to see me. But I feel even better when people no longer need my help – and better still when they don't need to see me in the first place.

That's where this book comes in. It's the 'Doctors' Book' in two senses. Unlike many self-help books, which are often written by non-doctors, and sometimes with an anti-doctor axe to grind, this one is largely written by doctors, although it embraces scores of tips from complementary therapists and other health professionals, too. And, because there's so much in the book that we doctors would love to shout about from the rooftops, but don't have the opportunity or time to, whether about staying healthy or treating illness yourself, it's a book written for doctors too.

They say that knowledge is power. When it comes to illness, I have no doubt that people who understand what is wrong with them, who know what can be done to help, and who have the power to do something about it themselves, are half way to getting better already. So I'm delighted to be associated with *The Doctors' Book of Home Remedies*: by sharing that knowledge, by bringing the best medical advice to everyone where and when they need it, this is truly a book worthy of a place in every home and every doctor's library.

And finally, a dedication:
This book is for my family, and for yours.

Stephen Amiel

Dr Stephen Amiel
London 2004

INTRODUCTION

When we decided to write the original *Doctors' Book of Home Remedies*, we knew we were tapping into a wide audience. Lots of people wrote to *Prevention* magazine with their own home remedies for everything from dandruff to ingrowing toenails. Many of the remedies made good sense, but some were, to be frank, pretty far-fetched.

We needed a home remedies authority, someone who could say, yes, it's fine to put aspirin on an insect sting; or no, don't tell people to apply a burning cigarette to an embedded tick. So we thought of doctors. They get constipation and insect bites, heartburn and haemorrhoids just like the rest of us. What do *they* do?

Luckily, doctors are as enthusiastic as their patients when it comes to home remedies. They are likely to have seen and heard everything – and to know what really works. We interviewed more than 500 doctors and other health professionals and gathered more than 2000 safe, effective self-care tips to create *The Doctors' Book of Home Remedies*.

In this edition, we've covered topics that reflect life today – such as hostility, burnout and road rage. These issues worry many of us, and there are things you can do about them without going to your doctor. Feeling angry? Pull into a lay-by and scream in your car – with the windows closed – for as long as you need to release pent-up hostility. Feeling burned out at work? Take a long lunch break once in a while: the place won't fall apart without you. And anyway, the doctor advises it.

There's a section on herb/drug interactions that you can look at for possible safety issues before trying a remedy – important in view of the fact that some herbal remedies are as powerful as conventional medicines. And we've included three special features: 'When to consult a doctor' gives vital advice about when it's *not safe* to treat yourself; 'Do just one thing' points out the self-help remedy most likely to give you immediate benefit; and 'Kitchen cures' offers simple treatments using store cupboard ingredients, such as applying diluted skimmed milk to sunburn or drinking sage tea to stop menopause-related night sweats.

Today, perhaps more than ever, people want to deal with their own health problems when it's practical to do so. That is, in part, because of the simple reality of living in today's hectic world. If you want to see your GP about a minor ailment, you'll be lucky to get an appointment the same day – but this book is on call 24 hours a day. We trust you will find it a valuable friend.

The Editors of *Prevention* Health Books

ACNE
15 remedies for smoother skin

Acne is very common among teenagers – about 80 per cent of young men and women develop pimples, half of them severe enough to require medical treatment. Adolescents get acne because hormones called androgens, which increase the amount of oil the skin produces, circulate at higher levels in their blood.

But teenagers aren't the only ones plagued by spots. Women whose hormones are fluctuating as a result of periods, taking the contraceptive pill, pregnancy or the onset of the menopause, for example, can also suffer from acne.

'Women can have pimples at 25, 35 and even older,' says dermatologist, James Fulton. 'My mother was still breaking out in spots when she was 62.'

Acne is a broad term covering a variety of symptoms including pimples, whiteheads, blackheads and skin cysts. It's a condition in which blocked skin pores result in spots that sometimes become inflamed.

Contrary to popular belief, eating chocolate or having dirty hair or skin do not cause outbreaks of acne. The condition is usually hereditary. If both of your parents had acne, the chances are that you will get it too. But if your sister is pimple-free while your face is a war zone, it may be because other factors have aggravated an acne outbreak. Common culprits include stress, sunbathing and changing seasons. Oral contraceptives and certain brands of make-up can also trigger acne. 'Working women may be especially vulnerable,' says Dr Fulton, 'if they're prone to stress and tend to wear a lot of make-up.'

So here's some advice for keeping your skin blemish-free.

Change your make-up. Dr Fulton believes that greasy make-up causes spots. 'The pigments in foundations, blushers, cleansing creams or moisturizers aren't the problem, and neither is the water. It's the oil. The oil is usually a derivative of fatty acids that are more potent than your own fatty acids. Use a non-oil-based make-up if you are prone to acne.'

Read the labels. Avoid cosmetic products that contain lanolins, isopropyl myristate, sodium lauryl sulphate, laureth-4, and D & C red dyes. Like oil, these ingredients are too rich for the skin.

Wash it off at night. Dr Fulton advocates simple soap and water. He says it's very important to wash your make-up off thoroughly every night

WHEN TO CONSULT A DOCTOR

A huge pimple on the end of your nose can make you feel horribly self-conscious. But acne can develop into something much more serious than a simple blemish.

The least problematic form of acne is the eruption of a few whiteheads and blackheads. At the other end of the spectrum, however, acne can cause severe inflammation that turns livid red or purple. This can result in permanent scarring. If you are worried about acne, see your doctor who will either give you something to help clear it up, or refer you to a dermatologist (skin specialist).

You may be prescribed a topical cream, gel or lotion with vitamin A or benzoyl peroxide to help unblock the pores and reduce bacteria. Or your doctor may decide that long-term low-dose antibiotics are the answer.

using a mild soap, and to rinse the skin carefully afterwards in plenty of fresh water.

Go for the natural look. 'Whatever make-up you use, the less you use of it, the better,' Dr Fulton advises.

Blame it on the Pill? Contraceptive pills can improve acne or make it worse – and acne often flares up 10 days or so after you've stopped taking the pill. Dr Fulton's research suggests that certain contraceptive pills containing combinations of levonorgestrel and ethinylestradiol or norethisterone acetate and ethinylestradiol can aggravate acne. If you're on the pill and have an acne problem, discuss it with your doctor. He or she may be able to offer you another brand or recommend a different method of contraception.

Dianette (cyproterone acetate and ethinylestradiol) is a hormone preparation for acne that can also be used as a contraceptive pill. Women with acne who want contraception may find this preparation particularly suitable.

Leave spots alone. Do not be tempted to squeeze pimples or white-heads. 'A pimple is an inflammation, and you might add to the inflam-mation by squeezing it,' says dermatologist Peter Pochi. You could also cause an infection: squeezing a whitehead can break open the wall of the skin pore, letting the contents leak on to the skin and cause a pimple. But, says Dr Pochi, gently squeezing a pimple with a little central yellow head releases the pus and can help the spot heal more quickly.

Otherwise, there isn't much you can do to a pimple to hurry its departure – most pimples last from one to four weeks, but they always go away eventually.

Attack blackheads. A blackhead is a very blocked pore. The material inside it is solid and the surface of the pore is widened. The black part of a blackhead is not dirt – in fact, dermatologists aren't really sure what it is. Dr Pochi recommends getting rid of a blackhead by squeezing the skin that surrounds it, and adds that this will not cause pimples.

Talk to your pharmacist. You can combat acne with over-the-counter products. The most effective ones contain benzoyl peroxide. 'The benzoyl part pulls the peroxide into the pore and releases oxygen, which kills the bacteria that aggravates acne,' says Dr Fulton. 'The benzoyl also suppresses the fatty acid cells that irritate the pores.'

Over-the-counter acne products come in various forms – gels, liquids, lotions or creams, such as Panoxyl acne gels and washes and the Oxy range. Dr Fulton believes that a water-based gel is least likely to irritate the skin. Put it on for an hour or so in the evening, but wash it off thoroughly at bedtime, especially from your neck and around your eyes.

Stop the spread of acne. Acne medication should be applied about 1cm around the affected area to help keep the acne from spreading: acne tends to spread across the face from the nose out towards the ears, and you need to treat beyond the red inflamed area. Unfortunately, says Dr Fulton, that spot cream won't fight the pimples you already have. But what it will do is act as a pimple preventative.

Give dry skin extra care. Acne products come in various concentrations, but this appears to have little to do with their effectiveness. Pharmacologist Thomas Gossel says that in most clinical trials, lower-strength products have proved as effective as higher-strength ones. What is important is to clean your skin thoroughly before applying any acne medication. Because dry skin can be sensitive to benzoyl peroxide, Dr Gossel recommends starting with a low-strength product first, and increasing the concentration gradually. And don't be alarmed if the product causes reddening of the skin: Dr Gossel says this is a normal reaction.

Try chamomile tea. Chamomile, widely available at supermarkets and health food stores, may be your best friend when it comes to clearing acne, says clinical herbalist Douglas Schar. Drinking the tea will stimulate the immune system; applying cooled tea will improve the health of your skin and pores. 'Two cups of chamomile tea per day, and a morning

How Hollywood hides spots

Pimples are bad enough for any of us, but they're disastrous if you're a film star. That tiny blackhead on your forehead? Put it on the big screen, and watch it grow to the size of a cauliflower. But when did you last see Julia Roberts or Colin Firth with a zit? Don't celebrities ever have spots? 'You bet they do,' says Hollywood make-up artist, Maurice Stein. 'The difference is, they can't let their pimples or any other blemish show.'

Stein has been a studio make-up artist for more than 30 years. Here are a couple of techniques that he's applied to 'the most expensive faces in the world.'

Go undercover. You can totally block out discoloration, whether it's pink, red, or purple, if you find a foundation make-up with a high enough pigment level, says Stein. The normal range for most foundations is 12 to 15 per cent. While you can't really tell the pigment level by looking at a product, you can tell by sampling it. Stein's advice is to 'take a drop and rub it on your skin. If it's so solid in colour that you can't see your own skin underneath it, then you know it has a high pigment level and will do a good job covering your blemish.'

Try it the stars' way. 'When I cover a pimple on an entertainer's face, I use two thin layers of foundation with a layer of loose translucent powder between each layer,' Stein says. 'This helps to set each layer.'

and evening wash with the same tea, will make a big difference in most cases,' says Schar.

Stay out of the sun. Because acne medications can cause adverse reactions to the sun, Dr Gossel advises keeping exposure to sunlight to a minimum.

Use one treatment at a time. If you have been using an over-the-counter acne product, mention it if your doctor gives you a prescription for your acne. Benzoyl peroxide is a close cousin to Retin-A and other products containing vitamin A derivatives, says Dr Gossel, and you must not use both at the same time.

ADDICTION
15 steps to recovery

Imagine a man who knocks back a few stiff drinks after work. Is he a 'pleasure' drinker or an alcoholic? What about the woman who raids the refrigerator when she's tired or depressed, or the people who spend hours sitting in front of the television?

Harmless diversions – or addictions?

Most people have some kind of addiction. They find something they like that makes them feel good, and they may use it again and again as a kind of coping mechanism, says Tom Horvath, who runs an addiction treatment centre.

We tend to think of addictions in their most severe forms: the drug addict who craves the next fix, for example, or the compulsive gambler who tips his salary into slot machines. But millions of us have milder addictions. We crave substances or experiences that make us feel good temporarily, but that often have harmful long-term consequences.

If you suspect that you have an addiction – to cigarettes, gambling, food or anything else – ask yourself this question: has your behaviour caused enough problems for you to consider stopping or cutting back? If the reply is yes, it's time to make some changes to break addiction's grip.

Start by listing pros and cons. It's difficult for most people to recognize that they have an addiction. One way to find out is to list the pros and cons of the behaviour that's worrying you.

The CAGE questionnaire

To find out whether or not you could have a drink problem, take this simple questionnaire test.

If your answer is 'yes' to two or more of the questions, it is highly likely (more than 90 per cent) that you have an alcohol dependency problem and should seek professional help, says family doctor Stephen Amiel.

C Have you ever thought you should CUT DOWN on your drinking?

A Have you ever felt ANNOYED by others' criticism of your drinking?

G Have you ever felt GUILTY about your drinking?

E Do you have a morning EYE OPENER?

First, write down all the things that you like about the substance or activity. If you drink, for example, the list might include things such as 'It helps me to unwind' or 'I like the feeling of euphoria'.

Second, write down the benefits of giving it up: 'I'd be more productive if I didn't drink' or 'I'd be less likely to row with my partner', or 'I'd like to stay healthy for my kids' sake'.

Now, compare the lists. Does it appear that the costs of your behaviour outweigh the benefits? Congratulations. You've just recognized that you have some problems – the first step towards making the necessary changes, says Dr Horvath.

And you've done it alone. You now need to decide when you're ready to make the necessary – and often difficult – changes to free yourself from addictions.

Cut down gradually – or stop completely. Some people wean themselves from addictions gradually – by initially smoking 10 fewer cigarettes each day, for example, or gambling once a week instead of every night. Others find it easier to stop just like that – in other words, go 'cold turkey'.

Both approaches can be equally effective. 'With weaning, people are generally less scared, so they're more motivated,' says Dr Horvath. Going cold turkey is harder to begin with, but it makes the whole process pass more quickly.

Distance yourself from cravings. Anyone who curtails addictive substances or behaviours will go through a withdrawal period. The cravings – for one more cigarette, one more drink, one more day at the racecourse – can be almost unbearably intense.

'I advise people to keep their cravings at a distance,' says Dr Horvath. In other words, acknowledge how you're feeling. Admit to yourself how uncomfortable you are. But don't give in. Distract yourself. Call a friend. Go for a brisk walk. Do the washing-up. Do whatever it takes to take your mind off the craving.

'Just because you have an itch doesn't mean you have to scratch,' he points out. Be strong. Individual cravings will disappear in minutes or even seconds, and the entire experience of cravings will often evaporate in a month or two.

Keep busy. 'A lot of people who make the commitment to quit doing something find themselves sitting at home all the time,' observes Peter DeMaria, a professor of psychiatry who specializes in substance abuse programmes.

If you don't keep busy – with exercise, hobbies or other activities that keep your mind and body active – you'll find yourself focusing more and

WHEN TO CONSULT A DOCTOR

Denial is one of the hallmarks of addiction. People with drug, alcohol or other addictions often insist that their behaviour is normal, even when the evidence of destruction is all around them.

Are friends, family members or work colleagues gently suggesting that you may have a problem? Listen to them. Look at your recent behaviour. Ask yourself if they are seeing something that you can't.

'Try to solve the problems on your own,' advises Dr Tom Horvath. 'Try cutting back or quitting entirely – and get the support of the people around you. If you've made one or several attempts that don't seem to be going far or fast enough, then it's time to get professional help.'

more on the cravings. Exercise can be especially helpful, says Dr De-Maria, because it's a way of reconnecting to healthy activities.

Get your mind racing. One way to distract yourself from cravings is to think about something – anything – at high speed. Count ceiling tiles as quickly as you can. Try reading book titles backwards. Do repetitious maths calculations in your head – such as subtracting seven from 1000, seven from 993, and so on.

When you do this type of thing quickly, says Dr Horvath, it completely occupies your mind, which helps you to get past the craving.

Avoid behaviour triggers. If you've just given up smoking, the last thing you need is an evening in a smoky pub. If you've been obsessed with the Internet, online Christmas shopping is probably not a good idea.

Alcoholics Anonymous (AA) and other self-help programmes teach members to avoid people, places or things that are associated with their addictions. 'Some people will alter their walking or driving routes in order to avoid parts of the city where they used to buy drugs, or to avoid people they used to hang out with,' says Dr DeMaria. 'With smoking, talking on the phone may be a trigger.'

You have to recognize what your triggers are and decide how best to respond when you're confronted by them. As time goes by, you'll find that addiction triggers will lose most or all of their pull. Even former alcoholics can go to pubs once they've truly kicked the habit.

Substitute good behaviours for bad ones. Avoidance is helpful in the early stages of fighting addictions, but no one can avoid all sources of temptation indefinitely. You can, however, develop substitute habits.

When you feel an urge for a cigarette, for example, chew gum. When the television beckons, read a magazine. After a while, your new habits will take the place of the old ones.

Make it harder to indulge. Addictions are grounded in habits, which means people sometimes indulge without really thinking about what they're doing. Smokers, for example, may find themselves three puffs into a cigarette that they don't remember lighting. People with eating problems may raid the biscuit tin without being consciously aware that they'd left the sitting room.

One way to break unconscious habits is to make them harder to practise. A smoker, for example, might put a packet of cigarettes inside a box and bind the whole thing with rubber bands. You still may decide to smoke, but at least you won't be doing it automatically.

The same approach works with other addictions. Turn off the computer when you sign off the Internet – and maybe even crawl under the desk to pull out the plug. Clear the house of alcohol, pornography or other forbidden things. Putting obstacles between you and your addiction will force you to think about what you're doing, which in turn will make the addiction easier to overcome, says Dr Horvath.

Find new sources of satisfaction. It's not enough merely to give up unhealthy behaviours. If you're going to be successful, you need to replace addictions with something positive.

'In order to develop new habits, you need gradually to change the sources of satisfaction in your life,' says Dr Horvath. This could be as simple as creating healthier lifestyle habits. Instead of spending the night in front of the television, for example, go to bed early and get more rest. You might focus more of your energy on eating healthy foods, exercising regularly, or even donating a few hours a week to a charity.

Learn from setbacks. Nearly everyone who struggles with addictions slips up occasionally. Expect it, says Dr Horvath. Don't be discouraged, and don't give up.

'When slips happen, ask yourself why they happened. Turn them into a learning situation,' says Dr Horvath. 'Persistence is the most important virtue. Everyone who keeps going is going to be successful. Eventually, you run out of ways to make mistakes.'

Get by with a little help from your friends. Giving up smoking or cutting down on alcohol can be a lonely business, says family doctor Stephen Amiel. And sometimes friends don't help when they offer you a cigarette or say, 'Go on, one more drink won't hurt'. Tell your friends what you intend to do, set a quit date when social, work or domestic pressures aren't so great, or maybe when you're due to go on holiday. Best of all try to get a friend or partner to give up with you, and get other friends to sponsor you for your favourite charity.

Reward your success. Think of the money you're saving by not smoking or gambling: try and set it aside each week for something special for you or your family, suggests Dr Amiel. A night out four weeks after quitting perhaps, or a holiday after six months. A couple getting through a carton of 200 cigarettes a week could save almost £5000 in six months – enough for a holiday in Florida for a family of four!

Nicotine replacement. Heavy smokers who want to go cold turkey but can't cope with the nicotine withdrawal cravings may benefit from a range of nicotine-containing products, says Dr Amiel. Gum, patches, nasal sprays and plastic cigarettes are now available on prescription from your doctor. You can tail off the strength of these over a period of weeks. Evidence suggests that these products work best in conjunction with smoking cessation groups or counselling.

Note: Check with your doctor first if you have heart disease, or are pregnant or breastfeeding.

Join a group. There are thousands of self-help groups for overcoming every sort of addiction – to alcohol, drugs, cigarettes, sex, overeating and gambling, to name just a few. Self-help groups are free and they can be very effective, either by themselves or in combination with some form of therapy, says Dr DeMaria. At self-help groups, you spend time with people in various stages of recovery. 'They've been through it all before, and they can act as role models and mentors.'

Do just *one* thing

Give up when you're pregnant. Most women realize that cigarettes, alcohol and drugs harm unborn babies in all sorts of ways, and make huge efforts to give up or cut down. It's a great opportunity to give up for good, says family doctor Stephen Amiel.

Think of it as the baby doing you a favour, as well as the other way round. Get your partner to help you by giving up too – that way your baby is more likely to come into a smoke-free, happier and healthier family.

If you have a smoking, alcohol or drugs problem, seek professional help as soon as you know you're pregnant or, better still, as soon as you know you want to try for a baby.

AGE SPOTS

8 ways to stop the spots

Age spots, commonly known as liver spots, are flat, rounded, brown areas that commonly appear on the backs of hands as well as on necks, faces and shoulders. The marks are nothing to do with age, says Audrey Kunin, a cosmetic dermatologist, but are in fact large, flat, sun-induced freckles.

'The reason they're called age spots is that they usually occur because of sun exposure over time – which means that for a lot of people they won't appear on their skin until they get a little older,' she says.

While age spots are common in older people, someone who's had significant sun exposure can get them as early as their late twenties or thirties. Sunlight contains ultraviolet (UV) rays that cause suntans and sunburn. As time goes by, this sun damage causes more pigment than normal to be deposited in the skin. This eventually leads to large, flat, brown freckles.

Age spots can look unsightly. And, if they change in size, they may actually be skin cancers, which is why it's worth having them looked at by a doctor. But, assuming that what you have are age spots, here are some tips on concealing or fading them, as well as preventing more.

Use a sunscreen. Because these brown blotches are caused by the sun's UV rays, limiting your exposure to the sun is the first important step in the battle against age spots. That means you should use a high factor sunscreen each and every time you go outdoors for any extended period of time, says dermatologist Ralph Daniel.

Even if you already have age spots, sunscreen keeps existing ones from darkening and helps to prevent more from popping up, says Dr Kunin.

Choose a good quality lotion with a sun protection factor (SPF) of at least 15. Apply it to exposed skin 10 to 15 minutes before you go outside, says Dr Daniel. Tests show that SPF 15 sunblock protects the skin against about 93 per cent of the sun's UV rays, he adds.

If you plan to spend most of the day on the golf course, tennis court or ski slope, use a sunscreen with an SPF of 30, says Dr Kunin. Ditto if you spend a lot of time on a boat or at the beach, because the sun reflects off the water. And since perspiration and water can wash off your sunscreen, be sure to reapply it regularly.

Wear a hat. Whether you're off to the beach or spending extended time in the midday sun, wear a cotton-lined sun hat with a brim at least 10cm wide to keep the sun off your face and neck, says Dr Kunin. This will give

WHEN TO CONSULT A DOCTOR

If your age spots have a mind of their own and don't respond to home remedies, or if you have an age spot that bleeds, itches, tingles or changes in size or colour, it's time to see your doctor. Some skin cancers, such as melanoma, can look like age spots.

you the protection needed to limit your chances of developing age spots.

Baseball caps, assuming they're worn with the peak in front, don't protect your ears, the back of your neck or even most of your face from full sun, says Dr Kunin. Straw hats don't usually offer much protection either – a straw hat that is loosely woven and unlined will let the sun shine straight through.

Protect your lips. The lips are an area that most people don't think about guarding from the sun. But age spots can pop up on your lips, too. Many women think that their lipstick will protect them. The sun, however, can often penetrate lighter shades, and lipstick typically wears off throughout the day leaving the lips naked and unprotected.

Apply either a lip balm or lipstick with an SPF of 15 to 30 before you go outside. If you still want to wear your favourite non-SPF lipstick, apply the lipstick over a layer of protective balm.

Shun the sun. Avoid the sun as much as possible during peak hours (from 10am to 4pm in summer or in hot climates, and from 10am to 2pm in spring, autumn and winter – even in temperate climates. This is when ultraviolet radiation is strongest, says Dr Kunin. If you have outdoor chores like gardening to do, aim to perform them early in the morning or in the evening. And remember that sunscreen is needed even in winter and on cloudy days.

Seek the shade. Since excessive sun exposure causes age spots, try and retreat to a shady spot on sunny days. At the beach or a barbecue, park yourself under a big umbrella. Also, whenever you're in the sun, wear tightly woven, light-coloured clothing if it's not too hot. This helps to keep UV rays from penetrating your skin. 'It sounds simple, but protecting yourself with sunblock or staying out of the sun are the two best ways to keep new age spots from cropping up,' says Dr Kunin.

Lighten up. If your age spots aren't too big or too dark, over-the-counter bleaching agents could help fade them, Dr Kunin says. Look for over-the-

Cut a few lemon slices and place them directly on your age spots for 10 to 15 minutes once a day, suggests dermatologist Audrey Kunin. 'The acid in the fresh lemon juice helps lighten the age spots in some cases.' It won't happen overnight, though. Dr Kunin says you should notice a difference in six to twelve weeks. Watch carefully, though. Overuse could cause the upper layer of skin to peel away.

counter products like Fade-out, which contain two per cent hydroquinone, the best-known active ingredient used in many types of bleaching agents. Hydroquinone lightens age spots until they become less noticeable or even disappear.

Apply the bleaching agent twice a day to your sun spots, carefully following the manufacturer's directions. Dab the cream directly onto the age spots with a cotton bud so that you don't bleach the pigment in unaffected areas.

'Be patient,' says Dr Kunin. 'You won't see results overnight. Lightening agents often take six to twelve months to do the job.' Stop the treatment when the age spots disappear, or the affected area may become lighter than your normal skin tone.

Cover up with make-up. If home remedies don't do the trick and you don't want to spend money on cosmetic treatments offered by dermatologists, such as a chemical peel or laser resurfacing, you can always reach into your make-up bag. 'Brown age spots can be concealed by applying a cream-based or water-based concealer,' says Dr Kunin. A lighter version of your skin tone does the best job of hiding age spots.

ALLERGIES

16 ways to alleviate the symptoms

Allergies are the result of an immune system run amok. They develop when your immune system overreacts to a normally harmless substance, such as pollen, cat dander or house dust mites. The problem is huge: there are 12 million hay fever sufferers in Britain, and pollen and other allergens cause a range of symptoms including sneezing, coughing, wheezing, chest tightness, difficulty breathing, itchy eyes and nettlerash (see *Rashes*, page 490), all of which may be allergy symptoms.

Allergies come in almost infinite variety. But most triggers, called allergens, stimulate the immune system through four basic routes: ingestion (eating peanuts or shellfish, for example), injection (such as having a penicillin jab), absorption through the skin (touching certain plants) and inhalation (breathing in pollen or house dust mites).

For food and drug allergies, and contact allergies, avoidance is the only option. But when you want relief from inhaled allergies, the answer is probably right under your nose, since house dust, pollen, cat dander (tiny flakes of dried saliva found on cat skin and hair) and mould are the most common triggers.

'You find a bit of everything in house dust,' says Thomas Platts-Mills, a professor of medicine who specializes in allergies and immunology. 'Different people are allergic to different things, but the single biggest cause of problems is the dust mite.'

The dust mite is an almost microscopic relative of ticks and spiders. But living mites are not the problem. People react, instead, to the faecal material that mites expel on carpets, bedding and upholstered furniture. The bodies of dead mites also trigger allergies.

Other common airborne allergens are equally hard to escape. Pollen fills the air almost everywhere with seasonal regularity. Mould grows wherever it's dark and humid – under carpets, in damp basements and in leaky garages and garden sheds. And with 7.7 million cats and 6.6 million dogs in Britain, it's not easy to escape pet dander. If you're sensitive to any of these allergens – probably because you've inherited the tendency – contact with them will trigger a sneezing, wheezing or itchy reaction.

Fortunately, there's much you can do to minimize the misery. The following doctor-tested and recommended tips will help you on your way to easier breathing and dry eyes.

Treat your symptoms. A certain amount of exposure to whatever bothers you is unavoidable. Over-the-counter antihistamines, available from your local pharmacist, work wonders on runny noses and red, itchy eyes.

Richard Podell, a professor of medicine, says that, for the most part, they do a good job. 'But,' he advises, 'if you have an allergy that persists for more than five to seven days, you should probably see your doctor.'

Some antihistamines are marketed as non-drowsiness inducing, but even these need to be used with caution when driving or operating machinery, and none should be mixed with alcohol, warns family doctor Stephen Amiel.

As with any over-the-counter medication, pregnant women should take advice from the pharmacist or their doctor. Avoid grapefruit juice if you are taking antihistamines containing terfenadine.

WHEN TO CONSULT A DOCTOR

Anaphylactic shock is an overwhelmingly severe allergic reaction that can occur occasionally in people, both with known allergies and without. Common culprits are wasp and bee stings, nuts or shellfish, but other allergens can cause it too in sensitized people.

Symptoms of anaphylactic shock include:

• sudden onset of swelling of the tongue, face, hands or neck;

• rapid onset of raised white or red blotches or welts (urticaria or 'hives');

• difficulty in breathing (with or without wheezing).

Anaphylactic shock is a medical emergency and if you think you or someone else is suffering from it, you should dial 999 and get immediate medical attention.

People at risk of further attacks, or those with very severe food or sting allergies can get adrenaline injections on prescription from their doctor: these can be self-administered to stop an attack in its early stages. Courses of desensitizing injections by hospital allergy clinics can also sometimes be arranged. Think about joining MedicAlert and get a bracelet to warn others that you have a potential problem.

You should also see your doctor if a less severe allergic attack does not respond to over-the-counter medications within a week, particularly if you have breathing problems or a bad rash.

Use your car's air-conditioning. If simply walking outside sets you wheezing and sneezing, imagine what tearing through pollen clouds in a car is going to do. If you are lucky enough to have air-conditioning in your car then use it. Of course, it's not the same as letting the wind rip through your hair, but remember, you're doing it for your health.

Consider an air filter. Keeping the air clean in your home can bring relief from pollen, mould and pet dander. HEPA (high-energy particulate-arresting) filters are the most efficient. When you use an air filter in your room, remember to keep the door closed so that the machine won't be overburdened with too much air to clean.

Air filters aren't much use against dust mites, however. The mites are relatively heavy and they hang in the air only for a few minutes or so and aren't floating around for the filter to draw them in.

Keep it dry. Keeping the air in your home dry will help put a stop to dust mite problems. Dust mites don't do very well in humidity below about 45 per cent, says Dr Platts-Mills. 'Generally, the drier, the better.' You can reduce humidity and condensation by improving ventilation (extractor fans and hoods, opening windows), and by using a tumble dryer with external venting, rather than putting damp clothes over radiators.

Structural damp needs more radical treatment. Speak to your landlord, council or housing association if you are unable to deal with it yourself: a letter from your doctor may help if your or your family's health is affected by damp housing conditions.

Try a dehumidifier. But remember to empty the unit's water frequently and clean it regularly so that it doesn't become a haven for mould. If a dehumidifier creates problems for a child or anyone sensitive to dry air, try putting a small room humidifier close to his or her bed.

Keep it clean. People with allergies fare better when dust and grime are kept to a minimum. Try not to use aerosol sprays or products containing harsh chemicals or scents that may irritate your airways. But your home will need more than a dusting with a dry cloth, which merely propels allergens into the air. Instead, wipe down hard surfaces and floors with a slightly damp cloth.

In humid areas like bathrooms wear rubber gloves and use a bleach solution, which will kill any mould. Add about a cup of bleach to a bucket of water, wipe surfaces with the solution, leave for five minutes and then rinse. Be careful not to splash bleach on fabrics or you'll damage them.

If you're allergic to house dust, pet dander or other household allergens, persuade or pay someone else to vacuum the carpets. The cost of hiring a helper is a small price to pay to avoid an allergic reaction.

Isolate your pets. More than 50 per cent of British households keep pets. But our furry friends trigger a staggering number of allergic reactions every year. Cat dander causes most of the problems, but dogs, birds, rabbits, horses and other pets with hair or fur also cause allergies in susceptible people. If you can't bear to part with your pet, make your bedroom a haven, sealed off from the rest of the house and forbidden territory for animals. All it takes to keep a dander allergy going is for a pet to walk through your room just once a week, observes Dr Podell.

Wear a face mask. Put on a mask when doing anything that's likely to expose you to an allergen that you know will cause you problems. A simple chore like vacuuming can throw huge quantities of dust and whatever else is in your home into the air, where it will hang for several minutes, says allergy specialist David Lang. Similarly, gardening can expose you to large volumes of pollen. A small mask that covers your nose and mouth, known as a dust respirator, can keep the allergen from reaching your lungs. An inexpensive version that comes highly recommended is made by 3M; the mask is available in hardware and DIY stores.

Enforce a no-smoking policy. Tobacco smoke is a significant irritant for the smoker and anyone else breathing nearby. Smoke can make allergies worse. You'll breathe more easily if you keep your home, office and car smoke-free zones.

Make your bed a mite-free zone. Encase your pillows and mattress in allergen-proof covers. These covers are widely available from department stores and bedding specialists. In order to create an effective barrier against dust mite allergens, the fabric weave needs to be tight (10 microns wide).

People on low incomes may qualify for a loan from the DSS Social Fund to buy a mattress cover, says Dr Amiel.

You can hoover mites from mattresses with a high filtration vacuum cleaner and make the environment less mite-friendly by removing the duvet and letting the mattress air regularly, so as to reduce the humidity in your bed.

Choose a hot wash for bed linen. Linens should be washed in water that is at least 60°C to rid them of dust mites and their waste. On most washing machines, this means selecting a hot wash, or a 'colourfast cottons' wash.

Get rid of your carpets. Carpets may look nice, but they make a perfect home for dust mites and mould. Tightly woven carpets also attract and retain pollen and pet dander. Even steam-cleaning may not help: 'It's not hot enough to kill the mites,' says Dr Platts-Mills. All steam cleaning really does is make it warmer and wetter underneath – creating an ideal climate for both mites and mould.

Buy cotton rugs. Replace your carpets with rugs, and you'll achieve two major benefits. Firstly, you'll eliminate your home's biggest collector of dust, pollen, pet dander and mould. Secondly, you'll make keeping your home allergen-free much easier.

Most cotton rugs can be washed at temperatures hot enough to kill dust mites. Furthermore, because of the rugs' loose weave, the floors underneath stay cool and dry, conditions distinctly hostile to mould and mites.

Mites simply can't survive on a dry, polished floor, says Dr Platts-Mills. 'It dries in seconds, versus days for a steam-cleaned carpet'.

Why homes became havens for dust mites

In the 1950s, housewives in Britain welcomed the vacuum cleaner with open arms. Before long, we couldn't live without one.

But the very technology that makes our lives easier today has indirectly contributed to a common medical problem: dust mite allergy.

The vacuum cleaner made fitted carpets more attractive than loose rugs. With central heating, homes tended to stay warm all year round. Add good insulation and 'economy' cool laundry cycles to the package and you end up with the perfect environment for dust mites.

Buy synthetic pillows. Dust mites are just as fond of synthetic (Hollofil or Dacron) pillows as those made from down, but synthetic pillows have one major advantage: you can wash them in hot water.

Minimize clutter. Dried flowers, books and ornaments collect dust and other allergens. Try to keep knick-knacks in display cupboards or drawers – or better still, rid your home of them entirely.

Bump them off with heat or cold. Soft toys and small cushions will benefit from a trip to the freezer for six hours a month, or the tumble dryer for an hour or so, says Dr Amiel. Both methods kill the house dust mite. Wash them afterwards if possible.

Make at least one room a sanctuary. Few people can afford air conditioning, or want to rip their wall-to-wall carpeting out of every room. But anyone can choose to make one room a sanctuary.

'Most people spend the largest part of their time at home in the bedroom,' says Dr Platts-Mills. Making just that one room an allergen-free area can do a great deal to alleviate the allergy.

Do it by air-conditioning the room in summer, sealing it from the rest of the house (by keeping the door closed), replacing carpets with laminated wood flooring or throw rugs, encasing bedding in allergen-proof cases and keeping the room dust-free.

ALOPECIA

13 ways to deal with excessive hair loss

Unlike other mammals, we humans don't rely on our hair to warm or protect us. But the multi-million pound hair care industry proves if nothing else how important our hair is to us. Hair, our crowning glory – or not – can influence our psychological, emotional and sexual wellbeing hugely. A new hairstyle, a bit of colour, or even a shampoo can make us feel a million dollars, but too much hair where we don't want it, or too little where we do, can blight our lives, male or female, young or not so young.

On average we lose 100 hairs per day. It's normal for some hair to come out in the shower or when we brush it: each hair on your head undergoes a cycle of growing, 'resting' and then falling out as another hair takes its place. Excessive loss of hair or baldness is known as alopecia. It can affect men, women and children and, though not life-threatening or painful, it can be very upsetting and affect your self-confidence, your relationships and your career.

Some hair loss occurs in both men and women as part of the normal ageing process, explains family doctor Stephen Amiel. Many of us are genetically programmed to lose more of our hair at an earlier age. This is the commonest type of alopecia, and is known as male pattern baldness (or androgenetic alopecia). Men, and women to a lesser degree, can both be affected. Most men will have lost some hair by the time they reach 60 – and in some, the process starts as early as 12. Hair thinning in women can also result from hormonal changes that occur in pregnancy, the menopause and when taking the Pill. In some women, high testosterone levels cause male pattern baldness.

Skin conditions such as psoriasis, eczema or fungal infections can cause hair loss, says Dr Amiel, as can certain medical conditions like thyroid problems or diabetes. And the physical stress of a severe illness, child-birth, a very high fever, sudden weight loss or an operation can cause temporary hair loss a few months later.

Emotional and psychological stress can trigger hair loss, too, and some people with psychological problems can absent-mindedly, or even deliberately, pull their own hair out.

Medical treatments can also cause alopecia: some (but not all) chemotherapy or radiation treatments for cancer cause hair loss, as do other drugs such as anticoagulants (warfarin) and anti-thyroid drugs.

More dramatic hair loss is seen in alopecia areata. This usually causes patches of hair loss on the scalp, face or eyebrows, but sometimes the whole scalp or even the entire body loses its hair (alopecia universalis).

The hair usually regrows after a few months, says Dr Amiel, but unfortunately this cannot be guaranteed. Here are some tips to help you make hair loss less of a problem.

Bide your time. If your hair loss was caused by an acute illness, childbirth or an operation, it is likely to be temporary and your hair will probably grow back on its own. Changing your hairstyle to cover the bald patches may help to make you feel better until it does.

Watch out for quackery. Cleopatra tried to cure Julius Caesar's baldness with ground-up burnt horses' teeth, bear grease, domestic mice and deer, says Dr Amiel. The ancient Egyptians also used hippopotamus and crocodile fat. Today's remedies may smell a little nicer, but most of them are just as ineffective and those that may help are *not* available on NHS prescription. *Caveat emptor* – buyer beware!

Try a magic potion. Minoxidil lotion (Regaine) works for about half of men (and women) with male pattern baldness, but it takes about four months to have a visible effect and must be continued indefinitely, as any new hair that does re-grow will fall out after treatment is stopped. It can be bought from pharmacies without a prescription.

Dare to go bare. Some people prefer to accept their hair loss and bare their head with pride. You might even want to go the whole hog and shave your head completely.

Opting for private treatment

Scalp surgery, which includes hair transplantation, scalp flaps and other procedures, has been used for a number of years but the results are variable, cosmetically. Complications like scarring and infection can occur, repeated procedures may be necessary and it is expensive.

Do your research carefully if you are considering these procedures.

Finasteride (sold as Propecia) is a tablet for men that causes some hair regrowth in half of those who take it and reduces hair loss in most of the remainder.

It must be taken continuously and although side-effects are uncommon, it can cause a reduction in sex drive. You will need to ask for a private prescription in order to buy it from a pharmacy.

WHEN TO CONSULT A DOCTOR

See your doctor if you think your hair loss is caused by stress or depression, or if your distress at your hair loss is affecting your physical or mental health. Your doctor can also help if your hair loss is due to a skin condition like a fungal infection or psoriasis, or to a treatable hormonal problem such as thyroid disease. Treating the underlying condition should stop hair loss and allow hair growth to return to normal.

If you have alopecia areata, your doctor will probably advise you to leave small patches alone, as the hair should regrow in time. You may be prescribed steroid creams, or your doctor might refer you to a dermatologist for injections of steroids into the affected skin (you may need several to see an effect). Occasionally, you may be offered an intramuscular steroid injection or a course of oral steroids if the loss is more extensive.

Women with male pattern baldness might be offered various hormones or other drugs to suppress or counteract the excess of testosterone. A combination of minoxidil and tretinoin (Retin-A) has also been shown by one study to be effective in male pattern baldness and alopecia areata in both women and men.

Make a styling change. Maximize the hair you have, suggests Dr Amiel. If you have white hair, add some colour so that it shows up better. If it's straight, a light perm will help to fill in the spaces. But be gentle – if your hair's already fragile, too many chemicals may be the last straw. Patches of alopecia areata can be concealed by a cunning cut.

Go for that hat. If you can't get the hairstyle you want, or if there just isn't enough hair to go round, buy turbans or hats to suit your mood, outfit or occasion.

Wigs don't have to look like rugs. There are some great wigs around – at a cost – but make sure you choose a reputable supplier. If you are having chemotherapy, you may be entitled to a wig at NHS expense, says Dr Amiel.

Double-sided adhesive wig tape will keep your wig secure even in the most turbulent of conditions.

If you know you're going to lose your hair, you can match your previous hair and style and get a suitable wig made beforehand. Or you could go for the style and colour you've always wanted but never dared to choose. Remember, there are no right or wrong choices: the most important thing is to do what you feel comfortable with.

Look after those locks. Avoid scraping your hair back or using tight hair rollers, as the pull on your hair can cause a type of hair loss called 'traction alopecia'. Also, hot oil hair treatments or the chemicals used in perms can cause inflammation of your hair follicles, which could lead to hair loss.

Beat the stress. Relaxation techniques or counselling may help if your hair loss has an emotional or psychological trigger, says Dr Amiel.

Try a herbal remedy. 'When large patches of hair suddenly drop off the scalp, it's a disturbing experience,' says clinical herbalist Douglas Schar. 'I find that alopecia, especially when of nervous origin, is often helped by regularly applying arnica cream.'

The cream is sold at health food stores, pharmacies and some supermarkets. Apply it twice a day to the bald areas. 'It's a little messy,' admits Schar, 'but it will stimulate the regrowth of hair.'

The low-down on supplements. Many companies selling hair loss cures and supplements claim that hair loss is due to some sort of dietary deficiency. In fact, you would have to be seriously malnourished, and effectively starving, to cause hair loss, says Dr Amiel.

Hair loss has often been blamed on iron deficiency anaemia, but dermatologists are divided as to the significance of this and are wary of reassuring women that if they take iron supplements their hair will return to normal.

Zinc, in oral or topical lotion form, is also said to benefit both male pattern baldness and alopecia areata. Such claims are based on very little scientific evidence, says Dr Amiel, and should be treated with caution. A balanced diet is more than adequate to provide all the nutrients, vitamins and minerals you need for healthy hair growth.

Join a self-help group. Hairline International – the Alopecia Patients Society (www.hairlineinternational.co.uk) – provides information and support for people who have lost or are losing their hair, or who are about to lose their hair as a result of chemotherapy.

ANAL FISSURES AND ITCHING

12 soothing solutions

Even though the symptoms are comparable – pain, bleeding and itching – the similarities between anal fissures and haemorrhoids (piles) are largely superficial. Haemorrhoids are generally swollen veins. In contrast, fissures are ulcers, or cracks in the skin that just happen to occur in the same general area.

Fissures are very much like those painful tears that sometimes develop in the corners of your mouth, says Byron Gathright, a specialist in colorectal medicine. Both the oral and anal variety occur where skin meets delicate mucous membrane. In the anus, a common cause of such tears is the passing of a large, hard stool.

New research points to anatomical problems that can contribute to chronic anal fissures, as opposed to isolated problems with the painful sores. Increased pressure in the internal anal sphincter muscle and reduced bloodflow to the area where fissures occur may make you more prone to chronic problems.

If you have fissures, you know these little sores can make your life – at least your sitting life – miserable. Take comfort in the fact that about 60 per cent of anal fissures heal within a few weeks. In severe chronic cases, surgery may be required, but this carries risks, including the possibility of faecal incontinence if the anal sphincter is injured. Fortunately, several non-surgical remedies exist to alleviate the pain and to prevent fissures from recurring. Here's what our experts suggest.

Soften stools with fibre and fluid. The anal opening was never meant to accommodate large hard stools. Generally a by-product of a low-fibre Western diet, rock-hard stools tug and tear at the anal canal, which can result in anal fissures as well as piles.

The solution? Change to a diet high in fibre and fluids that will produce soft stools. Eating more fruit, vegetables and whole grains, and drinking six to eight glasses of water a day are the best remedies and preventive measures you can take for anal fissures, says Dr Gathright. Once your stools are soft and pliable, your anal fissures should begin to heal on their own.

Try petroleum jelly. Eating more fibre will soften your stool, but you can also protect your anal canal by lubricating it before each bowel movement. A little Vaseline inserted about 1cm into the rectum may help

WHEN TO CONSULT A DOCTOR

Fissures generally don't require special medical attention unless they persist. 'The important thing with fissures is not to put off dealing with them forever – an ulcer that doesn't heal may be a cancer,' says obstetrician and gynaecologist Lewis Townsend. 'If you have fissures that don't heal within four to eight weeks, get them looked at.'

A bloody or mucus discharge from the anus should also be checked out, says family doctor Stephen Amiel, as this may occasionally be due to a more serious condition like colitis, diverticular disease or cancer.

the stool to pass without causing any further damage, says colorectal surgeon Edmund Leff.

Keep cool, dry and clean. Wash the anal area morning and night, and after every bowel movement, advises family doctor Stephen Amiel. Toilet paper alone leaves tiny, highly irritant traces of faeces on the sensitive skin around the anus, especially if you've got skin tags from previous fissures or external piles.

Moistened toilet paper or dermatological creams like aqueous cream work well. Be gentle but thorough when you dry; dab, don't rub, and if the pain or itching is really bad, use a hair dryer on a cool setting. Unscented talcum powder may help to reduce sweating and friction during the day, says Dr Amiel. Wear loose-fitting cotton underwear and don't get too hot in bed at night.

Avoid diarrhoea. It may seem odd, but not only can hard, constipated stools worsen anal fissures – so can diarrhoea. Watery stools soften the tissues around them, and they also contain acid that can burn the raw anal area and give you a form of 'nappy rash' to add further misery to your condition, says Marvin Schuster, a specialist in digestive disorders.

Don't scratch. Anal fissures may be itchy as well as painful, but using sharp fingernails on your tender anus can tear at the already sore tissue, says family doctor John Lawder.

Scratching also releases histamine-like chemicals into the skin, causing more inflammation and setting up an itch-scratch cycle, adds Dr Amiel. Keep your nails short if you find you tend to scratch in your sleep. If things get really desperate, sit on an ice pack! A pack of frozen peas or coffee beans wrapped in a small towel will mould to your contours and bring relief within a minute or so.

Lose weight. The more weight you carry, the more likely you are to sweat. Sweat in your anal area slows down healing, says Dr Lawder.

Soak in a hot bath. Warm water helps to relax the muscles of the anal sphincter and reduces much of the discomfort of fissures, says Dr Leff. But avoid bubble bath, bath salts and perfumed salts, says Dr Amiel, as these can all make soreness and irritation worse.

Steer clear of certain foods. While no specific food causes fissures, some foods may be excessively irritating to the anal canal as they pass through the bowels. Beware of spicy and pickled foods, says Dr Schuster.

Buy yourself a special pillow. Alleviate the pain associated with sitting on a fissure by buying a liquid-filled pillow from a specialist medical supplier, says Dr Lawder.

Wipe gently. Rough toilet paper and overzealous wiping slows down the healing of anal fissures. Use only white, unscented, high-quality toilet paper. Perfumes and dyes can further irritate the already irritated area, says Dr Lawder. You can soften toilet paper by dampening it under the tap before wiping.

Substitute facial tissue. The best toilet paper isn't toilet paper at all. Facial tissues coated with moisturizing lotion offer the least amount of friction to your sore bottom, says Dr Lawder.

Try ointments or suppositories. Your pharmacy will have a range of ointments or suppositories containing anti-inflammatory, local anaesthetic and mild steroid combinations. Used morning and night, and after bowel movements, these can soothe, relieve pain and reduce the urge to scratch, says Dr Amiel.

ANGINA
15 long-life strategies to protect the heart

More than a few people have confused the symptoms of angina with those of a heart attack. Angina isn't quite that serious, but it's close. Think of it as a heart *warning*.

Angina (the full name is angina pectoris) occurs when the heart gets insufficient blood and oxygen, which may result in temporary nausea, dizziness, or a burning or squeezing pain in the chest. Angina itself isn't a disease. It's a symptom of underlying problems, usually coronary artery disease.

'When you have chronic angina, you're at a much higher risk of having a sudden cardiac event, such as a heart attack,' says David Capuzzi, an expert in cardio-vascular disease prevention. 'Unfortunately, most people who experience acute cardiac events do not have prior angina to warn them.'

Anything that increases the heart's demand for oxygen, such as exercise or emotional stress, can trigger bouts of angina. The attacks normally last less than five minutes and are unlikely to cause permanent damage to the heart. The underlying problems, however, can be life-threatening.

The discomfort of angina can be relieved with nitroglycerine, beta-blockers or other medicines that dilate arteries or reduce the heart's demand for oxygen. In addition, it's essential to make some lifestyle changes to reduce attacks and prevent the problem from getting worse.

Keep cholesterol under control. Along with other fatty substances in the blood, cholesterol slowly accumulates on the linings of arteries and restricts blood-flow to the heart. If you're having episodes of angina, it probably means fatty build-ups have reached dangerous levels, says heart specialist Howard Weitz.

Keep your total cholesterol no higher than 5.2 millimoles per litre of blood (5.2mmol/L) – the maximum safe upper limit. An average healthy blood cholesterol is where total cholesterol is around 5.2mmol/L, and high-density lipoprotein, or HDL (the so-called 'good' cholesterol) is 1mmol/L or greater. Apart from the use of prescription medication, reducing the amount of saturated fat in your diet is one of the most effective ways to control cholesterol.

Saturated fat is mainly found in red meats, rich puddings, butter and hard cheeses such as cheddar, and snack foods. If you have high cholesterol levels, limit red meat to no more than twice a week and avoid snack foods made with butter or other fats, says nutritionist Kristine Napier.

Eat healthy meats. If you're a meat lover, keep your red meat lean, says family doctor Stephen Amiel. Better still, try low-cholesterol red meats like venison, or eat chicken – breast without the skin is best. Grill rather than fry, or if you must fry, use oils low in saturates and drain well on crumpled kitchen towel.

Feed on fish. Fish is really good for you: oily fish such as fresh tuna, mackerel, sardines or salmon won't put up your cholesterol, and the omega-3 oils they contain can actually protect your heart. Try and eat oily fish at least twice a week, advises Dr Amiel.

WHEN TO CONSULT A DOCTOR

Most people with angina have a form called chronic stable angina. This means that it occurs in predictable ways when they are active – during exercise, for example, or at times of emotional stress – with the pain lasting five minutes or less. Most chronic stable angina can easily be managed with medication and lifestyle changes.

Unstable angina, on the other hand, is much more serious. The discomfort can occur out of the blue, even when you're resting, and the pain may last 20 minutes or more.

'If there is any change in your usual pattern of angina – if symptoms such as pain or shortness of breath get more intense or insistent, dial 999 – you need to get to a hospital casualty department straight away,' warns David Capuzzi, a specialist in heart disease prevention.

Before the ambulance arrives, take 300mg of soluble aspirin straight away. Keep a supply of 300mg aspirin tablets in your cupboard, or take four of your 75mg aspirins in one go. Aspirin thins the blood and can help to dissolve blood clots that may be blocking circulation to the heart. It's important for people with angina or other evidence of coronary disease always to have chewable aspirin to hand.

Choose low-fat dairy produce. Stick to skimmed or semi-skimmed milk and, instead of butter, use margarines which are low in saturated fats, such as those made from sunflower or olive oil, says Dr Amiel. Some spreads and yoghurts, such as Flora Pro-Activ and Benecol, contain plant sterol ester extracts, which actually help to lower blood cholesterol levels over time.

Increase the fibre in your diet. Found in whole grains, pulses, fruits and other plant foods, fibre helps to prevent cholesterol from passing through the intestinal wall into the bloodstream. High-fibre foods are also filling, which means you'll naturally eat smaller amounts of other, fattier foods, Napier says.

Eat vegetarian. A meat-free diet isn't for everyone, but it's an ideal way for those with angina to partially control the underlying coronary artery disease. Not only is a vegetarian diet low in fat – watch the cheese though! – it also provides lots of antioxidants – chemical compounds that help to prevent cholesterol from sticking to artery walls. 'Diet alone can lower cholesterol by up to 20 per cent,' says Dr Weitz.

Most non-vegetarians, too, could still eat more fruit and vegetables, says Dr Amiel. Eating at least five portions (fresh, cooked, canned, dried, juiced – it doesn't matter) every day is one of the best ways to avoid heart disease, and probably cancer and diabetes as well.

Exercise often. Exercise is an important factor in preventing heart disease. Dr Weitz advises people to try and exercise for 20 to 30 minutes six or seven days a week.

It's important to talk to your doctor before starting an exercise plan if you experience angina. You will be advised to build up your fitness gradually – by starting with short walks or swims, for example, and increasing the exertion over a period of weeks or months. 'We worry about the weekend warrior who tries to get all of his exercise at once,' says Dr Weitz.

Exercise later in the day. 'Don't sprint or do any heavy lifting or other stressful exercises in the morning,' Dr Capuzzi advises. Morning can be a risky time for people with angina because fight-or-flight hormones, such as cortisol and noradrenaline, rise overnight and peak in the morning, he says. The levels stay high until about noon, and intense morning exercise is probably not a good idea for most patients with angina.

Be careful too on very cold days when angina symptoms are more easily provoked. Shovelling snow counts as exercise! Ease into the morning, and follow your doctor's advice.

Eat light meals. Large meals are a common angina trigger because blood diverted to the intestine during digestion is then not available to the heart, explains Dr Weitz. Many people can avoid discomfort by eating five or six smaller meals a day rather than two or three large meals.

Maintain a healthy weight. Those extra pounds that tend to accumulate over the years put an incredible load on the heart. For one thing, the heart has to work harder to supply blood to all that extra body tissue. Additionally, being overweight can result in raised cholesterol levels, which makes it harder for blood to circulate. And being overweight also makes you more prone to diabetes, which can itself damage your coronary arteries.

Stay away from smoke. Whether you smoke yourself or are exposed to secondhand smoke on a regular basis, now is the time to clear the air. Smoking even one cigarette temporarily reduces your heart's supply of oxygen, which can result in painful angina.

Take aspirin. If your stomach can handle it, experts generally agree that, if you have angina, taking one low-dose (75mg) aspirin tablet a day is good protection. It won't stop the pain of angina, but it does reduce the risk of blood clots that can lead to heart attacks. In fact, taking an aspirin each day can reduce the risk of coronary heart disease by 28 per cent.

Go nuts for vitamin E. Vitamin E is an antioxidant nutrient. Antioxidants help to prevent a process called oxidation, in which unstable oxygen molecules in the blood damage cholesterol, making it more likely to stick to arteries and reduce blood flow to the heart. Good dietary sources of vitamin E are nuts, vegetable oils, green leafy vegetables and some fortified cereals. Don't overdose on vitamin E, though, advises Dr Amiel. Recent evidence suggests that vitamin E supplements are ineffective compared with dietary sources and high doses may do more harm than good. Vitamin E is particularly helpful for smokers or those with diabetes, who are especially vulnerable to oxidation, says Dr Capuzzi.

Get extra vitamin C. Like vitamin E, vitamin C is an antioxidant that helps to prevent cholesterol from accumulating in the arteries. There's plenty of vitamin C in many fruits and vegetables, particularly citrus fruits and tomatoes. Vitamin C is easily destroyed by cooking or prolonged storage, though. So serve fruits and vegetables raw whenever possible; steam, boil, or simmer foods in a minimal amount of water, or microwave them for the shortest time possible; cook potatoes in their skins; refrigerate prepared juices, and store them for no more than two to three days. As with vitamin E, don't overdose on vitamin C: supplements are rarely necessary. High doses of vitamins E or C can increase oxidative stress and may do more harm than good.

Reduce stress in your life. Emotional stress is an inevitable part of daily life, but when tension and anxiety soar, the body's demand for blood and oxygen increases, which can result in angina. Exercise is an excellent way to reduce stress. Some people meditate. Others practice yoga. Experiment a bit and find out what works best for you.

ANXIETY

21 ways to control excessive worrying

Anxiety, or hand-wrenching, tummy-turning worry, is a natural reaction to some of life's most challenging situations.

A little bit of anxiety can be good. It helps to motivate you to meet a deadline, pass a test, or deliver a well-crafted presentation at work. It also keeps you from walking head-on into danger. As part of the fight-or-flight response, anxiety causes your heart rate to increase and your muscles to tense should you need to act.

At its extreme, however, worry runs amok. Once it begins to interfere with everyday life, worry is considered an anxiety disorder. At least one person in 10 in the UK will have their lives turned upside down by anxiety. Anxiety disorders include panic attacks, generalized anxiety disorder, phobias, post-traumatic stress syndrome and obsessive-compulsive disorder. Sufferers need medical attention and sometimes prescription drugs.

Millions of people fall somewhere in between these two extremes, however. They worry too much but don't have an actual disorder. Chronic worriers are capable of functioning from day to day, but anxiety eats away at their emotional and physical health. Edward Hallowell, a psychiatrist, calls this 'persistent toxic worry'.

'We virtually train ourselves to worry, which only reinforces the habit,' he says. 'Worriers often feel vulnerable if they're not worrying.' But if you worry too much, there are good reasons to stop: excessive worry or anxiety is associated with increased risk of depression, heart disease and other medical conditions.

Overleaf are some tips for tackling excessive worry.

WHEN TO CONSULT A DOCTOR

The line between normal worrying and an anxiety disorder can be hard to define. 'If your life is restricted by anxiety, seek medical attention,' advises psychiatrist Bernard Vittone. Also see a doctor if you:

- experience more than one panic attack a month or fear having a second attack;
- are nervous or anxious most of the time, particularly if your worry is attached to situations that would not make other people anxious;
- frequently experience insomnia, shakiness, poor concentration, tight muscles or heart palpitations;
- feel nervous in or avoid facing particular situations, such as crossing bridges or going through tunnels;
- take refuge from fear or worry by using drugs, including alcohol, or over-eating;
- can't stop obsessing or ruminating about the past;
- are in an emotional crisis, and the support of caring friends, family or clergy doesn't seem to help;
- fear you might harm yourself or others.

Breathe. 'Regulating the breath is the most effective anti-anxiety measure I know,' says Andrew Weil, a professor of medicine. Dr Weil advocates the yogic relaxing breath. Simply inhale through your nose for four seconds, hold your breath for seven seconds, and exhale through your mouth for eight seconds. Practise this technique throughout the day for about a minute at a time.

Make contact. Feeling connected reduces anxiety. The more isolated you feel, the more likely you are to worry, says Dr Hallowell, who recommends daily doses of human contact. Go to a restaurant, a supermarket or a library and start a conversation with someone, or call a friend or relative.

Meditate. Do some sort of meditative activity for at least 15 minutes, up to three or four times each day. Research shows that meditation can significantly lower anxiety. Find a quiet environment, clear your mind and actively relax, says psychiatrist Bernard Vittone. 'Focus on a mantra or make your mind a blank slate, whatever works for you.'

Stay in the present. Focus on what's happening now, not on the past or the future. Take one day, one hour – or even one minute – at a time, advises Dr Vittone.

Don't be a victim. If you're worried – about your job, health or finances, for example – devise a plan to solve potential problems. Don't be a passive victim, says Dr Hallowell. Taking action reduces anxiety: organize a job appraisal with your boss, book a check-up with your GP, or open a savings account.

Get the facts. Exaggerated worry often stems from a lack of information, explains Dr Hallowell. If your boss snubs you in the hall, you may worry that you're not doing a good job. But the boss may have been pondering a personal matter, not even aware that you were there.

Reduce distractions. People who are too anxious need to decrease stimulation, says Dr Vittone. Eliminate some of the racket vying for your attention. Turn off the car radio, don't answer the telephone

KITCHEN CURES

To calm yourself before bedtime, reach for a glass of warm milk. 'The old wives' remedy of drinking warm milk really does help,' says psychiatrist Bernard Vittone. Milk contains the amino acid tryptophan, which is known to have a relaxing effect.

Cut down on caffeine

Nothing is worse for anxiety than caffeine, says psychiatrist Bernard Vittone. Found in foods like chocolate; drinks such as coffee, tea, colas and energy-boosting drinks; and over-the-counter medicines such as cough syrups, nasal decongestants and cold remedies, caffeine affects neurotransmitters in the brain, causing anxiety. Research shows that people who are predisposed to anxiety and those with panic disorders are especially sensitive to caffeine's effects.

Caffeine is deceptive, says Dr Vittone. When you drink a cup of coffee, for example, you're likely to feel more vivacious for up to an hour. Two to 12 hours after that, caffeine's anxiety-producing effects kick in. Because of this delayed reaction, people rarely connect anxiety to their morning cup of coffee.

If you consume a lot of caffeine, try this test: abstain from coffee and other caffeine-containing foods and drinks for two weeks. Then, drink three cups of coffee in one sitting and see how you feel. You'll probably notice a tightening of muscles, worry, nervousness or apprehension several hours later.

'I really advocate trying to cut out caffeine completely,' Dr Vittone says. If that's asking too much, then limit coffee, tea or colas to one cup a day.

at home, take a lunch break away from your office – and away from your mobile phone.

Take a 'news fast'. Turn off the television and resist reading a newspaper. Taking a break from the news for a few days can help to decrease feelings of anxiety and may help to reduce personal worries, says Dr Weil.

Imagine the worst. Ask yourself, 'What's the worst that could happen?' 'How bad would it be?' 'What's the likelihood of it happening?'

The worst thing that can happen usually isn't that bad, Dr Vittone says. What's more, it seldom happens. Later, you may even wonder why you were worried at all.

Write it down. Putting your anxious thoughts down on paper can help to defuse them and restore calm, says Dr Weil.

Prepare to sleep. Before going to bed, give yourself time to unwind and

Choosing a therapist

If you suffer from anxiety your GP can refer you to a counsellor or psychologist for cognitive behaviour therapy. Alternatively, you may decide to consult a therapist independently, which will mean paying someone for their time and expertise.

• Try to obtain a personal recommendation – or ask your GP whether the therapist you are considering has a good reputation.

• Ask to see evidence of the therapist's qualifications.

• Determine how much the treatment will cost before you begin – some therapists are very expensive.

• During your first session, think about how comfortable the therapist makes you feel. If by the end of the session you feel more hopeful and empowered, you have probably found someone who can help you.

relax, says Dr Vittone. Spend 30 to 50 minutes doing something quiet and stress-free before bed. Read a light novel or watch a television comedy, and avoid doing any active tasks such as washing-up or ironing.

Laugh at yourself. Dr Vittone explains that seeing the funny side of a situation immediately defuses the threat. So take another view of your worries. Ask yourself 'what's funny about this situation?' or 'when I think about this in two years, will I laugh?'

Share your worry. Never worry alone. 'When we talk about our worries the toxicity dissipates,' says Dr Hallowell. Talking it through helps us to find solutions and to realize that our concerns aren't quite so overwhelming.

Let it go. Chronic worriers have a tough time letting go. You may cling to worry as though it will cure the problem, Dr Hallowell says. It won't. So practise, practise, practise. Train yourself to let go. He suggests meditation or visualization, but you can develop your own technique.

One of his patients 'sees' worries in the palm of her hand and blows them away. Another takes a shower and 'watches' his worries go down the drain. 'Don't feel like a failure if you can't do it at first,' he says. 'Keep practising.'

Handle with less care. Stop treating yourself as fragile. If you believe that you're fragile, it becomes a self-fulfilling prophecy. Instead, learn to make anxiety a stimulus and not a handicap. If you're about to give a speech, for instance, see it as a thrill instead of a threat.

Find your challenge. Anxiety often arises when people have too many things going on at once. Instead of viewing your busyness as negative, think of life as action-filled, rich or challenging. If you are bringing up a family, for example, think about how one day you'll really miss your children's presence at home. The way you interpret things makes all the difference, says Dr Vittone.

Avoid alcohol. Beer, wine and other alcoholic drinks can exacerbate anxiety. 'Alcohol reduces the anxiety when you first take it in,' says Dr Vittone. 'But when it wears off, it has the opposite effect.' People are often more anxious the day after a night of heavy drinking, he says. Avoid alcohol, or limit consumption to one or two drinks a day.

Try soothing valerian. Anxiety is nothing new. From earliest times, people have looked for herbs to take the edge off. According to clinical herbalist Douglas Schar, the safest, most reliable and most readily available natural anxiety melter is valerian.

Ideally, you should use the herbal medicine while you are resolving the source of your anxiety. 'The herb is best taken in capsule form,' says Schar. 'Take it three times a day if you are going through a bad patch, or on the spot if an anxiety attack overtakes you.'

ASTHMA
26 steps to better breathing

Many people think of asthma as a childhood illness rather than one that's a particular problem for adults. But the National Asthma Campaign's statistics show that 5.1 million people in the UK are being treated for the condition – one child in eight, and one in every 13 adults.

Asthma is rarely serious enough to require hospitalization. It may cause only occasional and short-lived symptoms, such as breathlessness, coughing or wheezing. But unless your asthma is well-controlled, it subtly interferes with normal activity and can quickly get out of hand.

Asthma occurs when the main air passages in the lungs, called bronchioles, become inflamed and overly sensitive to 'triggers'. During attacks, the lungs produce extra mucus and the bronchiole walls narrow, making breathing difficult.

No cure for asthma exists yet, but nearly everyone can dramatically reduce – and maybe even eliminate – their symptoms. Even if you currently use prescription drugs to treat your asthma, you may be able to reduce the dose or frequency by more than 50 per cent if you make certain changes to your lifestyle. Here are some approaches recommended by doctors.

Look into allergies. More than 80 per cent of adults with asthma have allergies that trigger or worsen symptoms. Thomas Plaut, an asthma specialist, believes that anyone who uses asthma medication every day should try and find out if they are allergic to anything (see *Allergies*, page 28). Think about when your symptoms occur and what you are doing at the time. Any patterns may help to indicate what you're allergic to. You might want to keep an asthma diary.

Keep a food diary. Food allergies are quite rare, but they're worth considering if you have asthma. For one thing, people with asthma tend to have more serious reactions to allergens in foods. And about eight per cent of those with severe asthma also have a food allergy, says Dr Plaut.

Almost any food can cause a reaction in someone with asthma. The main culprits are preservatives and additives, such as the sulphites added to some wines, beers, dried fruit and frozen foods.

If you write down everything you eat for a month or two and jot down the dates of asthma attacks and the severity of symptoms, you'll get a good idea of whether anything in your diet is contributing to the problem.

Avoid pollen. Pollen is a major asthma trigger. Plants pollinate at specific times of the year, so once you know which pollens are your triggers, take steps to avoid them. Stay indoors on summer mornings until about 10am if you can, and on warm, dry, windy days, for example, when pollen counts tend to be highest. During the warmer months, keep your windows closed.

Grass pollens are the main seasonal allergens in Britain, reaching peak levels in May, June and July. Local television and newspaper weather reports give daily pollen counts, so you'll know when it's a good idea to stay inside. Earlier in the year, allergies are more likely to be caused by tree pollens. And in autumn, moulds and fungi can cause problems.

Open the bathroom window. Mould is a common asthma trigger, and it thrives in bathrooms and other high-moisture areas. Good ventilation is essential. Use the extractor fan or open the window whenever you bath or shower to help remove the moisture that mould needs to thrive.

And after a shower, try wiping the bathroom tiles dry. It takes about 30 seconds, gets rid of excess moisture and is a good way of preventing mould, says Dr Plaut.

Wash your pets every week. Dogs and cats are loaded with dander – tiny flakes of dried saliva found on animal skin and fur that can provoke asthma attacks. Some people with asthma who are allergic to pets will need to find new homes for them. At the very least, bath your pets once a week – with or without shampoo – to remove dander.

Open windows when you cook. Strong food smells – from a smoky frying pan, for example, or the pungent oils in raw onions and garlic – can irritate the airways and trigger asthma attacks. Open the window or use an extractor fan when you cook to help waft the odours outside.

Keep dust under control. It's impossible to eliminate all dust, but the more you get rid of, the less likely you are to have asthma attacks, says Dr Plaut.

A few times a week, run a damp cloth over picture frames, windowsills and other areas where dust accumulates. Mop vinyl and wood floors, and use a vacuum cleaner equipped with a HEPA (high-energy particulate-arresting) filter (Dyson produces various models), which traps dust particles and keeps them from being breathed in.

Do just *one* thing

If you take medication for asthma control, get in the habit of using a peak-flow meter. Available from pharmacists, or on prescription from your doctor, it's a device that measures the speed at which air leaves the lungs. The meter is an invaluable way to detect the airway narrowing that occurs before an asthma attack. Treating asthma as early as possible can help to prevent emergencies.

A reading of between 80 and 100 per cent of your normal peak flow indicates that your breathing is healthy, says Dr Thomas Plaut. Lower scores may mean that you need higher doses of medication or that your asthma isn't adequately controlled.

It's also important to keep a daily diary that lists the following: peak-flow levels, the frequency and severity of symptoms, how often you are using medicines, and possible triggers you've been exposed to. By looking at the diary regularly, Dr Plaut says you will be able to detect factors that cause your asthma to worsen – and those that cause it to improve.

Get rid of dust mites. Despite the name, these microscopic creatures thrive on dead skin cells, not dust. They are a common asthma trigger, and because people shed millions of skin cells every day, dust mites cannot be totally eliminated. They can be reduced, however.

Vacuuming the house – not just the floors but also the upholstery – goes a long way towards reducing mite populations. It's also important to wash sheets, pillowcases and bathroom towels at least once a week. Use water that's 60°C or hotter to kill adult mites as well as the eggs, says Dr Plaut.

'It's also important to encase pillows and mattresses with covers made specifically to act as a barrier against dust mites,' he adds. Anti-allergy covers are available in the bed linen sections of larger department stores.

Make your house a smoke-free zone. Cigarette smoke is extremely irritating. It not only triggers asthma attacks but also can increase the risk of asthma in children.

If you are a smoker, try and quit: use nicotine patches, prescription drugs or join a support group. Let everyone know that smoking is banned in your house.

Feast on flavonoids. To fight the inflammation that accompanies asthma, eat foods rich in flavonoids – these are tiny crystals in fruits and vegetables that give them their blue, yellow or reddish hues. Good sources include citrus fruits, grapes, apples, onions, plums, grapefruit, cherries, blackberries, bilberries and blackcurrants.

Flavonoids not only strengthen the capillary walls, they are also antioxidants, which means they help to protect the membranes in the airways from damage by pollution. Eat a couple of servings of flavonoid-rich foods every day.

Take magnesium. Extra magnesium may help to decrease muscle tension and reduce airway spasms, explains Kendall Gerdes, an expert in environmental medicine. Fresh fruit and vegetables, and wholemeal bread, are good dietary sources of magnesium.

If increasing your intake of these does not help your asthma, try supplements (but don't stop the fruit and veg!). Take 100 to 500mg one to three times a day. Because high doses of magnesium (350mg or more) can cause stomach cramp, wind or diarrhoea in some people, Dr Gerdes suggests starting with the lowest dose and increasing it gradually until you experience these side-effects. Then cut back the dose until problems subside.

Note: If you have heart or kidney problems, talk to your doctor before taking magnesium supplements.

WHEN TO CONSULT A DOCTOR

The symptoms of asthma are often subtle at first, but they can get much worse very quickly. Any changes in your usual breathing patterns need to be checked by a doctor.

If you're already being treated for asthma, see your doctor if you find you need to use your asthma medication more frequently. Also, if your wheeze, cough or shortness of breath gets worse even after the medicine has been given time to work, you need to call your doctor. If ever you have an attack, it means the asthma isn't as well-controlled as it should be.

Supplement with quercetin. Quercetin is a flavonoid extracted from certain fruits and vegetables, such as apples and onions, that helps inhibit the allergic reaction that can lead to asthma. Take 250mg of quercetin (available in health food stores) per day, advises Elson Haas, a health and nutrition specialist.

Note. Because asthma is a serious, highly individual condition, it's a good idea to talk to your doctor before making any changes to your treatment, he adds.

Stay active. An active lifestyle can help to control asthma much better than a sedentary one. Physical activity helps to improve lung capacity and may enable people to use lower doses of medications or to use them less often. Anyone with asthma should discuss an exercise programme with his or her doctor.

Exercise in warm weather. Breathing in cold air – when cycling or skiing, for example – can irritate the airways and trigger asthma attacks. When exercising outdoors, make sure you wear a mask to create a reservoir of warm air, advises Dr Plaut.

If you notice that you have more asthma attacks during the cold months, consider changing your activities. Swimming is especially good because the moist air soothes the airways and reduces the risk of attacks.

Change your breathing style. Most people breathe using only their chest muscles. This makes it difficult to empty air from the lungs completely. For those with asthma, it's important to use the diaphragm as well. This large muscle between the chest and abdomen adds power to your breathing and helps to remove 'used' air from the lungs, which can reduce feelings of breathlessness, explains Dr Plaut.

KITCHEN CURES

If you or anyone in your family has asthma, put fish on the menu at least twice a week.

Fatty fish such as tuna, salmon and mackerel contain beneficial fats called omega-3 fatty acids. Asthma is an inflammatory disease, and the omega-3s help to damp down many of the body's processes that create inflammation.

It takes practice to get in the habit of diaphragmatic breathing (also called abdominal breathing). Several times a day, lie on your back with one hand on your belly and the other on your chest. As you breathe in, the hand on your belly should rise slightly, while the hand on your chest should barely move.

Take up a wind instrument. Playing an instrument like the oboe, saxophone or trumpet requires abdominal breathing, Dr Plaut says. Even if you aren't especially musical, it's great practice for breathing muscles.

Practise stress control. Yoga, self-hypnosis, deep breathing and other techniques for reducing stress are helpful for asthma because they help the airways to open more fully, says Dr Plaut.

Wash your hands often. Asthma attacks tend to surge in the autumn and winter, when people get more colds. Even a mild case of the sniffles can make asthma harder to control. Viral infections commonly trigger asthma attacks.

Cold viruses can survive for hours on doorknobs, hand-rails and even money. Washing your hands often – at least every few hours – will flush away the viruses before they have a chance to take hold.

Beware of aspirin and ibuprofen. About five per cent of people with asthma are sensitive to aspirin, ibuprofen and related pain relievers, known as nonsteroidal anti-inflammatory drugs (NSAIDs), says Dr Plaut. For those who are sensitive, an asthma attack or other respiratory problems can begin within two hours of taking the drugs.

If you need long-term pain relief – because of arthritis, for example – your doctor may advise you to switch to paracetamol or other analgesics that are less likely to trigger asthma attacks.

Don't put up with heartburn. The upward surge of stomach acids that cause the telltale pain of heartburn can also trigger asthma attacks. One of the best ways to prevent heartburn is to eat four or more small meals daily, instead of two or three large meals, Dr Plaut advises. Also, don't eat just before bedtime.

To help prevent stomach acid from going 'upstream', raise the head of your bed 10 to 15cm by putting blocks under the legs of the bed.

You can also quell heartburn with over-the-counter antacids, or talk to your doctor about acid-suppressing drugs such as cimetidine (Tagamet) or ranitidine (Zantac).

Sniff salt and water. Sinus infections are common in Britain, and the inflammation and mucus drainage can make asthma worse. Sinusitis often requires treatment with antibiotics, but you may be able to prevent infections by flushing your sinuses at home, says Dr Plaut.

Mix ½ teaspoon of salt into a cup of warm water. Pour a little of the solution into your cupped palm and snort it up one nostril while holding the other nostril closed. Then repeat with the other nostril. People who get frequent sinus infections should repeat this treatment once a day.

If you get infections less often, it's fine to flush the sinuses only when you have a cold or when your allergies are worse than usual.

Act quickly if asthma strikes. Don't ignore early signs of asthma attacks, even if the symptoms – wheezing, coughing, or faster breathing – seem mild at first.

Use your reliever inhaler promptly. It will help to reverse airway narrowing before the attack gets more serious, says Dr Plaut.

Buy or make a spacer. A spacer fits on to your inhaler and improves the delivery of inhaled medication to your lungs by up to 30 per cent, says family doctor Stephen Amiel. It is an inexpensive plastic device available from your pharmacist or on prescription from your doctor.

At the beginning of an asthma attack, try several puffs of your reliever inhaler via the spacer, one puff each minute or so.

If you haven't got a spacer, cut a hole just big enough for your inhaler nozzle in the bottom of a polystyrene cup or plastic bottle. Position the cup over your nose and mouth while you press the inhaler, or close your lips around the neck of the bottle.

Keep track of inhaler 'puffs'. If you use medication to control asthma, the worst thing is to discover that your inhaler is empty when you need it.

To prevent that happening, put a piece of masking tape on the inhaler and make a mark on the tape every time you use it.

ATHLETE'S FOOT

16 ways to get rid of it

You don't have to be an athlete to catch athlete's foot. The fungal infection, which is caused by an organism that lives on the skin and breeds best under warm, moist conditions, can be caught simply by letting your bare feet touch damp floors in changing rooms, swimming pools and bathrooms. But even though these balmy climates encourage the growth of the fungus, sweaty trainers are more often the culprit.

Athlete's foot (or *tinea pedis*) causes a flaky, sometimes itchy, and sometimes red rash. In most people this is confined to the spaces between the toes, but it can spread and affect more of the foot. In some people the skin becomes very sore and even bleeds. The condition may be worsened if it becomes infected with bacteria that take advantage of the damaged skin.

Creams, powders and sprays to treat athlete's foot can mostly be bought over the counter. They work by killing the fungus and need to be used until the skin appears normal, and then for a further two weeks to eradicate all the remaining fungal spores. Meanwhile, here are some tips on dealing with an active infection and ways to guard against a repeat.

Baby your foot. Athlete's foot can come on suddenly and may be accompanied by oozing blisters and an intermittent burning sensation, says family doctor Frederick Hass. When you're going through this acute stage, baby your foot. Keep it uncovered and rest it. Although the inflammation itself is not dangerous, it can get worse, leading to a bacterial infection if you're not careful.

Try an old-fashioned remedy. A time-honoured remedy is soaking the feet in potassium permanganate solution, says pharmacist Sue Livingston, but beware – the solution can stain the feet brown.

Soak in a salt bath. Soak your foot in a mixture of two teaspoons of salt per 500ml warm water, says chiropodist Glenn Copeland. Do this for 5 to 10 minutes at a time, and repeat until the problem clears up. The saline solution provides an inhospitable atmosphere for the fungus and lessens excess perspiration. What's more, it softens the affected skin so that antifungal medications can penetrate deeper and act more effectively.

Medicate your foot. Now's the time to apply an over-the-counter antifungal medication, such as miconazole and clotrimazole: brands include Daktarin and Canesten AF, which are available as creams, powders or

WHEN TO CONSULT A DOCTOR

How do you know if that red, itchy area between your toes is a true case of athlete's foot? According to dermatologist Thomas Goodman, the rash probably isn't athlete's foot if:

- it is on a child's foot. (It is very rare for a child below the age of puberty to have a fungal infection of the foot.)
- it is on top of the toes. (Eruptions on the tops of toes and the top of the foot are probably some form of contact dermatitis caused by shoes.)
- the foot is red, swollen, sore, blistered and oozing. See a doctor, because you may have an acute form of dermatitis.

You cannot assume that athlete's foot will go away of its own accord, says chiropodist Suzanne Levine. An untreated fungal infection can lead to cracks in the skin and possibly a nasty bacterial infection. Signs of bacterial infection include:

- inflammation that makes it very painful to walk;
- swelling in the foot or the leg at any time during a bout of athlete's foot, and a raised temperature;
- pus in the blisters or in the cracked skin.

sprays. Your pharmacist will be able to advise you. Dermatologist Thomas Goodman recommends that you lightly apply the medication to the area and rub in gently. Continue two or three times a day for four weeks (or for two weeks after the problem seems to have cleared up).

Treat between your toes. For athlete's foot between your toes, says Dr Goodman, try applying Driclor (aluminium chloride hexahydrate). Marketed for excessive perspiration of the feet, Driclor is available from pharmacies. This will not only kill fungus but also help to dry the area, discouraging regrowth. Apply between your toes two or three times a day. Continue for two weeks after the infection clears up.

Note: Don't use aluminium chloride on cracked or raw skin – it will sting like mad. Heal the cracks first with an antifungal agent.

Scrub away dead skin. When the acute phase of the attack has settled down, says Dr Hass, remove any dead skin, which houses living fungi that can reinfect you. 'At bath time, work the entire foot lightly but vigorously with a bristle nail brush. Pay extra attention to spaces between toes – use a small bottle brush there.' But if you scrub your feet in the bathtub, be sure to shower afterwards to wash away any bits of skin that could attach themselves to other parts of the body and start another infection.

Pay attention to toenails. Toenails are favourite breeding grounds for the fungus, says Dr Hass. Scrape the undersides of your nails clean at least every second or third day. Use an orange stick or wooden match rather than a metal nail file, which could scratch the nails and provide niches for the fungus to collect in.

Keep applying cream. Once your infection has cleared up, help to guard against its return by continuing to use (less often) the antifungal cream or lotion that cured your problem, says Dr Goodman. This is especially wise in warm weather. Use your own judgement as to how often to use it; from once a day to once a week is fine.

Choose proper shoes. Avoid plastic shoes and footwear that has been treated to keep water out, says Dr Copeland. They trap perspiration and create a warm, moist spot for the fungus to grow. Natural materials such as cotton and leather provide the best environment for feet, while rubber and even wool may induce sweating and hold moisture.

Change shoes often. Don't wear the same shoes two days running, says chiropodist Dean Stern. It takes at least 24 hours for shoes to dry out thoroughly. If your feet sweat heavily, change your shoes twice a day.

Keep shoes dry – and clean. Dust the insides of your shoes frequently with antifungal powder or spray. Another good idea, says chiropodist Neal Kramer, is to spray some disinfectant on to a rag and use it to wipe out the insides of your shoes every time you take them off. That will kill any fungus spores.

Air your shoes. Dr Hass recommends giving your shoes a little time in the sun to air out. Remove the laces and prop each shoe open. You should even leave sandals outdoors to dry between wearings. And wipe the undersides of their straps clean after wearing to remove any fungi-carrying dead skin. The idea is to reduce even the slightest possibility of reinfection.

KITCHEN CURES

For fungus between the toes, apply a baking soda paste, suggests chiropodist Suzanne Levine. Add a little lukewarm water to a tablespoon of baking soda. Rub the paste on to the fungus, then rinse and dry thoroughly. Finish the treatment by dusting with cornflour.

Socks matter, too. If your feet sweat heavily, says Dr Hass, change your socks three or four times a day. And wear only clean cotton socks, not those made from synthetic fibres. To kill fungus spores, says Dr Kramer, wash your socks twice in extra-hot water. Afterwards, be sure to rinse them thoroughly as detergent residues can aggravate your skin problem.

Powder your toes. To keep your feet as dry as possible, allow them to air-dry for 5 to 10 minutes after a shower or bath before putting your socks and shoes on, says dermatologist Diana Bihova. To speed up drying, hold a hair dryer about 15cm from your foot, wiggle your toes and dry between them. Then apply powder. To prevent making a mess with loose powder, put it in a plastic or paper bag, then put your foot into the bag and shake it well.

Cover up in public places. You can decrease your exposure to athlete's foot, says Dr Goodman, by wearing flip-flops in areas where other people go barefooted. That includes gyms, spas, health clubs, changing rooms and even around swimming pools. If you are prone to fungal infections, you can pick them up almost anywhere damp – so be vigilant.

BACKACHE
20 ideas to ease the pain

More than 11 million working days are lost each year in Britain as a result of back pain. It is estimated that four out of five of us will suffer from back pain at some time in our lives. It is most common among people of middle age, although younger men and women can also be affected.

There are two forms of back pain: acute and chronic.

Acute Back Pain

Acute pain comes on suddenly and intensely. It's the kind you usually experience from doing something that you shouldn't be doing or from doing it the wrong way. The pain can come from sprains, strains or pulls of muscles in your back. It may be extremely sore for several days, but doctors say that you can be free of the pain, without any lasting effects, by following these self-help tips.

Stay active. Forget the old adage about getting plenty of bed rest. Researchers at the University of Texas school of nursing found that patients who exercised returned to work more quickly than those who didn't.

WHEN TO CONSULT A DOCTOR

Simple mechanical back pain rarely needs a doctor's attention, and x-rays are actively discouraged. However, there are a number of 'red flag' symptoms, warning signs or factors, says Stephen Amiel, a family doctor. If you have back pain and any of the following applies, you should definitely consult your doctor soon.

- The pain is constant and getting worse, or is no better after 4–6 weeks.
- You continue to have great difficulty bending forwards.
- You get back pain for the first time before the age of 20 or after the age of 55.
- The pain follows serious trauma such as a road traffic accident.
- The pain is in the upper part of the spine.
- You have had cancer in the past or at present.
- You are on steroids.
- You have anorexia or osteoporosis.
- You are a drug abuser, or have HIV.
- You are generally unwell in yourself or have recently lost significant amounts of weight.
- You have developed problems in your nervous system (e.g. numbness, loss of power, difficulty with opening your bowels, passing urine etc.).
- You have developed an obvious structural deformity of your spine.

If you must go to bed, keep it brief. 'Most people think that a week of bed rest will take away the pain,' says back expert David Lehrman. 'But that's not so. For every week of bed rest, it takes two weeks to rehabilitate.'

A study conducted at Texas University bears this out. Researchers studied 203 patients who attended a walk-in clinic complaining of acute back pain. Some were told to rest for two days, others for seven days. There was no difference in the length of time it took for the pain to diminish in either group, reports one of the researchers, Dr Richard Deyo. But those who got out of bed after only two days returned to work sooner.

Put your pain on ice. The best way to cool down an acute flare-up is with ice, says pain researcher Ronald Melzack. It helps to reduce swelling and the strain on your back muscles. For best results, he says, try massaging the site of the pain with an ice pack – or a bag of frozen peas – for seven or eight minutes. Do this every few hours for a day or two.

Try some heat relief. After the first day or two using ice, doctors recommend that you switch to heat, says chiropractor and physiotherapist Milton Fried. Take a soft towel and put it into a basin of very warm water. Wring it out well and flatten it so that there are no creases in it. Lie on your stomach, with pillows under your hips and ankles, and fold the towel across the painful part of your back. Put some cling-film over the towel, and then put a heating pad, set on medium, on top of the plastic. If possible, place something on top that will create pressure, like a phone book. 'This moist heat will help to reduce muscle spasms,' he explains. You will probably need to enlist a friend to help you with this.

Use heat and cold. If you can't make up your mind which feels better, it's okay to use both methods, says orthopaedic specialist Edward Abraham. It may even have an added bonus: 'an intermittent regime of heat and ice will actually make you feel better,' he says. 'Do 30 minutes of ice, then 30 minutes of heat, and keep repeating the cycle.'

Stretch to smooth a spasm. Stretching a sore back will actually enhance the healing process, says Dr Lehrman, by helping the muscle to calm down more quickly than by simply waiting for it to calm down on its own. He recommends the following stretch for lower back pain: gently bring your knees up from the bed and to your chest. Once there, put a little pressure on your knees. Stretch, then relax. Repeat.

Roll out of bed. Every morning when you get out of bed, doctors advise that you roll out – carefully and slowly. 'You can minimize the pain of getting out of bed by sliding to the edge of the bed,' says Dr Lehrman. 'Once there, keep your back rigid and then let your legs come off the bed first. That movement will act as a springboard, lifting your upper body straight up off the bed.'

Chronic Back Pain

For some people, back pain is chronic, an ongoing part of everyday life. For whatever reason, the pain lingers on for what can seem like an eternity. Other people experience recurring pain: any little movement can set it in motion. The following tips are particularly helpful for those with chronic pain, although people with acute pain can benefit.

Support your mattress. The object is to make sure your bed doesn't sag in the middle when you sleep on it, says Dr Fried. A large, sturdy board – such as an old tabletop or a sheet of 18mm MDF – between the

Exercise the pain away

Exercise may be the last thing you want to think about when your back aches, but specialists say that exercise is the best thing for chronic back pain.

Exercise can be especially beneficial for people who suffer from back pain every day, especially if the pain varies throughout the day, says back specialist Roger Minkow. If you are under a doctor's care for back pain, ask before you begin any exercise programme.

Here are some exercises recommended by doctors.

Semi-press-up. Lie on the floor on your stomach. Keep your pelvis flat on the floor and push up with your hands, arching your back as you lift your shoulders. Do this once in the morning and once in the afternoon to strengthen your lower back.

Move into a crunch. While on the floor, turn over onto your back and do what's called a crunch sit-up. Lie flat with both feet on the floor and your knees bent. Cross your arms and rest your hands on your shoulders. Lift your head and shoulders off the floor as high as you can while keeping your lower back on the floor. Hold for one second, then repeat.

Swim on dry land. Lie on your stomach and raise your left arm and your right leg. Hold for one second, then alternate with your left leg and right arm as if you were swimming. This will extend and strengthen your lower back, says Dr Minkow.

Get into the pool. Swimming in a warm pool is regarded by most doctors as the best exercise for the back – it is even recommended for acute lower-back pain. Breast stroke can be a problem though, if you try to keep your head out of the water all the time by arching your back.

Exercise pedal power. 'Ride a stationary bike with a mirror set up so that you can see yourself,' says Dr Minkow. 'Be sure to sit up straight without slouching. If you have to, raise the handlebars so that you're not bent forward.'

Know your limit. If the exercise you're doing hurts or aggravates your condition, says Dr Minkow, don't do it anymore. 'You're not going to improve anything by gritting your teeth and doing one more repetition. If you feel fine the day after or two days after you exercise, then it's safe to continue exercising.'

mattress and the divan base will prevent the mattress from sagging.

Prolong the life of your mattress by turning it regularly (watch your back, though!) and change it after a maximum of ten years.

Drown pain with a waterbed. An adjustable waterbed that doesn't make a lot of waves is excellent for most types of back trouble, says Dr Fried. Dr Abraham agrees. 'In waterbeds, you get an equalized change in the pressure on various segments of your body,' he says. 'You can lie in one position for the whole night because of this.'

Become a 'lazy S' sleeper. A bad back can't stomach lying face down. 'The best position for someone resting in bed is what we call the lazy S position,' says Dr Abraham. 'Put a pillow under your head and upper neck, keep your back relatively flat on the bed, then put a pillow under your knees.'

When you straighten your legs, your hamstring muscles pull and put pressure on your lower back, he explains. Keeping your knees bent puts slack into the hamstrings and takes the pressure off your back.

Sleep like a baby. Sleep on your side in the foetal position for a good night's rest. 'It's a good idea to stick a pillow between your knees when you sleep on your side,' says Dr Fried. 'The pillow stops your leg from sliding forward and rotating your hips, which puts added pressure on your back.'

Take aspirin or ibuprofen every day. Doctors say that this can help to keep back pain at bay. Back pain is often accompanied by inflammation around the site of the pain, says Dr Fried, and simple over-the-counter anti-inflammatory drugs, such as aspirin or ibuprofen, can help to take it away. This can even help when the inflammation is quite severe. Paracetamol is not as effective because it is not an anti-inflammatory drug.

Note: Anti-inflammatory drugs can irritate the stomach lining and cause internal bleeding, says family doctor Stephen Amiel. If you suffer from frequent indigestion, heartburn or stomach ulcers, or you are over 75, you should not take these drugs without consulting your doctor first.

Take nature's anti-inflammatory. If you're looking for a natural anti-inflammatory, try willow bark (*salix alba*), which can be bought as a tincture or in capsule form in health food stores. 'Willow is a natural salicylate, the active ingredient that gives aspirin its anti-inflammatory power,' says Dr Fried. 'Taken after meals, it shouldn't hurt your stomach, and it works very well on mild to moderate back pain'. But, as with anti-inflammatory drugs, don't take willow if you suffer from stomach ulcers or heartburn.

Visualize yourself pain-free. The middle of the night can be the worst time for pain: it wakes you up, and it keeps you awake. Anaesthetist Dennis Turk recommends using a technique known as visualization at times like these. 'Close your eyes and imagine a lemon on a white china plate. See a knife next to it. See yourself picking up the knife and slicing the lemon. Hear the sound it makes cutting through. Smell the aroma. Bring the lemon up to your face and imagine its taste.'

The idea is to bring as much detail to the image as possible. The more involved the image is, the more you are engaged with it and the quicker you will become distracted from the pain.

Learn how to look after your back. It's often said, 'You're as old as your back', yet so many of us misuse our backs horribly, says Dr Amiel. Chronic back pain is often a result of poor posture, bad lifting and sitting habits, and tension.

Learn how to lift heavy objects using your legs, arms and back properly, says Dr Amiel. Check that your computer workstation and chair are adjusted to your dimensions and have a 10-minute break from your screen every hour you work at a computer.

Speak to your employers if you need training in lifting or different equipment to work with. And don't slouch for hours in a sagging armchair watching television.

Car seat comfort

Does your back cause you pain every time you get in the car? The seat could be the problem. While there are many possible causes of back pain, most people have what is called mechanical back pain – or pain related to sitting, standing, lifting or bending, says Dr Roger Minkow, who designs seats for aeroplane and car manufacturers.

'Test sit' a new car. Next time you change your car, test for seat comfort as well as driveability, suggests back specialist Roger Minkow. Adjust the seat so that your legs are slightly bent when you push on the pedals. The back of the seat should push against your lower back around your waist. It's a good idea to rent the same make and model for a weekend and go for a long drive to see how comfortable the seat is.

Inflate a pillow. If you are not in the market for a new car, an inflatable cushion is a cheap fix for mechanical back pain, says Dr Minkow. Cushions are available in health catalogues or online – try www.thebackshop.co.uk.

Don't over-inflate the cushion: it should feel floppy and just fill the space in the curve of the lower back, putting the spine into 'neutral' and preventing slouching.

Try the Alexander technique. Dr Amiel suggests taking a course of lessons to learn the Alexander technique. This shows you how to let go of unnecessary tensions, and how to use your body – particularly your back – to help you perform everyday activities as you were designed to.

Or learn to untie muscle knots with tai chi. Tai chi is an ancient Chinese discipline of slow, fluid movements. 'It's a great relaxation method that helps the muscles in your back,' says Dr Abraham, who uses the method himself. 'There are a lot of breathing exercises and stretching activities that foster a harmony within the body'. Tai chi takes time and self-discipline to learn, but Dr Abraham says that it's well worth it.

BAD BREATH
17 ways to overcome it

In Roman times, people used sticks for toothbrushes and tooth powder so abrasive that it ground away the surface of the teeth, exposing the pulp. When their teeth hurt, they applied olive oil in which earthworms had been boiled... After all that, it's probably safe to say they had bad breath.

Today, dental hygiene is big business. But people still worry about their breath. The good news is that for the most part – with proper dental care – bad breath, also called halitosis, can be avoided. Here's how.

Don't eat garlic. Certain tastes and smells recirculate through the essential oils that they leave in your mouth. Depending on how much you eat, the odour can remain for up to 24 hours, no matter how often you brush your teeth. Foods to avoid include raw onions, hot peppers and garlic.

Get rid of garlic breath. If you need to get rid of that garlicky breath, try one of these remedies, suggests family doctor Stephen Amiel: chew fresh parsley (see *Kitchen Cures* box, page 67), munch a coffee bean or chew a lemon wedge.

Give up smoking. Yet another reason to kick the habit – a smoker's breath can smell like the bottom of an ashtray to a non-smoker, says Dr Amiel.

Avoid smelly salami. Spiced meats such as pastrami, salami and

WHEN TO CONSULT A DOCTOR

If your halitosis lasts for more than 24 hours without an obvious cause, make an appointment to see your dentist or doctor, advises dentist Roger Levin. It could be a sign of gum disease, gastrointestinal problems or a more serious underlying condition. Bad breath can also be a sign of dehydration or zinc deficiency, or it can be caused by certain prescription drugs, including penicillamine (used to treat rheumatoid arthritis) and lithium, a drug used in bipolar disorder.

pepperoni also leave oils behind long after you have swallowed them. If an occasion calls for sweet-smelling breath, avoid these meats for 24 hours beforehand to keep them from talking for you.

Say 'no' to strong cheeses. Camembert, Roquefort and other ripe cheeses are called strong for good reason – they get hold of your breath and don't let go. Other dairy products may have the same effect.

Beware pungent fish. Some fish, particularly anchovies, but also the tuna in your packed lunch, can leave a lasting impression.

Stick with water. Coffee, beer, wine and whisky top the list of liquid offenders. Each leaves a residue that clings to the plaque in your mouth and infiltrates your digestive system. Every time you breathe out, you expel traces back into the air.

Carry a toothbrush. Some odours can be eliminated – permanently or temporarily – if you brush your teeth immediately after a meal.

The main culprit in bad breath is a soft, sticky film of living and dead bacteria that clings to your teeth and gums, says dentist Eric Shapira. That film is called plaque. At any time, there are 50 trillion of these microscopic organisms loitering in your mouth. They sit in every dark corner, eating each morsel of food that passes your lips, collecting little smells and producing little odours of their own. As you exhale, the bacteria exhale. So brush away the plaque after each meal and get rid of some of the breath problem.

Rinse out your mouth. Even when you can't brush, you can rinse. Take a sip of water after meals, swish it around and wash the smell of food from your mouth, says dentist Jerry Taintor.

Chew a mint or some gum. A fresh breath mint or minty chewing gum is just a cover-up, good for a short interview, a short ride in a small car – or a very short date.

Gargle a minty mouthwash. If you need a confident 20 minutes of freedom from bad breath, gargling with a simple minty mouthwash is a great idea. But like Cinderella's ballgown, when your time is up, the magic will be gone, and you'll be back to talking from behind your hand again.

Choose a mouthwash. Many modern mouthwashes contain antibacterial chemicals so they should improve gum disease and mouth odour. They are most effective when used before bedtime. Medicinal-tasting mouthwashes contain essential oils such as thyme, eucalyptus, peppermint and wintergreen, as well as sodium benzoate or benzoic acid. Red and spicy mouthwashes may contain zinc compounds. Both types neutralize the odour-producing waste products of oral bacteria. Gargle with the mouthwash, sticking your tongue out at the same time, and then spit the mouthwash out.

Brush your tongue. 'Most people overlook their tongues,' says Dr Shapira. 'Your tongue is covered with little hair-like projections, which under a microscope look like a forest of mushrooms. Under the caps of the "mushrooms", there's room to harbour plaque and some of the things we eat. That can cause bad breath.'

'Whilst brushing your teeth is a must for everyone, not everyone needs

KITCHEN CURES

Eat your parsley. Parsley adds more than a decorative green garnish to your plate; it's also a breath-saver because it contains chlorophyll, a known breath deodorizer. So pick up that sprig and chew it thoroughly. Or put a few handfuls (and maybe add some watercress to the mix) into a juicer. Sip the juice any time you need to refresh your breath.

Think 'spice is nice'. Several other herbs and spices in your kitchen are natural breath enhancers. Carry a tiny plastic bag of cloves, fennel or anise seeds to chew after strong smelling meals.

Try a herbal gargle. Make a mouthwash using extracts of sage, calendula and myrrh gum (all available from health food stores) in equal proportions and gargle with the mixture four times a day. Keep the mouthwash in a tightly sealed jar at room temperature.

How to test your breath

How bad is your breath? If you don't have a friend to tell you the truth, there are a couple of ways you can test your breath, says dentist Eric Shapira.

Cup your hands. Breathe into them with a deep 'haa-a-a'. Then sniff. If it smells rank to you, then it's deadly to those nearby.

Floss. Not to clean your teeth, although that's a good idea, but to find out just how bad your breath might be. Pull the floss gently between your teeth and then sniff some of the gunk you unearth. If it smells bad, you smell bad.

---

to brush their tongue,' says Dr Amiel. 'Unlike the teeth, your tongue is moving all the time and is continually bathed with saliva, so it's self-cleaning. But give it a try if you have a bad breath problem.' Sweep the top surface of the tongue gently with a soft toothbrush or ice lolly stick.

Try a herbal double. Bad breath usually results from sub-clinical infections in the mouth and gums, and the problem is easily cleared up, says herbalist Douglas Schar. Use a combination of goldenseal and echinacea to make your breath safe for public consumption.

Echinacea tablets, taken according to directions on the label, get your immune system working in the oral cavity, clearing out odour-producing bacteria. Goldenseal tincture keeps gum-disease-producing bacteria under control: mix half a teaspoon in half a cup of water, and gargle before bed. This double whammy really does the trick.

BED-WETTING
8 ideas for dry nights

In Britain, around 15 per cent of all five-year-olds wet the bed, and two-thirds of these are boys. Even teenagers can be affected, with around two per cent of 15-year-olds regularly wetting the bed. Bed-wetting, known medically as enuresis, has a number of causes. It often happens simply because the child sleeps so deeply that he does not wake when his bladder is full. Other causes include an overproduction of urine at night and slow physical development. From the age of four, anxiety may also play a role. Finally, genetics may be to blame: 70 per cent of bed-wetting children have a parent or sibling who had a similar problem. And in 1995, Danish scientists identified an area on human chromosome 13 that is at least partly responsible for bed-wetting. The good news is that almost all children eventually grow out of bed-wetting, with a spontaneous cure rate of about 15 per cent per year. Meanwhile, try these remedies.

Be realistic. If your child wets the bed, just keep calm and change the sheets, advises childcare expert Anne Price. The problem will eventually go away by itself. 'Children don't do it on purpose,' she says. 'So don't praise them when they are dry or punish them when they are wet.'

Change for the better. To help minimize psychological stress, Price recommends arranging the bedroom so that the child can change the sheets himself. If you leave out a plastic-backed bed protector (Pampers do packs of disposable ones), a child who has an accident can lay it over the wet patch and go back to bed. Leave out some dry pyjamas too.

Make it easier to get to the loo. Sleeping in a top bunk or in a cabin bed, dark corridors or a trek up or downstairs to the toilet can discourage a child from venturing to the loo in the middle of the night. Let your child sleep on the lower bunk bed, says family doctor Stephen Amiel. Leave a light on or a torch within easy reach, or leave a potty under the bed.

Don't restrict fluids. This is a natural temptation, says Dr Amiel, but children should have plenty of fluids throughout the day – about eight drinks in all. A last drink can be about an hour before bed, but avoid night-time drinks or foods containing natural diuretics – tea, coffee, cola and chocolate.

Reach for the stars. Although some experts prefer to avoid reward systems (see above), there are children who respond really well to schemes like star charts: a star for every dry night, with a reward for achieving a certain number over a period of time.

Make the rewards achievable and worthwhile, without being excessive, says Dr Amiel, and don't punish a wet night. As things improve, the target can be set a little higher by negotiation.

Consider an alarm. 'Bed-wetting alarms can work,' says urologist Bryan Shumaker. 'But you'd better have patience. The alarm is loud, and the chances are it'll wake up everybody in the house when it goes off.'

Bed-wetting alarms emit a buzzing or ringing sound when the child is wet. The theory is that the sound will condition him to wake up when he needs to pee. Eventually, wetting will cease, and a full bladder will trigger the child to wake up and use the potty or toilet. Most children respond

WHEN TO CONSULT A DOCTOR

Remember, bed-wetting is normal in many children, even at five, says family doctor Stephen Amiel. If your five-year-old child has never been reliably dry at night, especially if other family members were similar, it's only a problem if you or your child allow it to be. Most treatment programmes start at age seven upwards.

Many children may wet the bed again for a little while when they are unwell or there is an emotional upset like moving house or changing class, says Dr Amiel. Night-time bed-wetting should be taken seriously, however, if it starts to occur regularly again following six months or more of dryness (so-called secondary enuresis).

Secondary enuresis may indicate urinary infection, chronic constipation, emotional distress or (in rare cases) sexual abuse. If your child is passing large amounts of urine throughout the day as well, diabetes and kidney disease may also need to be excluded, although the child is likely to be unwell in other ways too.

If your child has never been able to achieve daytime dryness either, your doctor may need to have the kidneys and bladder investigated for structural or neurological abnormalities.

Drugs are available for bed-wetting children over six. The antidiuretic desmopressin may be especially helpful for special occasions like a sleepover or camp, says Dr Amiel, and can be administered orally or by nasal spray. Imipramine and nortriptyline (also used as antidepressants, though their action here is different) are effective, too, when given regularly.

to this strategy within a couple of months, says Dr Shumaker.

Today's alarms are much smaller and more sensitive to wetness than the original bulky mats and pads of a few years ago. They run on hearing-aid batteries and have moisture sensors that are simply attached to the child's pants. Research shows that children trained using an alarm have a relapse rate of just 10 to 20 per cent, and most of these children achieve lasting success second time round.

Alarms are the recommended treatment for motivated families where the child is seven or older, says Dr Amiel. Your doctor, or perhaps the school nurse, can refer you to a specialist enuresis clinic or paediatrician.

Boost bladder muscles. If your child goes to the toilet fairly frequently during the day, then he may benefit from bladder-stretching exercises, suggests paediatric nurse Linda Jonides. She recommends giving your child lots to drink during the daytime, and then practising bladder control by holding off going to the loo for as long as possible.

Practise patience and love. The vast majority of children outgrow bedwetting, and by the time they reach puberty, fewer than one or two per cent will still wet the bed, says Dr Shumaker. So be patient and supportive. No child wants to wet himself. It's unpleasant, uncomfortable and cold. All your child needs is patience and support.

BELCHING
6 ways to lessen burping

Belching is often caused by swallowing air, known medically as aerophagia. Everyone carries about 250ml of air and other gases in the gastrointestinal tract. Yet the body is constantly acquiring air and other gases throughout the day – either through the mouth or by producing its own. In all, it works out to more than 2.5 litres of gas in 24 hours. That's about 2 litres more than your body can contain, so it constantly seeks ways to release the excess. One of those ways is by belching.

Fizzy drinks and beer are guaranteed to cause problems, but your saliva also contains tiny air bubbles that travel to your stomach with every swallow. And those of us who swallow air along with our food are asking for trouble.

However, belching is a problem that appears to be easily cured. Most of us can, with practice, control the amount of air we swallow and save our visits to the doctor for something more important. Here's what to do.

Become aware of air. You can swallow up to 150ml of air every time you swallow, says gastroenterologist André Dubois. People who are nervous often do this. Some people are compulsive swallowers and create a problem simply by swallowing too much saliva. 'You can improve this by learning to control your swallowing reflexes,' he says. 'This is best done by becoming aware of it. Ask your friends or relatives to tell you if they notice you swallowing a lot. You probably won't notice it in yourself.'

Once you're aware of an excessive swallowing habit, you will automatically curb it, says Dr Dubois. There are also some personal habits you can change to help you take in less air.

• Avoid carbonated drinks.

• Eat slowly and chew your food completely before swallowing.

WHEN TO CONSULT A DOCTOR

Chronic belching is rarely due to any disease. See your doctor though if you think it's part of a general anxiety problem that you can't get on top of, or if you have other gastrointestinal problems like persistent heartburn, indigestion, weight loss or change in bowel habit.

- Always eat with your mouth closed.
- Avoid chewing gum.
- Do not drink out of cans or bottles, and do not drink through a straw.
- Avoid foods with a high air content such as beer, ice cream, soufflés, omelettes and whipped cream.

Keep the exit closed. There's a one-way valve (the lower oesophageal sphincter) that prevents the contents of the stomach from coming up into the gullet. Avoid foods that relax this valve: onions, tomatoes, mint and alcohol.

Curb a nervous habit. Chronic air swallowers can belch for ever, since belching tends to promote more belching. But even chronic swallowers can be helped. Marvin Schuster, a psychiatrist and specialist in digestive disorders, sometimes prescribes a pencil for patients who swallow air and start bloating up during tense situations. Clamping your teeth around a pencil, a cork or your finger keeps your mouth open and makes swallowing difficult, he says.

Cut down on fats. We can all eat a little too much a little too quickly and burp, says nutritionist Dr Samuel Klein. But that's different from people who are chronic belchers, who belch hour after hour, day after day. For those people, it may help to eat fewer foods that produce upper digestive system gas. Those foods include fats and oils such as salad dressings, butter, margarine and soured cream.

Burst bubbles with soothing antacids. To help alleviate a problem that already exists, digestive specialists sometimes recommend over-the-counter antacids such as Asilone. This contains dimethicone, a drug that relieves the symptoms of excess gas. 'Dimethicone breaks large bubbles into small bubbles in the stomach, which may decrease belching,' says Dr Klein. But it won't reduce the amount of gas in the gut.

Ginger – a tried and tested herbal cure. Next time you're at the supermarket, pick up some fresh root ginger (in the produce section near garlic and chillis), or some powdered ginger from the spice rack. A cup of ginger tea taken after a meal will help to cut gas production and thereby reduce belching, says herbalist Douglas Schar. Use a teaspoon of grated fresh ginger or half a teaspoon of dried powdered ginger in a cup of hot water and sweeten to taste.

BITES, SCRATCHES AND STINGS

20 tips for avoiding – or relieving – the pain

Most insect bites and stings are minor annoyances that itch like mad and produce nasty little lumps that fade away in a few days. Even nips from your dog or cat rarely cause real injury. But on those occasions when the bite is a little worse than the bark – or the buzz – doctors suggest the following tips.

Flies and Mosquitoes

Flying insects like mosquitoes and horseflies can make you pretty uncomfortable when they decide to munch on you. Here's what to do.

Disinfect the bite. Flies and mosquitoes can spread diseases. So wash the bite area thoroughly with soap and water, says Claude Frazier, an allergy specialist. Then apply an antiseptic.

Rub in an aspirin. Herbert Luscombe, a dermatologist, recommends that you moisten your skin and rub an aspirin tablet over the bite as soon as possible after you're bitten. The aspirin helps to control inflammation.
    Note: Ignore this tip if you're allergic to aspirin.

Herbal magic. As summer approaches, and the stingers and biters come to life, there are two herbal remedies people need to keep on hand: echinacea and marshmallow.
    Echinacea was used by Native Americans to treat all kinds of venomous bites, including those of the rattlesnake, while marshmallow is an ancient British remedy for soothing bee and wasp stings. Both work a charm, according to clinical herbalist Douglas Schar, when a flying insect attacks. Buy the tincture of either herb from a health food store, put it

into a small spray bottle, and hit any bite with a blast of spray. Bites will itch less, swell less and are less likely to become infected.

Relieve the itching. Fly and mosquito bites can result in swelling and intense itching that can last for three to four days. Dr Frazier recommends the following to control these symptoms.

- An oral antihistamine (ask your pharmacist to recommend an over-the-counter allergy or cold remedy).

- Calamine lotion.

- Ice packs.

- Salt (moisten it to a paste with water and apply it to the bite).

- Baking soda (dissolve one teaspoon in a glass of water. Dip a cloth into the solution and place on the bite for 15 to 20 minutes).

- Epsom salts (dissolve one tablespoon in a litre of hot water. Chill, then apply as above).

Practise prevention. The hotter the weather is, the more active flies and mosquitoes seem to be. Mosquitoes, in particular, are at their worst in damp areas, such as near ponds or in marshes. Some species are especially bothersome late in the day and are attracted to outdoor lighting after dark. So don't let your guard down at sunset.

If you are outside after dusk on a summer evening, wear light- or neutral-coloured clothes with long sleeves, trousers, and avoid strong perfumes, advises family doctor Stephen Amiel. Spray your bedroom with fly spray or use a plug-in insecticide, close the windows and door and turn the light off while you are out. On your return, if your windows don't have mosquito screens, open them in the dark, then draw the curtains before turning on the light so as not to attract flying insects. Citronella candles and mosquito coils may be helpful outdoors. In badly infested areas, or if you are particularly sensitive to mosquito bites, consider using a mosquito net impregnated with DEET. You may be able to avoid a bite in the first place by using the repellents below.

DEET. Dr Frazier recommends any commercial repellent containing N,N-diethyl-m-toluamide (DEET). Apply generously over all exposed skin, but be careful around the eyes – it can sting badly if perspiration carries it into the eyes. Don't use insect repellents under clothing either. And make sure DEET-containing repellents used on

WHEN TO CONSULT A DOCTOR

Any bite could develop complications. Stay alert for these potential problems.

Infection. Examine the wound periodically. If it gets red, painful, or hot, infection has probably developed. Get professional help.

Rabies. When abroad, be aware of rabies, which can be carried by any warm-blooded animal. If you're bitten, see a doctor as soon as possible for treatment. Once symptoms of the disease develop, the condition is fatal.

Malaria. Travellers who've returned from a malarial zone and develop a flu-like illness, with headache, high fever, rigors, sweats and muscle pains should see their doctor as soon as possible, and mention their travel history. Some of the most dangerous forms of malaria can take up to a year to produce symptoms, especially in those who've taken some malaria prophylaxis.

Lyme disease. The first sign of Lyme disease is often a characteristic rash and a raised temperature. The time between a tick's bite and the first sign of symptoms is usually 7 to 14 days but it may be as short as 3 days or as long as a month.

Crush injury. Sometimes a large dog, such as a German shepherd, will bite without breaking the skin. If you can see bite marks on both sides of an extremity, there may be internal damage. Get the bite looked at at the nearest hospital A&E department.

Bites to the head, hand or foot. If a dog bites you in any of these places, or if the wound is deep and gaping, see a doctor. Antibiotics are often required for puncture wounds which may look small on the surface but which may be teeming with bacteria deeper inside. Gaping wounds may need stitching, glueing or taping.

Cat bites. Cat bites are particularly prone to infection and should be looked at by a doctor. If you're just scratched by a cat, don't phone your doctor unless you suspect that the wound is infected.

Pre-existing chronic disease. If you have diabetes, lung disease, liver disease, cancer, AIDS or any condition that makes it hard for you to fight infection, see a doctor.

children don't contain more than 10 per cent DEET. The chemical, absorbed through the skin, can be harmful to children. Also, don't allow children to handle insect repellents, and don't apply repellent to a child's hands. Instead, apply it to your hands, then rub it on the child's skin.

Chlorine bleach. Dr Luscombe recommends bathing in a very diluted solution of chlorine bleach before going outside. Use liquid
bleach that contains 5.25 per cent sodium hypochlorite. Mix two
capfuls of the bleach in a tub of warm water. Soak in it for 15 minutes. Be very careful not to get the solution near or in your eyes. The
repellent effect should last for several hours.

Bath oil. Certain bath oils, such as Alpha-Keri and Avon's Skin-So-
Soft, have a repellent effect, Dr Luscombe says.

Vicks VapoRub. Some people report success with this strong-
smelling ointment, says Dr Luscombe.

Take vitamin B₁. Some studies suggest that high doses of vitamin B_1
(thiamin) can prevent mosquito bites, says Dr Amiel. A 300mg
tablet daily (lower doses for children, and not for children under
two), changes the odour of the skin after about two weeks. This is
apparently imperceptible to humans but repels mosquitoes.

Ticks

Few of us worry about the likelihood of being bitten by a diseased tick in
the UK, but the problem is becoming more common. Ticks are commonly
found in long grasses, fields where sheep or deer have been grazing,
moorland and woodland – so campers and hikers in areas like the Lake
District always run the risk of getting ticks.

Deer and sheep ticks transmit Lyme disease, and doctors say that there
are now a few hundred cases in the UK each year. Named in 1977 after
doctors discovered arthritis in a cluster of children in and near Lyme,
Connecticut, the disease can trigger a rash, fever, fatigue, headache,
muscle aches, and painful joints.

If you know you have been bitten by a tick, see your GP as soon as
possible. If caught early, Lyme disease is treatable with antibiotics; late
stage Lyme disease is less easy to treat.

Here's what you need to know so you're prepared.

Be vigilant. Summer is the height of tick season, though ticks pose a risk
from early spring until autumn. If you're spending any time outdoors,
especially in wooded or grassy areas – even grassy dunes – take the following precautions.

- If you're in an area known for ticks, leave as little skin exposed as possible, says professor of medicine, Joseph Benforado. Wear long trousers,
knee-high socks and long sleeves.

- Before going to bed at night, says Dr Benforado, inspect your body for any ticks. Be aware that certain species of tick are quite small and easily missed.

Ease it out. Ticks pose a special problem because they dig into your skin and hold on for dear life. Trying to brush away a tick as you would a fly has no effect. And forcefully plucking it out may leave its mouthparts embedded, setting the stage for infection. So use a gentler approach.

Clean the area with alcohol. Then, using blunt tweezers, grasp the tick as close to the skin as you can, says Dr Amiel. Pull steadily up and out, without twisting or squeezing too hard.

Don't use a lighted cigarette or match, he warns – the heat may cause the tick to embed itself even further into the skin.

Clean the bite. Once you've removed the tick, wash the bite area with soap and water, says Dr Frazier. Then apply iodine or another antiseptic.

Dogs and Cats

Twenty people a year die from infections caused by animal bites, most of them children. Around 200,000 dog bites occur each year in the UK, and 10,000 of these require hospital treatment. Cat bites are less common, but are four times more likely to cause infection. Here's what to do if you are bitten.

Assess the damage. Seek medical help for all but the most minor wounds, say doctors.

Thoroughly wash the bite. Animal bites – especially from cats – can transmit infections, says public health expert Stephen Rosenberg. He advises cleaning the wound thoroughly with soap and water to remove saliva and any other contamination. Wash for five full minutes.

Control bleeding. If there is any minor bleeding, cover the entire wound with thick sterile gauze or a clean cloth pad, says Dr Rosenberg. If you have nothing suitable to use as a bandage, thoroughly cleanse your hand and press it firmly against the wound. You may also put some ice against the pad (not directly onto the skin) and, if possible, raise the wound above heart level to help stop bleeding.

Bandage the area. When the bleeding has stopped, cover the bite with a sterile bandage or clean cloth. Tie or tape it loosely in place.

Reduce pain. Use aspirin or paracetamol to reduce pain. Keep the area raised above heart level and apply ice if there is any swelling.

Note: Do not give aspirin to anyone under 16.

WHEN TO CONSULT A DOCTOR

Bee stings can kill. A normal bee sting produces pain for a brief time and swelling that usually lessens in a few hours. But more severe symptoms may indicate an allergy (see *Allergies*, page 28), which can lead to deadly anaphylactic shock. Be on the look-out for chest tightness, a swollen itchy rash (known as urticaria or hives), nausea, vomiting, wheezing, hoarseness, dizziness, swollen tongue or face, fainting or shock. The more rapidly symptoms appear, the more life-threatening they are.

Most people who know that they have a severe allergic reaction to bee stings carry a ready-filled adrenaline injector with them at all times. If these symptoms appear, use the kit as quickly as possible. Then rush the victim to the nearest hospital or doctor. If no kit is available, apply an ice pack if possible, and dial 999.

Have a tetanus jab. Any animal bite or contaminated wound can lead to tetanus, says Dr Amiel. It is now considered unnecessary to have a tetanus booster if you are bitten, *provided you have had five tetanus injections at any time in your life.* Most children will have had four by the time they start school, and a fifth is given in their teens. But as routine immunization only started in 1961, many adults may not have complete immunity.

If you have not had five tetanus injections, or you are unsure, get a booster as soon as possible after being bitten, advises Dr Amiel. You may also need treatment with tetanus immunoglobulin, an antiserum. Fully immune people only require this with a very tetanus-prone wound, such as one contaminated with stable manure.

Insect Stings

Bees, wasps and their kin inject venom into the skin when they sting. That leads to pain, redness, and swelling at the site of the sting. Discomfort can last from several hours to a day, depending on what stings you and how many insects attack. Here's what do to if you're stung.

Identify your attacker. Knowing what you've been stung by can provide a clue to treatment – and help you to avoid more stings. A bee, which has a fuzzy, golden-brown body, can sting only once. That's because its barbed sting remains embedded in your skin. Without its sting, the bee dies.

Wasps and hornets, on the other hand, have smooth stings that can sting you repeatedly. So be prepared to run.

Act fast. The key to effective treatment is quick action. The faster you apply some sort of first-aid treatment, the better your chances of controlling pain and swelling.

Remove the sting. If you've been stung by a bee, remove the sting as soon as possible. Otherwise, the venom sac attached to it will continue to pump for two to three minutes, driving the sting and its poison deeper into your skin. But be careful not to squeeze the sting or the sac – doing so will release more poison into your system.

'Scraping the sting out is the best approach,' says insect expert Edgar Raffensperger. Use your fingernail, a nail file or even the edge of a credit card to gently scrape under the sting and flip it out.

Relieve the pain. At this point, your wound is still throbbing, so you want to deaden the pain fast. The following substances are effective – but for them to work, you must act quickly after being stung.

Cold. An ice pack, or even just an ice cube, placed over the sting can cut down on swelling and keep the venom from spreading, says Dr Luscombe.

Heat. Ironically, says Dr Luscombe, heat can also make you feel better by neutralizing one of the chemicals that causes inflammation. Take a hair dryer and aim it at your sting.

Aspirin. One of the simplest, most effective things you can do, says Dr Luscombe, is to apply aspirin. Moisten the sting, then rub an aspirin tablet into it. The aspirin neutralizes certain inflammatory agents in the venom.

Note: Don't try this tip if you're allergic to aspirin.

Baking soda. Dr Frazier recommends applying a paste of baking soda and water.

Meat tenderizer. 'An enzyme-based meat tenderizer breaks down the proteins that make up insect venom,' says David Golden, a professor of medicine. You have to use it straight away for it to be effective, however.

Activated charcoal. 'A paste of powdered activated charcoal will draw the poison out very quickly, so the sting won't swell or hurt,' according to Richard Hansen, author of *Get Well at Home*. Carefully open a few charcoal capsules and remove the powder. Moisten with water and apply to the sting. The charcoal works best if it stays moist, so cover it with gauze or plastic wrap.

Mud. If you don't have anything else handy, says Dr Hansen, you can mix a little clay soil and water into a mud paste. Apply as you would the charcoal, cover with a bandage or handkerchief, and leave it on until the mud dries.

Take an antihistamine. An over-the-counter oral antihistamine may help to relieve pain. Parents can give children an antihistamine-containing cough syrup, such as Benylin. The antihistamine has a mildly sedative effect and also lessens the swelling, throbbing and redness caused by the insect venom.

Don't get stung in the first place. A bit of prevention can save you a lot of pain later. Here are three ways to minimize your chances of getting stung.

Wear white. Stinging insects prefer dark colours. That's why bee-keepers generally wear pale khaki, white or other light colours.

Don't smell too tempting. Avoid perfume, aftershave or any other fragrance that will make a bee confuse you with a flower.

Use a bath oil. Certain bath oils repel stinging insects, says Dr Luscombe. Skin-So-Soft from Avon and Alpha-Keri have helped a lot of people. Rub the oil onto exposed skin before going out.

BLACK EYE

8 ways to clear up the bruise

'Black eye' is something of a misnomer. 'Navy blue eye' or 'rainbow eye' might be better. Whether you've run into a door frame or been punched, blood instantly fills the space beneath your eye. And because the skin here is so thin, the pooled blood beneath is easily seen as a very dark blue. Over the week or so that most black eyes take to heal, the blood is slowly reabsorbed into the body, evolving into a kaleidoscope of colours that actually signifies healing.

Over the centuries, there have been a host of weird and wonderful treatments for black eyes, ranging from leeches to liver to raw-steak compresses. They all share the same goal: to reduce swelling. But there are plenty of efficient ways to achieve that objective in a less disgusting manner. Here are some to try.

Pack it in ice. A cold pack keeps the swelling down and, by constricting the blood vessels, helps to decrease the internal bleeding.

Jack Jeffers, an ophthalmologist who specializes in sports injuries, recommends applying an ice pack for the first 24 to 48 hours. 'If your eye is swollen shut, use it for 10 minutes in every two hours on the first day,' he advises. To make an ice pack for the eye, put crushed ice in a plastic bag and tape the bag to the forehead. This keeps the ice from putting pressure on the eye. Alternatively, use a packet of frozen peas.

Try what boxers use. When a professional fighter gets a shiner, trainers apply what looks like a small metal iron, says David Smith, an eye specialist who has cared for hundreds of boxers with eye injuries. 'It is extremely cold, and they use it to control the immediate haemorrhage so that the swelling is minimized.' You can use the same sort of treatment by getting a chilled drink can and holding it against the eye intermittently (5 to 10 minutes in every 15 minutes) until you can get some ice onto it. 'Make sure the can is clean and then hold it lightly against your cheek, not your eye. Do not put any pressure on your eyeball.'

Go for green ice. Parsley, an old folk remedy for bruising, has anti-inflammatory and anaesthetic properties. And doctors recommend ice for treating bruises because it causes blood vessels to narrow, which reduces swelling. To make this remedy, mix two handfuls of fresh parsley with about two tablespoons of water, whizz it together in the blender, and freeze the mixture in an ice cube tray. Wrap the cubes in a soft cloth before applying them to your eye socket for 15 to 20 minutes.

Turn to a botanical. Herbal experts recommend both creams and gels made from the bright flowers of the arnica plant, and bromelain tablets, made from an enzyme found in pineapple, as remedies for bruises. You can find these products in health food stores.

Try some herbal witchcraft. The old English herbals are filled with references to people 'that have been hit by a cart, fallen from a tree or dry beaten' – in other words, had big bruises – and the herbs that quickly soothe a bruise. Traditional British remedies for a black eye are marigold or oak tincture. Another good remedy, from Native Americans, is witch hazel. If you are unlucky enough to get a black eye, hit the health food store, advises clinical herbalist Douglas Schar, and buy a tincture of one of the herbs mentioned. Mix the tincture 1 to 5 with distilled water, and apply generously and frequently on a cotton wool ball.

WHEN TO CONSULT A DOCTOR

Black eyes shouldn't be taken lightly, as they can involve serious internal eye injuries, including retinal detachment and internal haemorrhages that may not be obvious at first.

Ophthalmologist Anne Sumers believes that anyone who sustains a black eye should be examined in an A&E department or by an ophthalmologist. 'Often, serious complications have no symptoms,' she says. Don't try to rinse an injured eye or prise a swollen eye open, she adds. Instead, until you can see a doctor, apply ice packs.

If you have difficulty in seeing, you need medical attention immediately, says Keith Sivertson, a specialist in emergency medicine. Here is his list of other red-alert symptoms:

- pain in the eye;
- sensitivity to light;
- blurred or double vision;
- the sensation of objects floating through your field of vision;
- one eye doesn't move as completely as the other;
- one eye protrudes more than the other;
- your two pupils are of different size or shape;
- there's blood in the white or the coloured part (iris) of the eye;
- your eyelid is cut or torn;
- there's a foreign body in the eye.

Be patient. Once the eye bruises, there's not much you can do except control the swelling. Even make-up can't disguise it completely, although a good foundation will help once any cuts heal, says Anne Sumers, an ophthalmologist with an interest in sports medicine.

Avoid aspirin. Aspirin is bad news for black eyes. Aspirin is an anti-coagulant, which means that it inhibits blood clotting – making it harder to stop the bleeding that causes the discoloration. 'You may end up with a bigger bruise,' says Dr Jeffers. If you do need pain relief, take paracetamol.

Don't blow your nose. If a severe blow caused your black eye (something more than just bumping into a door), then blowing your nose could cause your whole face to swell up. 'Sometimes the injury fractures the bone of the eye socket, and blowing your nose can force air out of your sinus adjacent to the socket,' says Dr Jeffers. 'The air gets injected under your skin and makes the eyelids swell even more. It also can increase the chance of infection.'

When to ask for help. If you or someone close to you has been hit in anger, don't keep it to yourself. Your black eye or your child's could lead to even worse injuries and psychological damage. See your doctor or health visitor; contact your local social services; or get in touch with your local police domestic violence or child protection unit. The Women's Aid National Domestic Violence Helpline number is 0845 702 3468. Or call the Domestic Violence Helpline 0870 599 5443 (24 hours) for support and accommodation information for women and children experiencing domestic violence.

BLISTERS
18 hints to stop the sting

Blisters are your body's way of saying it's had enough. Be it too much friction or too much ambition, a blister – much like a muscle cramp or a stitch in your side – is designed to slow you down.

Though the following remedies deal with blisters on your feet, many of these recommendations can be applied to friction blisters on the hands or any other part of the anatomy where your body has said 'slow down'.

Blister Treatment

Here are some suggestions from the experts on dealing with the discomfort of blisters you already have.

Make a decision. Once you have a blister, you have to decide what is the best thing to do with it. Should you protect it and leave it alone, or should you prick it and drain the fluid? It depends on the size of the blister, says Suzanne Tanner, who practises sports medicine. 'A purist will probably tell you not to prick it, because then you don't run any risk of infection. But I think for most people that's just not very practical.'

Our experts say that you should prick large, painful blisters but leave smaller, painless blisters intact. If you have a big blister on a weight-bearing area, you have to drain it, says chiropodist Clare Starrett. 'They can get so full that they become like a balloon.'

Also, blisters likely to break on their own should be drained. Then at least you can control when and how the blister is opened, instead of leaving it to chance.

Be wise and sterilize. If you choose to drain a blister, first clean the blister and surrounding skin and sterilize your 'instrument', be it a needle or razor blade. 'I recommend alcohol to clean both,' says podiatrist Nancy Lu Conrad.

Other doctors advise sterilizing your instrument with a flame instead of alcohol. Simply heat the needle or razor blade with a match until it glows red. Then let it cool down before allowing it to touch your skin. Either method kills germs, and both are equally recommended.

Keep the skin on. Once you drain your blister, experts recommend leaving on the skin that goes over the top. The biggest mistake people make when treating their own blisters is that after draining them, they pull off the 'roof', says Richard Cowin, a foot surgeon. Think of the roof as nature's bandage. 'If you remove it, you're going to end up with a very red, raw, sore area,' he says. 'But if you leave it on, it'll eventually harden up and fall off by itself, significantly reducing your recovery time.'

Keep the dressing simple. After you've treated the blister, you need to keep it covered and protected while it heals. Though gauze pads and special plasters may be the first thing you'd expect a chiropodist to reach for, our experts suggest a much simpler approach. 'My first choice is a simple adhesive plaster,' says Dr Cowin. Gauze pads, however, are recommended for blisters that are just too big for a normal plaster to cover. Keep in place with waterproof adhesive tape.

Use Second Skin for a second wind. If you've treated and covered your blister and you can't wait for it to heal completely before returning to an active lifestyle, then try Spenco's Second Skin dressing, a spongy material that absorbs pressure and reduces friction against blisters and surrounding skin. Dr Conrad says that many athletes apply petroleum jelly to blisters and tape Second Skin over the top.

Give it some night air. Most doctors suggest removing the dressing at night to let the blister get some air. 'Air and water are very good for healing,' says Dr Cowin, 'so soaking it in water and keeping it open to the air at night is helpful.'

Change wet dressings. Though some doctors say that you can leave a dressing on for two days without causing any problems, all agree that if a dressing gets wet for any reason, it should be replaced. That means that you may need to change it quite often if your feet sweat heavily or if you do any activity that will make the dressing sweaty and damp.

WHEN TO CONSULT A DOCTOR

See your doctor at the first sign of infection, advises podiatrist, Nancy Lu Conrad.

'A good rule of thumb is that most wounds, no matter what they are, should get better each day,' adds foot specialist Clare Starrett. That rule holds for blisters as well, she says, pointing out that the classic signs of infection are redness, swelling, heat and increased pain.

'A blister is definitely infected when the fluid coming from it is not clear like water or when it smells unpleasant,' adds Dr Starrett. 'That's the time to seek medical help.'

Blister Prevention

Prevention is always better than cure, so here's what the experts recommend to stop blisters from developing in the first place.

Choose your shoes. It sounds obvious, but the more your shoes resemble the size and shape of your feet, the less likely they are to cause blisters, says family doctor Stephen Amiel. Shoes that are too narrow or pointed will pinch and damage your feet, while shoes that are too big will rub as your foot moves within them, and cause blisters. Make sure your new shoes are comfortable and snug from the word go – don't believe the salesperson who says they'll give. Be especially careful when buying shoes for children; check your child's shoe size every three months or so.

Toughen up your feet. If you're planning to do a lot of walking, toughen up the skin of your feet by walking around barefoot at home, or, even better, go for long walks barefoot on a sandy beach, advises Dr Amiel. Some walkers swear by surgical spirit: rub your feet with it daily for two weeks beforehand. Don't go walking in brand new boots, and keep your feet dry.

Listen to your feet. Friction blisters take a while to develop, so if your feet begin to feel uncomfortable, take notice and change your footwear, says Dr Amiel. Some people with diabetes or neurological problems may have reduced sensation in their feet and may miss the warning signs. If you have such problems, or if you have problems with the circulation to your feet (peripheral vascular disease), it is vital that you wear well-fitting shoes, and see your doctor at the first sign of blisters, discoloration or ulcers on your feet.

Cotton on to acrylic socks

There's an ongoing debate in the sock world that could have far-reaching consequences for countless blister-footed athletes – from weekend walkers to Olympic marathon runners. The cause of the 'friction' among foot care specialists is a study showing that acrylic socks may actually be better at preventing blisters than socks made of cotton or other natural fibres.

For years, most chiropodists recommended natural fibres and materials – think cotton socks and leather shoes.

But new research shows that cotton socks produce twice as many blisters in runners as acrylic socks and that the blisters formed by cotton socks are usually three times as big as those produced by their acrylic counterparts.

'As a veteran long-distance runner and someone who treats runners for blisters every day, the results don't surprise me in the least,' says the study's author, Douglas Richie, a chiropodist specializing in sports foot care. 'I am well aware that cotton fibre becomes abrasive with repeated use and that it loses its shape when wet. The shape of a sock is critical when it's inside a shoe.

'Many people equate acrylic with a silky, nylon-like fibre,' he says, 'but spun acrylic feels exactly like cotton and maintains its soft, bouncy texture even when wet.'

According to Dr Richie, other synthetic fibres, such as polypropylene and polyester, can work as well as acrylic fibres in keeping the foot warm and dry. And the non-blistering property of synthetic fibre holds true for any type of sporting activity, whether it's walking, running, tennis or aerobics.

Try a heel pad. Blisters that appear on the back of the foot usually result from the shoe's heel counter hitting the back of the heel in the wrong area, says Dr Cowin. 'All you usually have to do is put in a heel pad at the back of the shoe,' he says. Heel pads are available from sports shops and online.

Keep your socks on. As a general rule, avoid going sockless. People who do this get blisters on the backs of their heels all the time, says Dr Cowin. If you want to flash some ankle without suffering the consequences, he suggests buying 'trainer socks' that only cover the foot.

Powder daily. Make powdering your feet part of a daily routine. 'When people come in with shoes that fit but that still give them blisters, I tell them to apply baby powder to their feet before putting on their socks,' says Dr Cowin. 'This helps the sock to glide over the foot and prevent blisters.'

Coat to protect. If you're planning a long walk, run, tennis match or whatever, guard against blistered feet in new shoes by coating blister-prone areas with petroleum jelly to reduce friction, says Dr Conrad.

Joseph Ellis, medical adviser to a company that makes running shoes, suggests using nappy rash ointment, which is even thicker than petroleum jelly. 'The thicker the better,' he says. For walkers or runners who insist on going without socks, greasing up blister-prone areas is highly recommended.

Try new socks for new shoes. If you have a new pair of shoes that are rubbing and causing blisters, the first thing to do is change to different socks, says Dr Ellis. He recommends acrylic socks – available in sports shops – because they're made in layers designed to absorb friction, so your foot doesn't.

Treat your feet to sports insoles. Our experts agree that good quality insoles, available from sports shops, are excellent for preventing blisters.

Beware the terrible tubes. While tube socks, those unformed heelless socks you can slip into without thinking, can be tempting, our experts advise against them. Dr Cowin warns that they never fit properly. 'You need a proper fitted sock to help prevent blisters,' he says.

BODY ODOUR
9 ways to feel fresh and clean

Some scientists believe that body odour is a vestige of our evolution. That is, the smells we emit from certain parts of our bodies, mainly our armpits and groin, may have once served to advertise our sexuality, says Nathan Howe, a dermatologist and zoologist who researches the way animals communicate by smell. 'Of course,' he adds, 'whatever purpose was served by body odour once upon a time is simply objectionable now.' Few would disagree with that. If you want people to want to be near you, don't stink.

Easier said than done? Actually, there are quite a few ways to tackle body odour and come up smelling of roses.

Scrub-a-dub-dub. The most basic way to keep body odour at bay is to wash yourself with soap and water, particularly in those areas of the body most likely to smell, such as the armpits and groin, says dermatologist Kenzo Sato.

Body odour is usually caused by a combination of perspiration and bacteria, he says. Washing with soap and water cleans both culprits away.

The best type of soap for a body odour problem is a deodorant soap because it hinders the return of bacteria. How often you need to wash depends on your individual body chemistry, your activities, your mood and the time of year. If you're not sure whether you're washing often enough, ask a friend. Remember that sweat glands and bacteria work at night as well as during the day, which could mean you need to shower both morning and night.

Wash more than your body. You can wash till your skin wrinkles like a prune, but you'll still smell bad if your clothes aren't clean. Seven days in the same shirt is guaranteed to cause offence to others, says dermatologist Lenise Banse. How often do you need to change into a clean shirt? It depends on you as an individual. A clean shirt each day is enough for most people, but in hot weather you may need more than one shirt a day.

Smelly feet can be a genetic problem, but changing your socks once or twice a day will really help. Wear shoes that let the air circulate, and give your trainers a regular wash in the washing machine, too.

Choose natural fabrics. Natural fabrics like cotton and linen absorb perspiration better than synthetic materials. The absorbed sweat is then free to evaporate from the fabric.

Play doctor. Sometimes, if you sweat a lot and have a tendency to smell, standard deodorant soap may not be adequate. In this case, try an antibacterial surgical scrub, such as Hibiscrub, sold over the counter in most chemists, says Dr Howe.

Anti-perspirants attack best. Commercial deodorants are effective at masking underarm odour in most people, says pharmacist Hridaya Bhargava. They leave chemicals on the skin that kill odour-causing bacteria, but they don't control perspiration. If you have a strong body odour, you may need an anti-perspirant. These are basically drugs, he says, that reduce the amount of perspiration that the body produces. Most anti-perspirants combine anti-perspirant with deodorant.

Make the French connection. Another option if you can't tolerate common deodorants and anti-perspirants is a French product called Le Crystal Naturel, says dermatologist Randall Hrabko. It's a chunk of

Frequent, heavy sweating can be more than embarrassing. It can be a sign that you have an overactive thyroid or low blood sugar. You may also have an abnormality in the part of the nervous system that controls sweating. More commonly, severe sweating can be a symptom of an anxiety state, panic or phobic disorder, of the menopause or of obesity. Some medications such as antidepressants and Parkinson's disease drugs can also cause severe sweating. In any case, check with your doctor.

Pathological sweating (hyperhidrosis) can be helped by aluminium chloride-containing deodorants, such as Anhydrol Forte or Driclor, which can be obtained over the counter or on prescription. Occasionally, your doctor may recommend referral for surgical removal or botulinum toxin injections of the sweat glands in your armpits. Specialists may also help sweaty feet and palms with a solution of glycopyrronium bromide.

mineral salts, formed into a crystal, which helps keep bacteria under control without irritating the skin. It can be bought from some department stores and pharmacies, and online.

Watch what you eat. Extracts of proteins and oils from certain foods and spices remain in your body's excretions and secretions for hours after eating them and can impart an odour. Fish, cumin, curry and garlic head the list, says Dr Banse.

Keep calm. 'Getting sexually excited or feeling anxious and nervous will make you perspire more,' says Dr Bhargava. If you anticipate that a situation is likely to upset you, no matter how much you meditate or practise deep breathing, use an extra blast of deodorant in the morning.

Flush your body. Assuming hygiene is not the issue, herbalist Douglas Schar has an interesting approach to body odour. 'Sometimes people produce bad smells because they aren't excreting waste through the usual systems. Often, herbs that stimulate waste excretion dramatically improve the way a person smells.' He recommends adding two items to your weekly shopping list: linden tea, from a health food store, and fresh chicory, from the produce section at the supermarket. Both of these will get the excretory system pumping waste out, says Schar. Try two cups of linden tea and a chicory salad four times a week.

BOILS

9 tips to stop an infection

A boil is an infection deep inside the skin that causes redness, pain, swelling and pus. Boils generally develop when staphylococcus bacteria invade the body through a break in the skin, a blocked sweat gland or an ingrowing hair. The body's immune system sends in white blood cells, which collect as pus, to fight the bacteria. A pus-filled abscess begins to grow beneath the skin surface, rising up red with pain. Sometimes the body reabsorbs the boil; other times the boil swells to an eruption before it drains and subsides.

Boils are uncomfortable and ugly. Sometimes they leave scars. Occasionally, they can even be dangerous. But for the most part, you can treat them safely at home. Here's how.

Apply heat. 'Applying a warm compress is the very best thing you can do for a boil,' says dermatologist Rodney Basler. The heat will cause the boil to form a head, drain and heal a lot faster. At the first sign of a boil, place a warm, wet flannel over it for 20 to 30 minutes three or four times a day. Change it a few times during each session to keep it warm. It's not uncommon for it to take five to seven days until the boil breaks on its own, he says. Make sure no one else uses the flannel.

Prevent a recurrence. It's important to continue the warm compresses for three days after the boil breaks, Dr Basler says. You have to drain all the pus out of the tissues. You may also want to cover it to keep it clean, but it's not critical. A plaster acts mainly to keep discharge off your clothes.

Lance the lesion. When the boil has come to a pus-filled head, if

KITCHEN CURES

According to folklore, many home remedies for boils are as close as your vegetable rack. The following remedies, recommended by naturopath Michael Blate, are variations on the warm flannel compress described above. They should be wrapped in thin muslin cloth and changed every few hours. Try:

- a heated slice of tomato;
- a slice of raw onion;
- crushed garlic;
- the outer leaves of a cabbage;
- a used tea bag.

WHEN TO CONSULT A DOCTOR

Some boils warrant medical attention. If bacteria from a boil enters your bloodstream, it can cause blood poisoning. Don't squeeze boils around your lips or nose as the infection can be carried to the brain.

Boils that should be treated by a doctor include those that:

• are in the armpits or groin, especially if they recur;

• are in the breasts if you are breastfeeding;

• are very tender or painful;

• occur under thick skin like that on your back;

• occur in someone very young, very old or sick.

If there are any red lines radiating from a boil, or if you have any symptoms such as a raised temperature, feeling shivery or swollen glands, you should see your doctor, says dermatologist Rodney Basler, because the infection may have spread.

People with diabetes are especially prone to dangerous boils, says dermatologist Adrian Connolly, and may need a course of antibiotics. Recurrent boils may also be the first sign of developing diabetes, or occasionally of other serious diseases.

it's a small boil with no sign of spreading infection, you may want to break it on your own so that you can choose when and where it breaks. Letting the boil break on its own can create more of a mess, because it often breaks while you're sleeping. To lance the boil, simply sterilize a needle with a flame, make a small nick in the head, and squeeze gently.

While some doctors worry that squeezing can drive the infection deeper into the skin, thus spreading it through the lymph system, in reality that rarely happens, says Dr Basler. 'In the clinic, we just squeeze the dickens out of them.'

Use an antiseptic if you want to. It's not really necessary to treat an opened boil with an antiseptic, because the infection is localized, Dr Basler says. 'The important thing is to keep it draining.'

Keep it localized. When a boil is draining, keep the skin around it clean, says dermatologist Adrian Connolly. Take showers instead of bathing to reduce the rare chance of spreading the infection to other parts of the body. And after treating a boil, wash your hands thoroughly before preparing food, as staphylococcus bacteria can cause food poisoning.

Set the stage for prevention. If you're prone to boils, you may be able to reduce their frequency by cleaning your skin with an antiseptic cleanser like Betadine, says Dr Connolly, as this will help to keep the staph population down.

Get the family checked. Recurrent boils sometimes come from a reservoir of staphylococcus bacteria, usually in the nose. These may lurk unnoticed in a member of your family who may not themselves be getting the boils. If you get recurrent boils, and other diseases have been excluded, ask your doctor or practice nurse about swabbing everyone's nostrils, including your own.

Ignore cysts. A boil is usually a cyst – an uninfected, fluid-filled mass – that has become infected. 'Messing around with a cyst is the easiest way to get a boil,' says Dr Basler. Leave cysts alone or have them surgically removed.

BREAST PAIN
14 hints to reduce discomfort

Benign breast changes may be as bewildering as they are uncomfortable, but they are not unusual – two out of three women will suffer from breast pain at some time in their lives. Tenderness is common during pregnancy and before menstruation. This tenderness occurs because of the natural cycles of the reproductive hormones, oestrogen and progesterone. These hormones trigger cell growth in the milk-producing glands that requires nourishment from blood and other fluids which fill the surrounding areas. These fluid-logged tissues can stretch nerve fibres, causing pain and tenderness.

Another cause of breast pain is fibrocystic changes, which include lumps and cysts. These changes usually affect the non-working areas of your breasts: the fat cells, fibrous tissues and other parts not involved in the making or transporting of milk. And frequently, breast pain is caused by the simple fact of wearing the wrong sized bra.

Try the following strategies to provide relief and promote healing.

Make sure your bra fits properly. Many women in their thirties and forties are still wearing the same size bra as they wore in their teens or twenties. If you suffer from breast pain, see a specialist bra fitter who will help to choose the right size and shape for you. A firm sports bra can help to prevent nerve fibres in the breast, already stretched by waterlogged tissue, from stretching further. Some women find that wearing the bra to bed at night helps, says Gregory Radio, obstetrician and gynaecologist.

Adapt your diet. Change to a diet low in fat and high in fibre by eating more whole grains, vegetables and beans. An American study found that women who maintained this kind of diet metabolized oestrogen differently. More oestrogen was excreted in the stools, leaving less to circulate, says women's health expert Christiane Northrup. And that means less hormonal stimulation of the breasts. You should also reduce your intake of animal fats in butter, cream and fatty meat. You may need to maintain this diet for several months before noticing any change.

Stay slim. Keep your weight within the healthy range for your height. For seriously overweight women, losing weight can help to relieve breast pain and lumpiness, says Kerry McGinn, a staff nurse who specializes in breast health.

In women, fat acts like an extra gland, producing and storing oestrogen. If you have too much body fat, you may have more oestrogen circulating in your system than is good for you. And breast tissue, says Dr Radio, is very responsive to hormones.

Get your vitamins. Be sure to eat plenty of foods rich in vitamin C, calcium, magnesium and B vitamins, says Dr Northrup. These vitamins and minerals help to regulate the production of prostaglandin E, which in turn reins in prolactin, a hormone that activates breast tissue.

Cut out margarine and other hydrogenated fats. Hydrogenated fats interfere with your body's ability to convert essential fatty acids from the diet into gamma linoleic acid, says Dr Northrup. This acid is important because it contributes to the production of prostaglandin E. And prostaglandin E may help keep prolactin, a breast-tissue activator, in line.

Keep calm. Adrenaline, a substance produced by the adrenal glands when we are under stress, also interferes with gamma linoleic acid conversion, says Dr Northrup.

Try evening primrose. Gamma linoleic acid is present in evening primrose oil capsules and these have been a popular remedy for cyclical breast pain for many years. But, says family doctor Stephen Amiel, research has not conclusively proven their benefit, and they are no longer available on prescription.

You can still buy evening primrose oil capsules, though. The recommended dose is two 500mg capsules four times a day for three to six months. After that time you can stop treatment, but expect the condition to recur any time from two months to a year later.

Cut out all caffeine. Caffeine's role in contributing to breast discomfort is not proven. Some studies say it does, other studies are inconclusive. Still, Thomas Smith, cancer surgeon and breast specialist, strongly recommends cutting out caffeine. 'I've seen women with pain and other symptoms of benign breast changes get markedly better after abstaining,' he says. But just cutting out coffee isn't enough. 'You really have to cut out all caffeine,' he says. That means forgoing cola drinks, chocolate, certain frozen desserts, tea and over-the-counter pain relievers that contain caffeine, such as Anadin Extra.

Give up pepperoni pizza. Highly salted foods make you bloated, says Yvonne Thornton, an obstetrician and gynaecologist. It is particularly important to restrict your salt for the seven to ten days before your period – in other words, before the monthly hormonal changes occur.

Stay away from diuretics. It's true that diuretics can help to flush fluid from your system. And that can help to reduce the swelling in your breasts. But the immediate relief comes at a price, says Dr Thornton. Overuse of diuretics can cause an imbalance in your electrolyte system and lead to dehydration and muscle weakness.

Apply cold or heat – or both. Kerry McGinn says that some women find relief by dipping their hands in cold water and cupping their breasts. Others get relief from using a heating pad or hot-water bottle or taking a warm bath or shower. And still others find that alternating heat and cold works best.

Reconsider the Pill. Some women find that the combined oral contraceptive pill improves breast pain, others that it makes the pain worse, says family doctor Stephen Amiel. Breast tenderness is common in the first few months of taking oestrogen-containing contraceptives, but almost always resolves spontaneously. If not, speak to your doctor or family planning clinic about a change of formulation. The progesterone in the pill may actually prevent benign breast disease.

Try massage to ease fluid accumulation. Some women find that gentle breast self-massage helps to ease extra breast fluids back into the lymph passageways, says Kerry McGinn. A technique developed by masseuse Carolyn Gale Anderson involves soaping the breasts, rotating the fingers across the surface in coin-size circles, and then using your hands to press your breasts in and then up.

WHEN TO CONSULT A DOCTOR

No two women's breasts are the same: some will be much lumpier than others, and your own breasts can change from week to week according to your cycle, and from year to year as you age, when you're pregnant, or when you're breastfeeding.

The important thing, says family doctor Stephen Amiel, is to know your own breasts. About 90 per cent of breast lumps are found not by doctors, nurses or mammograms, but by women themselves.

The UK's NHS Cancer Screening programme no longer recommends a rigid monthly breast self-examination. Rather, you should become familiar with the shape, look and feel of your own breasts (soaping yourself in the bath is as good a way as any) at any time of the month.

You should report any of the following changes in your breasts without delay:

- a lump, lumpy area or area of thickening in the breast or armpit that seems different from the other side, especially if new;
- dimpling or puckering of the skin;
- a change in the appearance or outline of the breast;
- any new discomfort or pain in one breast, particularly if new or persistent;
- any discharge, rash, or change in shape of the nipple;
- any new veins standing out on one breast.

All women over 50 should participate in the regular NHS breast-screening programme, advises Dr Amiel.

But remember, he adds, most breast lumps, especially in younger women, turn out to be benign. However, you can only be sure by going to your doctor, who can arrange for you to be seen quickly by a specialist if there is any doubt. Simple tests (a mammogram, ultrasound and/or fine needle biopsy) can often be done all together on the same day.

Is the pain an emotional message? The first thing Dr Northrup looks at is what is going on in a patient's life, and specifically to do with the issues of nurturing or being nurtured. 'I often see tears,' she says.

Breasts are a highly charged symbol of nurturing for women, she says. 'You know that tingling feeling that accompanies the letdown of milk? Some women who have gone through the menopause still feel that when they hear a baby cry. That's how closely linked our breasts are to our emotions.'

BREASTFEEDING
18 problem-free nursing ideas

Breastfeeding is a wonderful way for mother and child to bond, and breast milk is nature's nearly perfect food. It not only contains all the nutrients that your baby needs, it also helps to protect your infant against infections. So much so, that the UK Department of Health now recommends that babies should, if possible, be fed only with breast milk until they are six months old.

Some studies show that breastfeeding significantly reduces the risk of stomach upsets and pneumonia during a child's first year, as well as allergies, ear infections and other illnesses even beyond the first year.

Less than an hour after birth, a full-term baby is physically able to nurse. With a little practice and sometimes a bit of help, both mum and baby can learn the age-old art of breastfeeding.

Breastfeeding is easy once you know how, says breastfeeding expert Julie Stock. And it's often easier than using bottles. For instance, while you feed your baby more often than infants given formula, you don't have to buy the formula or prepare the bottles. And even if you were to dash out without baby's changing bag, you'd at least have a supply of milk on board.

Here's what our experts advise to make breastfeeding trouble free.

Establish your milk supply. To get your baby accustomed to feeding and to establish your milk supply, try to avoid giving your baby bottles, even of water or expressed breast milk, in the first three to four weeks, and don't give your baby a soother unless he or she has a very strong sucking reflex.

Respect your body. 'It's unnecessary for a nursing mother to experience breast pain while nursing,' says Julie Stock. Seek help from a midwife, health visitor, breastfeeding counsellor or doctor if you do.

Mouth wide open. Be sure your baby's mouth is open wide before putting him to your breast; he should latch on to the nipple so that at least two centimetres of the areola is in his mouth.

Leave the baby on the same breast as long as he is sucking effectively, which means swallowing every suck or two. If you see him drifting off to sleep, wake him up, burp him and switch sides. Let him feed on the second side for as long as he wants. In general, feeding time varies from 20 to 30 minutes, Stock says.

Nurse from both breasts during each feed. Nurse on one side until the baby appears to be losing interest, says Stock. Then offer your baby the other side. Next time you feed, start with the side you ended with the time before. To avoid confusion between feeds, pin a safety pin on the side of the bra where you need to start the next feed.

Nurse often. New mothers are often amazed at how often a baby wants to suckle. In the very early days, life can seem to be one endless feed. Most new mums expect a routine more appropriate to bottle-feeding. But you'll probably find yourself nursing 8 to 12 times a day in the early weeks, says Stock.

Human milk is easily digested, so a baby needs to nurse frequently, explains Carolyn Rawlins, an obstetrician and breastfeeding expert. That in turn helps to create a strong bond between mother and child.

Don't try to toughen your nipples. Massage or manipulation to toughen your nipples won't help and could even do some damage, Dr Rawlins says. 'If you position your baby correctly, you won't have any nipple soreness at all.'

Use breast shells for inverted nipples. It's best to start using these during the sixth or seventh month of pregnancy. The gentle suction from a breast shell helps to pull inverted nipples out. But don't use them for more than 15 to 20 minutes a day, says Dr Rawlins.

Don't use soap. 'Use absolutely no soap on your nipples because it dries them out,' warns Dr Rawlins. The little bumps around the areola are glands that produce an antiseptic oil. So you don't need soap.

Let your nipples air-dry. Be sure to air-dry nipples before you cover them, says Stock. And don't use any breast pads that hold moisture, such as those backed with plastic.

Use your milk to help heal sore nipples. 'Ninety-five per cent of nipple soreness results from the position in which the baby sucks,' says Stock. The pain stops once you correct the problem, though the damage may take a little more time to heal. To speed healing, air-dry your nipples when you finish a feed, express a little bit of milk, and dab it on to your nipples. Milk left at the end of the feed is very high in lubricants and contains a natural antibiotic.

Wear the right nursing bra. The best way to choose a nursing bra is to buy a cup size larger and a bra size bigger than your maternity bra, says Stock.

WHEN TO CONSULT A DOCTOR

If your breast feels sore and inflamed, you have a temperature or you have flu-like symptoms, see your doctor. You may have mastitis, a breast infection.

Mastitis is usually treated with antibiotics. If that's what your doctor prescribes, be sure to finish the course of tablets even if the symptoms have already disappeared. This will help to prevent recurrent infections.

Meanwhile, you can help to speed up healing on your own by going to bed, drinking lots of clear fluids and nursing more frequently, says obstetrician and breastfeeding expert Carolyn Rawlins. Don't stop feeding. Your milk isn't infected, and if you stop feeding while you have mastitis, it could trigger a breast abscess.

'I wouldn't buy too many bras in the beginning,' she says. 'It's best to wait and see.'

Here are other tips for selecting a good bra.

- Choose cotton rather than synthetic fabric.

- Make sure the opening for feeding is large enough not to put pressure on any part of the surrounding breast: this could lead to blocked milk ducts.

- Try on the bra to make sure you can easily open and close the cup with one hand. This makes life much easier as it leaves the other arm free to hold the baby and allows you to be discreet.

- Be sure that the straps are broad and comfortable and the bra isn't too tight around your ribs.

Stay alert for blocked ducts. Tight clothes, your own anatomy, tiredness or going any length of time without nursing can cause blocked milk ducts. A blocked duct can lead to infection if not dealt with promptly.

KITCHEN CURES

Cool with cabbage leaves. Some breastfeeding experts recommend using raw green cabbage leaves to soothe engorged breasts. Apply clean, chilled, or room-temperature inner leaves of the cabbage as compresses, changing them every two hours or so, or when they wilt. Use only until any engorgement subsides. Overuse can lead to a reduction in milk supply, according to some reports.

'If you feel a hard, painful-to-touch spot anywhere on the breast, get rid of it by using warmth,' says Stock. Massage the breast, starting at the chest wall and working your way downwards with a circular motion.

Most important, however, is to allow your baby to nurse on that side frequently, she says. 'Baby's sucking will help to clear a duct faster than anything else. Usually, it clears up within 24 hours.'

Try warm compresses to relieve full breasts. If your baby is not keeping up with your milk production and you get uncomfortably full, put some warm wet compresses on your breasts, says nurse practitioner Kittie Frantz. This opens the ducts so that the milk flows more freely. Nurse the baby more often and longer, and drink plenty of fluids so that you urinate every hour.

Control leaking. Most breastfeeding mothers leak from time to time – usually when they hear their, or anyone else's baby crying. If you feel milk leaking from your breasts, take the heel of your hand and press the nipple into your chest. If you leak a lot, buy some reusable breast pads that you can wash yourself. Pure cotton pads work well.

Stop smoking. Yet another reason to give up the habit! Smoking reduces your milk supply and reduces the amount of vitamin C you pass to the baby, says family doctor Stephen Amiel. Smoking just before breastfeeding can delay milk 'let down', and your milk will taste strongly of nicotine. If you can't give up,

Do just *one* thing

Position your baby correctly. Our experts are unanimous that this is the key to problem-free feeding. Nurse practitioner Kittie Frantz, who runs a breastfeeding clinic, says: 'The baby should face you completely: head, chest, genitals, knees. Hold the baby so that the buttocks are in one hand and the head is in the bend of your elbow. Let your other hand slip under your breast, with all four fingers supporting your breast. But don't put your fingers on the areola (the darker area around the nipple).

'Now tickle the baby's lower lip with your nipple to get the mouth to open wide. When the mouth opens wide, pull the baby's body straight in quickly so that the mouth fixes on the areola.' The nipple should be deep in the baby's mouth, adds obstetrician Carolyn Rawlins. 'Then there is no movement of the nipple when the baby sucks.'

If the baby isn't sucking properly, put your finger in the corner of his mouth to break the suction and reposition him.

then don't stop breastfeeding, but try to avoid smoking for at least half-an-hour before feeding.

Don't drug your baby. Remember that a number of drugs pass into breast milk and may affect your baby, says Dr Amiel. If you need to see your doctor for any reason, mention the fact that you are still breast-feeding, and if you are buying over-the-counter medication, tell the pharmacist.

Note. Alcohol and 'recreational' drugs can also pass via breast milk to the baby.

BRONCHITIS

10 tips to stop the cough

Bronchitis is an infection and inflammation of the lining of the bronchial passages, the airways that connect the windpipe to the lungs. It is often triggered by an upper respiratory infection, and if it doesn't improve, bronchitis can lead to pneumonia. In many ways, bronchitis is a lot like a cold. It's usually caused by a virus says Barbara Phillips, a lung specialist. 'So antibiotics won't do much good. Sometimes, though, bronchitis is caused by bacteria, and in that case antibiotics will work.'

Acute bronchitis usually goes away by itself in a week or two, she says. But people with chronic bronchitis can cough and wheeze for months. Although you have to let acute viral bronchitis run its course, there are things that you can do to breathe more easily while you have it.

Stop smoking. It's the most important thing to do, especially if you're a chronic sufferer. Quit smoking, and your chances of ridding yourself of bronchitis go up dramatically. 'Ninety to 95 per cent of chronic bronchitis is due directly to smoking,' says lung specialist Daniel Simmons.

If you've smoked for a long time, some of the damage to your lungs may be irreversible, but the fewer years you've been smoking, the more likely it is that you will make a complete recovery, says Gordon Snider, who also specializes in lung disorders.

Become active about passive smoking. Avoid people who smoke, and if your partner smokes, get him or her to stop. Other people's smoking could be causing *your* bronchitis. Exposure to second-hand smoke – known as passive smoking – can result in bronchitis.

Keep the drink flowing. Drinking lots of clear liquids will help the mucus to become more watery and make it easier to cough up, says Dr Phillips. 'Four to six glasses a day will do a good job of breaking it up.'

Warm liquids or plain water are best. 'Avoid caffeine or alcoholic beverages,' says Dr Phillips. 'They are diuretics; they make you urinate more, and you actually lose more fluids than you gain.'

Breathe in warm, moist air. Warm, moist air helps to vaporize mucus. If you have phlegm that is thick or difficult to cough up, a vaporizer will help to loosen the secretions. As a cheaper alternative to a vaporizer, try boiling an electric kettle in your bedroom, says family doctor Stephen Amiel. Leave the lid off so it doesn't switch itself off, but watch carefully that it doesn't boil dry, and keep it well away from children or the very frail. You could also stand in your bathroom, close the door and run your shower, breathing in the warm mist that steams up your bathroom.

Sit over the sink. Dr Snider advises inhaling steam from the bathroom basin. 'Fill the sink with hot water, put a towel over your head and the

Antibiotics generally aren't the answer

At the first sign of a nasty cough, combined with a sore throat and chest, wheezing, tiredness and a raised temperature – all of which are symptoms of bronchitis – people tend to ask their doctors for antibiotics. Generally, though, antibiotics are a waste of time because up to 95 per cent of all cases of bronchitis are caused by viruses, which antibiotics won't touch. Bacteria trigger only a small proportion of acute bronchitis infections.

Doctors are often reluctant to prescribe antibiotics because there's little evidence that they shorten the course of the illness or ease its symptoms. There is some evidence, however, that bronchodilators – asthma drugs that open the airways – can relieve symptoms.

Researchers found that patients who used bronchodilators were more likely to stop coughing within a week of starting the medication compared to those who took a placebo. The patients who used bronchodilators also returned to work sooner than those given the placebo. But doctors advise that bronchodilators are most likely to work in patients whose bronchial passages are inflamed.

Bronchodilators usually come in the form of inhalers.

WHEN TO CONSULT A DOCTOR

Bronchitis requires a doctor's attention when:

- you think your baby or young child may have it;
- your cough is getting worse, not better, after a week;
- you have a fever or are coughing up blood;
- you have pain in your chest when you take a deep breath;
- you are bringing up yellow or green phlegm throughout the day, especially if you are a non-smoker;
- you get recurrent attacks of cough and wheeze (asthma may be the cause here);
- you are older and get a hacking cough on top of another illness;
- you are short of breath and have a very profuse cough;
- you are elderly;
- you have heart or lung disease.

sink, creating a tent, and then inhale the steam for five to ten minutes every couple of hours.'

Don't expect too much from expectorants. There is no scientific evidence that any medicine loosens or dries up mucus, says Dr Phillips. Drinking fluids is the best way to loosen secretions.

Listen to your cough. 'If you have a productive cough, one in which you cough up phlegm, you don't really want to suppress it completely, because you won't be coughing up the stuff your lungs want to get rid of,' says Dr Simmons. His advice is to put up with it the best you can.

On the other hand, if your cough is nonproductive – that is, you're not coughing anything up – then it's a good idea to take a cough medicine designed to suppress a cough. The most effective over-the-counter one is pholcodine.

Focus on prevention. Infants, young children, smokers, people with heart or lung disease and the elderly are more likely to develop bronchitis. They are also more likely to have a case of bronchitis that worsens into pneumonia. People who are vulnerable should avoid strenuous outdoor work and exercising on days when air pollution is high.

Have your flu jab. If you have chronic bronchitis, make sure you get a flu jab every autumn. Flu jabs are also recommended if you are over 65, if you have asthma, heart disease, immune suppression or other serious chronic illness. A one-off vaccine against pneumococcal pneumonia is also recommended for these groups, and for everyone over the age of 75.

Keep liquorice tea in the larder. 'I've worked in London, the capital city of respiratory disease,' says clinical herbalist Douglas Schar, 'so I'm used to treating bronchitis.' Bronchitis is rife in London and most big cities worldwide, according to Schar. The best herb for treating bronchitis, he says, is liquorice, and the best form is liquorice tea, available from health food stores. You can use it to treat an active case or to stop one from taking hold. Three cups of liquorice tea a day can make a big difference. If you are prone to bronchitis, keep some in the larder and start taking it at the first sign of trouble.

BRUISES
7 healing ideas

Unless you wrap yourself in cotton wool, you'll never be bruise-proof. But you can lessen the likelihood of large bruises, and shrink and heal the ones you occasionally incur. Here's how.

Chill bruises. Use an ice pack to treat any injury that might lead to a bruise, advises casualty consultant Hugh Macaulay. Apply an ice pack – or a bag of frozen peas – wrapped in a thin cloth to protect your skin, as quickly as possible following the injury. Keep the ice in place for 15 minutes. If you suspect the bump will blossom into a severe bruise, continue this ice treatment every couple of hours for the first 24 hours. Allow your skin to warm up naturally and don't apply heat between ice packs.

Cooling constricts blood vessels, and that means less blood spills into the tissues to create a bruise. A cold pack also minimizes swelling and numbs the area, so it won't hurt as much as a bruise left unchilled.

Follow ice with heat. After 24 hours, use heat to dilate blood vessels and improve circulation in the area, says dermatologist Sheldon Pollack.

Prop your feet up. Bruises are little reservoirs of blood. Blood, like any liquid, runs downhill. If you do a lot of standing, blood that has collected

Keep parsley-packed ice cubes in your freezer for an instant bruise remedy. Herbalist Sharleen Andrews-Miller suggests putting a handful of parsley and ¼ cup of water in a blender or food processor. Whizz it to a pulp, fill an ice cube tray half full with the mixture and freeze. When needed, wrap the ice cubes in muslin or a thin cloth and apply them to the bruise. Parsley is a cooling herb that decreases inflammation and reduces pain, she says.

As a bonus, when you're cooking you can take a parsley cube out of the freezer if you want to add a little parsley to a soup or a sauce.

in a bruise will seep down through your soft tissues and find other places to puddle.

Boost your vitamin C. Studies show that people who lack vitamin C in their diets tend to bruise more easily. Vitamin C helps to build protective collagen tissue around blood vessels in the skin, says Dr Pollack. Your face, hands and feet contain less collagen than, say, your thighs, so bruises in those areas are often darker, says Dr Macaulay. We also lose our ability to renew collagen as we age: this is one reason why older people bruise more easily.

Increase your dietary vitamin C intake by eating more fruit and vegetables. Citrus fruits, kiwi fruit and tomatoes are particularly rich in vitamin C; fortified cereals and potatoes are also good sources, says family doctor Stephen Amiel. Remember that vitamin C does not survive lengthy cooking or storage. Eat fresh fruit and vegetables as soon as possible after buying, and microwave or steam vegetables rather than boiling them.

Vitamin C supplements (maximum 500mg three times a day) are rarely necessary if you have a healthy diet, says Dr Amiel, but if you bruise easily and other causes have been ruled out, give them a try.

Watch those medicines. People who take aspirin to protect against heart disease and those taking blood thinning drugs will find that a bump turns into a bruise very easily.

Steroids such as oral prednisolone can cause bruising with prolonged use: be careful too about using stronger steroid creams on eczema or psoriasis for longer than recommended, and don't use them on the face, advises Dr Amiel. The steroids contained in some inhaled preparations for asthma and hay fever only rarely get into the body in sufficient quantities to cause bruising. Other drugs such as anti-inflammatories and antide-

WHEN TO CONSULT A DOCTOR

Sometimes bruises are a sign of illness. So if you bruise easily and can't work out why, talk to your doctor. Some blood disorders can cause unexplained bruises. Also, AIDS can cause purplish bumps that appear to be bruises but which don't heal and disappear.

Purpurae are small purple marks on the skin – tiny bruises that can appear spontaneously. Occasionally they may indicate septicaemia caused by one of the bacteria (meningococcus) responsible also for meningitis. If you or your child develops spontaneous purpurae or larger bruises, especially in association with fever, drowsiness, vomiting, stiff neck or headache, seek **immediate** medical attention.

The glass test. If you think a rash may be caused by purpurae, press the side of a glass firmly against the skin. *With purpurae, the rash doesn't fade.*

pressants can occasionally inhibit clotting under the skin and cause larger bruises. Alcoholics and drug misusers tend to bruise easily, too. If you take medicine that might cause easy bruising, talk to your doctor about the problem.

Treat belated bruises. You don't have to bump in order to bruise. If you notice bruises a day or two after exercising, use heat to begin the healing process.

BURNOUT
18 routes to revival

Burnout starts insidiously: the feeling that the work will never be done, relationships at work aren't what they used to be, the job isn't fun anymore. The symptoms of burnout may be both emotional and physical, and they evolve so gradually that they're often hard to recognize at first. Loved ones and colleagues may be the first to notice.

Feelings of excessive responsibility and lack of a sense of control contribute to burnout, which in turn can contribute to serious medical problems, including high blood pressure, gastrointestinal disorders, coronary artery disease and sleep problems, says Dr Peter Moskowitz, a specialist in stress management.

The emotional signs often begin first. 'You may feel irritable, finding that you have less ability to deal with minor problems at home and at work,' he observes. People under stress may begin to quarrel with colleagues, experience road rage during the drive home, or pour an extra drink before dinner. They may show signs of depression – struggling to get out of bed in the morning – or symptoms of anxiety – lying awake at night.

Later, physical signs appear, such as headache, stomach pain, backache, chronic fatigue and a general just-been-run-over-by-a-bus feeling.

Who is at greatest risk of burnout? Surprisingly, workers who burn out are often the most highly motivated, dedicated people at work. 'You can't burn out unless there's been a fire in the first place,' explains Dr Moskowitz. Some people may experience burnout as disillusionment with a job that no longer seems as challenging as it once did.

Other people at risk are those who worry excessively or who put work before themselves or their families. 'These people don't manage stress well, and don't have a well thought-out plan for looking after themselves and balancing their lives,' says Dr Moskowitz. 'They don't realize that lifestyle balance is the most potent form of stress management available.'

Downsizing, layoffs, mergers, short-term contracts and the constant demand for higher productivity are all taking their toll on British workers, with a staggering 3 in 10 employees suffering from mental-health problems. It is estimated that about 80 million days a year are being lost in the UK to stress – at a cost of £5.3 billion.

Fortunately, burnout isn't inevitable. There are many positive steps you can take to revitalize your outlook on your job, your relationships – and your life. Here are a few strategies that our experts recommend.

Set yourself a goal. If you're not satisfied in your job, view it as a stepping-stone to something better. 'If you're in a bad position but you're en route to a goal that means something to you, it's much easier to endure,' says psychologist Karen Bierman. She asks people to think about where they're heading for in life, and then to make a plan to get there.

Keep your perspective. Many people who get burned out simply take their jobs and bosses too seriously, adds Dr Bierman. 'What the boss says or does carries far more weight than it should.' To combat this tendency in yourself, try to be your own compass. Listen to your boss, but use your own judgement about how you can best do your job.

Reframe your thoughts. You can't always control what happens around you, but you can control how you respond to those events, says Jack Singer, an industrial psychologist who specializes in burnout. If redundancies in your company have led to a heavy workload for you, remind yourself that you were valuable enough to keep in the first place. Give yourself credit for being able to handle more work than you used to. Feel good about doing the best job you can.

Dig into your work. 'Don't sit there fretting about how much there is to do, procrastinating out of fear that you'll never get it done,' Dr Singer adds. Get organized and set goals at the beginning of each day, doing the toughest tasks first and crossing off items on a list as you complete them. Build small rewards into your day, such as enjoying a cup of tea or a walk around the building, as you accomplish what you set out to do.

Forget work-ethic clichés. Many people have a message in their heads that repeats, 'if a job's worth doing, it's worth doing well' or 'don't do anything by halves'. Push the Stop button, Dr Bierman says. 'Let's face it. Some tasks aren't worth 100 per cent effort.'

Take paperwork, for instance. This often deserves to be done halfway at best. Give yourself the right to differentiate between what is worth doing well and what is worth doing well *enough*. Remember, the best can be the enemy of the good.

Make your work space somewhere you like to be. Hang up cartoons that make you laugh, display pictures of people you love or pin up postcards of places you like.

Laugh. Humour and laughter lower blood pressure and boost immunity, says Dr Singer. 'Every time you laugh, it's a way of exercising your internal organs.' He recommends putting a 'fun quotient' into every office. Whether this means keeping a book of cartoons beside your phone to flip through when you're on hold, getting everyone to bring in baby photos of themselves, or offering a booby prize for the week's worst joke, it doesn't matter. All you need is a reason to laugh.

Practise time management. Melissa Stöppler, a stress-management expert, encourages people to learn to double-task to save time and combat burnout. Sort out your post while waiting on the phone, or do the ironing while catching up on the news. Save time by combining jobs and never doing just one thing when you go out of the house. Always keep a supply of stamps, greetings cards and ingredients for a quick supper. Minimize waiting time by booking appointments for first thing in the morning.

Just say no. People sometimes feel burned out because they are simply too overloaded. Dr Stöppler recommends examining all of your 'extra' responsibilities, such as coaching the kids' football team, running the mums' and toddlers' group, or participating in focus groups at work. Drop those that have become chores or obligations. Don't take on anything new without first asking yourself, 'Will I enjoy this activity?' Make your initial response to all new requests, 'I'll think about it' – which will give you time to do just that.

Tell a friend. Find a sympathetic ear and talk about your feelings, says Dr Bierman. Explaining your situation and getting some friendly support can help to relieve the pressure.

Look after your health. Physical ill-health can contribute to a feeling of burnout, as well as the other way round. See your doctor if you think you may have an underlying physical problem, or if you are smoking too much, using stimulant drugs or drinking to excess as a way of trying to cope. You can also use the opportunity to have your blood pressure checked perhaps, or to discuss healthy lifestyle options.

Exercise often. Regular exercise combats burnout by reducing stress. It also boosts your resistance to disease, lowers your blood pressure, lowers your cholesterol levels, helps to control body weight and helps to lift depression. Exercising at least three days a week for 30 to 60 minutes at a time is especially important for people who feel frazzled and burned out, so make this a priority, recommends Dr Moskowitz.

Eat well. You cannot have control over all of the stresses that make you feel burned out, but you do have control over what you eat. Eat a low-fat, high-fibre diet. You'll gain a sense of satisfaction knowing that you're doing the best you can for your body, and you may even lose some weight into the bargain.

Get restful sleep. Let go of the day's worries and unfinished business. Tell yourself that you will make decisions tomorrow, after a good night's rest. Visualize one of your favourite holiday resorts or a peaceful scene from a film. Imagine yourself in that place as you drift off to sleep. Avoid alcohol, tobacco and exercise for at least one hour before you go to bed. Dr Moskowitz advises investing in a firm comfortable mattress, too.

Develop self-awareness. If you want to take care of yourself, Dr Moskowitz recommends some form of calm reflection daily. Relaxation techniques that foster health, healing, and self-awareness include prayer, meditation, yoga, tai chi and breathing exercises.

Try different approaches until you find the form of relaxation that suits you best, suggests Dr Stöppler. Some, such as tai chi, involve both physical and mental exercises, while others, like meditation, rely chiefly

WHEN TO CONSULT A DOCTOR

Many people can follow a few self-help steps and are soon able to make changes for the better, developing either a new sense of challenge and satisfaction from their jobs or the courage to move on. Sometimes, though, burnout can become a destructive force that requires professional guidance, says psychologist Karen Bierman.

There may be external clues that you need help, such as being given a poor job appraisal, taking a lot of time off sick or having a major fight at home. Or the clues may be internal, such as feeling depressed or anxious.

If your behaviour, your anxiety or depression interferes with your daily life or persists despite any self-help efforts, then talk to your doctor, says Dr Bierman.

on mental discipline. One way to begin, she says, is to set aside quiet moments every day in a place free of distraction where you can breathe deeply, relax your muscles and reflect on a simple message such as 'I am calm and relaxed'.

Practising a relaxation technique should never become a chore crammed into a packed schedule but, rather, should be a respite to which you look forward, Dr Stöppler stresses.

Deepen your relationships. People who feel burned out often take out their frustration on those who love them most. That's like shooting yourself in the foot, because time devoted to enriching relationships with family and friends will help to soothe feelings of burnout, says Dr Moskowitz.

Get a life and a community. Seek out some like-minded people with whom you can share part of your life. This could mean pursuing a hobby, finding a place of worship or doing voluntary work. 'Connecting with people gives you a wonderful source of support and encouragement and make you more resilient to stress,' Dr Moskowitz observes.

Be brave – take risks and move on. If you've established that the source of your unhappiness is your job, and you can't change or delegate the tasks that trouble you most, have the courage to find another job that suits you better. 'It's scary, and it involves risk, but your risk will be rewarded tenfold,' promises Dr Moskowitz. 'Nothing changes without some pain. With risk comes personal growth and renewal.'

BURNS

13 treatments for scalds to skin or mouth

When you accidentally catch your wrist on the oven shelf, spill hot soup into your lap or get a face full of steam on taking the lid off a microwaved dish, you need to put the fire out – fast! Likewise, taking a gulp of scalding coffee or biting into a pizza straight from the oven can cause a horrible burn and needs quick action. Here are some tried and tested coolers.

Burns on the Skin

Douse that flame. 'The first and most important thing is to stop the burning process,' says emergency medicine expert William Burdick. Cool your burns with lots and lots of cold water – 15 to 30 minutes' worth or until the burning stops. But *don't* use ice or iced water – they could make your burn worse.

'If it's a contact burn, run the injured part under cold water,' says Dr Burdick. 'If it's hot grease or splattered hot material like battery acid or soup, remove the clothing that's saturated first, wash the grease off your skin, then soak the burn in cold water.' If the clothing sticks to the burn, rinse over the clothing, then get to the nearest casualty department. Do not attempt to pull the clothing off yourself.

Once you've got rid of the heat, you're halfway to healing. The coolness stops the burn from spreading through your tissue and works as a temporary painkiller.

Leave butter for your bread. You wouldn't try to smother a fire with a giant slab of butter, would you? The same goes for a burn. Fat on a burn can hold the heat in your tissue and make the burn worse. It also might cause an infection. Don't use other folk remedies either. Vinegar, potato peelings and honey won't help.

Cover the burn and then do nothing. After you have cooled and cleaned the burn, gently wrap the area in a clean, dry cloth, such as a thick gauze pad. Then, for at least the next 24 hours, leave the burn alone. Burns should be allowed to begin the healing process on their own.

Help it to heal. Starting 24 hours after you burn yourself, wash your injury gently with soap and water or a mild antiseptic solution once a day, suggests John Gillies, an A&E technician. Keep it covered, dry and clean between washings.

Soothe with aloe. Two to three days after your burn, break off a fresh piece of aloe and use the plant's natural healing moisture, or squeeze on an over-the-counter aloe cream. Both have an analgesic action that will make your wound feel better.

Make soothing solutions. When your burn starts to heal, break open a capsule of vitamin E and rub the liquid onto your irritated skin. It feels good and may help to prevent scarring. Don't apply vitamin E oil to broken skin, though. Or reach for an over-the-counter remedy such as the after-sun cooler Solarcaine (not suitable for children under three).

Leave blisters intact. Those bubbles of skin are nature's own best bandages, says Gillies. So leave them alone. If a blister pops, clean the area with soap and water, then smooth on a little antiseptic ointment and cover.

Burns in the Mouth

Reach for water. If you burn your mouth sipping a scalding cup of coffee or other hot food or drink, rinse your mouth and gargle with cool water for five to ten minutes. Avoid hot foods and drinks for several days.

Apply some ice. Putting an ice cube in your mouth straight away brings down the temperature, eases the pain of the burn, and helps to control the swelling, says dentist Kimberly Harms, much like plunging your hands into cold water after burning them. Just pop a piece of ice into your mouth and suck.

Cool with ice cream. A scoop of ice cream can help to put out the fire on the roof of your mouth, says dentist Van Haywood. Or try an iced milkshake.

Gargle with salt water. Rinsing your mouth with a warm salt-water solution – ½ teaspoon of table salt mixed into 250ml of warm water – cleans the area and helps to heal the burn, says dentist John Caimi.

Avoid crunchy and hot foods. Change your eating habits for a few days, suggests Dr Haywood. Avoid hot spicy foods for a few days and foods with sharp edges like crisps. Eating bland soft foods while the burn heals is a must.

Learn from your burn. Next time, beware when you order pizza, gulp hot coffee or eat just-microwaved food. The latter is important because microwaved foods often cook unevenly, so the outside may feel cool but

WHEN TO CONSULT A DOCTOR

You can usually treat first degree burns yourself. Most second degree and all third degree burns should be treated by a doctor. See a doctor, too, for burns on people over 60. This is how to tell the difference between first, second and third degree burns.

- First degree burns, like most sunburns and scalds, are red and painful.
- Second degree burns, including severe sunburn or burns caused by brief contact with electric hotplates, tend to blister and ooze and are painful.
- Third degree burns are charred and white or creamy coloured. They can be caused by chemicals, electricity or prolonged contact with hot surfaces. They are not usually painful because nerve endings have been destroyed, but they always require a doctor's care.

Other burns that call for urgent medical attention include:

- burns on the face, especially around the eyes or mouth;
- any burn associated with shortness of breath, in case of inhaled flame or fumes;
- any burn you aren't sure is first degree or relatively mild second degree;
- any burn or scald bigger than your hand or, in the case of a child, theirs;
- burns that show signs of infection, including a blister filled with greenish or brownish fluid, or a burn that becomes hot again or turns red;
- any burn that doesn't heal within ten days to two weeks;
- chemical or electric burns. Corrosive chemical burns can burn through several layers of skin and tissue. If you are burned this way, immediately flush cool running water over the burned area for 15 to 20 minutes.

If you are going to see a doctor about a burn, wash it, but don't apply any ointments, antiseptics or sprays, advises A&E technician John Gillies. You may, however, wrap the affected area in a dry, sterile dressing. Remove anything – e.g. shoes, bracelets, watches or rings – that may restrict bloodflow to an injured area.

For severe burns that damage several layers of skin or destroy underlying blood vessels or nerves, dial 999 immediately. While you wait for the ambulance, raise burned areas above the heart and cover with a clean sheet to reduce any loss of body heat.

the middle might be scalding. 'Let pizza or other hot foods cool for a minute or so before you take your first bite,' advises Dr Haywood.

BURSITIS
10 ways to ease your pain

Bursitis is an inflammation of the fluid-filled sacs in the joints, called bursae, that ensure the body's movements are smooth and friction-free. You have more than 150 of them nestled in your shoulders, knees and other joints. Bursitis pain flares whenever repeated movement stresses a specific joint, such as a long day of tennis or golf causing intense shoulder pain.

Bursitis strikes, it retreats, it strikes again. The acutely painful stage of bursitis lasts four to five days, sometimes even longer. The on-again, off-again nature of acute bursitis is aggravating for people with the condition and frustrating for those trying to determine what type of treatments actually work.

At the moment, there is no 'cure' for bursitis. Until medical researchers come up with one, here are some tried-and-tested remedies that may bring temporary relief from this painful condition.

Rest is best. The first thing you do with any joint pain is rest, says physiotherapist Alan Bensman. 'Stop the activity that's causing the pain and rest the joint. Forget that old sports adage about working through the pain.'

Immobilize and ice. If the joint is hot, reach for ice, says chiropractor Allan Tomson. 'Alternate 10 minutes of ice, 10 of rest, 10 of ice, and so on.' As long as the joint is hot, avoid applying heat to it.

Attract relief with opposites. Once the joint cools down and if the pain or swelling is not terribly acute, Dr Tomson sometimes recommends cold-and-hot combination treatments – 10 minutes of ice, followed by 10 minutes of heat, followed by 10 minutes of ice, and so on.

Take painkillers. Ibuprofen, an anti-inflammatory painkiller, can be very effective, says Dr Bensman, and for those who can tolerate it, aspirin is also a useful anti-inflammatory. Paracetamol provides pain relief but it does not have the beneficial anti-inflammatory property. If you're not sure which painkiller is best for you, discuss the options with your doctor.

Soothe the pain with castor oil. When the pain is no longer acute, Dr Tomson recommends a castor oil pack, which is as simple to make as it is effective. Spread castor oil over the afflicted joint. Put a soft cotton wool cloth over the oil and then apply a heating pad.

Apply a soothing balm. Alternative remedies can speed up relief when used with standard treatments, says Alison Lee, a specialist in pain management. One remedy worth trying is Tiger Balm, a Chinese massage cream containing menthol, which may ease bursitis pain when used once or twice a day. If you can't find Tiger Balm in your health food store, you can make a homemade balm by mixing water and turmeric powder (a spice used in curry recipes) into a paste. Apply once or twice a day.

Gently move the joint. Once the pain is no longer acute, gentle exercises are a good idea. If elbow or shoulder pain is the problem, doctors recommend swinging the arm freely to relieve the ache. Exercise for only a couple of minutes at a time to begin with, but do it often during the day.

You want to maintain a range of movement, says orthopaedic surgeon Edward Resnick. 'You don't want a stiff shoulder, but you don't want to overstretch it either.' He recommends bending forward and supporting yourself with your good arm and hand on a chair. Allow the painful arm to drop downward, then swing this arm backwards and forwards, then from side to side, and finally in circles, both clockwise and anti-clockwise.

Some experts recommend doing soothing exercises in the bath or a swimming pool. Float your sore limb on the surface of the water, then move it gently, without pushing it.

Stretch. The importance of exercise following a bursitis attack cannot be overemphasized. Our experts all recommend stretching techniques to return full, normal movement to the joint.

One effective stretch for stiff shoulder joints is called the cat stretch. Get down on your hands and knees. Put your hands slightly forward of your head, then keep your elbows stiff as you stretch backward and come down on your heels.

Another stretch involves standing facing a corner and walking your fingers up the wall in the corner. 'The object is to try and get your armpit into the corner,' says Dr Resnick.

Try a natural anti-inflammatory remedy. Flaxseed oil (also called linseed), which contains omega-3 fatty acids known to reduce inflammation, is sometimes recommended for people with recurrent bursitis. Add one to two tablespoons to your salad dressing.

Note: Prolonged or excessive use of flaxseed products can affect your potassium levels, warns family doctor Stephen Amiel, so if you are on medication for blood pressure or your heart, moderate your use of flaxseed and mention it to your GP. You may also get flatulence or diarrhoea.

WHEN TO CONSULT A DOCTOR

Though it can be very painful, bursitis may subside with just a little TLC. But if it's due to an infection or gout, you need to see a doctor. How can you tell? If the joint is tender, warm and red, those are warning signs. But sometimes those symptoms are not evident even if you have an infection, so it is best to ask for your doctor's advice when you have a flare-up of bursitis.

Be patient. Bursitis generally takes about ten days to heal – sometimes more, sometimes less. If all else fails, doctors promise that time will eventually heal the wound.

CALLUSES AND CORNS
16 ways to smooth and soothe

Those little bumps and lumps that make your feet look ugly are piles of discarded dead skin cells – calluses and corns formed by friction and irritation from the everyday wear and tear from shoes, or adjacent bones on the same foot. Not only are they unsightly, they can also be quite painful.

'Calluses are your body's way of protecting you from pressure,' says chiropodist Neal Kramer. 'When the pressure gets extreme, the callus gets thicker and thicker. If it develops a hard core, it becomes a corn. Soft corns, which form between toes and remain soft from foot perspiration, happen when two bones from adjacent toes become over friendly. The skin between them thickens in an attempt to protect you from the constant pressure.'

'People can live with calluses more easily than with corns,' says Richard Cowin, a foot surgeon. 'If you get painful corns on your toes, it's like having a bad toothache. It can ruin your day.'

So if you want to start every day on the right foot, try these tips.

Stay away from sharp instruments. First and foremost, say the experts, don't play surgeon. Resist the temptation to pare down calluses and corns with razor blades, scissors or other sharp instruments.

'Bathroom surgery is extremely dangerous,' says foot expert Nancy Lu

Conrad. 'It can lead to infections and worse. I've seen horrible things happen to people who thought they could be their own surgeons.' And people with diabetes should *never* treat their own foot problems.

Pad the area. It's best to take action against a callus *before* it has the chance to become a corn. An easy way to take pressure off a callus, says Elizabeth Roberts, a professor of chiropody, is to place a little gauze or absorbent cotton over the area, then cover it with a thin piece of moleskin. She recommends removing the covering each night, as well as when bathing, so that the skin can breathe and excessive moisture doesn't accumulate under the pad.

When you remove the moleskin, be sure to hold the skin of the sole of your foot taut while you *slowly* pull the moleskin back towards your heel. If you pull quickly or in the opposite direction, you could tear the skin.

Customize your insoles. Here is an easy way to modify insoles to relieve pressure on calluses, recommended by chiropodist Mark Sussman. Buy a pair of foam-rubber insoles and wear them for a week. Your calluses will leave impressions, indicating the areas of greatest stress and showing you the areas *around which* each insole needs to be built up to even out the pressure.

If the callus is in the middle of the ball of your foot, cut 5mm-thick foam or felt into two strips (each 1cm wide by 5cm long). Glue them on either side of the depression. Take another strip (5cm wide by 5cm long), and position it behind the depression. If the callus is off to one side, use appropriate combinations of strips. When you wear the insoles, the pads will redistribute weight away from the callus and give relief.

Be a little abrasive. Before treating a callus, soak your foot in comfortably hot water for several minutes. Then, says Dr Cowin, use a callus file or pumice stone to lightly roughen the area and rub off the top layers of skin. Finish by applying some hand cream, such as Aquadrate or Eucerin, which contain 10 per cent urea and help to dissolve hard skin. If you have bad calluses, make this part of your daily routine after showering or bathing.

But, he warns, don't use abrasive action on hard corns, as that will make the area very tender and more painful than it was before.

Take five. Here's another way to soften stubborn calluses. Crush five or six aspirin tablets into a powder. Mix into a paste with ½ teaspoon each of water and lemon juice. Apply to the hard-skin spots on your foot, then put your foot into a plastic bag and wrap a warm towel around everything. The combination of the plastic and the warm towel will help the

WHEN TO CONSULT A DOCTOR

People with diabetes or any kind of reduced feeling in their feet should never treat themselves, says Neal Kramer, a chiropodist. Diabetes affects tiny blood vessels throughout the body, including those in the feet. That leads to decreased circulation, which reduces the ability of wounds to heal and resist infection.

'Anyone with a circulation disorder is okay if his or her skin remains intact,' says Dr Kramer. 'But any kind of cut or opening in the skin can become very dangerous.' People who don't feel pressure or pain all that well may not know when they cut themselves, or may not be aware of the severity of an injury – and could end up with a nasty infection.

paste to penetrate the hard skin. Sit still for at least 10 minutes. Then unwrap your foot and scrub the area with a pumice stone. All that dead, hard, callused skin should come loose and flake away easily.

Note: Don't try this tip if you are allergic or sensitive to aspirin.

Leave some calluses alone. Sometimes a little hard skin is good. 'People who go barefoot a lot develop calluses across their soles,' says Dr Frederick Hass, a GP. 'They protect the skin from rough terrain or ground heat. If sufficiently developed and toughened, they can even ward off cutting by sharp objects. These calluses are rarely painful.'

Sometimes a callus develops as a safeguard against an ingrowing toenail. As the sharp-edged nail bites into the adjoining tissue, the skin thickens and hardens to prevent further intrusion. Should you develop this kind of callus, leave it alone, says Dr Hass.

If it becomes painful, you can get temporary relief by soaking your foot in warm, soapy water, but don't ever attempt to trim it. If it becomes too painful, ask your doctor to refer you to a specialist who can sort out the ingrowing nail.

Work fast to prevent a corn. If your callus treatment has been unsuccessful and the pressure is extreme, the callus will get thicker and thicker. Once it develops a hard core, it becomes a corn.

It's best to take action when a corn first takes shape, says Dr Hass. At that point, a corn is a hardening small circle of skin that causes little or no pain. Massage the area gently with lanolin as soon as you can to soften the corn and make it less responsive to pressure, then pad it to relieve pressure.

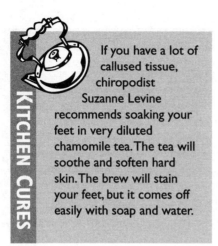

KITCHEN CURES

If you have a lot of callused tissue, chiropodist Suzanne Levine recommends soaking your feet in very diluted chamomile tea. The tea will soothe and soften hard skin. The brew will stain your feet, but it comes off easily with soap and water.

Avoid medicated pads. 'I don't recommend corn plasters or any other over-the-counter medications,' says Dr Kramer. 'They are nothing more than acid, which doesn't know the difference between corns and calluses and normal skin. So although they may work on your corn or callus, they will also eat away normal skin, causing burning or even ulcers.'

If you *must* use corn plasters or other over-the-counter salicylic acid products, available as liquid, ointment or discs, be sure to follow the advice of chiropodist Suzanne Levine: apply *only* to the problem area, not the surrounding skin. If treating a corn, first put a doughnut-shaped non-medicated pad around the corn to shield adjacent skin. Never use any of these products more than twice a week, and see your doctor if there's no sign of improvement after two weeks.

Enjoy a good soak. 'Your corn pain may be coming from a bursa, a fluid-filled sac that becomes inflamed and enlarged at the site between the bone and the corn,' says Dr Levine. 'For temporary relief, soak your feet in a solution of Epsom salts and warm water,' she advises. This will shrink the bursa sac and take some pressure off nearby sensory nerves. But if you then put tight shoes back on, the bursa will soon swell up again. (See also *Bursitis*, page 113.)

Make horseshoes. To cushion corns, says Dr Roberts, don't use corn pads with an oval opening. The oval will cause pressure on the surrounding area, making the corn or callus bulge into the opening. If you have that type of pad, cut a wedge out of it to make a horseshoe shape. Position the pad far enough behind the corn so that as you walk – if your foot slides forward in your shoe – the pad won't rub against the corn it is supposed to protect.

Get spot relief. Even better than a corn pad, says Dr Roberts, is a spot-shaped plaster, which also has the advantage of a sterile gauze centre. But avoid adhesive bandages that have to be wrapped right round your toe. Their bulk may lead to irritation and discomfort.

Give soft corns space. Soft corns – the ones that form between two toes – require different care from ordinary corns. Because soft corns are caused by bones from two adjacent toes rubbing together, says Dr Cowin, you need to use something soft to separate the toes. You can buy toe separators or toe spacers, which are simply little pieces of foam that you place between the toes.

Stretch your shoes. Calluses and corns are often caused by shoes, so making some simple adjustments to your shoes may help to ease your pain. Stretching your shoes may help to remove the pressure that caused the friction.

Some shoe repairers offer a stretching service, or you can use this home method suggested by chiropodist Marvin Sandler. Apply a leather-stretching solution (your local shoe repairer should stock this) to your shoes. This allows the leather fibres to stretch while you walk. Apply the solution many times, and walk in the shoes – while the leather is still wet – until they feel comfortable.

Watch out for high heels. A lot of problems in women are the result of wearing high heels, says Dr Conrad. In a court shoe, your foot slides right to the front of the shoe, cramming everything into a space that is too small.

Lace-ups are a better bet – they keep the back of the foot firmly in the shoe and stop the foot from slipping forwards and putting pressure on the ball of your foot and your toes as you walk.

To avoid problems, says Dr Cowin, wear well-fitting shoes that don't have exceptionally high heels. 'For special occasions, high heels won't hurt,' he says, 'but flatter shoes are better for everyday wear.'

Get a proper fit. 'The most important thing when buying a shoe is fit,' says foot specialist Terry Spilken. 'Whether a shoe costs £15 or £150, if it doesn't fit properly, it's going to cause problems.

'Make sure the shoes are the right length; you want a thumb's-width distance from the end of your longest toe to the end of your shoe. (And your longest toe isn't necessarily your big toe.) You should also have enough width across the ball of the foot, and enough room in the toe so that there's no pressure across the toes.'

Look for natural materials that breathe, like leather, advises Dr Spilken. And remember that it's just as bad for your feet to buy shoes that are too big as ones that are too small. 'If the shoe is too big, your foot will slide in it and create friction. That friction can cause a callus or corn just as easily as a tight shoe pinching.'

CARPAL TUNNEL SYNDROME

13 coping techniques

The bane of office workers, waiters, carpenters and journalists, carpal tunnel syndrome is a painful reminder of how much many of us depend on our hands to earn a living. At first, symptoms include numbness, tingling, loss of strength or flexibility and pain. Yet carpal tunnel can progress over time, with a small percentage of patients developing permanent injury. That's why it's best to deal with symptoms quickly.

Most people with carpal tunnel syndrome recover completely and avoid injuring themselves again by changing the way they work. What's more, those with carpal tunnel can make changes to ease the pain.

Carpal tunnel syndrome isn't something that happens overnight. It's a cumulative trauma disorder that develops over time when your hands and wrists perform repetitive movements.

Think of the Dartford Tunnel. Imagine how hard it is to try to get through it during rush hour as multiple lanes of traffic fight to squeeze into two-lane tubes. The small carpal bones at your wrist, overarched by a tight fibrous band, form the carpal tunnel, which can be a lot like that tunnel under the Thames during rush hour. When you use your hand in repeated motions – writing, typing or hammering – the tendons, which run like lanes through your wrist, swell and compress the median nerve that runs to your hand.

Median nerve compression can also arise from any other condition causing swelling, irritation or thickening of the synovial membranes that surround the tendons and produce the lubricating synovial fluid. These conditions include previous fracture of the carpal bones or wrist, underactive thyroid, diabetes, rheumatoid arthritis, menopause and pregnancy.

Women are twice as likely as men to experience carpal tunnel syndrome. Symptoms normally affect one hand but can be present in both, says neurologist Colin Hall. 'Sometimes the affected hand will feel numb or tingle, or feel like it's fallen asleep.' The median nerve doesn't supply your whole hand, though, so, in carpal tunnel syndrome, your little finger and the side of your ring finger next to it are unaffected.

Here are some suggestions for dealing with that feeling when it comes.

Go round in circles. Susan Isernhagen is a physiotherapist who specializes in reducing work-related injuries and rehabilitating those who have been injured. 'When the tingling begins, it's time to do some hand exercises,' she says. One of these is a simple exercise that rotates the wrist.

WHEN TO CONSULT A DOCTOR

Wrist and hand pain are not always caused by carpal tunnel syndrome – they could be a symptom of other illnesses, says physiotherapist Susan Isernhagen. 'If you get a crackly or crunchy feeling in your wrist when you exercise it, that's not a sign of carpal tunnel syndrome,' she says. 'It may be a symptom of osteoarthritis.' Ask your doctor to look at it.

For severe or persistent carpal tunnel syndrome, your doctor may prescribe a course of diuretics to relieve fluid overload, arrange for you to have an anti-inflammatory cortisone injection into the carpal tunnel, or refer you to an orthopaedic surgeon for consideration of an operation known as surgical decompression.

Move your hands around in gentle circles for about two minutes. 'This exercises all the muscles of the wrist, restores circulation, and gets your wrist out of the bent position that normally brings on the symptoms of carpal tunnel syndrome.'

Raise your hand. Get those hands off the keyboard and up into the air. 'Raise your arm above your head and rotate your arm while rotating your wrist at the same time,' says Isernhagen. This gets your shoulders, neck and upper back in a better position and relieves the stress and tension.

Take a break. 'Rest your hands on a desk or a table and then rotate your head for about two minutes,' recommends Isernhagen. 'Bend your neck backwards and forwards, then tip your head to either side. Then do some neck turns, looking over your right shoulder, then over your left.'

Make exercise as routine as eating. It's important to exercise and relax all the muscles that are giving you problems every day, even when you're not in pain, Isernhagen says. Practise exercises like those described above at least four times a day.

Take painkillers. 'To reduce pain and inflammation, take a nonsteroidal anti-inflammatory like aspirin or ibuprofen,' says orthopaedic surgeon Stephen Cash. Don't take paracetamol, though. 'Paracetamol reduces pain,' he says, 'but it doesn't do anything for inflammation.'

Put the pain on ice. 'Cold packs will help to bring down any swelling,' Isernhagen says. Don't wrap your wrist in a heating pad as that just increases the swelling.

The vitamin B₆ debate

Doctors first recommended vitamin B₆ supplementation for carpal tunnel syndrome 30 years ago. But there is much debate as to the vitamin's usefulness.

Several books recommend taking 100 to 200mg vitamin B₆ per day to ease symptoms. But prolonged use at this dosage can actually cause nerve damage: the recommended daily consumption of B₆ for women is just 1.2mg, and for men 1.4mg.

Critics say that large doses of vitamin B₆ are not only useless in the treatment of carpal tunnel syndrome, they can also be dangerous.

Because vitamin B₆ can be toxic at high doses, it should be taken only under the supervision of a doctor.

Hands up. Keep your hands above shoulder height when you take a break from work, says Isernhagen. 'Sit with your elbows supported on your desk or propped on the arms of your chair. Keep your hands pointed upward.'

Put the squeeze on your pain. Making squeezing movements with your fingers will help to relieve the tingling, says Isernhagen. Press your fingers into your palm, then stretch them right back and hold. Repeat.

Keep your hands on the bed. Keep your arms close to your body and your wrists straight while sleeping. 'If you let your hand drop over the side of the bed, it can increase the pressure,' Isernhagen says. And if you are woken in the night by the pain in your hands, try doing the exercises that you do during the day. You could also place a pillow beside you in bed, so that your wrist can be slightly elevated.

Don't bind the wrist. You don't want to tie up traffic in your wrist. Avoid wrapping your wrist with a support bandage, because you could bind it too tight and cut off the circulation, says Isernhagen.

Use the right grip. If you have to carry anything with a handle, make sure the grip fits your hand. If the grip is too small, build it up – try using the rubber strip used to bind tennis racquet or cricket bat handles, available in sports shops. If the grip is too large, get another handle, advises Isernhagen.

Handle with care. 'Don't concentrate pressure at the base of the wrist when using hand tools. Use your elbow and shoulder as much as possible,' recommends Isernhagen.

CHAFING

9 ways to rub it out

For many years, a university wrestling team had trained in cotton shirts. Then the training uniform changed. The students were given hardwearing 50 per cent polyester, 50 per cent cotton practice shirts. They were economical and would last for ever – and not lose their colour. But the players soon complained that the shirts rubbed, leaving their skin sore and chafed. And even though they were washed every day, the fabric stayed rough and abrasive.

Chafing increases the chances of infection, and after a while, several team members had had herpes simplex infections on their faces or necks. The following year, the team went back to all-cotton shirts. There were few rashes; herpes infections dropped. So, if something rubs and leaves a rash, look for an alternative.

Wear natural fibres. The wrestlers' problems were caused by the heavy duty, synthetic-blend shirt. When the team switched back to 100 per cent cotton, the rashes cleared up.

Wash before you wear. Wash any new exercise clothes before you wear them, says Richard Strauss, a specialist in sports medicine. Washing can soften fabric enough to reduce chafing.

Wrap it up. People who are overweight or who have big thighs, which make chafing more likely, may find relief by using elastic bandages around the parts of their legs that rub, says Tom Barringer, a GP. The bandages shield the skin when your thighs rub together, and instead of skin against skin, the rubbing will be fabric against fabric. Make sure the elastic bandage is secure so that it doesn't move across your skin.

Keep it tight. A pair of athletic tights or Lycra cycling shorts are snug, yet they stretch and cause no friction against the skin, says Dr Barringer.

Put cotton first. When your sportswear is made of a potentially abrasive fabric, wear cotton underwear to keep the fabric from your skin, says

Dr Strauss. 'Lots of sportsmen don cotton underpants and wear their supports on top,' he says.

Grease your body. Petroleum jelly between your thighs, around your toes, under your arms – anywhere you chafe – acts as a lubricant, helping the rubbing skin to glide instead of chafe, says Robert Boyce, an expert in exercise physiology.

Sprinkle on talcum powder. An old standby for chafing, talcum powder works as a lubricant in the same way as petroleum jelly. It helps the skin slip past skin without catching and rubbing.

Protect it with a plaster. You can stop small areas from chafing with an adhesive bandage. Runners, for instance, put plasters over their nipples to prevent irritation from rubbing against running shirts.

Try another sport. Overweight exercisers may find chafing a problem until they lose weight, says Dr Boyce. His advice is to change sports while your skin heals. If you have sore spots from walking, try a stationary bicycle. If the bicycle causes problems, try swimming – a virtually chafe-free sport.

CHAPPED HANDS
23 soothing tips

Sometimes it seems there's nothing more painful – or unattractive – than chapped hands. Blame it on ageing and the weather. As you age, your body produces less of the oil you need to keep skin smooth and supple. When you add the low humidity of cold winter days and central heating indoors, you have a recipe for dry and irritated skin. But there are many soothing solutions for turning rough, dry hands into something soft enough to hold.

Keep away from water. Basically, if you have chapped hands you want to avoid water at all costs, says Joseph Bark, a dermatologist. 'Consider water to be as bad as acid for your hands.

'Repeated washing removes the skin's natural oil layer, which allows moisture within the skin to evaporate. And that's extremely drying.' Always think twice about washing your hands unnecessarily.

WHEN TO CONSULT A DOCTOR

If you have splits and cracks on your hands, or if what you think are chapped hands begins with little blisters along the sides of the fingers, you have hand eczema, and you should see your doctor, advises dermatologist Joseph Bark.

Other signs may indicate that what you have is more than a case of chapped hands. If after two weeks of self treatment your hands don't clear up, again, see your doctor. You may have a fungal infection or psoriasis of the hands.

Dermatologist Diana Bihova warns that people like doctors, nurses, chefs and housewives – whose occupations require them to immerse their hands in water for prolonged periods – can easily contract monilial paronychia, an annoying fungal infection involving the skin around the cuticle. Bar staff who handle beer, which is yeasty, are particularly susceptible. When the infection strikes the finger's protective nail fold, it becomes red, swollen and painful.

Just wash your palms. 'When you have to wash your hands often, try to do just the palms,' recommends dermatologist Diana Bihova. 'You can wash the palms much more often than the backs of the hands, which have thinner skin and dry out easily.'

Use cleanser, not soap. 'Instead of using soap, clean your hands with an oil-free skin cleanser such as Cetaphil,' says Dr Bark. 'Rub it onto the skin, work it into a lather, then wipe it off with a tissue. It's a wonderful way to wash skin without any irritation whatsoever.'

Try the bath oil treatment. Taking the no-soap idea one step further, dermatologist Rodney Basler recommends washing your hands with bath oil. They may not feel as clean as they do when you use soap, but they won't dry out.

Use a moisturizer. Use a good hand cream every time you wash your hands and at bedtime. 'Its strength should depend on the severity of your chapping,' says Dr Basler. 'Lotions are the least moisturizing, followed by creams and then ointments.'

Avoid hot air dryers. If the toilet at work has a hot-air dryer instead of towels, bring in a towel from home, advises Dr Bihova. 'Hot-air blowers are associated with chapped hands. If you have to use one, keep your

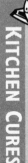

'If you want the cheapest home remedy going, use cooking margarine,' says Dr Bark. It coats the skin and keeps water locked in. The key is to use very little and rub it in well so that your hands don't feel greasy.

'You don't have to buy expensive creams to get good results,' agrees dermatologist Howard Donsky. Cheap alternatives for people with dry and normal skin include cocoa butter, lanolin, petroleum jelly and light mineral oil.

hands at least 20cm from the nozzle and dry them thoroughly.'

Soak those hands. Although in general you should keep your hands out of water, sometimes a therapeutic soak is helpful. For an inexpensive way to achieve the moisturizing effects of skin creams, simply soak your hands in warm water for a few minutes. Then pat off excess water and apply vegetable or mineral oil to the damp surface to seal in moisture, says Howard Donsky, a dermatologist.

In the same vein, Dr Basler recommends soaking your hands in a water-and-oil solution. 'Use four capfuls of a bath oil that disperses easily in water (Alpha-Keri works well) in 500mls of water. At the end of the day, soak for 20 minutes to get oil back into the skin. That alone will help chapped hands.'

Double up. 'When applying any type of lotion or cream, use what I call Bark's double-layer application technique,' says Dr Bark. 'Put on a very thin layer and let it soak in for a few minutes. Then apply another thin layer. Two thin ones work much better than one heavy one.'

Try lemon oil. 'To smooth and soothe irritated hands, mix a few drops of glycerin with a few drops of lemon essential oil (both are available from health food shops). Massage this into your hands at bedtime,' says skin-care specialist Lia Schorr.

Wear protective gloves. Lots of unexpected things around the house can irritate chapped hands. Dr Bihova recommends wearing plain white cotton gloves for doing any kind of dry work. 'That includes reading the newspaper and even unpacking your shopping.' Any friction against skin already dry, cracked or red will aggravate it. Cotton gloves let skin breathe and at the same time absorb any moisture that accumulates so it won't irritate your skin.

'Cotton gloves also keep the skin clean so you don't have to wash your hands as often and risk perpetuating the problem,' says dermatologist

Nelson Novick. 'If you need to get an extra-good grip on something, use leather gloves,' adds hand model Trisha Webster.

Mix rubber and cotton. 'For wet work, it's extremely important to wear cotton gloves underneath the rubber ones,' says Dr Novick. That's because perspiration, lotions and medications on your hands accumulate inside the gloves and may become irritating quite quickly.

If the cotton gloves get wet, change them immediately. Otherwise, replace them with a fresh pair every 20 minutes. 'I don't recommend rubber gloves with built-in cotton linings, because it's very difficult to wash them,' he says. 'But you can wash cotton gloves in a mild detergent.'

Dr Bihova agrees. 'The biggest mistake women make when they have hand problems is wearing just rubber gloves. That only makes the hands worse. The rubber traps moisture, stops the skin from breathing and creates too much friction.'

Model your hands after hers

When your fingers are your fortune, you take good care of them. Trisha Webster is a professional hand model whose hands appear in many jewellery and cosmetic ads. How does she keep her hands looking young?

Stop problems before they start. 'I try to keep my hands out of water at all costs,' says Webster, 'which is why I always let someone else do the washing-up (well, it's one of the reasons!).

'When I can't avoid getting my hands wet, such as in the bath, I always moisturize them straight afterwards. It takes just a few minutes for the moisture that's accumulated in the skin to evaporate. When that happens, your hands are drier than they were before.'

Get protection. 'I never go outdoors in the winter without protecting my hands. That means putting on a good layer of moisturizer and then gloves.'

Use sun sense. 'A long time ago, I stopped going out in the sun, because it dries and ages hands.'

If you're not ready to give up the sun, dermatologist Diana Bihova suggests using a moisturizing sunscreen on your hands. 'Sunscreens moisturize hands and keep them looking younger, so make their use an everyday habit,' she says. 'But avoid gels and alcohol-based sunscreens because alcohol is drying. Also, products containing the active ingredient PABA can be irritating if you have sensitive skin.

Prevention is your best solution

Chapped hands are easier to prevent than to treat. Here are some ways to do that.

Stay out of hot water. A good rule of thumb is to avoid hot water, detergents and strong household cleaning products.

Avoid soap. Because chapped hands occur when oil is removed from the skin, don't use harsh soaps. Choose a mild soap, preferably one with cold cream in it. Dr Bark often recommends Dove, 'virtually the mildest soap there is.'

Put moisture into the air. 'Skin moisturizes itself from the inside out,' says Dr Basler. 'If there's moisture in the air, not as much will be drawn out through the skin. So it's a good idea to use a home humidifier.'

Pamper your hands. 'When you apply moisturizer to your face in the morning, immediately apply some to your hands. At night do the same, advises Dr Bihova. 'That keeps them supple and helps them to resist chapping. Twice a day is a must, but also do it whenever you wash.'

Wear gloves to bed. Here's a soothing treatment from dermatologist Thomas Goodman. Wear cotton gloves to bed, having first moistened the fabric with about a teaspoon of petroleum jelly so that the gloves won't absorb the cream from your hands. Then apply hand cream at bedtime and slip on the gloves. Leave them on overnight.

Ask someone to wash your hair. 'Believe it or not, even shampoo can make tender hands feel worse,' says skin specialist Stephen Schleicher. 'Either let someone else shampoo your hair or wear plastic gloves.'

Beware of handling food. 'The juices of raw meat and vegetables

KITCHEN CURES

To remove the top layer of dead skin cells from chapped hands, skin-care specialist Lia Schorr suggests this treatment.

Put a cupful of uncooked porridge oats in a blender and process to a very fine powder.

Put this in a large bowl, and rub your hands in the powder, gently removing dry skin. Rinse with cool water, pat dry and apply plenty of hand cream.

Wait two minutes and apply more cream.

– potatoes, onions, tomatoes or carrots – can be very toxic to skin, especially if it's already irritated,' says Dr Goodman. 'So wear tissue-thin plastic gloves when handling food.' Dr Schleicher warns against squeezing oranges, lemons or grapefruit with bare hands. 'They're terribly irritating and will dry your hands further.'

CHAPPED LIPS

11 tips to stop the dryness

Those who have chapped lips know that they can quickly turn a smile into a scowl. Peeling and inflamed lips, known medically as cheilitis, can be caused by cold, dry weather and exposure to the sun, or allergic reactions to lipstick, toothpaste, food or drink can make your lips peel. Try some of these soothing remedies to take the pain out of smiling.

Try the palm or balm solution. 'The best way to deal with chapped lips is to avoid the dry, cold weather that can cause them in the first place,' says dermatologist Joseph Bark. 'But as heading for the tropics is not too practical for most people, you can head for the chemist instead.' Buy some lip balm. Then, before you go outside – and several times while you're out – coat your lips with it. As lips don't keep anything on them very well, reapply the balm every time you eat, drink or wipe your mouth.

Occasionally, very sensitive lips can react to the balm itself, especially if it contains lanolin or chemical flavourings and perfumes, says family doctor Stephen Amiel. Try a hypo-allergenic lanolin-free type if you think you are affected. Good old petroleum jelly may not taste as nice but it works just as well for many people.

Use a sunscreen. 'Remember, too, that the sun can burn lips at any time of year,' says Dr Bark. He recommends buying a lip balm with built-in sunscreen of at least sun protection factor (SPF) 15.

Dermatology professor Nelson Novick agrees: 'Sun damage to the lips can cause dryness and scaliness. It is especially bad for the lower lip, which bears the brunt of ultraviolet rays.'

Wear lipstick. A creamy lipstick helps to soothe lips that are already chapped, says make-up expert Glenn Roberts. 'In fact, just wearing lipstick gives some protection and may help to prevent chapping in the first place.'

'I believe that wearing lipstick is one of the reasons women seldom get

WHEN TO CONSULT A DOCTOR

Chapped lips are unlikely to be due to a serious medical problem, says family doctor Stephen Amiel. But if you have angular cheilitis, you ought to check with your doctor that you're not anaemic.

If thrush is the cause, you'll need treatment with nystatin lozenges or liquid, or miconazole gel. Sometimes oral thrush can occur following a course of antibiotics or prolonged use of inhaled steroid asthma inhalers, but if you get oral thrush for no obvious reason, you should definitely see your doctor, as occasionally it can be an early sign of diabetes or immune deficiency.

lip cancer,' says Dr Bark. 'In 14 years of practice, I've treated perhaps one or two women for lip cancer but literally hundreds of men.'

Be wise. Cracking and scaling of the lips, particularly at the corners (angular cheilitis) can sometimes be due to deficiencies of iron or B vitamins, especially riboflavin (vitamin B$_2$), says Dr Amiel. There's plenty of iron in meat, poultry, fish, fortified cereals, apricots, chocolate and red wine. The iron in beans, lentils and soya is poorly absorbed on its own, so, if you're relying on these foods for extra iron, eat plenty of vitamin C-containing fruit and vegetables to help its absorption. Good dietary sources of riboflavin are dairy products, meat, poultry, fish, whole grains and leafy green vegetables.

Look out for thrush. Soreness and cracking of the lips at the corners can be features of thrush, a fungal infection caused by *Candida albicans*, says Dr Amiel. Babies can get this, especially if they use a dummy and dribble a lot. Older people with poorly fitting dentures, ground down or missing teeth, can also get it, as the corners of the mouth fold inwards, forming moist crevices in which candida can flourish.

Look for thrush in your baby's mouth: you may see a white adherent coating on the tongue and white spots with a red background on the inside of the cheeks. Sterilize dummies and teats well to avoid re-infection, advises Dr Amiel. Visit your dentist to check your dentures: they too need to be sterilized well.

Drink up. Moisturize your lips from the inside out by drinking extra fluids in winter. 'I recommend a glass of water every few hours,' says dermatologist Diana Bihova. Another way to help counter dry lips is to humidify the air at home and at work.

Chapped lips are commonly seen in children with high temperatures, adds Dr Amiel, partly as a result of dehydration. Make sure they get plenty of extra fluids, cool them down by opening windows, using a fan or tepid sponging, and give them paracetamol or ibuprofen to bring their temperature down.

Mind your own beeswax. 'To my mind, the single best product for chapped lips is Carmex,' says dermatologist Rodney Basler. 'It's an old-fashioned product that comes in a little tin and contains, among other things, beeswax and phenol. No prescription medication is better than that.' Carmex is sold in pharmacies.

Stop licking. Chapped lips are a dehydration problem, according to Dr Basler. 'When you lick them, you briefly apply moisture, which then evaporates and leaves your lips feeling drier than before. And saliva contains digestive enzymes. OK, they're not very strong, but they don't do sore lips any good.'

'Licking chapped lips can lead to something called lip-licker's dermatitis,' warns Dr Bark. 'It's usually seen in children but can occur in adults, too.' What happens when you lick your lips is that you remove any oil that might be on them from surrounding areas. (The lips themselves don't have any oil glands.) Soon, you're licking not just your lips but also the area around them. Eventually, you end up with a red ring of dermatitis around your mouth.

Don't use toothpaste. Allergy to flavouring agents in toothpaste, sweets, chewing gum and mouthwashes can cause chapped lips in some people, says dermatologist Thomas Goodman. Tartar-control toothpastes are even worse than normal ones for drying lips. Stop using toothpaste, he suggests. Instead, use a toothbrush alone or a brush dipped in baking soda.

Think zinc. 'Some people have a tendency to dribble in their sleep, which can dry out lips or aggravate ones that are already chapped,' says Dr Novick. Stop the problem by applying a protective layer of zinc oxide ointment every night.

Rub a finger against your nose. 'This is what I tell people who work outdoors and may not have anything else to hand,' says Dr Bark. 'Rub your finger on the side of your nose. Then rub it around your lips. It picks up a little of the oil that's naturally there. It's the kind of oil our lips are looking for anyway, and they usually get it from contact with adjacent skin. You couldn't get much more of a home remedy than that.'

COLD SORES
18 tips to heal herpes simplex

Around 80 per cent of the adult population in the UK have antibodies against the herpes simplex 1 virus (the cold sore virus) in their blood. Generally, they were exposed during childhood to the highly contagious herpes virus that causes cold sores – this is different from the herpes virus that causes genital herpes.

Normally, after an initial outbreak the virus lies dormant in nerve cells, but occasionally it becomes reactivated. When that happens, you may experience an unpleasant sensation of numbness, tingling, burning or itching on your lip or the skin around your mouth before a cold sore appears.

There are a number of steps you can take to minimize the pain of a cold sore and to speed up its healing.

Treat it fast. The most effective treatment for a cold sore is an antiviral cream called acyclovir 5 per cent (Zovirax), says family doctor Stephen Amiel. This is available both on prescription and over the counter from pharmacies. As soon as the first symptoms appear, apply the cream to the area five times a day for five days. It usually cuts the length of the outbreak and limits pain. 'You need to work fast, though,' says Dr Amiel. 'Acyclovir will only work if started within 24 hours of the onset of the tingling that precedes the sore.'

Let it be. If a cold sore isn't really bothering you, just leave it alone, says James Rooney, a virologist who specializes in oral medicine. Make sure you keep the sore clean and dry.

Replace your toothbrush. Your toothbrush can harbour the herpes virus for days, reinfecting you after the present cold sore heals. Researchers at the University of Oklahoma in the USA exposed a sterile toothbrush to the virus for 10 minutes. Seven days later, half of the disease-producing viruses remained, says Richard Glass, a professor of dentistry.

Dr Glass recommends that you throw away your toothbrush when you notice you're just beginning to get a sore. If you still develop the cold sore, throw your toothbrush away after the blister develops. That can prevent you from developing multiple sores. And once the sore has healed completely, replace your toothbrush again. He says that patients who tried this method found it significantly reduced the number of cold sores they typically experienced in a year.

Don't keep your toothbrush in the bathroom. A damp toothbrush in a moist environment like a bathroom is a perfect environment for herpes simplex virus. That moisture helps to prolong the life of the herpes virus on your toothbrush, so Dr Glass recommends keeping your toothbrush in a dry place.

Use small tubes of toothpaste. Toothpaste can transmit disease, too, says Dr Glass. Buy small tubes so that you replace them regularly.

Protect with petroleum jelly. You can protect your cold sore by covering it with petroleum jelly, says Dr Glass. But don't dip the finger you used to touch your sore back into the jelly. Better still, use a clean cotton bud.

Zap it with zinc. Research shows that zinc, applied the minute you feel that tingling, helps to speed up healing time. Try Lypsyl Cold Sore Gel, available from pharmacies, which contains one per cent zinc sulphate.

Take lysine supplements. Dermatologist Mark McCune advises patients who have more than three cold sores a year to supplement their daily diets with 2000–3000mg of the amino acid lysine, available from health food stores. He also recommends that they double up on the dosage when they feel the itching and tingling that signals the development of another cold sore. Don't take amino acids without your doctor's advice, however: amino acids may not be suitable if you have liver or kidney problems, or if you are pregnant or breastfeeding. And as with all such supplements, there is no official guarantee of safety, purity or effectiveness.

Not all studies have found lysine helpful for people with cold sores. But in one, admittedly small, study of 41 patients, Dr McCune and his colleagues found that a daily dose of 1248mg of lysine helped subjects to cut the number of cold sores they had in a year. Good food sources of lysine include dairy products, potatoes, fish, pork and brewer's yeast.

Identify the pattern. What was going on in your life just before you got your last cold sore? What about the cold sore before that? If you do some detective work, you may work out what triggers your cold sores. If you can find out when you are most prone to cold sores, take lysine supplements when you're most vulnerable, says Dr McCune. Common triggers include stress, menstruation, sunlight, fatigue, another minor illness and a variety of foods.

Freeze it. Some of Dr Rooney's patients apply ice packs when they first feel the tingling. 'I'm not sure that it works, but if I were to speculate, I'd

WHEN TO CONSULT A DOCTOR

If a cold sore becomes pus-filled or develops a golden-coloured crust spreading into the surrounding skin, see your doctor, advises virus expert James Rooney. You probably have a bacterial infection, impetigo, which will benefit from a course of antibiotics.

Your doctor may also prescribe a course of oral aciclovir as an alternative to ointment, says family doctor Stephen Amiel. This will usually be too late for the current attack, but frequent sufferers may want a course to keep in reserve. There is some evidence that oral treatment is more effective than ointment at reducing the duration of symptoms. Occasionally, a low dose of aciclovir, taken daily for several months, may be prescribed if your life is being made a complete misery by cold sores, says Dr Amiel.

If your general immunity is low, either because you are on drugs like steroids or chemotherapeutic agents for cancer, or because of something like HIV/AIDS, the herpes virus can spread rapidly and cause a life-threatening infection, says Dr Amiel. Seek medical help urgently if you are in an at-risk group and you develop a herpes infection.

If you suffer from severe eczema, you should also see your doctor as you are also more at risk of a herpes infection spreading rapidly.

Rarely, the herpes virus can cause meningitis or encephalitis even in otherwise well people. Symptoms can include fever, fits, headaches, personality change or coma.

say that ice decreases inflammation,' he says. 'And if inflammatory substances aid the reactivation process, this could help.'

Dab on witch hazel. Other patients claim that breaking a sore and using witch hazel or alcohol to dry it really helps, says Dr Rooney.

Numb it. Most over-the-counter products, like Colsor or Carmex, contain some emollient to reduce cracking and soften scabs, and a numbing agent like phenol or camphor. Phenol may have some antiviral properties, too, says Dr Rooney.

Block sun and wind. Protecting your lips from damage through sunburn or wind exposure was cited by all our experts as a key to preventing cold sores.

Avoid arginine-rich foods. The herpes virus needs arginine as an essential amino acid for its metabolism. So cut out arginine-rich foods, which include chocolate, cola drinks, peas, grain cereals, peanuts, gelatin, cashews and beer.

Perfect your coping skills. Studies have shown that stress can trigger recurrences of the herpes simplex virus. High levels of stress are not necessarily the culprit, says Cal Vanderplate, a psychologist who specializes in stress-related disorders. 'How you cope with the stress – how you perceive it – is what's important.'

His number one stress-buster is maintaining a loving social support system. 'A sense of control is also very important. If you take a positive attitude towards your health, you'll have more influence over your symptoms.'

Relax. By the time your cold sore erupts, it's too late to do anything about the stress that triggered it, says Dr Vanderplate. But you may be able to reduce the severity of the outbreak by doing some relaxation exercises, such as yoga, visualization or meditation.

Exercise. There is evidence that exercise helps to boost the immune system, says Dr Vanderplate. The stronger your immune system, the better able it is to defend you against viruses. Exercise is also a super way to relax, he says.

Don't worry about how it looks. No one likes getting a cold sore. But if you have one, focusing on it and worrying about how you look can make it worse. 'Tell yourself that it is just like a pimple,' says Dr Vanderplate, 'and it won't interfere in your life in any way.'

COLDS
29 remedies to win the battle

If colds are so common, why isn't there a cure? The answer is about simple mathematics. As many as 200 viruses are responsible for the millions of colds we get each year, thwarting scientists' ability to concoct a cure that will work against them all.

Antibiotics, highly effective at knocking out bacterial infections, are useless against colds, which are caused by viruses. So most people live with the sniffles and aches, perhaps take an over-the-counter remedy or two, and hope the symptoms will disappear in the usual week or so.

But there's a lot you can do to get through a cold more comfortably, doctors say. Some remedies may even help you get over it more quickly. Here's how.

See if vitamin C works for you. 'Vitamin C works in the body as a scavenger, picking up all sorts of rubbish – including virus rubbish,' says family doctor Keith Sehnert. Vitamin C may also help to ease coughing, sneezing and other symptoms, although scientific studies produce mixed results when the vitamin is put to the test. One summary of 30 studies, published in 2000, found 'a consistently beneficial but generally modest therapeutic effect on the duration of cold symptoms'. On average, vitamin C reduced the number of days people experienced cold symptoms by 8–9 per cent.

You're certainly going to do yourself no harm by taking plenty of vitamin C in your diet, even if it doesn't stop your cold in its tracks, says family doctor Stephen Amiel. Citrus fruits, tomatoes and kiwi fruit are particularly good sources.

If you are going to take vitamin C, experts recommend that you take about one gram a day. To help maintain levels of vitamin C throughout the day, take half of the recommended dose in the morning and half at night.

Zap it with zinc. Sucking on zinc lozenges can cut colds short, from an average of eight days to an average of four, according to US researchers. Volunteers sucked on four to eight lozenges a day, each containing 13.3mg of zinc. Other studies, though, showed no significant benefit when zinc preparations were compared with placebo (dummy) tablets.

Zinc can also dramatically reduce symptoms such as a dry, irritated throat, says Elson Haas, who specializes in preventive medicine. 'It doesn't work for everyone, but when it works, it works,' he says.

There are many brands of zinc lozenges available that come in various flavours. But before choosing a brand, check the label. Some lozenges contain more zinc than others. Always follow the directions on the label, and don't take more than the recommended amount.

Taking more than 25mg of zinc a day can impair immunity and cause nausea, vomiting dizziness or anaemia. High doses over an extended period of time can hinder your ability to absorb copper, another vital mineral. And don't take vitamin C and zinc at the same time, as the two bind together making the zinc less effective.

Wash your hands of colds. A large study of US naval recruits showed that those who washed their hands at least five times a day (under orders!) had half the amount of respiratory illness as those who didn't. Colds are most commonly caught from touching contaminated surfaces and then touching your nose or mouth, says Dr Amiel. Remember, an uninhibited sneeze expels millions of cold viruses from the nose at about 70 mph: these viruses can survive for several hours on skin, clothes, books, door handles and escalator handrails. Wash your hands whenever you think of it, especially after travelling on public transport.

Eat a good breakfast. A balanced breakfast can go a long way towards helping to keep colds at bay, according to a British study. Researchers have found that people who regularly eat breakfast report the fewest number of colds and illnesses, perhaps because breakfast is an indicator of a healthy lifestyle.

Be positive. A positive attitude towards your body's ability to heal itself can actually mobilize immune system forces, says family doctor Martin Rossman. He teaches this theory by getting his patients to practise imagery techniques to fight colds.

Relax completely and 'imagine a tiny tornado decongesting your stuffed-up sinuses,' he suggests, 'or an army of microscopic cleaners mopping up germs with buckets of disinfectant.'

Rest and relax. Extra rest lets you put all your energy into getting well. It can also help you to avoid complications like bronchitis and pneumonia, says Samuel Caughron, a professor of medicine.

Take a day or two off work if you're feeling really bad, he advises. At the very least, slow down your everyday activities and reorganize your time. 'Trying to keep up with your normal routine can be draining because, when you're not feeling well, your concentration is down, and you'll probably need to double the amount of time it takes you to do things,' he says.

Stay at home. When you're ill, socializing can wear you out physically,

---

KITCHEN CURES

An old-fashioned folk remedy has now been proved to work: a cup of hot chicken soup can help to unblock your nasal passages. Researchers in Florida found that hot chicken soup increased the flow of nasal mucus. Nasal secretions act as a first line of defence in clearing germs from your system, scientists say.

Garlic and onions are recognized antivirals, so use plenty of both in your salads when you have a cold. Finally, adding spice to your food in the form of cayenne or chilli peppers will further help to clear your nasal passages.

compromising your immune system and causing your cold to linger, says Timothy Van Ert, a specialist in preventive medicine. Stay at home and snuggle up. Your friends, colleagues and fellow commuters will also thank you for not sharing your cold with them.

Keep warm. Wrap up against the cold, advises Dr Sehnert. This keeps your immune system focused on fighting your cold infection instead of displacing energy to protect you from the cold.

Take a walk. Light exercise improves your circulation, helping your immune system to circulate infection-fighting antibodies, says Dr Sehnert. Do gentle exercises indoors or take a brisk half-hour walk, he suggests. But don't take any strenuous exercise, he warns, which could wear you out.

Feed a cold – lightly. The very fact that you have a cold in the first place may suggest that your diet is putting a strain on your body's immune system, says Dr Haas. Counteract the problem, he advises, by eating fewer fatty foods, meat and milk products, and more fresh fruit and vegetables.

Drink lots of fluids. Drinking six to eight glasses of water, juice, tea and other mostly clear liquids a day helps to replace important fluids lost during a cold, and helps to flush out impurities that may be weakening your system. 'Remember – dilution is the solution to pollution,' says Dr Haas.

Stop smoking. Smoking aggravates a throat already irritated by a cold, says Dr Caughron. It also interferes with the infection-fighting activity of cilia, the microscopic 'fingers' that sweep bacteria out of your lungs and throat. So if you can't kick the habit for good, at least do so while you have a cold.

Ease a sore throat. Gargle morning, noon and night – or whenever it hurts most – with salt water, Dr Van Ert advises. Fill a 250ml glass with warm water and mix in a teaspoon of salt. The salt water will soothe a sore throat.

A herbal double. Echinacea and goldenseal represent a two-pronged attack against coughs and colds, says clinical herbalist Douglas Schar. Coughs and colds are caused by viruses. Echinacea is a powerful immune-system stimulant which increases the number and activity of the white blood cells responsible for keeping viral infections under control. It clears up the root of the problem.

Goldenseal has an anti-inflammatory action on the mucous membranes, which reduces congestion. In addition, it has broad-spectrum antibacterial action that reduces the incidence of secondary infections, such as sinusitis, bronchitis and tonsillitis, which can follow a cough or cold.

Used together, these two herbs can help coughs and colds to pass uneventfully. The herbs are sold separately or as combination capsules. Start taking them as soon as you feel a cough or cold coming on and continue until you have been clear of symptoms for a week, says Schar.

Sip a hot toddy. Clear your stuffed-up nose and help yourself to a good night's sleep by drinking a hot toddy – a hot drink consisting of whisky or rum, water, sugar and spices – or half a glass of wine before bedtime, suggests Dr Caughron.

Another popular recipe is a measure of whisky, a teaspoon or two of honey and the juice of half a lemon topped up with boiling water. Don't imbibe any more alcohol than that, however, since too much can put a strain on your system, making recovery more difficult.

Drink tea at bedtime. For a good night's sleep, brew a cup of relaxing hops, valerian or linden to bring on deep relaxation and a recuperative sleep. A good night's sleep does a lot to clear a cough or cold, says Schar. Sweeten the tea with honey, which adds its own antiviral and antibacterial activity to the brew.

Drink liquorice root tea. Soothe your sore throat and quieten a cough with liquorice root tea. Liquorice root contains compounds which act as anti-inflammatories, taking the redness and pain out of a sore throat. In addition, it is rich in compounds proven to quieten coughing.

Buy powdered liquorice root at a health food store and add half a teaspoon to a cup of boiling water. 'In my experience, three cups a day, sipped gingerly all day long, really makes a difference,' says Schar, 'especially to that irritable coughing that keeps you awake at night.'

Breathe steam. Taking a steamy shower can help to clear congestion, says Kenneth Peters, who specializes in headache management. Or fill a bowl with boiling water, drape a towel over your head and the bowl creating a tent, and inhale the steam until it subsides. This also relieves a cough by moistening a dry throat.

Adding a few drops of olbas oil, menthol-and-eucalyptus or Friar's balsam to the hot water may help ease congestion further, says Dr Amiel, but the steam's the main thing.

Note: Be extremely careful with the boiling water, warns Dr Amiel. Sit at a table, don't use it in bed. Most pharmacies sell a two-handled beaker,

WHEN TO CONSULT A DOCTOR

Millions of people consult their doctor each year with colds. Apart from recommending symptomatic relief remedies and rest, doctors can do nothing but offer sympathy, says family doctor Stephen Amiel – and even that may be in short supply on a winter Monday morning! Speak to your doctor though if:

• your cold and cough symptoms are not beginning to improve after a fortnight;

• you develop shortness of breath, wheezing, or chest pains when you breathe deeply;

• you are producing excessive amounts of green, yellow or bloody phlegm;

• you have a fever above 38°C (101°F) for more than three days;

• you have a fever above 39.5°C (103°F);

• you have a fever which returns after a few days of being normal;

• you develop earache or a discharge from your ear;

• you have persistent green or yellow nasal catarrh, headache or bloody nasal discharge, suggesting a secondary bacterial sinus infection;

• you have persistent loss of appetite.

In general, says Dr Amiel, get a doctor's advice earlier for small babies and frail older people, especially if they are not drinking good amounts of fluid; also for people with asthma, chronic bronchitis, diabetes, or immune systems suppressed by illness or drugs like steroids.

rather like a baby's feeding mug, with a face mask attachment to provide a safe steam inhalation alternative.

Keep the night air moist. You may find that putting a humidifier next to your bed at night helps to keep the airways clear, allowing you or a child to sleep more peacefully. Otherwise, take the lid off your electric kettle and let the water almost boil away, filling the room with steam. Keep well out of reach of children and frail adults.

Use petroleum jelly on a sore nose. Relieve a nose made raw from blowing by applying a lubricating layer of petroleum jelly around and slightly inside your nostrils, suggests Dr Peters.

Take the medicine. Don't let your cold symptoms keep you from getting a healing night's sleep. Many cold remedies are available without a prescription. Some treat specific symptoms. Others contain a combination of drugs – plus alcohol, in some cases – aimed at treating a wide range of symptoms. These combination drugs, however, can have many uncomfortable side effects like nausea and drowsiness.

If you need to take medicines during the day, take those that treat only the symptoms you are experiencing. Be sure to follow the instructions carefully, advises pharmacist Sue Livingston.

- For relief of the body aches or fever that can accompany a cold, take aspirin, ibuprofen or paracetamol. *Don't* give aspirin to children under 16 as, in rare cases, it can trigger fatal liver failure (Reye's syndrome).

- To stop sneezing and dry up your runny nose and watery eyes, take an antihistamine such as cetirizine (Zirtek) or loratidine (Clarityn) – both non-sedating, or chlorpheniramine (Piriton) – which has a sedating effect. Antihistamines block your body's release of histamine, a chemical that causes these symptoms. Ask your pharmacist for advice: some antihistamines cause drowsiness, so save these for bedtime or at least for when you won't be driving or doing anything that requires coordination.

- Nasal sprays and drops, such as Otrivine or ephedrine, are effective decongestants. However, they shouldn't be used for longer than three days. Over-use can have a rebound effect, and make your nose even more blocked than it was before.

- To relieve a tickly cough, try cough drops and syrups. Look for products that contain cough-suppressants, such as Robitussin Dry Cough Syrup and pholcodine linctus.

- Lozenges can also combat coughs. Some, including Dequacaine, Tyrozets and Merocaine, contain anaesthetics that slightly numb your sore throat, thereby relieving your need to cough.

- Menthol or camphor rubs have a soothing, cooling effect and may relieve congestion and help you to breathe more easily, especially at bedtime. Apply Vicks VapoRub or a similar product to your bare chest before going to bed.

Don't spread your germs. When you need to cough, go ahead and cough. When you need to blow your nose, go ahead and blow. But cough and sneeze into disposable tissues instead of setting germs free in the environment, Dr Van Ert advises, then promptly throw the tissue away and wash your hands. This will help to prevent your healthy friends and family from catching your cold.

CONJUNCTIVITIS
9 remedies for pink-eye

Conjunctivitis is inflammation of the conjunctiva, a membrane that lines the inside of the eyelids and covers the white of the eye. Red and irritated, infected eyes feel as if they're being scratched by stray grains of sand. There's often a discharge, too. The culprits are viruses, bacteria or allergies. While conjunctivitis won't threaten an adult's sight, it's unsightly and uncomfortable. Here's what you can do.

Wash the red away. 'A warm compress applied to the eyes for 5 to 10 minutes three or four times a day will make you feel better,' says paediatric ophthalmologist Robert Petersen.

Keep eyes clean. Conjunctivitis often gets better by itself, says Dr Petersen. To help the healing process, keep your eyes and eyelids clean by using a cotton wool ball dipped in cool boiled water to wipe the crusts away.

Make your own tears. 'If you add a pinch of salt to a cup of boiled water, you can make a saline solution the same strength as tears,' says family doctor Stephen Amiel. 'This has a mild antiseptic action and is more effective than water on its own.' Wipe outwards from the corner of the eye next to the nose, says Dr Amiel, and be sure to discard each piece of cotton wool after a single sweep across the eye.

Use baby shampoo. Adults who habitually get a lot of discharge and crusting along the lid margins – a condition known as blepharitis – should bathe their eyes twice a day with very hot tap water, using a clean flannel or cotton wool ball, says Dr Amiel. This softens the crusts and allows natural oils to flow from the eyelid glands. You should also make a solution of one part baby shampoo to 10 parts warm water and, using a clean cotton bud (at least one for each eye), rub the solution into the base of the eyelashes twice a day.

Sodium bicarbonate is an effective alternative. Dissolve a pinch of bicarbonate in a cup of boiled water to make a solution that will last for a week

Throw in the towel. Throw your towel, flannel and anything else that comes in contact with your eyes into the wash. 'This infection is highly contagious. Don't share a towel or flannel with anyone, because it will easily spread the disease,' says Dr Petersen.

WHEN TO CONSULT A DOCTOR

Conjunctivitis is an easily treatable problem that will usually go away on its own in about a week. You should, however, avoid taking a wait-and-see attitude. See your doctor if:

- after five days the infection is getting worse, not better;

- you have a red eye that is associated with significant eye pain, change in vision, or a large amount of yellow or greenish discharge;

- redness is caused by an injury to your eye. Infections can get into the eye if you've scratched the cornea, leading to an ulcer, loss of vision, or even loss of your eye, warns paediatric ophthalmologist Robert Petersen. Corneal infections aren't always triggered by injuries, though. Sometimes the herpes simplex virus from a cold sore on the mouth is spread when you touch your eye;

- your eyes are gritty and seem persistently drier than normal. This can sometimes be a symptom associated with more generalized conditions such as rheumatoid arthritis, sarcoidosis or lymphoma.

Don't chlorinate your eyes. Does swimming in a pool leave your eyes pink? The chlorine added to swimming pools can cause conjunctivitis, but without the chlorine, bacteria would grow – and that could cause it, too, says Dr Petersen. He suggests that anyone susceptible to conjunctivitis should wear tight-fitting goggles while in the water.

Cool down allergic conjunctivitis. If you survive summer swimming but not summer pollen, your conjunctivitis may be caused by an allergy. Eyes that itch like a mosquito bite and have a stringy discharge are probably affected by allergic conjunctivitis, says ophthalmologist Daniel Nelson. Take an over-the-counter antihistamine, he advises, 'and use cold, not warm, compresses. A cold compress will really relieve the itch.'

And whatever you do, avoid the temptation to rub your eyes, says Dr Amiel. You'll release more

KITCHEN CURES

Cool as a cucumber. 'Cucumber can work wonders for itching eyes,' says family doctor Stephen Amiel. Cut thin slices from a refrigerated cucumber, put one over each eye and leave in place for a few minutes.

histamines from the inflamed conjunctivae and just make the itching worse.

Use ointment at night. 'Germ-caused conjunctivitis intensifies when your eyes are closed. That's why it tends to get worse at night when you are asleep,' says Dr Petersen. He suggests that you put any prescribed antibiotic ointment in your eyes before you go to bed, so as to prevent crusting.

Simple eye ointment is available over the counter, says Dr Amiel, and can be used instead if your conjunctivitis doesn't require antibiotic ointment from your doctor.

CONSTIPATION

16 solutions to a common problem

More than three million people in the UK suffer from constipation once a month or more. Bowel habits are often the subject of humour, but constipation is no joke for sufferers. Women appear to experience more constipation than men, and older people more than younger people. It can cause abdominal discomfort and bloating, and make you feel sluggish and miserable.

There are many causes of constipation including a lack of dietary fibre, insufficient liquid intake, stress, certain medicines, lack of exercise and bad bowel habits, says Paul Rousseau, a geriatrician. We take a look at all of these factors, and suggest ways to remedy the situation.

Determine if you really are constipated. We are regularly bombarded with laxative advertisements that give the impression that a daily bowel movement is vital to good health. But that just isn't so, says Marvin Schuster, who specializes in digestive disorders.

Many people think they're constipated when they are not. In reality, the need to defecate varies greatly from individual to individual. For some of us, a bowel movement three times a day is normal; others go three times a week.

Fine-tune your fluid and fibre intake. Our experts agree that the first thing you should do if you're constipated is to check your diet. The foremost menu items for battling constipation are dietary fibre such as fruits, vegetables, beans and other pulses, and liquids, essential for keeping the stool soft and helping it to pass through the colon.

How much liquid and how much fibre do you need? Let's start with the liquid. A minimum of six glasses of liquid, and preferably eight, should be part of every adult's diet, says nutritionist Patricia Harper. While any fluid will do the trick, the best is water, she says.

Eat lots more fibre. According to the British Nutrition Foundation, most people in the UK do not eat enough fibre. The average intake is 12g per day, while the recommended adult intake is 18g per day. And if you suffer from constipation you should consume even more – up to 30g a day, suggests Harper.

Whole grains, fruits and vegetables are the best fibre sources. It's not difficult to increase your fibre intake if you choose foods carefully. A bowl of breakfast bran cereal can provide as much as 13g, and other high-fibre foods are cooked dried beans, prunes, figs, raisins, popcorn, oats, pears and nuts.

Get your whole grains by switching to wholemeal bread and pasta (there's even a high-fibre white bread to fool the kids!). One word of warning, though: increase your fibre intake gradually so as to avoid bloating and wind. Some people are intolerant of bran and get bloated however gradually they introduce it. Substitute other high-fibre foods if you are affected.

Keep herbs as a second string. 'There is nothing natural about being constipated,' says clinical herbalist Douglas Schar. 'Birds and hedgerow creatures don't suffer from the problem – but then they don't eat processed foods!' More often than not, our problem is rooted in bad eating and can be corrected with dietary changes.

'My rule is diet first, herbal remedies second,' says Schar. View herbal remedies as 'constipation crisis medicine', not daily fare. For the occasional case of constipation, dandelion, yellow dock and senna pods will do the job. Buy them at the health food store, and follow the directions on the label.

Make time for exercise. Exercise is not only good for your heart, it's also good for your bowels. In general, regular exercise tends to combat constipation by moving food through the bowel faster, says Edward Eichner, an expert in the effects of exercise on the human body.

Go for a walk. Any form of regular exercise tends to ease constipation, but the one mentioned most often by our experts is walking.

Walking is particularly helpful for pregnant women, many of whom experience constipation as their inner workings are compressed to accommodate the growing foetus. Anyone, including mums-to-be, should walk a hearty 20 to 30 minutes a day, suggests obstetrician Lewis

Townsend, but pregnant women should take care not to get too breathless when they walk.

Learn new habits. Throughout our lives, many of us condition ourselves to go to the bathroom not when nature calls but when it's convenient. Ignoring the urge to defecate, however, can eventually lead to constipation.

It's never too late to improve your bowel habits, says Dr Schuster. 'The most natural time to go to the toilet is after a meal,' he adds. So pick a meal, any meal, and every day following that meal sit on the toilet for 10 minutes. In time, says Dr Schuster, you will condition your colon to act as nature intended.

Slow down and take it easy. When you're frightened or tense, your mouth becomes dry and your heart beats faster. Your bowels stop up as well. 'It's part of the fight-or-flight mechanism,' says family doctor John Lawder. If you think that tension is the cause of your constipation, make time to relax, perhaps by listening to relaxation tapes.

Have a laugh. It may sound funny, but a good belly laugh can help with constipation in two ways. It has a massaging effect on the intestines, which helps to foster digestion, and it's a great stress reliever, says Alison Crane, an expert in therapeutic humour.

Try and avoid laxative tablets. Chemical laxatives often do what they're intended to do, but they're terribly addictive, warns Dr Rousseau. If you take too many and your bowel gets used to them, your constipation can get worse. When should you take laxatives from a bottle? 'Almost never,' he says.

Not all laxatives are the same. In most chemists, next to the chemical laxatives you'll find another category of laxative, often labelled 'natural' or 'vegetable' laxatives, whose main ingredient is usually crushed psyllium seed – also known as ispaghula.

This is a super-concentrated form of fibre, which, unlike the chemical laxatives, is non-addictive and generally safe, even if taken over long periods, says Dr Rousseau. He stresses, however, that these must be taken with lots of water (read the instructions on the package), or they can gum up inside you.

Try one doctor's special recipe. Psyllium-based laxatives can be expensive. So make your own by buying psyllium seeds in a health food store and crushing them yourself. Grind two parts psyllium with one part flax and one part oat bran (also available in health food stores) for a

WHEN TO CONSULT A DOCTOR

Constipation is not usually serious. A change in bowel habit towards constipation is usually less significant than a change towards diarrhoea, especially in older people. You should see your doctor, however, if symptoms are severe or disabling, last longer than three weeks, or if you find blood in your stool. Although it's rare, constipation can be a sign of a serious underlying disorder, such as hypothyroidism, depression, cancer of the rectum or of the colon. You should also see your doctor if your constipation accompanies a distended abdomen, as this may indicate an intestinal obstruction.

super-high-fibre concoction. 'Mix the ingredients with water, and eat a little of the mash every night at around 9 o'clock,' says Dr Lawder.

Review your medicines and supplements. Several medicines can bring on or exacerbate constipation, says Dr Rousseau. Common culprits include antacids containing aluminium or calcium, antihistamines, certain anti-Parkinson drugs, calcium supplements, codeine or morphine-based painkillers, phenothiazines (a group of tranquillizers), sedatives, and tricyclic antidepressants (such as imipramine and desipramine). If you think prescribed medications are causing your constipation, don't stop taking them before discussing your concerns with your doctor.

Beware of certain foods. Some things may constipate one person but not another. Milk, for instance, can be extremely constipating to some, while causing diarrhoea in others. Foods that tend to produce gas, such as beans, cauliflower and cabbage, can be problematic for people whose constipation is part of an irritable bowel syndrome (IBS).

You should suspect IBS and avoid gas-producing foods if your constipation is variable, alternates with diarrhoea, if your stool is frequently pellet-like, and you have occasional mucus in your stool. **Don't** diagnose yourself with IBS if you're over 40 when you get the symptoms for the first time, and **never** assume it's IBS if you pass blood as well as mucus (see *Irritable Bowel Syndrome*, page 359).

Don't strain. Forcing a bowel movement is unwise. You risk giving yourself haemorrhoids (piles) and anal fissures, which are painful and can also aggravate your constipation by narrowing the anal opening. Straining can also raise your blood pressure and lower your heartbeat, which can be dangerous, especially for the elderly.

Get fast relief – once in a while. If you're really miserable, nothing works faster to move your bowels than a suppository. For occasional use, these are perfectly all right, says Dr Rousseau. Don't use them too often, though, or you risk creating a lazy colon, exacerbating your constipation problem. Choose a glycerol suppository as opposed to any harsher chemical alternatives.

COUGH
20 throat-soothing strategies

Coughing is the body's way of removing irritating substances from the airways. But too much coughing can make it impossible to sleep or even to relax. Some people have even broken ribs during severe coughing fits.

Mucus-filled 'productive' coughs are usually caused by allergies, colds or other respiratory tract infections. Build-up of mucus in the airways makes it hard to breathe, and the body responds by trying to remove it. 'Dry' coughs, on the other hand, are caused by irritation due to smoking, for example, or from inhaling fumes, dust or other airborne irritants.

Most coughs clear up on their own within a week to 10 days. In the meantime, here are a few ways to reduce the discomfort and help the cough to pass more quickly.

Enjoy slippery elm lozenges. Available in health food stores and some chemists, slippery elm is loaded with a substance that soothes the throat and helps to reduce coughing. The lozenges even taste pretty good, says paediatrician Stuart Ditchek. Take up to five or six lozenges per day.

Try this slippery solution. The next time you have a wracking cough, try this helpful formula, suggests Dr Ditchek. Add a teaspoon of slippery elm powder or liquid to two cups of hot water. Stir in a tablespoon of sugar, add a sprinkling of cinnamon, and drink.

Drink as much water as you can. The body naturally loses fluids when you have a cold or flu. In addition, the accompanying congestion forces mouth breathing, which increases throat dryness and coughing, says Anne Davis, a specialist in respiratory medicine. Try and drink at least eight glasses of water a day. This will moisturize tissues and help to calm the cough.

Another good reason for drinking more water is that moist mucous

WHEN TO CONSULT A DOCTOR

Most coughs are caused by viruses: they will go away on their own and will not be helped by antibiotics. Viral coughs can persist for up to four weeks or more after a cold, so there's no need to go to the doctor if you're generally in good health and are free of other symptoms. More persistent coughs may, however, be due to heartburn or to more serious illness, including pneumonia, chronic obstructive airways disease, asthma, heart failure and, occasionally, cancer or tuberculosis (TB).

Do see the doctor if:

• your cough is not improving after four weeks;

• the cough is associated with wheeze, shortness of breath or swelling of the ankles;

• you have sharp chest pains, especially on breathing in;

• you are producing excessive amounts of green, yellow or bloody phlegm;

• you have a fever above 38°C (101°F) for more than three days;

• you have a fever above 39.5°C (103°F);

• you have a fever which returns after a few days of being normal.

As with colds, get a doctor's advice earlier for small babies and frail older people, especially if they are not drinking good amounts of fluid; also for people with known asthma, chronic bronchitis, diabetes, or immune systems suppressed by illness or drugs like steroids.

membranes are better able to resist the viruses that cause colds. 'If mucus is too thick, it doesn't work as well,' says Dr Davis.

Sip ginger tea. Ginger acts as a potent natural anti-inflammatory herbal agent. Most people use ginger tea to soothe their painful throats, although fresh ginger from the vegetable section of your local supermarket is also good.

Try zinc lozenges. The research isn't conclusive, but some studies suggest that sucking on zinc lozenges can reduce the discomfort of a scratchy throat. Don't take more than the recommended dose as zinc can be toxic in large amounts.

Take vitamin C. Nothing prevents the occasional cold, but studies have shown that taking vitamin C at the first sign of infection can cut the severity of symptoms, including cough, by about 50 per cent, says Dr Ditchek. Megadoses, popular a few years ago, are no longer widely advocated. While the recommended daily amount (RDA) for vitamin C is 60mg, higher doses of between 100 and 500mg per day may be helpful.

Alternatively, increase the intake of vitamin C in your diet, suggests family doctor Stephen Amiel. Fruits are the best source, especially citrus, tomatoes, kiwi and berries; one 100g guava provides a staggering 200mg of vitamin C on its own.

KITCHEN CURES

'One thing that can trigger coughs is throat irritation,' says respiratory specialist Anne Davis. Sucking on boiled sweets or barley sugar increases saliva flow.

The combination of saliva and juices from the sweets soothes irritated tissues, she explains.

Add some echinacea. Available in health food stores and most pharmacies, echinacea helps the immune system to fight cold viruses. It's also an effective way to reduce the duration and severity of coughs and other cold symptoms, says Dr Ditchek. Take 12 drops of echinacea tincture four times a day. In capsule form, take one or two capsules three or four times per day for 10 days to two weeks.

Note: People with allergies and auto-immune diseases are advised not to use this remedy.

A spoonful of honey. A cup of chamomile tea works well, especially if it's flavoured with honey and lemon. Hot liquids are soothing when you have a cough, says Dr Davis. Adding honey to the tea may provide extra relief because the thick sweetener calms irritated tissues and cough receptors in the throat.

Eat raw or lightly cooked garlic. It's rich in chemical compounds that help to inhibit cough-causing viruses in the respiratory tract, says Dr Ditchek. Garlic is a wonderful natural antibiotic that can assist in fighting off colds and common upper respiratory infections. Try eating two to four garlic cloves a day. Or take garlic capsules, following directions on the label.

Drink chicken soup. And be sure to add lots of hot, pungent spices like pepper, garlic and curry powder. The warm fluid and the spices will help to break up stagnant mucus in your lungs, and these natural expectorants will help to get rid of mucus.

Humidify the airways. Once or twice a day, take a long, hot shower or bath. Or plug in a room humidifier. Breathing steam reduces airway irritation and makes mucus easier to cough up. If you don't have a humidifier, fill your room with steam by boiling an electric kettle with the lid off until it's almost boiled dry, says Dr Amiel. You'll need to keep a close eye on it and keep it well out of the reach of small children and the frail elderly. You could also make your own little steam tent or buy a steam inhalation device from the pharmacy (see *Colds,* page 135).

Humidifying the air is also a good way to prevent cough-causing colds and other infections, says Dr Ditchek. Air that is too dry takes moisture from the nose, throat and lungs, making it easier for viruses to take hold.

Avoid cigarette smoke. Even if you don't smoke yourself, breathing second-hand smoke almost guarantees that you'll get an irritated throat. Smokers often have persistent coughs because the body responds to the irritation by producing enormous amounts of mucus, says Dr Davis.

If you are a smoker, the best thing that you can do is give it up. Ask friends or family members who smoke to do so away from you.

Consider a cough suppressant. Cough suppressants should be used only if you have a dry cough, Dr Davis says. Productive coughs should be encouraged, not suppressed, as it is important to clear secretions from the airways.

Over-the-counter medicines that help to blunt the 'cough reflex' in the brain include pholcodine, and medicines containing dextromethorphan such as Benylin Dry Cough and Meltus Dry Cough. Doctors usually recommend these products only for temporary relief – when a cough keeps you up at night, for example.

Use an expectorant. One way to make productive coughs even more productive is to take an over-the-counter expectorant that contains guaifenesin, such as Robitussin Chesty Cough. Expectorants make mucus thinner and easier to expel, says Dr Davis.

Do just *one* thing

Most coughs are the body's way of getting rid of debris and mucous secretions. You don't want to interrupt that normal process. What you do want to do is reduce the discomfort. For 'productive' coughs, blowing your nose frequently helps to eliminate mucus before it has a chance to stimulate the cough reflex, says paediatrician Stuart Ditchek.

For 'dry' coughs, drink plenty of broth, tea or other warm fluids, which soothe the throat and reduce irritation.

Don't tolerate heartburn. It's a common cause of persistent coughs, says Dr Ditchek. The same stomach acids that cause heartburn (also called gastroesophageal reflux) can also trigger coughing fits when the acids irritate the oesophagus or airways. If you cough mainly at night, after meals or while lying down, there's a good chance that stomach acids are to blame.

One of the easiest strategies to keep stomach acids where they belong is to raise the head of your bed by putting wood blocks or old phone books under the legs. It also helps to eat four or five small meals a day instead of two or three large meals. Finally, stay on your feet – or at least sit upright in a chair – for at least two hours after eating. Avoid food triggers, such as dairy produce, that aggravate symptoms.

If you want to try a herbal heartburn remedy, suck on liquorice lozenges. Take two lozenges before meals. Have your blood pressure checked if you plan to use this remedy for more than a few days, advises Dr Ditchek.

If the coughing persists and you are taking an ACE inhibitor (a drug for high blood pressure, also commonly taken by people with heart problems and diabetes), talk to your doctor about possibly trying a different antihypertensive drug, says Dr Davis. ACE inhibitors can cause a cough.

Get allergies under control. If you're sensitive to pollen, mould or other allergens, even brief exposure can stimulate mucus production – followed by days or weeks of coughing as your body tries to remove it, says Dr Ditchek.

Once you know what you're allergic to, avoidance is the best approach. If you get hay fever, for example, avoid pollen by staying indoors during the morning and evening hours, when pollen counts are highest. For quick relief from symptoms, take an over-the-counter antihistamine.

Get some rest. It's the oldest – and probably the most ignored – advice for fighting cold symptoms like coughing. You may want to keep going, but you must try and get some rest, Dr Davis says. Otherwise, that minor cold and cough might progress to something a lot more serious.

Add a pillow or two. An extra pillow or two will help to reduce the amount of coughing caused by post-nasal drip, where catarrh from a cold or allergy trickles down into the back of the throat, triggering the cough reflex, says Dr Amiel. It will also help night-time cough associated with chronic bronchitis, asthma and heart failure. If your cough is caused by heartburn though, you're better off raising the head of the bed by putting something under the legs.

CUTS AND GRAZES

9 ways to make it better

While boys and girls seem to have a monopoly on cuts and grazes, adults get their share, too. A finger gets in the way of a knife slicing onions. A backpack carelessly tossed in the front hall causes a nasty fall. And every winter, ice lurks like a sinister joker waiting for victims who fall, ripping their trousers and tearing their skin at the same time. Life may be full of accidents. Luckily, our kitchen and medicine cabinets are filled with the tools to deal with them.

Stop the bleeding. The fastest way to stop bleeding is to apply direct pressure. Place a clean, absorbent cloth over the cut, then firmly press your hand against it. If you don't have a cloth, use your fingers. If blood soaks through your first cloth, add a second one and press steadily. Add new pads over old ones because removing a cloth may tear off coagulating blood cells.

If applying pressure doesn't stop the bleeding, raise the limb to heart level to reduce the pressure of blood on the cut. Continue applying pressure. This should stem bleeding.

Strap it up. When the bleeding stops or slows down, tie the wound firmly with a cloth or wrap it with a crepe bandage so there is pressure against the cut, but do not cut off circulation, says A&E technician John Gillies.

Apply extra pressure. If the cut continues to bleed, it is more serious than you thought, and you probably need to see a doctor immediately. Until you get medical help, find the pressure point nearest to the cut between the wound and your heart.

Pressure points are places you might think of when taking a pulse: inside your wrists, inside your upper arm about halfway between the elbow and armpit, and in the groin where your legs join your torso. Press the artery against the bone.

Stop pressing about a minute after the bleeding stops. If bleeding starts again, reapply pressure.

Don't use a tourniquet. With most everyday cuts and scrapes, first aid is enough. Tourniquets can be dangerous. 'If you apply a tourniquet, the person may end up losing that limb because you cut off all circulation,' warns Gillies.

What makes paper cuts so sore?

Schoolchildren, office workers and paper pushers of any kind will all agree – even though they're small, paper cuts can be really painful. What is it about them that prompts normally demure professionals to utter expletives that would make an ex-con blush? In a word, particles.

If you cut yourself shaving, the razor makes a clean cut, leaving behind few, if any, particles that trigger pain. But a paper cut leaves paper fibres coated with chemicals from the papermaking process. These fibres and bacteria remain in the wound, triggering pain receptors in the skin.

Clean the wound twice a day. This is important to prevent infection and to decrease the chance of permanent discoloration. Wash the area with soap and water or just water, says A&E doctor Hugh Macaulay. The idea is to dilute the bacteria in the wound and remove dirt. If you don't remove stones or sand from a cut, they can leave pigment under the skin.

Keep it damp. When exposed to air, cuts form scabs, which slow down new cell growth, says Patricia Mertz, a dermatologist. She recommends a plastic dressing similar to food wrap, such as vapour-permeable films and membranes like Opsite or Hydrofilm. They come in all sizes. Or ask you pharmacist for for gauze impregnated with petroleum jelly. Both

Peeling off the plaster

Do you – or your children – hate taking sticky plasters off? Then follow these tips.

- Use a tiny pair of scissors to cut the padded part from the sticky sections. Pull this gently away from your graze. Then remove the sticky strips.

- If your scab is stuck to the pad, soak the area in a weak solution

of salt in warm water. Be patient: the dressing will come away.

- If a plaster is stuck to the hairs on your arm, leg or chest, pull in the direction of hair growth. Use a cotton wool ball soaked in baby oil or surgical spirit to wet the adhesive before pulling it from the skin.

WHEN TO CONSULT A DOCTOR

First aid isn't always enough. The following signs mean you need to see a doctor.

- Bleeding is bright red and spurting. You may have punctured an artery.
- You cannot wash all the debris out of the wound.
- The cut or graze is on your face or any other area where you want to minimize scarring.
- Your wound develops any red streaks or weeps pus, or the redness extends more than a finger's width beyond the cut.
- The wound is large and you can see down into it. It may need stitches.
- You've lost sensation or movement in a cut finger. You may have cut a nerve or tendon.
- You've cut yourself on an object possibly contaminated with HIV or hepatitis. After washing the cut very thoroughly with soap and water, or alcohol, and encouraging it to bleed for a little while, go to your nearest accident and emergency department, where preventive treatment and/or immunization can be given. If you can transport it safely, take the object with you, so that it can be tested for viruses.

types of dressing trap healing moisture in the wound but allow only a little air to pass through. Cells regenerate more rapidly when moist.

Do you need a tetanus jab? It is now considered unnecessary to have a tetanus booster if you are cut, provided you have had five tetanus injections at any time in your life, says family doctor Stephen Amiel. Most children will have had four by the time they start school, and a fifth is given in their teens. But as routine immunization only started in 1961, many adults may not have complete immunity.

If you have not had five tetanus injections, or you are unsure, get a booster as soon as possible after being cut. You may also need treatment with tetanus immunoglobulin, an antiserum. Fully immune people only require this with a very tetanus-prone wound, such as one contaminated with stable manure.

Try one of nature's medicines. 'Herbal medicine offers a kaleidoscope of first aid remedies,' says clinical herbalist Douglas Schar. 'My favourites are echinacea, yarrow, witch hazel and calendula. All of these herbs contain anti-inflammatory and antimicrobial compounds. Even better, they also contain compounds which speed up the healing process.' Buy any of the above in tincture form, says Schar, put it in a small spray bottle, and when domestic misadventure strikes, spray the cut or graze thoroughly. He recommends spraying three times a day until the wound has completely healed.

An ounce of prevention. Many cuts around the home can be prevented, says Dr Amiel. In the kitchen, keep knives sharp – they're safer that way. Store them properly, not loose in a drawer with other things. Keep the handles dry and clean and always cut away from the body on a proper cutting surface. Never place knives blade upwards in a dishwasher, or leave them at the bottom of a washing-up bowl. Wrap broken glass and opened tins up carefully in several layers of newspaper.

Wear protective gloves in the garden and be especially careful clearing rubbish outside your home, or letting your children play near rubbish: there may be discarded needles, razor blades and so forth among the debris which, apart from cutting you or your child, may occasionally be contaminated with the hepatitis or HIV virus.

DANDRUFF
16 tips to stop flaking

Dandruff is the most common scalp complaint seen by hairdressers. Just about everyone has the problem to some degree, often leading to a scratch-and-itch cycle, says dermatologist Maria Hordinsky. Ignoring the condition lets the scaling build up. That, in turn, can cause itching, which can lead to scratching. Scratching too vigorously can wound the scalp and leave it open to infection. This vicious cycle can be avoided, however, with some simple home remedies.

Shampoo often. The experts are unanimous: wash your hair often – every day if necessary. 'Generally, the more frequently you shampoo, the easier it is to control the dandruff,' says dermatologist Patricia Farris.

Start mild. Often a mild, non-medicated shampoo is enough to control the problem. Dandruff is frequently caused by an oily scalp, says hair-care specialist Philip Kingsley. Washing daily with a mild brand of shampoo, diluted with an equal amount of water, can control the oil without aggravating your scalp.

Then get tough. If normal shampoos aren't doing the job, switch to an antidandruff formula. Dandruff shampoos are classified by their active ingredients, which work in different ways. Those with selenium sulphide or zinc pyrithione work fastest, says dermatologist Diana Bihova, slowing down the rate at which scalp cells multiply. Those with salicylic acid and sulphur loosen flakes so that they can be washed away easily. Those with antibacterial agents reduce bacteria on the scalp and the chance of infection. Those with tar retard cell growth.

Use a coal tar shampoo. 'For very stubborn cases, I recommend tar-based formulas,' says Dr Farris. Lather with a tar shampoo and then leave it on for five to 10 minutes so that the tar has a chance to work. Most people rinse dandruff shampoos off too quickly. Brands include T Gel and Polytar.

Don't be too harsh. If tar-based shampoos – or any other dandruff preparations – are too harsh for everyday use, alternate them with your usual shampoo, says Dr Farris.

Don't mix black with blonde. If you have fair hair, think twice about tar-based shampoos. In rare instances, they can give white, blonde, bleached or tinted hair a temporary brownish tinge, says Dr Farris.

KITCHEN CURES

Thyme, a common kitchen herb, is reputed to have mild antiseptic properties that can help to alleviate dandruff, says hairstylist Louis Gignac. Make a rinse by simmering four heaped tablespoons of dried thyme in 500ml of water for 10 minutes. Strain the brew and allow it to cool. Pour half the mixture over clean, damp hair, making sure the liquid covers the scalp. Massage in gently. Do not rinse. Save the remainder for another day.

Lather twice. Always lather twice with a dandruff shampoo, says dermatologist Jeffrey Herten. Work up the first lather as soon as you get into the bath or shower so that the shampoo has plenty of time to work. Leave it on until you've almost finished. Then rinse your hair very thoroughly. Follow that with a quick second lather and rinse. The second rinse will leave just a bit of the medication on your scalp so that it can work until your next shampoo.

Cap it. Dr Bihova has a different approach to improving the effectiveness of medicated shampoos. After you've worked up a lather, put on a shower cap over your soapy hair. Leave it on for an hour, then rinse thoroughly.

WHEN TO CONSULT A DOCTOR

Severe scaling of the scalp may have a number of causes. Classic dandruff is a form of seborrhoeic eczema, which can spread to the neck, eyebrows and face. It seems a yeast may be implicated in this condition, and your doctor may give you a prescription for an antifungal, ketoconazole, as a shampoo (also available over-the-counter) or cream. You may also need a short course of a steroid-containing scalp application.

Psoriasis may also cause flaky patches on the scalp which may be mistaken for dandruff. The scaling may be more localized than in dandruff, and the patches tend to be thick and hard. Psoriasis often runs in families and other parts of the skin are usually affected as well. Tar or salicylic acid shampoos are available on prescription, but you may also need a steroid-containing scalp application, or calcipotriol (Dovonex) scalp application (see *Psoriasis*, page 460).

Occasionally, shampoos are the problem, rather than the solution. You may develop an allergic reaction to chemicals in the shampoo, or to the chemicals in certain hair colourings. The onset is usually quite dramatic and the scalp may burn, redden or even blister. You may need a prescription for steroids, antihistamines and sometimes an antibiotic if there is secondary infection.

Switch shampoos. If you've found a brand of shampoo that works well for you, keep using it, says dermatologist Howard Donsky. But remember that your skin can adapt to a shampoo's ingredients, so it's a good idea to change your brand every few months to maintain its effectiveness.

Massage it in. When shampooing, says Dr Farris, gently massage your scalp with your fingertips to help loosen scales and flakes. But don't scratch your scalp, or you may end up with sores that are worse than the dandruff.

Get into condition. Although dandruff shampoos are effective on your scalp, they can be harsh on your hair, says Dr Farris. So use conditioner after every shampoo to counteract their effects.

Let the sun shine. 'A little sun exposure is good for dandruff,' says dermatologist Joseph Fowler. That's because direct ultraviolet light has an anti-inflammatory effect on scaly skin conditions. And it may explain why dandruff tends to be less severe in summer. But be sensible. 'You have to balance the sun's benefit to your scalp against its harmful effects

Although excess scalp oil can cause problems, an occasional warm-oil treatment helps to loosen and soften dandruff scales, says dermatologist Jeffrey Herten. Heat a little olive oil until just warm. Wet your hair (otherwise the oil will soak into your hair instead of reaching your scalp), then apply the oil directly to your scalp with a paintbrush or a cotton wool ball. Section your hair as you go so that you treat just the scalp. Put on a shower cap and leave it on for 30 minutes. Then wash out the oil with a dandruff shampoo.

on your skin in general,' Dr Fowler advises. Limit your exposure to the sun to 30 minutes or less per day, and wear sunscreen on exposed skin.

Calm down. Don't overlook the role that emotions play in triggering or worsening skin conditions like dandruff and other forms of dermatitis. Stress often makes them worse, says Dr Fowler.

So if your emotions are strained, look for ways to counteract stress. Exercise. Meditate. Get away from it all. And don't worry so much about your dandruff.

Try some herbal magic. When dandruff is serious there is usually an underlying problem with the scalp, says clinical herbalist Douglas Schar.

Oregon grape tincture, added to your favourite shampoo, will make a big difference by correcting the abnormal skin condition at the root of the dandruff problem. You'll need to use your home-medicated shampoo for at least two weeks before you begin to see a difference.

DENTURE PROBLEMS

13 ideas for a more secure smile

False teeth were invented by the Etruscans in central Italy nearly 3000 years ago. They made dentures out of ox teeth, held together with highly visible gold bands. For Etruscans, wearing dentures was nothing to be ashamed of – it was actually a status symbol.

False teeth have come a long way since then. Today, there are numerous choices in dental ware, including partial and full dentures, those that can be removed, and those that are implanted into the bone like real teeth.

All dentures take some getting used to, says George Murrell, a dentist who specializes in fitting false teeth. He and other specialists have some suggestions.

Look in the mirror. Smile. Frown. Be happy. Be sad. Be serious. Practise moving your teeth and lips in private so that you'll be more confident in front of other people, says Dr Murrell.

Practise talking. Wearing dentures is like having an artificial limb, says dental surgeon Jerry Taintor. You have to practise using it to use it well. Recite vowel sounds and consonants. Read aloud to yourself. Listen to your pronunciation and your diction, and correct anything that doesn't sound right.

Make a video of yourself. A video could help in more ways than one. It would give you a stranger's-eye view of how you look. And you could show the tape to your dentist, who might find the images useful for deciphering problems in your jaw muscles or lip movements.

Watch out for toothpicks. Those tiny wooden spikes are dangerous for denture wearers, says Dr Taintor. 'You lose a lot of your tactile sense with dentures, so you could easily bite through a toothpick without realizing it, and the spike could get lodged in your throat.'

Use an adhesive. If your new teeth are a less-than-perfect fit, there's nothing wrong with using a denture adhesive during the adjustment period, says Dr Taintor. It's when you have to use the adhesive all the time that you need to have the plate refitted. You can buy over-the-counter denture adhesives – a type of soft paste that forms a vacuum between your gums and your dentures – in any chemist.

Massage your gums. Place your thumb and index finger over your gums (index on the outside) and massage them, says dentist Richard Shepard. This promotes circulation and keeps your gums healthy and firm.

Start soft and slow. No, you're not doomed to baby foods for the rest of your life, but start with soft food, says Dr Taintor. If you gradually increase the texture and hardness of your food, your gums will become accustomed to the dentures and and your ability to use them will improve.

Get those new teeth clean. If you have dental implants, you need a twice-a-day cleaning routine just as when you were caring for your original teeth, says Dr Murrell. 'We can do beautiful dentistry, but it won't last if it isn't taken care of.'

Scrub with soap and water. When you have finished eating, take out your dentures and scrub them with plain soap and lukewarm water.

Baby your mouth. 'Babies are born with plaque in their mouths,' says dentistry professor Eric Shapira. 'Even if you have no teeth, you need to wash your gums to remove the plaque.' Use a soft brush and gently brush your gums, but don't brush hard enough to make your mouth sore. A good clean reduces the likelihood of bad breath and helps your gums to stay healthy.

Try lozenges. One common complaint among denture wearers, says Dr Murrell, is excess saliva during the first few weeks of wearing dentures. Solve this problem by sucking on lozenges frequently for the first couple of days. This helps you to swallow more often and gets rid of excess saliva.

Rinse with salt water. To help clean your gums, rinse your mouth every day with a glass of warm water mixed with a teaspoon of salt, says Dr Taintor.

Give your gums a rest. When you can, take your teeth out and give your gums a break, says Dr Taintor.

DEPRESSION
29 mood lifters

According to the Department of Health, around 20 per cent of women and 14 per cent of men in the UK suffer from depression at any one time. The Mental Health Foundation puts the figure even higher, saying that symptoms affect a staggering one in four British adults. 'We have a range of emotions, and feeling depressed at times, for short periods, is quite normal,' says psychiatrist Bernard Vittone.

If you and your doctor agree that your depression is mild, there are many ways recommended by experts to boost your mood. Even if you are being treated for chronic or severe depression, the following strategies may help.

Learn about depression. Read books, listen to tapes or watch videos. Education helps you to realize that you're not alone and that the condition you have is really very common, says psychiatrist Edward Hallowell.

Express yourself. The opposite of depression is expression. The blues often result from a pattern of suppressing and then repressing our feelings, says Dr Hallowell. Release your feelings through art, music or anything creative.

Get out of the house. Aim for a few hours out every day, says Dr Vittone. Being in the same place too long, particularly if you're alone, breeds depressive thoughts and symptoms. Visit the library, go shopping, see a film. Stimulation is important for people with depression, he says. Researchers think that stimulation keeps the brain's feel-good neurotransmitters like serotonin flowing.

Be with friends. Socialize at least twice a week, advises Dr Vittone. Don't just plan meetings, business lunches or telephone conferences. Get together with people to talk, laugh and relax. You'll be stimulating those feel-good neurotransmitters. Although researchers aren't sure how socializing affects nerve chemicals, says Dr Vittone, they do know that the chemicals are helpful.

Have a giggle. Watch a comedy on television, see a funny film or watch some live stand-up comedy. Happiness is contagious, says Dr Vittone.

Let it be. It's okay to feel anything, says Dr Hallowell. There are no 'bad' feelings. Accepting how you feel helps you to get past it. Similarly, remind yourself that feelings change and that you will survive.

Take time to heal. Be patient with yourself. Sometimes you'll take a step forwards; on other days you'll take two steps backwards. Healing never occurs in a straight line. Tomorrow is another day to try again.

Stick to a routine. Alternating rest with activity brings healing by restoring the body's natural rhythms. Go to sleep at the same time and get up at the usual time every day. When your inner world is chaotic, maintaining a routine gives you some sense of order, says Dr Hallowell.

Sleep. Lack of sleep may cause depressive symptoms, such as lack of concentration and low energy, or exacerbate existing depression. Gauge how much sleep you need by how rested you feel.

Be an optimist. Be optimistic, even if you don't believe it at first, says

WHEN TO CONSULT A DOCTOR

See a doctor if you are depressed most of the time for two weeks or longer, even though you haven't experienced a significant loss, such as the death of a loved one. Also seek help if you have experienced a loss and your depression continues for several months or if you have intermittent bouts of depression for more than two years. And have a check-up to rule out other possible illnesses such as hypothyroidism or anaemia.

Symptoms of a depressive illness include feeling hopeless, helpless, sad or blue; losing interest in previously enjoyable activities; or an inability to be cheered by normally happy events. Other signs include insomnia, changes in appetite, low energy, poor concentration, irritability, a negative attitude and frequent guilty feelings. But be aware that symptoms of depression and anxiety (see *Anxiety*, page 44) often overlap.

Don't delay seeking help for someone who is having persistent thoughts of, or is making plans for, self-harm or suicide.

Dr Vittone. Your attitude is likely to become a self-fulfilling prophecy. If you expect a positive outcome, you're more likely to act in ways that make that happen, and other people are more likely to react positively to you. The way we think directly affects our moods, he says.

Keep up-to-date. Tune in to the television or radio news. Pick up a newspaper or magazine. Keeping up with current events helps you to feel more involved in life around you, says Dr Vittone. But there is one proviso: limit watching or reading about traumatic events to half-an-hour at a time. Watching too much bad news isn't good for you.

Don't decide now. Keep decision making to a minimum when you're feeling low. You make less considered or wise decisions when you are depressed than when you're feeling good.

Forgive yourself. Even with mild depression, temporary forgetfulness and clumsiness are common. You might mislay your keys or drop a glass. Try to laugh at silly mistakes – your nervous system is simply not at its best.

Have a massage. When you're feeling low, you may feel as though your mind and body are disconnected. The healing touch of massage – once a week if possible – helps to reconnect mind, body and spirit, says Dr Hallowell.

Do just *one* thing

Get going. Depression causes a huge amount of inertia. It makes it hard even to get out of bed in the morning. Fight it by getting moving. Exercise helps to banish the blues, says psychiatrist Bernard Vittone.

Walk, jog, cycle, swim or join an aerobics class at a local fitness centre. Aim for 20 to 30 minutes' activity, four or five times a week.

Or try yoga, tai chi or stretching about three times a week to loosen your body, relieve stress and get you smiling again. Even better, do a bit of both.

Some doctors believe that exercise, especially aerobic exercise, produces endorphins, the body's natural antidepressants. 'We don't really know why exercise works,' says Dr Vittone. 'We just know that it does.'

Discover your spiritual side. Research shows that spirituality can improve mood, whether you pray, go to religious services or read inspiring words.

Don't blame yourself. No matter what mistakes you think you've made, forgive yourself. Treat yourself with kindness, and never give in to regret. Everybody has failures. Guilt is form of self-punishment: you don't deserve it.

Try holiday therapy. Consider taking a break, says Dr Vittone. Even three days by the sea can be enough to jolt you out of a mild depression. Alternately, take mini-breaks during the day. When your mood is low, give yourself a lift by finding a minute or two to picture somewhere you'd like to be. Mentally immerse yourself in the sights, sounds, feelings and scents of that special place.

Think about the good things. Remind yourself what's good in life. Every day, try noting down five things for which you're grateful. 'Try to find things, little or big, that you appreciate,' says Dr Vittone. When we feel low, we tend to overlook the good things in life.

Make someone's day. One way to feel good about yourself is to make someone else feel good. Pay a compliment, let someone out in front of you in busy rush-hour traffic or smile at a stranger. 'You'll feel better,' says Dr Vittone, 'and the other person will feel good, too.'

Look forward. Try to organize at least one event at the end of each week that you can look forward to with enthusiasm. Plan a day out, a shopping trip or dinner at a favourite restaurant. When you feel low, think about your plans.

Eat healthily. Eat a balanced diet rich in complex carbohydrates (fruit, vegetables and whole grains), lean protein and some fat. These foods provide the nutrients our bodies need to produce the necessary chemicals that help to maintain normal moods, says Dr Vittone. Don't eat too much or too little of anything. Moderation is the key.

Take vitamin B. A lack of B vitamins is sometimes associated with depressive symptoms such as fatigue, poor concentration or moodiness. Take a multivitamin/mineral supplement that's high in the Bs, including folic acid, B_6 and B_{12}. Folic acid may even increase the effectiveness of antidepressant medicines, says Dr Andrew Weil, author of *8 Weeks to Optimum Health*. He advises choosing a supplement that contains about 400 micrograms of folic acid.

Try St John's wort. Many studies show that this herbal remedy (also known as hypericum) improves mild depression. But do not use St John's wort and antidepressants at the same time. That is overkill, says clinical herbalist Douglas Schar, and can cause problems.

The best plan is to try taking St John's wort for a couple of months. If it does not help, then consider talking to your doctor about prescription antidepressants.

Note: If you are on prescription medications, speak to your doctor before taking St John's wort as it may react with other drugs including warfarin, digoxin, oral contraceptives and drugs for epilepsy.

Or a herbal pick-me-up. Depression is often a symptom of burnout (see *Burnout*, page 105) adds Schar. You have been doing too much for too long and have simply run out of steam. More than depressed, you are depleted. If you think that this may be the case, Schar suggests taking daily doses of energy-boosting herbs like Siberian ginseng or astragalus.

Avoid alcohol. Alcohol is a central-nervous-system depressant. After a drink, you may feel better at first. But later, depression may

KITCHEN CURES

Eat lots of sardines, trout, mackerel, wild salmon, kippers and other fish from cold northern waters, says Dr Weil. These fish are high in omega-3 fatty acids. Some research shows that low levels of these fatty acids may underlie some psychiatric illnesses, such as depression. 'Evidence suggests that the rising levels of depression in the Western world in recent decades may be related to a low omega-3 intake.'

worsen, leading to a vicious cycle of drinking to chase away the blues, followed by more depressive feelings, followed by more drinking. Limit alcohol to one or two drinks at a time, Dr Vittone says, and don't drink every day.

Don't exceed the recommended limit of 14 units a week for women, and 21 for men. A unit (10g of alcohol) is equivalent to a small glass of wine, half a pint of standard strength beer or a single pub measure of spirits. And remember, if you are already taking antidepressants, you should try to avoid alcohol altogether.

Beware of drugs. Illegal drugs are very bad news for depression. So-called 'soft' drugs like ecstasy and cannabis can be as bad as the 'harder' drugs like amphetamines ('speed'), cocaine and heroin in triggering serious depressive symptoms and illness.

Spruce yourself up. Spend time on grooming says Dr Weil. Buy an outfit that suits you. It will give you a positive outlook and make you feel better.

DERMATITIS AND ECZEMA
23 clear-skin remedies

Eczema is sometimes called 'the itch that rashes'. This is because, rather than being a rash that itches, the reverse is true: scratching produces the rash. While eczema may look different from person to person, it usually shows up as dry, red, extremely itchy patches on the skin.

An estimated one in 12 adults and one in eight children in the UK will have eczema at some time in their lives.

Although scientists still do not fully understand what causes eczema, it appears to be an abnormal inflammatory response of the immune system in response to an irritant – anything from house dust mites to rough fabrics to detergents.

This so-called atopic eczema or dermatitis runs in families and is often associated with other atopic conditions like asthma and hay fever. In babies the rash can be anywhere, including the face and behind the ears, but in older children, the skin creases are most often affected. Two thirds of children will grow out of eczema by their teens and it's rare for an adult to develop atopic eczema for the first time.

Some people can learn to avoid triggers, but for many the best strategy is to control the itching and dryness that usually accompany these skin conditions. The experts tell us that, in general, the best way to treat the itching of eczema at home is to keep any patches of dry skin moist and well-lubricated. For that reason, many of the remedies offered in *Dry Skin* (see page 204), may help with this problem as well.

Beware of dry air. Eczema is aggravated by dry air, especially in winter in centrally heated homes and offices. As dry air tends to aggravate the itching of eczema or dermatitis, keeping indoor air moist should be a priority for sufferers and their families, says dermatologist Howard Donsky.

One way of tackling dry air is to buy a humidifier. You'd need a really big unit to tackle the whole house, so instead, try sleeping next to a humidifier.

Make bathwater lukewarm. A lukewarm bath helps to clean and moisturize the skin without overdrying it. Steamy baths or showers, or those that last longer than 10 minutes, will aggravate the condition.

When drying yourself, pat rather than rub with a towel. And always remember to use a moisturizer within three minutes of getting out of the bath or shower.

Moisturize. Moisturizing after washing is more important than what sort of soap you use, but most dermatologists advise against using normal, and particularly perfumed, soap: even baby bath products can irritate sensitive babies' skin.

There are a number of soap substitutes that your pharmacist, health visitor or doctor can advise you about. You may need to experiment with different types. And you can bath as often as you like if you moisturize, says dermatologist Hillard Pearlstein. 'Dry skin results from water loss, not oil loss, and the oil in moisturizer holds the water in.' Try an aqueous cream, emulsifying ointment or E45 cream, available from pharmacies.

Take an oatmeal bath. For an additional soothing treat, Dr

KITCHEN CURES

Cold, wet compresses can help to soothe and relieve the itching associated with eczema that gets so bad that it begins to ooze. 'I tell people to try cold milk instead of water,' says dermatologist John Romano. 'It seems to be a lot more soothing.'

Pour milk into a glass with ice cubes and let it sit for a few minutes. Then soak a gauze pad in the milk and apply it to the irritated skin for two to three minutes. Keep wetting the cloth and repeating the process for about 10 minutes.

WHEN TO CONSULT A DOCTOR

When eczema is severe or widespread, and lotions, home remedies and over-the-counter medications don't relieve the itching, see your doctor. Many prescription medicines can help. A doctor will also be able to rule out other causes for your eczema. Lupus, an auto-immune disorder, is one such disease. Lupus leaves a patchy, red skin rash, roughly resembling a butterfly, on the cheeks or bridge of the nose. As one patch heals, a new one forms. These sores itch and form scales. A person with lupus may experience severe joint pain, fever and lung inflammation. Exposure to sunlight, certain drugs or an emotional crisis typically trigger lupus attacks. If you recognize these symptoms, see your doctor.

Also, if oozing eczema, also known as weeping eczema, does not respond quickly to cold compresses applied several times a day, or if your eczema appears to have become infected, see your doctor.

Donsky recommends adding colloidal oatmeal bath products like Aveeno colloidal bath additive to the bath, and even using oatmeal as a soap substitute. The term colloidal simply means that the oatmeal has been ground to fine powder that will remain suspended in water. Pour two cups of colloidal oatmeal (available at chemists) into a bath of lukewarm water. For use as a soap substitute, wrap some colloidal oatmeal in a handkerchief, bind a rubber band around the top, dip it in water and use it like a flannel.

Avoid antiperspirants. Metallic salts such as aluminium chloride, aluminium sulphate, and zirconium chlorohydrate are the active ingredients in many antiperspirants, and these can cause irritation in people with sensitive skin. 'Usually it's the antiperspirant, as opposed to the deodorant, that's irritating,' says Dr Donsky. Look for products that contain aluminium zirconium, such as Sure Ultra, and silicone-related moisturizers like dimethicone in some of the Nivea range, advises pharmacist Sue Livingston.

Cool with calamine. Calamine lotion is good for many types of rashes that ooze and need to be dried out, says dermatologist John Romano.

Choose comfortable cotton. Cotton clothing worn next to the skin is much better than polyester and, in particular, it's better than wool, says Dr Romano. The best advice is to avoid synthetic fibres or itchy fabrics as well as tight or badly fitting clothes.

Put your diet to the test. According to Dr Pearlstein, food allergies can play a big role in atopic dermatitis during childhood. They are intimately related before a child reaches the age of six, he says, but you can take charge of an infant's diet and do much to help his or her skin.

Eggs, orange juice and milk have all been implicated as eczema triggers in children. But, says Dr Pearlstein, you shouldn't cut out these foods wholesale. Talk to your GP about trying an elimination diet. Such diets seem to work best in infants less than two years old, he says. 'After the age of six, we've found that food plays a minimal role for most people.'

For adult patients, Dr Pearlstein leaves diet adaptation largely up to the individual. If you think that any food you eat has an adverse effect on your skin, avoid it and see what happens, he says. If your problem clears up, you may have a food allergy.

Is it a nickel rash?

Eczema, or atopic dermatitis, is one type of skin rash, and doctors aren't quite sure what causes it. Another type, called contact dermatitis, is obviously caused by contact with an irritant. One increasingly common type is nickel rash.

Nickel dermatitis occurs 10 times more often in women than in men and is often triggered by ear-piercing. Strangely, having the ears pierced can cause rashes in other areas of the body whenever the person comes into contact with nickel-containing metal. Suddenly, bracelets, necklaces and watches that you have worn for years can bring on a contact rash.

If this is happening to you, the following tips might help.

Buy stainless steel studs. Newly pierced ears should be studded only with stainless steel posts until the earlobes heal (this usually takes about three weeks).

Stay cool. Because sweat plays a big role in nickel rash – it leaches out the nickel in nickel-plated jewellery – stay out of the sun if you're wearing this type of jewellery. Or don't wear it at all if you're going anywhere hot.

Go for gold. Buy only good quality gold jewellery, says dermatologist Howard Donsky. If it's less than 24-carat gold, there is some nickel in it; the lower the carat, the higher the nickel.

Look at your diet. Some dermatologists advise nickel-sensitive patients to watch what they eat.

Having observed that nickel dermatitis can occur without any apparent contact with the metal, the doctors advise people to avoid apricots, chocolate, coffee, beer, tea, nuts and other foods high in nickel.

Prevention begins in infancy

Women who have atopic dermatitis may wish to protect their newborn babies from the condition.

Researchers in Israel analysed 18 scientific studies and found convincing evidence that, in families with a history of atopic dermatitis, exclusively breastfeeding in the first three months of life can protect infants from developing the condition during childhood. The preventative role of breastfeeding was less strong in the general population, and negligible in babies with no immediate relatives who had suffered from atopic dermatitis.

Try boosting your omega-3 intake. Salmon, mackerel and other oily fish contain omega-3s and other essential fatty acids that may help to prevent allergies and inflammation, both of which are associated with eczema.

Avoid quick changes in temperature. 'If you have eczema,' says Dr Donsky, 'then rapid temperature changes can be a problem.' Going from a warm room out into cold winter air can trigger itching. Wearing layers of cotton clothing and avoiding hot baths or showers are good ways to protect yourself.

Read labels for urea. 'Emollients that contain urea are pretty good for relieving the itch of eczema or dermatitis,' says Dr Pearlstein. 'Urea is a sloughing agent. We usually use it when the skin is thickened from rubbing and scratching.' Urea-containing products worth a try, says Sue Livingston, are Calmurid, Aquadrate or Eucerin. All are available from pharmacies.

Beware of baby lotions. Baby lotion isn't always the best thing for childhood eczema, says Dr Romano. 'It has a high water content, which can further dry and irritate the skin as it evaporates.' Furthermore, some of the fragrances and active ingredients in baby lotions (lanolin and mineral oil) are common causes of skin allergy.

Instead, says Sue Livingston, use simple emollients like aqueous cream, emulsifying ointment and E45 cream.

Drink Oregon grape tea. Oregon grape root, sold in health food stores, is amazingly effective in the majority of cases, says clinical herbalist Douglas Schar. Add one tablespoon of the dried root to 250ml of boiling water and simmer for 10 minutes. Strain and drink every morning. Don't be disappointed if the results aren't immediately apparent. You need to give the remedy at least three months to have a significant effect on your skin.

Chronic dermatitis, eczema and psoriasis will all improve when the herb is used for long periods of time, says Schar. Usually the tea is enough. However, in severe cases, or to speed up the cure, applying Oregon grape cream will also help. The cream is available at many health food stores.

Be careful with Chinese herbs. A few small trials in the west have shown some benefit from the use of traditional Chinese herbs in reducing the inflammation of eczema. The herbs are brewed up as a tea or mixed into a skin cream. However, there have been reports of liver damage from some herbal preparations and also of strong steroids being secretly mixed into 'herbal' creams. It's best to avoid these preparations unless you get them from a licensed practitioner or dermatologist.

Try antihistamines. Antihistamines reduce classic allergy symptoms like headaches, runny nose and itching. And over-the-counter antihistamines can also be good for eczema, says Dr Romano. They reduce itching by preventing histamine from reaching and swelling sensitive skin cells. Follow label directions and be aware that some antihistamines cause drowsiness.

Wash once, rinse twice. When you do the washing, you must make sure the detergent is rinsed out thoroughly, says Dr Romano. 'Don't use too much detergent, and always use a second rinse cycle to get all the soap out.'

Enzyme-containing biological detergents are best avoided if you have sensitive skin. If you want to use a fabric softener, buy one recommended for sensitive skins.

Look after your eyes. In a 20-year study of 492 people at the Mayo Clinic in Rochester, Minnesota, in the USA, 13 per cent of those with atopic dermatitis developed cataracts. There is undeniably a higher incidence of cataracts in people with atopic dermatitis, says Dr Pearlstein. So see your ophthalmologist regularly.

DIABETES

39 ways to regulate blood sugar

Most people never give it a second thought – the food they eat is transformed into energy and that's that. Their bodies do all the work for them, digesting the food and converting carbohydrates into a type of sugar, called glucose, that enters the bloodstream. Next, the pancreas kicks out insulin, a hormone that travels through the body, attaching to receptors on the outsides of cells. Once attached, insulin acts like a key that 'unlocks' the cell so that glucose can enter it and be used for energy. If the body doesn't need the sugar for energy, it stores it as fat. Usually, this process hums along like a well-oiled machine. People only notice the process when it breaks down.

The monkey wrench that interrupts the flow is diabetes. Nearly 1.4 million people in the UK have been diagnosed with the condition, and doctors think that there are probably a million more undiagnosed cases. Almost one in ten adults over 65 will develop Type 2 diabetes, and the condition is even more common in people of African, African-Caribbean and Asian origin.

Diabetes, also known as diabetes mellitus, comes in two forms. Type 1, or insulin-dependent diabetes, is believed to be an auto-immune condition in which the pancreas fails to manufacture insulin. Though onset can occur at any age, patients are usually diagnosed in childhood or as young adults and require daily insulin injections throughout their lives.

The vast majority of diabetics have the other form of diabetes, type 2 or non insulin-dependent diabetes. This usually develops in adults over 40, but unfortunately more and more children and younger adults also are developing type 2 diabetes. This is thought to be due to the epidemic of obesity amongst children in western societies, a result of too much junk food and too little exercise. In this case, the pancreas produces insulin, but the body does not use it properly, and the pancreas goes into overdrive to make up for this 'resistance'. In time, the pancreas cannot make enough insulin to make up for the insensitivity, and diabetes follows. Inactivity, ageing, obesity or a diet high in saturated fats can all contribute to insulin resistance.

With either form of diabetes, glucose builds up in the bloodstream. Left untreated, this can lead to serious complications such as blindness, stroke, kidney failure and heart disease. But the good news is that type 2 diabetes can often be controlled through simple measures. Losing weight, eating wisely, taking enough exercise and reducing stress can all improve blood glucose levels. Even people whose diabetes requires medication will maintain better glucose control if they adopt a healthy lifestyle.

WHEN TO CONSULT A DOCTOR

Diabetes is a serious illness that requires a doctor's care, even when it is controlled. Consult a health care professional before making any changes to your diet or exercise routines.

However well you feel, you should see your doctor once or twice a year at least, so that your long-term glucose control, your kidneys and your cholesterol level can be checked, your blood pressure measured, and your circulation, skin and nervous system checked. Some men with diabetes get problems with erections, and this is a good opportunity to discuss ways of dealing with this. You will also need an annual eye check from a specialized optometrist or eye specialist, and may need to see a chiropodist and dietician on a regular basis, too.

Three complications of diabetes require prompt medical attention: severe hyperglycaemia, hypoglycaemia and ketosis.

Hyperglycaemia is when your blood sugar spikes high. Signs that your blood sugar is too high include frequent urination, fatigue, unexplained weight loss and increased thirst. You should get in touch with your doctor if you can't reduce it, says diabetes expert Christopher Saudek.

Hypoglycaemia is when blood sugar drops too low. Symptoms include shakiness, dizziness, headache, confusion, sudden mood changes – often unusual aggressiveness – and a tingling sensation around the mouth. Many people with diabetes requiring insulin, and some who are on tablets, have periods of hypoglycaemia, but you should see a doctor if symptoms are severe or occur frequently (see box, 'Coping with a hypo', page 179).

Ketosis is a serious, potentially fatal condition that occurs when ketones – acids that build up in the blood – become dangerously high and poison the body. Warning signs include sweet-smelling breath (reminiscent of pear-drops or nail varnish remover), loss of appetite, increased thirst, frequent urination, fatigue, nausea and vomiting. Ketosis occurs only in people with type 1 diabetes, not in those with type 2.

Looking after yourself when you have diabetes is not only about keeping your glucose levels down, though. Just as important, you need to pay attention to the other big risk factors for heart disease: high blood pressure, high cholesterol and smoking. Here is some helpful advice.

Beat diabetes to the punch. Many people have Type 2 diabetes for years without even realizing it, says family doctor Stephen Amiel. 'Sometimes it only comes to light when complications like a heart attack or loss of vision develop. If you're overweight, or you have a strong family history of diabetes, or you come from an at-risk ethnic community, or you had high blood sugar levels in pregnancy, ask your doctor to check your blood sugar on a regular basis.'

Yet another good reason to quit smoking. There's evidence that smoking increases your risk of developing diabetes by increasing insulin resistance, says Dr Amiel. It's also a major risk factor in its own right for heart disease, circulatory problems and kidney disease – all conditions which people with diabetes are more prone to. So if you have diabetes, make a very special effort to quit (for helpful advice on quitting, see *Addiction*, page 21).

Nurture Good Nutrition

No one nutrition prescription can apply to everyone with diabetes, says Marion Franz, a nutritionist who specializes in diabetes management. 'Each person with diabetes should have a diet plan that suits him or her individually.' That involves considering what ethnic or cultural foods you prefer, what other health worries you may have (high cholesterol or high blood pressure, for example), and what changes you are realistically prepared to make.

Watch your sugar. Sugar is not a forbidden food for people with diabetes, says Dr Franz. But it's worth remembering that sweets, chocolate and foods containing sugar are often high in calories and low in nutritional value.

Do just *one* thing

Lose weight. The most effective thing that an overweight person with type 2 diabetes can do is to lose weight, says diabetes expert Christopher Saudek. Losing excess pounds is sometimes all it takes to bring blood sugar under control. How much weight you need to lose varies for each individual, but even small drops can yield big results.

You don't have to be stick thin, and you don't have to reach an ideal body weight, says nutritionist Carla Miller. Losing just 5 to 10 per cent of your body weight may be enough to gain glucose control. Of course, you'll have to maintain that weight loss, or your blood sugar will rise again. That's why how you trim down is important.

Avoid fad diets, advises Dr Saudek. Most are difficult to maintain and some are not healthy. Your best bet is to combine exercise with a low-calorie diet.

Talk to a doctor, clinic nurse or dietitian and work out the right combination for you.

Eat fewer fats. Keeping fats to about 30 per cent of your total calorie intake can reduce your chance of developing high cholesterol and heart disease.

Eat even fewer saturated fats. Saturated fats, from fatty meats, cheese and butter should account for only 10 per cent of your total daily calorie intake. Switching to a diet higher in monounsaturated fats, found in olive oil, grapeseed oil and nuts, may help to reduce insulin resistance, according to diabetes researcher Harry Preuss. Choose low-fat dairy products and lean meats, and avoid hydrogenated fats such as found in many margarines, and coconut oil or palm oil, found in manufactured biscuits, cakes and pies.

Avoid fad high-protein diets. Because foods high in animal protein, such as meats and cheeses, tend also to be high in fat and cholesterol, limit proteins to between 10 and 20 per cent of your diet. You might lose weight following popular high-protein, low-carbohydrate diets, such as the Atkins diet, but keeping it off will be a problem. You're better off eating a balanced diet that you can live with, says Dr Franz.

Eat less salt. Diabetes and high blood pressure sometimes go hand in hand, and people with diabetes can be more sensitive to the effects of excess sodium, says Dr Franz. Cut down on salt by adding less to your cooking and at the table, and by checking food labels for sodium. Avoid obviously salty foods like olives, crisps and salted nuts.

Feast on fibre. One small study of 13 people who ate 25g each of soluble and insoluble fibre – a total of 50g a day – found that they were able to achieve a 10 per cent drop in blood sugar levels.

While that's encouraging news, Dr Franz warns that, from a practical standpoint, 50g a day may be a bit tough to stomach. 'We really don't know if, in the long term, people can eat enough fibre to influence blood glucose levels,' she says.

Nevertheless, high-fibre diets have other health advantages. They slow down the absorption of fats and carbohydrates, reducing their adverse effects on the glucose-insulin system. Also, high-fibre foods tend to be very filling, so you eat less. Eat lots of whole grains, beans, lentils and vegetables.

Drink alcohol in moderation. You needn't give up alcohol the moment you're diagnosed with diabetes. Moderate drinking has been shown to lower the risk of heart disease and may actually improve insulin sensitivity, according to some studies. To realize such benefits, however, don't drink too much. Three units of alcohol a day is the upper limit for men, and two units for women. A unit is a glass of wine, a single measure of spirits or a half pint of beer or lager. People with diabetes should never drink on an empty stomach as alcohol can cause blood-sugar levels to plummet dangerously low.

Get the family involved. Carla Miller, a nutrition expert, studied the eating patterns and food choices of 45 men and women with type 2 diabetes for a year. She found that those with the best blood-sugar control were men whose wives prepared low-fat meals and went for regular walks with them. On the other hand, women without that level of support from another person didn't have good glucose control. Worst off were women who prepared low-fat meals for themselves but made separate meals for their families. The moral of the story is to enlist your family's support and eat more healthily – together.

Plan ahead. Diabetes requires a pretty intensive lifestyle overhaul, acknowledges Dr Miller. You need to exercise, eat healthily and monitor your blood sugar, which requires a lot of organization and time. In her study, Dr Miller found that the people most successful at controlling their blood-sugar levels were those who did a lot of meal preplanning. Decide at the beginning of the week what meals you want to eat, and then shop for those foods. If you take packed lunches to work and keep healthy snacks to hand, you'll be less likely to eat high-fat meals or sugary snacks.

Consult a dietitian. A dietitian or nutritionist can design you an individual nutrition plan. That is especially important if you have other health issues, such as high cholesterol and high blood pressure, to consider, says Dr Miller. Book several appointments so that you can gradually incorporate any changes.

Get Your Heart Pumping

In addition to dietary changes, experts recommend regular exercise for people with diabetes. Exercise acts just like medicine, explains Robert Hanisch a physiologist and expert in diabetes management. It lowers blood sugar as muscles turn glucose into energy. Obese people with type 2 diabetes who exercise regularly achieve better glucose control. Furthermore, studies show that increased physical activity, including walking, can reduce the risk of heart attack, stroke and other complications in people with diabetes.

Even people dependent on insulin injections or oral medicines can reap the benefits of exercise. 'At the very least, they will need less medication. And the results are immediate,' says Hanisch. Check your blood glucose immediately before and after exercise. There will be individual variations, but on average there is a one to two per cent drop in blood sugar for every minute you exercise. That means 10 minutes of aerobic exercise will usually cut blood sugar by 10 to 20 per cent. The glucose will remain lower until the next meal or snack.

Check with your doctor before beginning any exercise programme. Here are some tips to get you going.

Start slowly. If you are not used to exercise, don't overdo it. Begin with a low-impact, low-intensity workout, such as walking. Walk at a comfortable pace, advises Hanisch. If you push yourself too hard, you won't find it enjoyable, and you'll be less likely to continue. 'Blood sugar can go down even when you are walking very slowly,' he says.

Five sessions a week. Consistency is the key, says Hanisch. Whether you walk, cycle, swim or jog, a routine you can manage five times a week will give the best results, producing a long-term change in your body. After two to three months of consistent exercise, you are likely to become more sensitive to insulin, and you will need less medicine.

Be a morning person. Exercise early in the day will help to keep blood sugar down all day long. You will still see fluctuations in glucose levels after meals, says Hanisch, but a 30-minute morning walk will keep levels 30 per cent lower than they might otherwise be.

Drink plenty of water. Dehydration can affect blood glucose levels, so staying well-hydrated during exercise is especially important for people with diabetes. Drink two glasses of water two hours before exercising, and take further sips during your routine.

Lift light weights. Weight training can help to build strength. But people with long-standing diabetes, and especially those with diabetes-related eye disease, need to limit themselves to many repetitions with very light resistance in the range of 500g to 2kg weights. Lifting heavy weights can injure a weakened retina. If a weight is light enough, you should be able to perform the correct strengthening techniques with minimal effort. If in doubt, use a lighter weight.

Take care of your toes. People who have diabetes-related foot problems such as peripheral neuropathy should take special care before they go walking or jogging. You may need advice from a chiropodist to ensure correct weight distribution (see box, 'Look after your feet', page 180).

Become Less Stressed

When something stressful happens and sends your emotions on a roller-coaster, your blood sugar goes along for the ride. That's because stress hormones like adrenaline increase blood glucose. 'Stress hormones mobilize glycogen that has been stored in the liver and metabolize it to glucose,' says psychiatrist Angele McGrady. The adrenaline and extra sugar released into the bloodstream give you a boost of energy.

If you were undergoing physical stress, such as being chased by a pack of wild dogs, you'd respond by running away, and the extra blood sugar would be used up, Dr McGrady explains. Today, however, most of our stresses are psychological. We sit and brood and don't use up that extra blood sugar.

Because their bodies don't metabolize glucose effectively, it's especially important for people with diabetes to try to decrease their stress levels. In a small study conducted by Dr McGrady, 18 people with diabetes reduced their blood-sugar levels by around 10 per cent through simple relaxation exercises.

Breathe deeply. Deep breathing is a good way to start, says Dr McGrady. Sit with your legs and arms uncrossed. Inhale deeply from your abdomen. Then breathe out as much air as possible, relaxing your muscles as you do. Continue this relaxed breathing for about 15 minutes.

Buy a relaxation tape. If you can't unwind, a relaxation tape can help. 'Most of us aren't used to sitting quietly with no thoughts in our heads,' says Dr McGrady. 'It's very helpful to have sound in the background.' Recordings of gentle sounds from nature, such as ocean waves, enable you to pace your breathing and set a tone for you to relax. Or choose a guided imagery tape, in which a soothing voice mentally shepherds you through a pleasant scene, such as a walk through a forest.

Focus on something pleasant. Guided imagery works because it uses your senses of recall and concentration to help you relax. You can achieve the same effect by looking at an art book or an illustration that you like. 'Look at the picture for several minutes, then close your eyes and recall as much as you can,' says Dr McGrady. 'If you do it often enough, you can eventually do it without even having the book in front of you.' You could put a peaceful scene on your screensaver, too.

Practise progressive relaxation. Tensing and relaxing the muscles in your body allows you to consciously control muscle tension.

First, lie on your back in a comfortable position. Then, begin deliberately tensing and releasing one set of muscles – the fist is a good place to start. Move upwards along your arms, to the neck, and face, and then down the back and legs.

Do not tense any muscle hard enough to cause pain. Tapes and CDs are available to talk you through this process.

Coping with a hypo

Hypoglycaemia is when blood sugar drops too low. Symptoms include shakiness, dizziness, headache, confusion, sudden mood changes – often unusual aggressiveness – and a tingling sensation around the mouth. Many people with diabetes requiring insulin, and some who are on tablets, have periods of hypoglycaemia.

If you have mild hypoglycaemia, take three glucose tablets, eat five or six boiled sweets or drink a small carton of of fruit juice. It's important to treat it immediately, as you can pass out if it gets worse.

If you are with someone who has diabetes and they become confused or drowsy, try and get something sweet into them quickly: it's safe to assume their glucose blood levels are too low rather than too high. If they're conscious and cooperative enough to swallow, give them some milk, lemonade or cola, or smear some honey, jam or syrup in their mouth. Some people carry a supply of a special gel, Hypostop, which can be used instead. Follow up the sugar with a longer-acting carbohydrate snack – some bread and jam or biscuits.

If the person is unconscious or nearly so, do not attempt to put anything in his or her mouth as there is a risk they'll choke. **Call for an ambulance immediately.** Some people have a supply of glucagon, a hormone which increases blood sugar levels. This can be given by a partner or carer as an intramuscular injection, but some training is essential beforehand.

Look after your arteries with low-dose aspirin. Aspirin reduces the risk of a heart attack by discouraging blood cells called platelets from sticking together in the arteries. It's even more effective for people with diabetes than for those without the condition. The usual dose is 75mg per day, but check with your doctor as to how much aspirin is right for you, says diabetes specialist Aaron Vinik.

Testing, Testing

Once you have been diagnosed with diabetes, testing your blood sugar becomes an integral part of your life. Here are some techniques.

Look for patterns. Monitor your glucose levels by recording your levels four times a day for several weeks, suggests Dr Miller. That helps you to

Look after your feet

Peripheral neuropathy is a complication of diabetes in which high blood sugar damages nerve cells over time, leading to a lack of sensation.

Because the nerves in the feet are the longest in the body, the feet are usually most affected by this condition, making them prone to injury and sores. Sores that don't heal properly can become ulcerated and infected and, in serious cases, may even require amputation.

An estimated six out of every 1000 people with diabetes will have a limb amputated – but the vast majority of these could be avoided. Here are some recommendations for protecting your feet.

See a chiropodist. Once you've been diagnosed with diabetes, have your feet checked frequently, recommends Marc Brenner, a chiropodist who specializes in diabetic foot problems. A chiropodist will determine if you have neuropathy and will help to care for your feet if you do.

Trimming toenails or treating your own calluses and corns, for example, can be dangerous for people with neuropathy and should be done by a foot specialist.

Keep them covered. Wear a good pair of socks. The best are made of a combination of cotton and synthetic material.

On very cold days, wear two pairs – a thin one next to your skin and a thick pair. 'The more insulation you have between your foot and the ground, the better,' says Dr Brenner.

---

spot patterns. Test first thing in the morning, one to two hours after meals and just before going to bed.

Monitor changes. When making changes in your diet, test immediately before a meal, then two hours after. Before a meal, levels should range between 4 and 6.5mmol/l (millimoles per litre). After a meal, levels should be no higher than 9mmol/l.

Ideal levels may vary from individual to individual, so consult your doctor, diabetic nurse or consultant about the best levels for you. You should also test more often when you're unwell, especially if you're on medication for diabetes. Your sugar control may also change when you're pregnant, so consult your doctor as soon as pregnancy is confirmed.

Test when you exercise. When beginning a new exercise routine, test immediately before and immediately after your workout, says Hanisch.

Be sure the shoe fits. Have your feet properly measured by a fitter, says Dr Brenner. Your chiropodist should be able to recommend a shoe shop that offers this service. Get your feet measured in the afternoon, when your feet are more likely to be swollen.

Trainers are fine. You probably won't need custom-made shoes. A high-quality trainer will serve you well. Look for ones with plenty of room in the toe; a removable insole if you need to fit in a custom-made orthotic insole; a padded, thick tongue; a cushioned heel; and cushioning on the ball of the foot.

Wear an orthotic. Your doctor may suggest that you wear an orthotic – a custom-made device that fits into your shoe. It keeps pressure off certain spots on the foot or spreads pressure across the entire foot. Your specialist will measure you if you need an orthotic.

Inspect daily. Check for swelling or sores using a large mirror to see all angles of the foot. Better still, ask a family member to look for you: ask him or her to touch your foot to make sure it's neither discoloured nor too hot – both signs of infection.

Take them swimming. If you have neuropathy, exercise is still important. Swimming is safest, says Dr Brenner, because there is no pressure on your feet.

Carefully dry your feet afterwards and sprinkle them with foot powder to avoid fungal or yeast infections.

If your blood sugar is low before starting – 4 to 6mmol/l – eat a piece of fruit or drink a small glass (125ml) of juice. Both contain about 15g of carbohydrates, which will raise your blood sugar by about 25 per cent. Do the same if your levels drop after exercise.

Do spot checks. Most people with diabetes habitually monitor first thing in the morning. That's not enough, says Dr Amiel. It's better to do several checks a day at different times *for a day or two every month* or so than a daily test at the same time: this gives you a better picture of what influences your blood glucose.

Blood sugar values should be 5 to 7mmol/l on average at bedtime.

Write it down. Keep a written record of your sugar levels, and note what and when you ate as well as when you exercised and for how long. This information can help your doctor to manage your care.

DIARRHOEA
23 strategies to deal with it

In the past when someone had diarrhoea, doctors whipped out their prescription pads and dispensed antidiarrhoeal medicine. Today, they think the best medicine is to simply let diarrhoea run its course, so to speak.

'Acute diarrhoea is one of your body's best defence mechanisms,' says medical researcher Lynn McFarland. 'It's your body's way of getting something nasty out of your system.' That thought may or may not be of much comfort to you right now, but it explains why doctors today prefer you to ride it out instead of automatically trying to halt this annoying, but hopefully short-lived, illness.

'I don't recommend antidiarrhoeal medication when a patient has acute diarrhoea unless there is an urgent need for control – like a very important meeting that just can't be missed,' says David Lieberman, a gastroenterologist. 'Otherwise, I think the purge is probably beneficial and helps to speed up recovery.'

With that approach in mind, most of the tips below are designed to help you weather the discomfort of diarrhoea and make a quick recovery, rather than try to halt the course of diarrhoea and risk prolonging the illness.

Is there a milk connection? A major cause of diarrhoea is intolerance to lactose, the sugar found in milk and other dairy products, says William Chey, a specialist in digestive disorders. This is especially common in people of African, Asian and Middle Eastern origin, up to 75 per cent of whom may have a degree of lactose intolerance.

'Lactose intolerance can begin in infancy, or it can kick in suddenly during adulthood.' One day you can be drinking milk, and the next thing you know you have wind, pain and diarrhoea. Temporary lactose intolerance can follow a bout of gastroenteritis, infection with gut parasites, or dietary iron deficiency.

The cure is to avoid lactose-containing foods, which means staying away from most dairy products, apart from yoghurt, some aged cheeses like Cheddar, and dairy foods specifically labelled lactose-free. Full-fat milk is better tolerated than skimmed or semi-skimmed. Hopefully this can be a temporary measure, until your gut recovers its ability to digest lactose.

Take the tolerance test. Given the dose-related nature of lactose intolerance, as well as its ability to kick in unexpectedly, how can you be sure that milk products are responsible for your tummy troubles?

WHEN TO CONSULT A DOCTOR

Diarrhoea should normally leave you only slightly the worse for wear. In infants, small children, elderly people, or those already sick or dehydrated from another illness, however, acute diarrhoea can be particularly severe and requires prompt medical attention.

Medical help is also needed if diarrhoea doesn't subside within a day or two, if it is accompanied by fever and severe abdominal cramps, or if it occurs with rashes, jaundice (yellowing of the skin and whites of the eyes) or extreme weakness. If you see blood, pus or mucus in the stools, see your doctor.

'The most immediate risk associated with acute diarrhoea is dehydration,' says gastroenterologist Harris Clearfield. 'So if an individual is having a major bout of diarrhoea and isn't taking in any food or drink, you could be looking at a medical emergency.'

Even if your diarrhoea isn't too bad, a change in bowel habit towards a looser, more frequent stool should be investigated if it persists for longer than six weeks. There may be a simple explanation, like a change in your diet or a bowel infection, but sometimes it could be the first sign of bowel cancer.

First, completely abstain from milk products for a week or two and see if that helps, says Dr Lieberman. If it does, then gradually add back milk products with the knowledge that at some point you may reach a level where the intolerance symptoms return. Once you know what that level is, you can avoid lactose-induced diarrhoea by eating fewer dairy products.

Look at your medicines. Antacids containing magnesium, like Maalox and magnesium trisilicate, are a common cause of diarrhoea, says family doctor Stephen Amiel. They stop water being reabsorbed from the gut, making the stool soft and watery. If you need an antacid, use one containing aluminium hydroxide, such as Gaviscon instead, he says. Pharmacist Sue Livingston suggests trying Asilone tablets or Aludrox liquid: 'these are less likely to cause diarrhoea,' she says, 'but they're also less effective.'

Other medicinal culprits include some antibiotics, quinidine, metformin, omeprazole and colchicine. Consult your doctor if you think these or any other medications may be causing you problems. If you develop diarrhoea when you are taking laxatives for constipation, speak to your doctor about changing the dose, or using a gentler preparation.

Occasionally, people who are extremely constipated develop so-called 'spurious' or overflow diarrhoea; frequent, difficult to control, watery stools which leak past the blockage. This may require an enema.

Large doses of vitamin C can be a culprit behind diarrhoea, too. Anything over the recommended daily amount of 60mg can cause diarrhoea in some people, but most of us are fine with up to 2000mg per day, as long as this is split up over the course of the day.

Eat a clear diet. 'Start with a clear-liquid diet,' says Dr Chey. 'By clear I mean chicken stock, jelly and other foods or fluids you can see through.' This helps your bowel to rest during the diarrhoea, rather than forcing your system to handle more than it can. After you've tested the waters with broth and jelly, you can gradually introduce rice, bananas, apple purée or yoghurt into your diet as your symptoms improve.

Breast milk is an exception to the clear fluid rule: if your baby has diarrhoea, you should continue breastfeeding, supplementing with a glucose-electrolyte solution like Dioralyte or Rehidrat, as advised by your doctor or health visitor.

Keep up your fluid intake. It doesn't really matter what you eat, says Dr McFarland. It's much more important to make sure your fluid intake is high. Though many people don't feel like drinking large amounts of liquids during bouts of diarrhoea, all our experts agree that increasing your fluid intake is vital to ward off dehydration.

Fluids that contain salt and small amounts of sugar are particularly beneficial, as they help the body to replace glucose and minerals lost during diarrhoea. A good rehydration fluid can be easily made by adding a teaspoon of sugar and a pinch of salt to one litre of water.

A more complex but better tasting mix can be made by adding a half teaspoon of honey and a pinch of salt to 250ml clear fruit juice. Stir well and drink often.

Older children and adults may prefer soft bottled drinks. Lemonade, cola, Lucozade or similar will do. Get the non-diet variety (you need the sugar), and stir out the fizz. 'The gas may add further explosiveness to a delicate situation,' says Dr Clearfield.

Or just buy Rehidrat or Dioralyte sachets from a pharmacy. These contain a balance of glucose and electrolytes to replace those your body is losing.

Avoid these foods. While eating may not be as important as drinking for riding out diarrhoea, some foods should be avoided. Obvious ones to decline include beans, cabbage and Brussels sprouts.

Other foods containing large amounts of poorly absorbed carbohydrates can aggravate diarrhoea. A short list includes bread, pasta and other wheat products; apples, pears, peaches and prunes; corn, oats, potatoes and processed bran. And, in case you fancied some soothing ice cream, all our experts say that you should avoid dairy products (with the exception of yoghurt) during a bout of diarrhoea. Even if milk products didn't trigger the diarrhoea, they tend to aggravate diarrhoea once you've got it.

Stay out of the kitchen. While we're still on the subject of food, any member of the family with diarrhoea should not prepare food for other members of the household until the diarrhoea subsides. Careful hand washing helps to keep a parasitic infection from spreading.

Note: If your job involves contact with large numbers of people or food handling, health and safety regulations may require that you stay away from work until all symptoms subside. Diarrhoea may be caused by a food poisoning bacteria like salmonella. If you're a food handler, you will need to have your stool tested by your doctor. Public health officials will need to be notified and will check you and your close contacts before you can return to work, even if you feel better.

A medicine for emergencies. Our experts insist that letting diarrhoea run its course is the best medicine. If, however, you absolutely have to go somewhere, and be in control while you're there, an over-the-counter product called loperamide, sold as Imodium or Diareze, is probably your best bet. 'Loperamide is very effective,' says Dr Clearfield. 'It works by causing the bowel to tighten up, and by doing so, prevents things from moving along.' Other products, such as Kaopectate or Pepto-Bismol, can be taken for mild diarrhoea.

Skip these food remedies. Things like pectin, acidophilus tablets, carob powder, barley, bananas, Swiss cheese, and a host of exotic foods, teas and other folk remedies have all been used as treatments for diarrhoea. 'They work to bind the bowel and slow down the course of the diarrhoea,' says Dr McFarland. But in his opinion, that's not necessarily what you want to do. You simply increase the time that whatever is causing the problem stays inside you. What you want to do is get it out.

Be careful on holiday. One way to ruin a holiday is to contract traveller's diarrhoea. Here are some tips for avoiding it.

- Avoid uncooked vegetables, especially salads, fruit you can't peel, undercooked meat, raw shellfish, ice cubes and drinks made from impure water (the alcohol in drinks won't kill bugs).

- Make sure that any plates and cutlery you use have been washed in purified water.

Traveller's diarrhoea

Montezuma's revenge, Delhi belly, Tiki trots. Whatever you call it, traveller's diarrhoea can dampen your spirits on even the best holiday.

The most common cause is the bacterium *Escherichia coli*. This widespread little organism normally lives in your intestines and performs a role in digestion. But foreign versions of *E. coli* – and to a foreigner, the British version is foreign – can give you diarrhoea by producing a toxin that prevents your intestines from absorbing the water you ingest in the form of fluid and food. And all that fluid has got to come out.

Shigella and salmonella bacteria can also cause traveller's diarrhoea, while a smaller number of cases are caused by rotavirus and the giardia parasite. Changes in diet, fatigue, jet lag and altitude sickness have all been blamed for traveller's diarrhoea, but up to half of all cases are unexplained. There are ways to help your body fight back. Here's what doctors suggest.

Drink water. Why, when your stools are mostly water, would the most important treatment be to drink plenty of the right fluids? Because dehydration, the loss of water and electrolytes, can kill.

'A lot of what you take in will be pumped straight out at the other end,' admits Thomas Gossel, an expert in toxicology. 'But you'll reach a point where you stabilize and begin retaining it. If you didn't replace any fluids at all, you could become dehydrated in a day.'

Look at your urine. The darker your urine, the more fluid you need. Urine should be clear or pale yellow. If very dark urine

- Drink only water that's been carbonated and sealed in bottles or cans. Clean the part of the container that touches your mouth with purified water. Boiling water for three to five minutes purifies it, as does adding purifying tablets.

- Drink acidic drinks like colas and orange juice when possible. They help to keep down *E. coli*, the bacterium responsible for most stomach upsets.

- Drink acidophilus milk or eat live yogurt before your trip. The bacterial colonies established in your gut before your trip and maintained during it will reduce the chance of a hostile bacterial invasion.

persists, especially if you have a pale yellow stool, you need to be checked for hepatitis

Use a rehydration solution. A great way to rehydrate is to drink an oral rehydration solution. These drinks contain sugar and salt and help to replace vital electrolytes lost through diarrhoea. They also help your intestines to absorb water. Over-the-counter rehydration sachets are widely available in the UK, so buy and take them with you. Brands include Rehidrat and Dioralyte.

Alternative drinks. If you didn't manage to pack any rehydration sachets, drink clear fruit juices or weak tea with sugar. Soft bottled drinks are fine, too, but stir the fizz out first.

Firm it up. Pepto-Bismol, an over-the-counter diarrhoea medicine, can be the traveller's friend. It makes stools bulkier and firmer, and kills bacteria. Don't worry if your tongue and diarrhoea turn black: it's a natural side effect of Pepto-Bismol.

Do a little coaxing. Natural fibre-based laxatives for relieving constipation, such as Fybogel and Isogel, also help with diarrhoea. Some can absorb up to 60 times their weight in water to form a gel in the intestine. You will still expel water, Dr Gossel says, but it won't be so runny.

Have a check-up. If symptoms persist on your return, you'll need to have a stool specimen checked by your doctor or local travel clinic. Without treatment, bacteria and parasites can be unwelcome souvenirs of your holiday for months.

Be careful if you're on the Pill. If you have very severe diarrhoea, you cannot rely on your contraceptive pill being absorbed in sufficient quantities.

You should, therefore, use additional precautions during recovery and for seven days afterwards. If the vomiting and diarrhoea occurs during the last seven tablets of your packet, the next pill-free interval should be omitted.

DIVERTICULOSIS
23 self-care techniques

Diverticulosis is a condition of the elderly population. It affects more than half of those over 60 in the UK, and almost everyone over 80. It is associated with the low-fibre diet of Western society – and the incidence is correspondingly lower in vegetarians, who eat more fibre, than in meat eaters.

The condition is characterized by tiny, grapelike pouches or sacs (diverticula) along the outer wall of the colon. These pouches show up on x-rays, but many people never have this area x-rayed and don't even know that they have the condition, says Samuel Klein, an expert in nutrition.

If your diverticula cause symptoms such as an alteration in bowel habit, abdominal pain, or rectal bleeding, you have diverticular disease. About 10 per cent of those with diverticulosis will get diverticulitis, a painful inflammation that can become serious. So having diverticulosis does not mean that you're destined for severe pain or a hospital stay. You can take an active role in treating and preventing diverticulosis, thus avoiding the pain of diverticulitis. Here are the experts' suggestions.

Eat more fibre. 'Diverticulosis has come about with the advance of processed foods – foods that are low in fibre,' says colorectal surgeon Paul Williamson. The average Briton eats about 12g of fibre a day, significantly less than the minimum 18g recommended by the British Nutrition Foundation.

Fibre helps to reduce tension on the colon and helps it to expand when eliminating waste. Fibre also draws water into the stool, making bowel movements softer and smoother. Wholemeal bread and bran cereals are excellent sources of bran fibre, which appears to be the most effective type of fibre in preventing diverticulosis. Sprinkling raw bran over foods such as soups or stews is also an option.

Vegetables and fruit are other good sources of fibre, although fruit and vegetable juices contain hardly any – so reach for an apple instead of its juice.

Eat processed foods in moderation. This is good general health advice, but it also applies to treating diverticulosis. If you eat a lot of low-fibre processed foods, says Dr Klein, you won't have room to eat the high-fibre foods you need.

Don't worry about eating seeds. Until recently, many doctors told

WHEN TO CONSULT A DOCTOR

If you live long enough, the chances are you will get diverticulosis. Even so, the odds are you won't get diverticulitis – a painful inflammation that is potentially serious. But you should be aware of the warning signs.

Fever and severe pain in the lower left area of the abdominal region are good indicators that diverticulosis has advanced to diverticulitis, says digestion expert Marvin Schuster.

This change shouldn't be taken lightly. It could be a rupture or bleeding, warns A&E doctor Albert Lauro. And although it doesn't happen often, people can die from diverticulitis.

So act on those warning signs and get to a doctor fast. And keep calm – the odds are still in your favour. Any infection can normally be treated with antibiotics, rest and diet says Dr Lauro.

You should never assume that abdominal pain, rectal bleeding or a change in bowel habit are due to diverticular disease. They may be, but your doctor will also want to rule out such conditions as colitis and cancer.

their patients to avoid tomatoes, strawberries and other foods with small seeds. They believed that the seeds could lodge in the diverticula and trigger inflammation. But research has shown no evidence to support the ban on seeds, and nutritionists point out that many of these foods are also good sources of fibre.

Increase your fibre intake slowly. Take six to eight weeks to gradually build your fibre intake up to 30g per day, Dr Klein suggests. 'You need time for your digestive system to adapt.' You will probably experience bloating and wind in the first few weeks, says Marvin Schuster, an expert in digestive disorders. But most people get over this.

If you can't get enough fibre in your diet, take a supplement. The best are psyllium seed (also known as ispaghula) supplements such as Metamucil, says Dr Schuster. They're natural, too.

Don't use suppositories. While they may offer a quick fix to constipation, suppositories aren't the best choice for stimulating bowel movements. 'Your system can get addicted to them,' Dr Klein explains. 'And then it becomes a vicious circle – you need more suppositories.' (See also *Constipation*, page 144.)

Drink lots of liquids. 'Drink six to eight glasses of water a day,' advises Dr Klein. Liquid is an important partner to fibre in combating constipation, which is associated with diverticulosis.

'If you have to strain a lot when having a bowel movement,' says Dr Schuster, 'you expand the little diverticula through the muscle walls of the colon.'

Go when you have to go. If you don't answer nature's call, you defeat the object of adding more fibre to your diet and drinking more liquids. Don't suppress the need to move your bowel, advises Dr Williamson.

Exercise. It tones more than your legs and hips. Exercise also tones the muscles in your colon and you don't have to strain as much, says Dr Klein.

Soothe your pain with heat. To relieve tenderness or cramping, hold a heating pad against the left-hand side of your abdomen.

Don't smoke. Harmful in so many ways, smoking may also aggravate diverticulosis, says A&E doctor Albert Lauro.

Drink in moderation. Alcohol in moderation – a drink or two a day – relaxes the colon and can improve the situation a little, says Dr Schuster.

Avoid caffeine. Coffee, chocolate, teas and colas all tend to irritate the colon, says Dr Williamson.

Look for a pattern. Certain foods may disrupt your bowel habits or cause loose stools, Dr Williamson says. Try to identify those foods and avoid them.

Take it easy with painkillers. Avoid over-using ibuprofen, a painkiller in the family of drugs

---

KITCHEN CURES

Digestion expert Craig Rubin recommends this homemade remedy for constipation, but it's useful for anyone who wants to add fibre to their diet. Mix 3 tablespoons of unprocessed bran and 3 tablespoons of apple purée with 2 tablespoons of prune juice. Refrigerate. Take 2 to 3 tablespoons of the mixture after dinner, then drink a full glass of water. If you need to, you can increase your dose to 3 to 4 tablespoons.

Whole prunes, prune juice and herbal teas are also effective natural laxatives. Specially formulated teas can be found in most health food stores.

Ways to add more fibre

Eating enough fibre is the most important thing you can do to treat and prevent diverticulosis. Here are some tips for making the transition to a high-fibre diet that don't involve sitting down to a bowl of raw bran.

- Make a habit of eating wholemeal bread instead of white bread.
- Feed your sweet tooth by eating fresh fruit for pudding.
- Eat more vegetarian meals.
- Leave skins on potatoes, apples, peaches and pears.
- Add dried fruits such as raisins and apricots to your meals.
- Substitute beans for some of the beef in curries or casseroles.
- Add pearl barley to vegetable soups.

known as nonsteroidal anti-inflammatory drugs (NSAIDs). These drugs inhibit prostaglandins, fatty acids that protect the cells in the intestinal tract. NSAIDs may also provoke bleeding from the diverticula. Codeine-containing analgesics cause constipation, so should be used sparingly if you have diverticulosis.

Regular use of paracetamol is also associated with increased symptoms of diverticular disease. One study of more than 35,000 men found that those who took NSAIDs or paracetamol more than twice a week were twice as likely to develop diverticular disease as men who didn't take the painkillers regularly.

DIZZINESS
17 tips to stop the spinning

Few sensations are more uncomfortable, and potentially dangerous, than dizziness. Older people experience dizziness or balance disorders more frequently, but these problems can affect people of all ages.

The word dizziness is used to describe a variety of feelings ranging from mild unsteadiness to severe vertigo, where people feel that the world is spinning. Inner-ear problems such as injury, viral infections, inflammation, debris in the inner ear and bleeding can all cause vertigo, says neurologist Terry Fife.

But not all dizziness is due to inner-ear problems. Dizziness may also result from poor circulation, side effects from medication, and a condition called postural hypotension, in which blood pressure temporarily drops when you're in an upright position or after you suddenly get up.

Dizziness often disappears on its own, but it can have long-term consequences, especially when it leads to a loss of balance and falls. 'People can become so frightened of falling that they stop being physically active,' says Dr Fife.

Here's what experts advise to control dizziness.

Stay still. If you feel an attack coming on stay absolutely still, without moving your head. Keeping still lets your blood pressure stabilize and helps the inner ear to regain its normal equilibrium. However, if you still feel dizzy, gradually **sit down** – it's a lot safer than trying to stay on your feet when the world is spinning. But take things carefully and avoid any sudden movements, as these may make you feel worse.

Reach out and touch something. When you feel an attack of dizziness or 'spinning' coming on, lightly rest your fingers on objects around you – a bookcase, for example, or a table or the back of a chair.

Spinning sensations occur when the brain receives conflicting messages, Dr Fife explains. Your eyes may be convinced that you're whirling, while your feet know very well that you're standing still. This conflict in sensations makes the vertigo worse. 'If you make contact with enough objects, your sensory nerves start to adjust,' he says.

Flex your legs. If you have postural hypotension, the blood tends to pool in the legs and feet. This causes a reduction in bloodflow to the brain, which can result in dizziness. 'Flexing your leg muscles before you stand up – by crossing and uncrossing your legs, for example – helps to push blood back into circulation,' says hospital doctor Joshua Hoffman.

Get up in stages. Don't leap out of bed in the morning. Instead, swing your legs over the side of the bed and rise to a sitting position. Wait for a minute or two, then slowly stand up. This gives your blood pressure time to adjust, which may prevent dizziness, says Dr Hoffman.

If you tend to feel dizzy getting out of bed in the morning, make sure there is a stable piece of furniture next to the bed for you to hold on to, or perhaps consider having a grab rail fitted.

Keep moving. It's normal for people who experience frequent dizziness to become increasingly afraid of falling. As a result, they become more and more sedentary. This reduces the ability of the brain to monitor and fine-tune the sense of balance – which will make falls even more likely.

WHEN TO CONSULT A DOCTOR

Everyone gets dizzy from time to time – when getting out of bed, for example, or standing up after working in the garden – and it isn't always a problem.

Uncomplicated vertigo may respond to medication, or you may need referral for further investigation and treatment. Many hospitals now have special falls clinics where your doctor can refer you if your dizziness is causing you to fall.

'If dizziness is mild, occurs rarely, and was clearly provoked by a particular activity, it is probably harmless,' says neurologist Terry Fife. Dizziness that occurs often, however, or is accompanied by other symptoms is potentially serious. Your doctor may want to check your blood pressure and pulse, rule out any neurological, inner ear or migraine-type problem, and check your blood for anaemia, diabetes or thyroid problems.

Dizziness and black-outs that occur especially when looking upwards may be due to compression in the neck of the circulation to your brain. It is important to see a doctor to rule out this possibility, too.

Dizziness that's followed by fainting could be a warning sign of heart disease. A stroke can also cause vertigo or dizziness, especially if you're also experiencing slurred speech, blurred or double vision, or numbness or tingling in the arms or legs.

If vertigo comes on completely out of the blue or is accompanied by any of these other symptoms, you need to see a doctor right away.

It's important to stay physically active to maintain muscle strength as well as balance, says Dr Hoffman. Take your usual walks. Go shopping. Ride an exercise bike. As long as you move carefully at 'high-risk' times – holding handrails when walking down stairs, for example, or moving slowly after changing position – you're unlikely to lose your balance.

Wear flat shoes. Apart from the fact that walking on heels is dangerous when the world seems to be spinning, flat shoes give you more contact with the ground. More contact makes it easier for your brain to process information about your posture. This prevents inner-ear confusion and can help to prevent falls, says Dr Fife.

Use a night-light. Darkness can be especially treacherous for those with inner-ear problems because the brain, which normally compensates for the lack of information from the ears by drawing on more information from the eyes, does not receive enough visual clues to help the body stay properly orientated. Simply using a night-light could help to prevent dizziness or falls, says Dr Fife.

'If you have significant inner-ear problems, never swim in the dark,' Dr Fife adds. 'When underwater, some people are unable to tell what's up and what's down. A few of my patients have nearly drowned because they could not tell which way to come up for air and kept groping at the bottom of the swimming pool, convinced that down was the direction to go to come up for air.'

Beware of thick carpets. Deep pile carpets may feel good underfoot, but the cushioning can make it harder for your body to stay properly orientated, says Dr Fife. This is because the soft surface makes it harder for the nerves in the feet to detect the changes in joint position used to maintain balance.

Fit grab rails in bathrooms. The bathroom is a high-risk area because the combination of slippery surfaces and off-balance movements – bending over to brush your teeth, for example – make falls more likely. And bathing or showering make blood vessels dilate and trigger a drop in blood pressure. If you move too quickly, your brain may not get enough oxygen and you'll feel light-headed and dizzy, says Dr Hoffman. So fit grab bars beside the bath, in the shower and next to the loo. Then you'll have something to hold if dizziness strikes.

Do just *one* thing

Know your dizziness triggers. Dizziness and vertigo that occur at predictable times – on getting out of bed first thing in the morning, for example, or when you suddenly change position – may indicate an easily treated inner-ear disorder.

A sudden drop in blood pressure can trigger dizziness, and this can be caused by a variety of things, including sudden temperature changes, such as when you go from a heated house out into cold winter air. Hunger is a trigger for some people, and having just eaten is a trigger for others. Hunger-related dizziness may be related to low blood sugar, while dizziness after a meal can be blamed on digestive processes that 'steal' blood from the brain, says neurologist Terry Fife.

If you've recently had a cold, don't be surprised if you start experiencing dizziness. Cold viruses sometimes travel to the inner ear and cause inflammation, damaging the inner-ear balance mechanism, and resulting in vertigo. The condition usually clears up within a few months.

Drink plenty of water. Our sense of thirst declines over time, which means older adults tend to run a little on the dry side. Even mild dehydration can cause drops in blood pressure that result in occasional dizziness, says Dr Fife.

Try to drink 8 to 10 glasses (250ml each) of water a day. 'Water is good, but when someone is dehydrated, sports drinks are even better,' says Dr Fife. They contain sodium and other electrolytes that help the body to retain fluids.

KITCHEN CURES

Dizziness is often accompanied by nausea. Ginger, a traditional remedy for sickness, has been shown to ease this nausea, says neurologist Terry Fife. Try fresh ginger, eaten by the slice or grated and used to make an infusion. Or take over-the-counter supplements, following label directions.

Reduce your salt intake. Attacks of vertigo that are accompanied by ringing or buzzing in the ears (tinnitus) and deafness may be caused by a condition called Ménière's disease, which occurs when fluid accumulates in the inner ear. If you have been diagnosed with this condition, then following a low-salt diet can help to reduce fluid build-ups that cause attacks of vertigo.

When buying packaged foods, check the labels for sodium content and look out for products labelled 'low sodium' or 'sodium-free'. It's fine to add a little salt to food at the table but don't use it during cooking. Adding salt to food during cooking imparts less flavour than when it is added at the table.

Consider motion-sickness remedies. If you experience dizziness associated with motion (car-sickness, air-sickness, sea-sickness), there are various over-the-counter medications available, such as Dramamine or Sea-Legs. Or your doctor may be able to give you a suitable drug on prescription. These medications help to reduce chemical signals from the inner ear to area of the brain that triggers vomiting. (See *Motion Sickness*, page 396)

Reduce stress. Doctors aren't sure why, but emotional stress tends to make inner-ear disorders worse. If you are experiencing vertigo or dizziness more than you used to and your doctor has ruled out some of the physical causes, it may be a sign that you need to unwind. Make time for long gentle walks. Practise deep breathing for a few minutes every day. Or simply let yourself relax and do nothing now and then.

Panic attacks are often associated with a feeling of dizziness due to over-breathing (hyperventilation). Breathing in and out steadily into a paper bag placed firmly over the nose and mouth is an effective way to combat this problem.

Make a list of the medicines you take. Then check it with your doctor, then with your pharmacist. Many prescription and over-the-counter drugs, including aspirin, antidepressants, antidiabetic drugs, tranquillizers and drugs for treating high blood pressure, can cause dizziness. Unsteadiness is also a common side-effect of sleeping tablets and is a significant cause of falls, particularly in the elderly. It may be worth considering other strategies to help you to sleep. However it is not a good idea to stop taking sleeping tablets suddenly: your doctor will be able to advise you on how to stop gradually. So, in some cases, changing your medicines may be all that's needed to reduce or eliminate dizziness.

Alcohol is a drug too. Dizziness and true vertigo are, of course, well-known effects of excess alcohol, as most of us have found out to our cost at one time or another. These effects can be particularly hazardous if you mix alcohol with many sorts of medication or 'recreational' drugs.

DRY EYES
18 moistening ideas

Dry eyes occur when the eyes don't produce enough tears to keep them moist and comfortable. 'Eye dryness is a common problem,' says Anne Sumers, an ophthalmologist. Half of all people over the age of 40 experience eye dryness in some form, whether it's an intermittent or a persistent problem. Dry eyes are a part of ageing, she says.

Blinking your eye creates a three-layered film of water, oil and mucus. At around 40, the tear glands begin to slow down, producing less of this soothing eye liquid. The problem is even worse for women after the menopause because hormone changes dry up secretions, including tears, says Dr Sumers.

Dry eye is a simple name for a complex and irritating condition that is characterized by redness, burning, itching, scratchiness and sensitivity to light. Although it's usually just another symptom of ageing, dry eye may also be caused by exposure to environmental conditions, injuries to the eye or general health problems. Sun, wind, cold, indoor heating and air conditioning, staring at computer or television screens, and even high altitudes can cause further discomfort if you experience eye dryness.

As well as postmenopausal women, people who are more prone to dry eye include contact lens wearers, people who have had laser eye surgery, and those with arthritis and diabetes. A wide variety of medications, including decongestants, antihistamines, diuretics, anaesthetics, antidepressants, drugs for heart disease, ulcer remedies, chemotherapy and drugs containing beta-blockers can slow down your tear production and cause dry eyes, says ophthalmologist Stephen Pflugfelder.

But whether your eyes are only slightly dry, or really uncomfortably scratchy, it is possible to get your tear ducts flowing again. Here's how.

Apply a warm compress. If your eyes become dry every now and then, place a warm compress on your eyelids for 5 to 10 minutes at a time, two or three times each day, suggests Dr Pflugfelder. This can stimulate tear flow.

Opt for ointment. To combat cases in which eye dryness gets unbearable while you sleep, apply a tear-replacement/moisture-sealing ointment at bedtime to help ease your pain, says Dr Sumers. These extra-thick, over-the-counter eye ointments contain white petroleum jelly and mineral oil, and they last longer than drops.

To apply the ointment, pull the lower eyelid down, look up and squeeze a dab of ointment in the trough between your lid and eye. Blink

WHEN TO CONSULT A DOCTOR

See your doctor if you've used artificial tears for a few days, and made other changes in your environment, but still don't notice any improvement in the dryness of your eyes, says ophthalmologist Phillip Calenda. Your doctor will examine you for local allergic or infective eye conditions, and perhaps review your medication. Parkinson's disease, thyroid problems, colitis and diabetes, as well as some forms of arthritis, may also be associated with dry eyes.

Your doctor may refer you to an eye specialist who can test the quality and quantity of your tear production and examine your eyes in more detail. If your dry eyes are thought to be due primarily to insufficient tear production rather than excess evaporation, the eye specialist can insert a tiny collagen plug into your tear duct, says ophthalmologist Anne Sumers. The plug helps to conserve the tears that you produce and also keeps any artificial tears in your eyes for longer. If this trial plug relieves your symptoms, a permanent but reversible silicone plug may be inserted, or the tear duct closed irreversibly by laser or cautery.

Do just *one* thing

Try artificial tears. Available over-the-counter, artificial tears help to soothe tender, gritty eyes, says ophthalmologist Anne Sumers. Artificial tears can be used throughout the day, and come in different thicknesses. Thinner versions are less likely to blur your vision or leave a residue on your eyelashes, but they require more frequent application. Experiment to find the formulation that's right for you. And choose a preservative-free brand, because some preservatives can be toxic and damage the surface of the eye.

Good choices include Viscotears or Tears Naturale.

Whatever type you choose, this is how to insert the eyedrops. Gently pull down the lower lid and squeeze the drops into the corner of your eye near your nose. Keep the eye closed for a minute to make sure the drops stay in the eye. Use them from once to 10 times a day, depending on how severe your dryness problem is.

to spread the ointment around. These thick ointments can blur your vision for a while, so they're best applied when you're already in bed, advises Dr Sumers.

Pop out those contacts. If your eyes are feeling dry and irritated, the last thing you need is something sitting in them, like contact lenses. A contact lens is basically a sponge, and it soaks up natural and artificial tears. When there are fewer tears in the eye, contacts can make the eyes even drier, more irritated, light sensitive – and red.

So pop out those contact lenses, put on your glasses for the rest of the day, and apply artificial tears as often as you need to, says Dr Pflugfelder.

Wear wraparound shades. Because wind and sun can further dry out your eyes, wear sunglasses for extra protection, preferably wraparound shades, which extend past the sides of your eyes, suggests Dr Sumers.

Stay out of the direct line of fire. A blast of heat or air conditioning may be just what the rest of your body needs to make a car journey more bearable, but a direct flow of hot or cold air to your eyes can make them even more irritated. If you have dry eyes, point your car's air vents downwards, says Dr Sumers. That way, you'll get the relief you need from the outdoor elements without causing your dry eyes any more misery.

The same principle applies when flying. Make sure that the overhead air vents aren't pointed directly at your eyes. 'Aeroplanes are notoriously dry environments,' says Dr Sumers, 'so don't make matters worse for your eyes by letting cool air blow directly onto your face.'

Get fresh. Open a window and let in some fresh air, suggests Dr Sumers. This will let some much-needed moisture into the room, which could do your dry eyes a world of good.

Bring in some greenery. Buy a houseplant or two and put them in rooms where you spend lots of time. They can increase the amount of humidity in a room.

KITCHEN CURES

Eat nuts. Some specialists believe that a deficiency of certain essential fatty acids (EFAs), specifically omega-3 and omega-6, may contribute to dry eyes. For a good source of omega-6 EFAs, eat 12 almonds or pecan nuts a day, plus plenty of whole grains and legumes. Omega-3 EFAs can be found in salmon, mackerel, sardines and herring, and walnuts.

Avoid a common mistake.
Many people who feel their eyes getting dry and itchy take an antihistamine. That simply makes already dry eyes even drier, says Dr Sumers.

Blink a lot. If part of your job description includes spending long hours in front of a computer screen, take occasional blink breaks, says ophthalmologist Phillip Calenda. The same applies if your leisure time is spent in front of a television screen By constantly staring at the screen, you don't blink as much as you should, which causes eye moisture to evaporate more quickly. Taking a blink break will help to restore the much-needed tear film over your eyes. Spending five minutes each hour looking into the distance instead of reading or doing other close work will allow the eyes to blink more.

Keep a level head. Dr Pflugfelder has another practical suggestion for people with dry eyes who spend a majority of their working day in front of a computer screen. 'Position your computer so that it's directly at eye level or so that you're looking slightly down at the computer screen,' he says. 'If you're looking up at your computer screen, your eyes will be more wide open and will dry out more quickly.' Eye experts recommend making the following changes to your workstation to minimize eye dryness and eyestrain if you work on a computer all day.

- Screen distance: sit about 50cm from the computer monitor, a little further away than reading distance, with the top of the screen at or below eye level.

- Equipment: choose a monitor that tilts or swivels and has both contrast and brightness controls.

- Furniture: make sure you have an adjustable chair.

- Reference material: put papers on a document holder so that you don't have to keep looking back and forth, turning your head and refocusing your eyes.

- Lighting: modify lighting to eliminate reflections or glare.

- Rest breaks: take rest breaks from time to time and blink often to keep your eyes from drying out.

Dry Mouth
19 mouthwatering solutions

For some people, the sensation of having a dry mouth is simply an infrequent nuisance. For others, it's quite a serious problem, says dentist John Caimi. Mouth dryness, known medically as xerostomia, can be really debilitating. If left untreated, it can lead to mouth sores, tooth decay and other oral health problems. Your mouth needs adequate saliva flow in order to coat and lubricate oral tissues, which in turn helps to prevent tooth decay and gum disease.

According to Dr Caimi, dry mouth affects a wide variety of people, including older adults whose mouths naturally dry out over time, as well as people who have diabetes, anxiety disorder or an autoimmune disease known as Sjögren's syndrome, in which a dry mouth occurs in association with dry eyes and other symptoms. In cancer patients, dry mouth is often the result of chemotherapy or radiation therapy.

Most often though, mouth dryness is a side-effect of prescription drugs or over-the-counter medication, says family doctor Stephen Amiel. Common culprits include blood pressure tablets (enalapril or captopril), antihistamines (such as cyclizine), antidepressants (such as amitriptyline or fluoxetine), codeine or morphine-containing analgesics and decongestants (such as pseudoephedrine hydrochloride).

As the population ages and prescription drugs become more common, dry mouth is becoming more widespread. Here are some suggestions to help relieve the dryness, protect soft tissue and prevent the tooth decay that results from having a dry mouth.

Chew sugarless gum. Chewing stimulates the salivary glands. Try sugarless gum that contains xylitol, a sweetening agent that reduces cavity-causing bacteria, says dentist Dan Peterson.

Sip water regularly. Take frequent sips of water throughout the day. Swirl it around in your mouth and through your teeth to combat the dry feeling, says Dr Caimi.

Drink eight 250ml glasses of water each day, says dental hygienist Anne Bosy. The more active you are, the more water you need. If you're working out in the gym, take a water bottle with you. If you have an all-day meeting, make sure there are jugs of water on the table.

Suck on some ice. Ice chips are another source of water, says Dr Caimi. But suck on the ice, don't chew it. Chewing ice can damage your teeth.

Rinse away the pain. Chronic dryness will make your mouth more easily irritated and sore, because one of the main jobs of saliva is to neutralize the erosive acids from plaque, according to Dr Caimi. Rinse your mouth out with a cupful of warm water into which you have mixed ¼ teaspoon of baking soda and ⅛ teaspoon of salt. This soothing combination neutralizes acids and draws out infection from gum tissues.

Suck sugar-free boiled sweets. Sucking hard sweets stimulates saliva flow, says Dr Peterson, who recommends citrus or mint-flavoured sweets.

Crunch crudités. Diets high in fibre and bulk also seem to stimulate salivary glands. Anne Bosy suggests eating fibrous foods, such as raw carrots, celery or apples at mealtimes and as snacks. These rough-textured foods also clean your tongue as you chew and swallow, which is good for overall oral hygiene.

Say no to sweets. Limit your intake of sweet, sticky, sugary foods if you're experiencing a dry mouth. Your lack of saliva will keep these foods stuck to your teeth, increasing your risk of cavities, says Dr Peterson.

Quench your thirst wisely. Alcohol and caffeine-containing drinks can make a dry mouth worse, says Dr Amiel, and sugary drinks will further damage teeth in a mouth that's often dry. So stick to water, sugar-free or milky drinks, or fruit juices that are not too acidic, like apple or pear juice. Lukewarm drinks are more effective than hot or cold drinks for quenching thirst and you should also avoid hot drinks if your mouth is sore.

Control your bad habits. Tobacco will make a dry mouth worse, says

WHEN TO CONSULT A DOCTOR

Regular dental check-ups are an important first line of defence against dry mouth syndrome, because your dentist will be better able to diagnose any problems in an earlier stage, when they can easily be corrected. Your dentist may also be able to recommend a fluoride mouth rinse or gel as an extra safeguard for your teeth, says dentist John Caimi.

If you notice a red, dry irritation in your mouth or a lack of saliva, see either a doctor or dentist. The sooner you get help, the better, because it's easier to correct the problem in an early stage.

A dry mouth may be the first sign of oral thrush, says family doctor Stephen Amiel. This yeast infection can result from the use of antibiotics or steroid-containing asthma inhalers, but occasionally signifies the presence of diabetes, immune deficiency or a blood disorder.

If you think that a prescription medication is causing a dry mouth, tell your doctor immediately, says Dr Caimi. In some cases, a different prescription or a simple adjustment in dosage may stop mouth dryness and the problems that can go with it.

Dr Amiel, as will many 'recreational' drugs like cannabis, ecstasy, cocaine, amphetamines and opiates.

Avoid irritants. Spicy or salty foods may cause pain in a dry mouth, says Dr Caimi, as can orange juice because of its high acid content.

Choose a high fluoride toothpaste. When saliva production is low, your risk of cavities and gum disease is high. Dr Peterson recommends brushing at least twice a day with an extra-strength fluoride toothpaste.

Here's a fluoride-treatment programme that Dr Peterson recommends for extra tooth protection. After brushing your teeth and just before you go to bed, apply toothpaste with your toothbrush or a cotton bud to gums and teeth. Let it sit for one minute, then swish for one minute to force the paste to cover all your teeth and gums. Then spit out all the excess paste, but don't rinse your mouth. Go to bed with the fluoride residue on these surfaces. Do this again in the morning, and don't eat or drink anything for 30 minutes after this routine. This procedure should be done once or twice a day for four to six weeks.

Watch out for foaming agent. If you have mouth dryness, avoid toothpaste that contains the foaming agent sodium lauryl sulphate, because it can irritate gum tissue, says Dr Peterson. Virtually all brands contain this ingredient, but health food stores sell various toothpastes without it. Ask in the shop for advice. A company called Bay House Aromatics sells toothpastes free of this additive. Find them at 88 St Georges Road, Brighton BN2 1EE, or online at www.bay-house.co.uk.

Use a mouthwash. Use an antibacterial mouthwash such as Corsodyl or Chlorohex, that doesn't contain alcohol or sugar, suggests Dr Caimi. Alcohol further dries out your mouth and can irritate already sensitive gum tissues, while sugar causes tooth decay and cavities, which you are more prone to if you have mouth dryness.

Change your toothbrush frequently. When your toothbrush has a build-up of toothpaste in between the bristles, it's time to buy a new one, says Anne Bosy. Over time, toothbrushes harbour bacteria and can infect your mouth with the bacteria that cause bad breath. Buy a new toothbrush every couple of months to keep bacteria and bad breath at bay.

Brush every time you eat. One of the main tasks of saliva is to dislodge trapped food morsels in your mouth, says Anne Bosy. So if you lack the normal amount of saliva, food particles can hang around for longer in your mouth and cause bad breath. The solution is to brush your teeth after every meal, morsel or midnight snack.

Soak your dentures. Dentures make people with dry mouths more susceptible to infection from yeast organisms, which adhere to the plastic. Soak your dentures overnight in a denture-soaking solution such as Steradent to prevent infection, says Dr Peterson. Rinse dentures thoroughly in the morning before putting them in.

Moisturize the air. Use a humidifier in your bedroom to get some moisture into the air and to cut down mouth dryness at night, says Dr Peterson. If you're a mouth breather, try to breathe through your nose at night to prevent saliva from evaporating while you sleep.

If you are breathing through your mouth because your nose is

KITCHEN CURES

Use sauces and gravies on foods to add more moisture, suggests dentist Dan Peterson. A dry mouth can make dry foods taste like sawdust. A little moisture makes foods much more palatable.

Drinking fluids frequently throughout a meal will increase the moisture content of your mouth, too, making food easier to swallow, and improving your sense of taste.

blocked, try using salt water nose drops, a natural decongestant, suggests Dr Amiel. Dissolve a level teaspoon of table salt in half a litre of water (or a generous pinch in a cup), tilt your head back slightly and put a little of the solution into each nostril. You could use an over-the-counter nasal decongestant for a few days, but overuse can make the problem worse. If nasal blockage is chronic or one-sided, see your doctor.

If all else fails, fake it. For better overall comfort and lubrication of your mouth, Anne Bosy suggests over-the-counter saliva substitutes in the form of rinses, gels and sprays for people who have chronically dry mouth or little or no salivary action. These saliva substitutes include many of the same enzymes and minerals as real saliva and help to keep mouth tissues lubricated. Use two or three times a day (one of those times being just before bedtime).

DRY SKIN AND WINTER ITCHING

10 ways to keep the moisture in

Often, winter means dry, itchy skin. But it doesn't have to. Even if you live in a cold, dry climate – or keep warm in a centrally heated home or an office with drying, warm-air heat – you can maintain healthy soft skin. Because the dryness results from a lack of *water*, not oil, all you need to do is replenish that moisture. Here are some moisturizing strategies.

Ignore the adverts. 'Nothing beats plain petroleum jelly or mineral oil as a moisturizer,' says dermatologist Howard Donsky. In fact, if you don't mind the greasiness, virtually any kitchen vegetable oil – such as rapeseed or sunflower oil – can be used to combat dry skin. They are effective, safe and pure skin lubricants – and cheap, too. They have one drawback, though. All tend to be greasy.

'People like things that smell good, feel good, and don't make them feel like an oven-ready chicken,' says dermatologist Hillard Pearlstein. So if you prefer an over-the-counter moisturizer, go for it. Just be aware that they're all basically alike; there is no scientific proof that any one product is better for you than another.

Use oatmeal to heal. Research suggests that people first discovered the skin-soothing effects of oatmeal nearly 4000 years ago. Many of us are still discovering it today. 'Oatmeal can work in the bath as a soothing agent,' says Dr Donsky. Just pour two cups of colloidal oatmeal (like Aveeno, available from pharmacies) into a bath of lukewarm water. The term colloidal simply means that the oatmeal has been ground to a fine powder that remains suspended in water.

'You can also use oatmeal as a soap substitute,' he says. Tie some colloidal oatmeal in a handkerchief, dip it in water, squeeze out the excess and use it as you would a normal flannel.

Don't try to drink dryness away. Many beauty writers recommend drinking 'at least seven or eight glasses of water per day' to keep your skin hydrated and prevent dryness. And while adequate water is essential for good health, don't believe the hype that you'll see results in your skin.

'If you're totally dehydrated, your skin will become dry,' says dermatologist Kenneth Neldner. 'But if you are normally hydrated, you cannot possibly counteract or correct dry skin by drinking water.'

Put water where it counts. 'The best way to get water into the skin is by soaking in it,' says Dr Pearlstein. He recommends a 15-minute soak in *lukewarm*, not hot, water. Forget the idea that you should bathe every day. The rule of thumb for dry skin is bathe less and use cooler water.

Lubricate the skin. 'Follow each bath with a moisturizer,' says Dr Pearlstein. 'The tendency is for all the moisture that has soaked into the skin to evaporate. If you bath frequently, a moisturizer is doubly important. The moisturizer is what holds the water in.' Many people think that moisturizer puts oil back into the skin, but that's not totally true. Instead, he says, moisturizers applied after the bath help to keep water in the skin and therefore prevent drying.

Dry yourself damp – then stop. 'It's much more effective to apply moisturizer to damp skin immediately after bathing than to put it on totally dry skin,' says Dr Neldner. That doesn't mean you have to hop from the bath or shower soaking wet and immediately apply lotion. But a couple of pats with a towel will make you as dry as you want to be before you apply lotion, he says. 'You're trying to trap a little water in the skin, and that's the fundamental rule of fighting off dryness.'

Select creamy soaps. Dr Pearlstein recommends that people with dry skin reach instead for creamy soaps like Neutrogena, Dove or Oilatum. These soaps have extra fatty substances – cold cream, cocoa butter, coconut oil or lanolin – added during the manufacturing process.

These fatty soaps may not clean quite as well, but they are less irritating to dry skin.

WHEN TO CONSULT A DOCTOR

If your dry skin becomes itchy, cracked, red and painful you may have atopic eczema or another form of dermatitis. Scratching will only make this worse, so, in addition to your creams and moisturizers, you may need antihistamines and steroid-containing creams or ointments from your doctor. Yellow, oozing areas may indicate a secondary bacterial infection requiring antibiotics.

If the skin has red and flaky patches, you may have psoriasis, seborrhoeic eczema or a fungal skin infection, all of which may respond to prescription medicines from your doctor.

Occasionally, dry skin may be an indication of an underlying condition like an underactive thyroid or diabetes.

Drying and wrinkling of the skin is a natural part of the ageing process, as our skin loses its ability to produce natural oils and collagen. In women, the decline in natural oestrogens at the menopause is partly responsible. Hormone replacement therapy may help menopausal dry skin: you should however weigh up with your doctor the wider risks and benefits of this treatment before opting for it.

Don't wash so often. If it's not dirty, don't wash it, advises Dr Pearlstein. 'Dermatologists see more problems from the overuse of soap than we ever do from the lack of it.'

Let a humidifier help. Dry skin and itching is exacerbated by central heating, says Dr Pearlstein. It can reduce indoor humidity to as low as 10 per cent, whereas 30 to 40 per cent is closer to ideal for keeping moisture in your skin. For that reason, our experts all recommend using humidifiers during those dry winter months – but with a proviso.

Humidifiers are like air conditioners – you would need a huge unit to humidify a whole house. Much better to put a small unit next to your bed, instead. If you use a humidifier in your bedroom, then close the door to keep moisture in. It might also help to leave the bathroom door open when you bath or shower. Every little bit of humidity helps.

Keep it cool. One good way to combat winter itching is to turn down the central heating thermostat. 'Keeping your house on the cool side in winter might help,' says Dr Pearlstein. 'That's because cool air has an anaesthetic effect – it makes your skin feel good.' When you overheat your house, blood vessels dilate, and when blood vessels dilate, the itching/tingling cycle begins.

EARACHE AND EAR INFECTION

29 ways to stop the pain

Earaches can be very painful and, unfortunately, they tend to occur at night. The explanation is a combination of anatomy and pressure. Eustachian tubes lead from the back of the throat to the middle ear, and blocked tubes are the most common cause of earache in children and adults.

During the day, you hold your head up and your eustachian tubes drain naturally into the back of your throat. Also, as you chew and swallow, the muscles of the eustachian tubes contract, opening them and allowing air into the middle ear.

But at night when you sleep and your head isn't upright, the tubes can't drain as easily. And you're not swallowing as often, so they aren't getting as much air. The air already in the middle ear is absorbed and a vacuum occurs, sucking the eardrum inwards. Several hours after you've fallen asleep, your eustachian tubes may become blocked, especially if you have a cold, sinus infection or allergy.

Sometimes earache signifies a middle-ear infection called otitis media. This condition is more common in children than adults, because as we grow, our eustachian tubes become narrower, longer and less prone to plugging up. Another reason children get ear infections is that the nerves to the area may not be fully developed in some babies, which can affect the eustachian tubes. And children in day nurseries are exposed to more colds, which can lead to ear infections.

In adults, a middle-ear infection arises when sinuses get blocked as a result of an allergy or a cold, or when the eustachian tubes get clogged during an aeroplane descent.

The usual symptoms of a middle-ear infection are pain and hearing loss, but adults and children can get ear infections without pain. Sometimes the eardrum perforates and the ear discharges mucus, pus or blood. The relief of pressure behind the eardrum often relieves the pain, and the perforation usually heals on its own. In fact most ear infections will heal just as quickly without antibiotics as with them, says family doctor Stephen Amiel, usually within a week to 10 days. Some studies suggest that pain is relieved a little quicker than with painkillers on their own, but antibiotics can cause side-effects of their own, such as diarrhoea.

Other things cause earaches, too. Infections of the ear canal, known as external otitis or swimmer's ear, can trigger pain. Atmospheric pressure from flying or deep-sea diving can cause ears to ache even if they aren't

WHEN TO CONSULT A DOCTOR

If you have earache, you need to see a doctor if the pain doesn't settle within a few days. But you should also make an appointment if you suffer from hearing loss or if your ears stay plugged up for more than a couple of days after a cold. You could already have an ear infection or fluid in the middle ear.

Ear infections rarely result in permanent hearing loss, says family doctor Stephen Amiel. Children with persistent fluid in the middle ear (glue ear) may be delayed in their language and educational development if the condition persists long-term. Doctors now recommend a wait-and-see policy for glue ear, as symptoms often clear up within a few months, and there's no evidence of benefit from medication.

Sometimes, a small operation is recommended, to insert grommets (tiny tubes to drain the fluid and allow air to circulate across the eardrum), and/or to remove the adenoids.

infected. Odd things, such as tiny clippings from a haircut, can fall into the ear canal and irritate your eardrum. Even odder things can find their way into children's ears: beads, peas and sweets are the most common. 'I've fished a good few things out of adult's ears too,' says Dr Amiel. 'Pen tops, pencil rubbers, cotton bud tips, and a wad of cotton wool that my patient said must have been there for at least fifteen years!'

Then there is referred pain – a problem that exists somewhere else – that makes your ears ache. These earaches can originate in your teeth, tonsils, throat, tongue or jaw.

When your ears ache, you need to see a doctor. But until you do, here are some quick pain stoppers.

Take painkillers. If you have an earache, take paracetamol or ibuprofen. A dose at bedtime may be enough to let you sleep.

Sit up. A few minutes upright decreases swelling and starts your eustachian tubes draining. Swallowing also helps ease the pain. If you can, prop your head up slightly while you sleep to get better drainage, says Dudley Weider, an ear, nose and throat specialist.

Have a drink. Swallowing triggers the muscular action that helps your eustachian tubes to open and drain, Dr Weider adds. Open tubes mean less pain.

Wiggle your ear. Here's a test to help determine whether you have otitis externa (an external problem like swimmer's ear) or otitis media (an internal middle-ear infection). Hold your ear, says Donald Kamerer, an ear, nose and throat expert. If you can wiggle it without pain, the problem is probably in the middle ear. If moving your ear causes pain, then the infection is probably in the outer ear canal.

Use warm drops. Stand a bottle of baby oil, olive oil or mineral oil in a bowl of hand-hot water, says Dr Weider. Leave it in the water until it reaches body temperature. Put a drop or two of oil into the offending ear to lessen the pain.

Note: If you think the eardrum may be ruptured or punctured – there is usually a discharge when this happens – then do not drop fluids into the ear.

Try a herbal approach. Earache is both painful and difficult to treat, says clinical herbalist Douglas Schar. This is because of the ear's structure – namely a complex collection of interconnected channels, which provide a perfect place for bacteria to hide. The solution, says Schar, is a herbal double whammy.

The first weapon is echinacea tablets, available from health food stores, pharmacies and some supermarkets. These will stimulate the immune system to clear the infection at the root of the problem.

The second weapon is the topical application of garlic or mullein oil. These oils have antimicrobial and anti-inflammatory properties, targeting the germs that cause the infection and the inflammation that causes the pain. You can buy garlic oil, mullein oil or a blend of the two in most health food stores. Apply two to four drops in the affected ear. Cover the ear with a little wad of cotton wool to stop the oil from running out. Apply more drops every six to eight hours, using fresh cotton wool each time.

According to Schar, this combination will speed up the healing of most ear infections; he recommends continuing the treatment for a week after the infection appears to have gone.

Note: If you think the eardrum may be ruptured or punctured – there is usually a discharge when this happens – then do not drop fluids into the ear.

Chew gum. Most people know this is one way to open their ears when flying, but have you considered it at midnight? The muscular action of chewing may open the eustachian tubes.

Yawn. Yawning moves the muscle that opens the eustachian tubes even better than chewing gum or sucking on mints.

Drying-out cures for swimmer's ear

All it takes to come down with a stubborn bout of swimmer's ear is the combination of ears and unrelenting moisture. It's like keeping your hands in dishwater. The skin gets macerated and leathery, says ear, nose and throat specialist Brian Hands. The ears are constantly bathed in water – swimming, showering, shampooing. Then you try and dry them with cotton buds. These take off the top layer of skin along with protective bacteria, allowing harmful bacteria to invade.

Swimmer's ear begins as an itchy ear. Left untreated, it can turn into a full-blown infection. The pain can be excruciating. Once infection sets in, you'll need a doctor's help and a course of antibiotics to cure it. But there are plenty of things you can do to stop the pain getting worse, and even more to stop it before it starts.

Try an over-the-counter remedy. Most pharmacists sell ear drops that can help to dry up swimmer's ear. If ear itchiness is still your only symptom, one of these preparations might rescue it from infection, says family doctor Dan Drew. Use it each time your ears get wet.

Plug up the problem. Wear earplugs when you swim, shampoo, or shower to keep the water out, says Dr John House, who looks after the US Olympic swimming team. Wax or silicone plugs that can be softened and shaped to fit your ear are available from chemists.

Swim on the surface. Even if you're battling swimmer's ear, you can keep on swimming, says Dr Drew. Swim on the surface, which will let less water into the ear than when you break the surface.

Soothe away pain with heat. Warmth – a towel straight from the tumble dryer, a covered hot-water bottle, a heating pad set on low – will help to ease the pain.

Leave earwax alone. Earwax harbours friendly bacteria and coats the ear canal, protecting it from

Don't grit your teeth. Referred earache can often result from spasm in the strong muscles around the temporo-mandibular joint, where your lower jaw articulates with your skull (see *Jaw Pain and TMJ Problems*, page 364). All sorts of things can cause this type of pain, says Dr Amiel. The list includes clenching your teeth, grinding your teeth at night, excessive gum chewing, nail biting or cradling a phone between your shoulder and the side of your head, a bad bite or dental malocclusion. Stress can make matters worse. See your dentist or doctor.

moisture, say Drs Kamerer and House. Cooperate with your natural defences by *not* cleaning the wax out.

Make substitute wax. Since the irritation of swimmer's ear wears away earwax, you can manufacture your own version using petroleum jelly. Moisten a cotton wool ball with the jelly, says Dr Hands, and tuck it gently, like a plug, just in the edge of your ear. It will absorb any moisture, keeping your ear warm and dry.

Use spirit or vinegar. Ear drops of white vinegar, surgical spirit or a mixture of the two will kill germs and dry your ears at the same time. Put your head down, with the affected ear up. Pull your ear upwards and backwards (to help straighten the canal) and squeeze a dropperful of vinegar into the ear canal. Wiggle your ear to get the liquid to the bottom of the canal. Then tilt your head the other way and let the vinegar drain out.

Note: Surgical spirit and vinegar treatments are for prevention, not treatment, of swimmer's ear, as they sting too much if the ear is already inflamed. Also, *never* put any fluids into an ear if you think the eardrum might be perforated.

Protect with baby oil. This can be a preventative solution before swimming. Apply as you would the spirit or vinegar.

Be careful where you swim. You are less likely to pick up bacteria in a treated pool than you are in a pond, says Dr Drew. Don't swim in dirty water.

Take out your hearing aid. If you wear a hearing aid, you can get swimmer's ear without going near the water. A hearing aid has an earplug effect, explains Dr Hands. It picks up moisture that lodges in the ear canal. And trapped moisture can breed the germs that brew an infection.

Take your hearing aid out of your ear as often as possible to give your ear a chance to dry out.

Hold your nose. If you're flying at 32,000 feet when your ears begin to ache, pinch your nostrils shut, take a mouthful of air and then, using your cheek and throat muscles, force the air into the back of your nose, as if you were trying to blow your fingers off the end of your nose. A pop will tell you when you have equalized the pressure inside and outside your ear.

Don't sleep during an aeroplane descent. If you want to sleep while flying, close your eyes at the beginning, not at the end of the trip. Rapid changes in air pressure occur during ascent as well, but ear pain tends to

Prevention — much better than cure

Ear infections are the most common cause of hearing loss in children. While you can't prevent ear infections, there are some things you can do that may help to reduce the chances of your child getting them.

Choosing childcare. Children exposed to large groups of other children are more likely to come into contact with the bugs that cause ear infections. Parents who need day care for a child prone to ear infections may want to consider a small setting, such as a childminder, rather than a nursery, until their child outgrows ear infections.

Breastfeed. Research shows that breastfeeding protects infants from otitis media. In one US study of 306 infants being seen in GP surgeries, twice as many formula-fed infants as breastfed infants developed an ear infection between the ages of six months and one year. In fact, formula feeding was the most significant factor associated with ear infections, even more important than being in a day nursery.

An earlier study of 237 infants in Helsinki, Finland, showed that 6 per cent of breastfed babies and 19 per cent of formula-fed babies had developed middle-ear infections by the end of their first year. By the age of three, only 6 per cent of those breastfed developed an infection compared with 26 per cent of those fed formula. Researchers believe that the difference is due to breastfed infants having an enhanced immune response to respiratory infections.

If you bottle-feed your baby, experts advise holding her in a fairly upright position during feeds so her head is above her tummy level. This position helps to keep the eustachian tubes from getting blocked, reducing the risk of ear infections.

Stop smoking. Smoking can push an adult with ear problems towards an infection by filling the air with irritants, which leads to eustachian tube congestion. Secondhand smoke can be just as hard on children prone to ear problems.

Beware of open fires. A smoky fire in your grate or wood-burner can fill the air with hard-to-breathe and hard-to-tolerate toxins.

Be patient. Children often outgrow ear infections by the age of three

be more acute during descent because atmospheric pressure increases as you get closer to the ground. You don't swallow as often when you're asleep, so your ears won't keep up with pressure changes during descent, and you might wake up in pain.

Head off trouble. Before you have a problem, use an over-the-counter decongestant. For instance, if you have to fly and you know your sinuses are going to back up and block your ears, take a decongestant or use nose drops an hour before you land, Dr Weider suggests. At home, if you have a stuffy head, use a decongestant at night before you get into bed to help avoid the middle-of-the-night ache.

Note: Nasal decongestants should not be used for more than a few days at a time – after a while you can't stop using them without causing rebound congestion.

Advice for swimmers. Like people who fly, scuba divers must be able to equalize the pressure inside their ears with that of the water around them, or they can experience ear trouble. Shallow diving is more likely to cause an earache because the greatest changes in air volume occur in relatively shallow water, less than 10m deep. Avoid super-snug earplugs and wet suits with tight-fitting hoods, which prevent equalization of pressure during descent, recommends family doctor Gary Becker.

For recreational swimmers, swimming on the surface puts less pressure on the eardrums than swimming underwater, says Dan Drew, a family doctor and keen swimmer. To avoid eardrum stress, don't dive deeper than a metre or so.

Avoid aggravating the situation. If you tend to get ear problems when you have a cold or an allergy such as hay fever, try to avoid or delay flying, and avoid diving until your head clears.

Nothing smaller than your elbow. Resist the temptation to poke around in an itchy or blocked ear with fingers, cotton buds or pencils, says Dr Amiel. You'll push any wax or debris further into the ear and risk damaging the ear canal or drum.

EARWAX
4 steps to clean ears

Earwax, also known as cerumen, protects your eardrum from dust and debris. Left alone, it does its job quite nicely, migrating harmlessly to the outer ear as it dries, only to be replaced by fresh wax that forms in the ear canal.

Occasionally, the wax forms a hard plug next to the eardrum that has to be removed by a doctor. The wax plug can cause partial hearing loss – which may be progressive, tinnitus (noises in the ear), earache or a sensation of fullness in the ear. These symptoms tend to arise quite suddenly, when water trickles behind the wax plug after swimming or washing your hair and is trapped against the eardrum. A wax plug can also trap bacteria, making infection more likely.

Here's how to prevent that from happening.

Stick nothing in your ear. Never put anything smaller than your elbow into your ear, is a motto that ear doctors swear by. Never stick anything sharp – a toothpick, a pencil tip, a paper clip – into your ear, because you could tear your eardrum. Don't use a cotton bud or finger either, says ear, nose and throat expert George Facer. You may think you're cleaning out your ear, but you are actually ramming the wax deeper so that it acts like a plug over your eardrum.

Drop in a softening fluid. Try olive oil, almond oil or sodium bicarbonate ear drops (5 per cent) in a dropper bottle from the pharmacy (these are very inexpensive and only contain sodium bicarbonate, glycerol and purified water). Some over-the-counter proprietary remedies contain organic solvents which can irritate the sensitive skin in the ear canal, and are best avoided.

Pour a generous amount of the softening liquid into the ear, says family doctor Stephen Amiel. Lie on your side for 10 to 15 minutes with that ear uppermost. Repeat on the other side if necessary. Hard wax may require treatment twice a day for several days. Remember that the liquid you pour in may settle behind the wax plug at first, making your symptoms temporarily worse.

Once the wax is soft, you're ready to rinse. Fill a bowl with body-temperature water. Then fill a rubber bulb syringe with the water and, holding your head over the bowl, squirt the water *gently* into your ear canal. The stream of water should be under very little pressure. Turn your head to the side and let the water run out. 'I've syringed my own ears with our turkey baster,' says Dr Amiel. 'It worked brilliantly. I popped the baster in the dishwasher afterwards and no-one was any the wiser!'

Note: No liquids at all should be used if there is a possibility that you have a perforation of the eardrum, warns Dr Amiel. See your doctor instead: you may need a referral to a specialist for suction removal of the wax.

Blow-dry your ears. Don't rub your ears dry, say doctors. Instead, dry your ears with a hair dryer or drop a little surgical spirit into each ear to complete the drying.

Do this once you have rinsed your ears to clean them, as described above, and also every time you shower.

Let nature do its work. A monthly ear wash is more than enough for anyone, says ear specialist David Edelstein. Wash more often, and you will wash away the protective layer of wax that is supposed to be there.

EMPHYSEMA
18 tips for easy breathing

Emphysema is almost always a degenerative disease, developing gradually after many years of exposure to toxins or smoke, which destroy the alveoli or small air sacs in the lungs. Over time, the lungs lose their elasticity making breathing difficult. Emphysema is usually seen in combination with chronic bronchitis: together, these conditions are known as chronic obstructive pulmonary disease (COPD).

Although it develops slowly, the toll emphysema exacts on the lungs is anything but minor. The alveoli, which normally stretch as they transport oxygen from the air to the blood, and then shrink as they force out carbon dioxide, lose their effectiveness. Patients with emphysema have difficulty exhaling because their damaged lungs trap air and cannot exchange stale air for fresh.

While there is no cure for emphysema, there are plenty of steps you can take to ease symptoms, prevent progression of the disease and enjoy life. Here's how to save your energy for the things you really want to do.

Stop smoking now! 'It's never too late to stop,' says Henry Gong, a specialist in preventive medicine. 'Even if you stop in your fifties or sixties, you'll help to slow down the deterioration of your lungs.' (See *Addiction*, page 21.)

Don't be a passive smoker. If the smoke from your own cigarettes can harm you, so can the secondhand smoke from your partner's cigarette or the air in a smoky pub. You can develop emphysema by inhaling the cigarette smoke from your smoking partner after decades of living together, says Dr Gong.

Avoid allergens. If you have known allergies that affect your breathing, it's doubly important to stay away from what causes them when you have emphysema, says Dr Gong (see *Allergies*, page 28).

WHEN TO CONSULT A DOCTOR

See a doctor if you experience any of the following symptoms:

• feeling confused or disorientated during an acute respiratory infection;

• sleepiness or slurred speech during an acute respiratory infection;

• blood or any other change in colour, thickness, odour or the amount of mucus that you cough;

• worsening shortness of breath, coughing or wheezing;

• waking up short of breath more than once a night;

• fatigue that lasts more than one day;

• ankles that stay swollen even after a night of sleeping with your feet elevated;

• needing to use more pillows or sleep in a chair instead of a bed so that you don't get short of breath;

• morning headaches, restlessness and dizzy spells;

You should have regular check-ups to review your medication and measure any changes in your breathing capacity. Your doctor may want you to see a specialist respiratory nurse or chest physician for more detailed investigation of your breathing and how different medications might help. The specialist might also assess you for home oxygen therapy if your blood oxygen levels are persistently very low.

See your doctor if you want help to quit smoking. Finally, you should make sure you get an annual flu immunization, and have a one-off immunization against pneumococcal pneumonia.

Control what you can. You can't repair your airways. What you can do, says lung specialist Robert Sandhaus, is increase how efficiently you breathe, use your muscles and approach your work. You can rearrange your kitchen, for instance, so that you can do in five steps what used to take 10. Or buy a small trolley to help with your housework. Little changes like these can save energy.

Exercise. All our experts agree that regular exercise is vitally important to people with emphysema. What kinds are best?

'Walking is probably the best overall exercise,' says professor of medicine, Robert Teague. You should also exercise to tone the muscles in your upper body. Try using 500g or 1kg hand weights, and work the muscles in your neck, upper shoulders and chest. This is important because people with chronic lung diseases use their neck and upper respiratory chest muscles more than other people. Dr Teague advises people with asthma and emphysema to swim, because the activity allows them to breathe very humid air.

Eat less – but more often. As emphysema progresses and there is more obstruction to airflow, the lungs enlarge with trapped air. These enlarged lungs push down into the abdomen, leaving less room for the stomach to expand. That's why six small meals will make you feel better than three large ones. Your best bet, says Dr Teague, is to eat high protein meals, as these supply a lot of calories and not much bulk.

Watch your weight. Some people with emphysema gain a lot of weight and tend to retain fluid, says Dr Teague. It takes more energy to carry extra body weight. The closer you are to your ideal weight, the better for your lungs. Other emphysema patients are very skinny, he adds. 'Because they have to breathe harder, they expend more energy.' If you are under-weight, eat more calories, especially in the form of high-protein foods.

Become a champion breather. There are several things you can do to get the maximum benefit from each breath you take.

Make your breathing uniform. When Dr Teague and his colleagues studied 20 patients with advanced emphysema, they found that even under normal conditions their subjects had very chaotic breathing patterns. 'We taught them normal breathing patterns, and it helped, at least in the short term.'

Breathe from your diaphragm. This is the most efficient way to breathe. Babies do it naturally. If you watch them, you'll see their tummies rise and fall with each breath.

To see whether you're breathing from your diaphragm or your chest, Francisco Perez, a neurologist, tells his patients to lie down, put phone directories on their stomachs, and see what happens to them when they breathe. If you are breathing from your diaphragm, the directory will rise with each intake of breath.

Keep those airways open. You can strengthen your breathing muscles by blowing out slowly through pursed lips for 30 minutes a day, says Dr Gong. Try to exhale for twice as long as it took you to breathe in. This will help you rid the lungs of stale air, so fresh air can get in.

Try vitamins C and E. Dr Sandhaus advises his emphysema patients to take a minimum of 250mg of vitamin C twice a day, and 350mg of vitamin E twice a day. But don't embark on any vitamin therapy without your doctor's okay. Dr Sandhaus believes that vitamins C and E may be helpful because they're antioxidants, which help to counteract the damage done by cigarette smoke.

Relax. If you see your disease as a threat, you will cause certain physiological mechanisms that can make your emphysema worse, says Dr Perez. 'When you're in a state of alarm, you demand a lot of oxygen. Alarm is created by the thought process, which you can control. That means you can also control the physiological mechanisms.

Sit up more in bed. People with emphysema usually find they sleep better if they are more upright in bed in a well-ventilated room. A triangular foam rubber wedge may work better than a pile of pillows: these can sometimes be obtained through your doctor, district nurse or chest clinic.

Wear loose clothes. Choose clothes that let your chest and abdomen expand freely. That means no tight belts, bras or underclothes.

Set small goals. One way to shift your focus from 'emphysema is incapacitating' to 'emphysema is something I have control over' is to set realistic small goals for yourself, says Dr Perez.

Exercise is a great way to boost your confidence, he says. Set yourself a goal based on physical evidence. Use charts and graphs to measure your progress. This gives you an objective measure of your ability to achieve something.

Join a support group. The British Thoracic Society encourages patients and their relatives to set up or join patient support groups. The groups are not run by doctors, though they may have access to respiratory specialists. The website (www.brit-thoracic.org.uk) has a list of UK support groups.

Ask a member of the family to be your coach. For those times when you're short of breath, it's really helpful to have a partner encourage and coach you through the episode, advises Dr Perez.

Don't isolate yourself socially. Some people with emphysema make pessimistic generalizations about their shortness of breath, says Dr Teague. They refuse invitations, because they're scared they might be out somewhere and get short of breath. Don't give up going to places you'd normally enjoy.

Pace yourself. Something people with emphysema have to learn to do is to take their time, says Dr Teague. 'You really can do what you want to do, but you have to do it at your own pace. That is not always an easy thing to do.'

Coordinate your breathing to your lifting. Lifting is easier if you lift while you exhale through pursed lips. Inhale while you rest. Also, if you have to climb stairs, climb while you exhale through pursed lips and inhale while you rest.

Don't use unnecessary sprays. You don't need to add to your respiratory problems by inhaling foreign substances. Use liquid or gel-type hair products and roll-on or solid deodorants. Avoid aerosol-spray household cleaners.

EYE STRAIN
10 tips to avoid it

People who spend as little as two hours a day staring at a computer screen can experience 'computer vision syndrome'. Symptoms include eye strain, blurred vision, headaches and dry eyes. Our eyes weren't designed to focus for hours on words on an illuminated background. If you find your eyes straining to read the paper or your vision blurring as you try to focus on your computer screen, here are some suggestions that may help.

Rest your eyes. Our experts say that it's the best way to relieve eye strain. And that's easier than you may think. 'You can do it while you're on the phone,' says ophthalmologist Samuel Guillory. 'If you don't need to read or write, just close your eyes while you're talking. People who practise this technique say that their eyes really feel better.'

Pay attention to lighting. 'It doesn't hurt your eyes to read in dim light, but you can strain them if the light doesn't provide enough contrast,' says Dr Guillory. 'Use a soft light that gives contrast, but not glare, when you read. And don't use any lamp that reflects light directly back into your eyes.'

Try reading glasses. You can buy impact-resistant, good-quality glasses quite inexpensively in chemists, says ophthalmologist David Guyton.

WHEN TO CONSULT A DOCTOR

Sometimes the cause of eye strain is a lot more serious than passing your 40th birthday. Strain can also be caused by eye misalignment, where one eye starts to turn in or out. This needs to be treated by an ophthalmologist who can suggest specific exercises, prescribe prism glasses or, if necessary, perform eye muscle surgery to realign the eyes. Other eye conditions, some general conditions and certain medications can also affect your visual acuity and cause eye strain.

• Eye conditions include: cataract (clouding of the lens); glaucoma (increased pressure within the eye, often familial); infections of the eye with viruses, fungi or parasites; injury to the eye surface; and clouding of the cornea following overuse of, or ill-fitting, contact lenses.

• General conditions which may be associated with changes in your vision include: diabetes; migraine; high blood pressure; thyroid disease; multiple sclerosis; AIDS; colitis; and some forms of arthritis.

• Medications which may cause blurred vision include: drugs used for urinary retention, prostate problems and incontinence; some antihistamines; digoxin; some anti-inflammatories; oral contraceptives; and tranquillizers.

If blurred vision or eye strain comes on suddenly for no obvious reason, is associated with pain in the eye (rather than irritation), redness, marked sensitivity to light or recent trauma, you need to see a doctor urgently, if necessary by going to your nearest A&E department.

Even if you have none of these other symptoms, you should see your optometrist and/or your doctor if your decline in vision cannot easily be corrected by glasses, or if you are taking medications or have other health problems that may be connected. Many cases of diabetes and high blood pressure, for example, only come to light when the eyes become affected.

The list is long, but the message is simple. If there is any doubt, seek professional advice.

Pick the right power. You are the best judge of which reading glasses work best for you. Choose the least powerful ones that let you read at the distance you want to, says Dr Guyton. 'If you buy glasses that are too powerful, you will see fine close up, but things will be blurred beyond that distance.'

Interrupt your work. Take hourly breaks if you use a computer for six

Insight with yoga

For Dr Meir Schneider, yoga wasn't only the key to gaining spiritual insight. It also was the key to simply gaining sight. Dr Schneider, who was born blind, claims that daily yoga exercises helped to cure his blindness. His vision is 20/60 and improving, he says. While it might be pushing scientific boundaries to say that yoga cures blindness, the following techniques may be helpful in handling eye strain.

Hands on eyes. 'Rub your hands together until they are warm.

Then close your eyes and put your palms over your eye sockets. Don't press on your eyes; just cover them. Breathe deeply and slowly and visualize the colour black. Do this for 20 minutes every day.'

Put your eyes 'on the blink'. Your eyes have their own masseuse – the eyelids. Make a point of consciously blinking your eyes 300 times every day, says Dr Schneider. 'Each blink cleanses your eyes and gives them a tiny little massage.'

to eight hours a day. Do some other work, get a coffee, go to the loo – just take your eyes off the screen for 10 to 15 minutes. Also, consider sometimes working from a printout instead of reading on-screen.

Darken your screen. Those aren't just letters and numbers on your screen. They're also tiny lightbulbs that send light directly into your eyes. You need to turn the wattage down, so to speak. 'Don't make the screen too bright,' advises Dr Guillory. 'Turn the brightness down to a dim level and then adjust the contrast to make up the difference.'

Work in the shade. When it comes to relieving eye strain, it's best to keep your computer in the dark. 'Shade your screen by creating a hood over it,' Dr Guillory suggests. 'Go to an art shop and buy a sheet of black cardboard. Put it on top of your monitor and fold both sides down over it. What you've done, essentially, is put your screen in a black box. So now you can turn the brightness down to a very low level.'

Brew a pot of eyebright tea. Cool it slightly and then soak a towel in the still-warm tea, says Meir Schneider, an expert in self-healing techniques. Lie down and place the warm towel over your closed eyes, leaving it there for 10 to 15 minutes. It will make your eye strain go away. Be careful not to get the tea in your eyes, though.

FATIGUE
37 energy-boosting hints

Everyone, at some time or another, feels tired. And who wouldn't like to have more energy than they have now?

The broad prescription from doctors is still the same: get plenty of rest, eat a balanced diet and exercise. But here, we go beyond these generalizations and offer more specific, high-energy suggestions.

Warm up. 'Give yourself an extra 15 minutes in the morning before you start your day,' says Vicky Young, an expert in occupational health. Then you won't start the day feeling rushed and tired.

Eat a three-piece breakfast. The three components of a good breakfast are carbohydrates, proteins and fats, advises family doctor Rick Ricer. You don't really need to *add* fat to your breakfast table. You will get plenty of fats, a good form of storable energy, in the proteins you eat.

A bowl of cereal (a complex carbohydrate) with milk (a source of protein) can get your day off to a good start. Wholemeal toast or muffins are also good complex-carbohydrate choices, and for protein you could add low-fat yoghurt or scrambled eggs.

But don't eat an ultra-high-carbohydrate breakfast laden with sugar. This can overactivate your insulin causing your blood sugar to drop, leaving you jittery and on edge. So resist that almond croissant on the way to work.

Plan the day. Take time each morning to set specific goals for the day, says David Sheridan, a doctor who works in local government. 'Decide what you want to do – don't let a routine control you.'

Tackle the source of the problem. Whether the problem is work or a family feud, you have to resolve it, says Dr Graham, former consultant to the US running association. If you can't resolve your problem, at least take a break from it. If you're trying to hold down a second job, resign. And if relatives or friends have overstayed their welcome, politely ask them to leave.

Switch off to turn on. Television is well known for lulling people into lethargy. Try reading instead, suggests Dr Ricer. It's more energizing.

Exercise for energy. 'Exercise actually gives you energy,' Dr Young says. Numerous studies back these words, including one by NASA, where more than 200 employees were put on a moderate and regular exercise programme. The results: 90 per cent said that they had never felt better, almost half said they felt less stress, and almost one-third reported that they slept better.

Dr Young recommends giving yourself a dose of energetic exercise – brisk walking is enough – three to five times a week for 20 to 30 minutes each time, and no later than two hours before bedtime.

Listen to your body. Despite all the good that exercise can do, it can also be addictive, and it can be harmful if you overdose. Listen to what your body is telling you. 'I really have to work at making myself take time off, and that a break will be good for me,' says endurance athlete Mary Trafton.

Tackle one thing at a time. Dr Sheridan advises making lists. People often feel tired when they think about all that they have to do, and they don't know where to start. Setting priorities and charting your progress as you make your way through the list will help you to remain focused and energetic.

Take one a day. If you're guilty of missing meals, dieting and not eating properly, Dr Young advises taking one multivitamin/mineral supplement a day. 'A lack of good nutrition can cause fatigue,' says Dr Ricer, 'and a supplement can help to make up for the missing nutrients. But don't expect a vitamin to give you instant energy.'

Herbal pick-me-ups. In the 1950s Russian researchers began looking for drugs that increased resistance to stress, strain and fatigue. They had war and famine in mind. In the process they discovered a group of herbal drugs which they dubbed adaptogens. Though designated for a different type of hardship, they really do help people to maintain an 'on-the-go' lifestyle, says clinical herbalist Douglas Schar.

If day-to-day living is making you feel tired and washed out, try herbal adaptogens like siberian ginseng, panax ginseng, rhodiola rosea or maca. These remedies will make your body better able to withstand stress and give you a steady supply of perky energy.

Teach your body to tell the time. Circadian rhythms act as our bodies' internal clocks, raising and lowering our blood pressure and body temperature at different times throughout the day. This chemical action causes the swings we experience – from feeling alert to feeling mentally and physically foggy.

So why are some people's natural peak times so inconvenient – like late at night? 'I think sometimes people, perhaps without even knowing it, work themselves into a particular time cycle,' says exercise physiologist William Fink.

Fink suggests changing your routine as much as is practically possible to complement your circadian rhythms. Start by getting up a little earlier or a little later – say, 15 minutes – until you feel comfortable. Keep it up until you achieve a routine that suits you.

Stop smoking. Doctors always advise giving up smoking, but add this to the list of reasons: smoking reduces the amount of oxygen available to your body. The result is fatigue. When you first give up, however, don't expect an immediate energy boost. Nicotine acts as a stimulant, and withdrawal will probably cause some temporary tiredness.

Make exercise an all-day activity. Whether you work out early, at lunchtime or in the evening, don't save all your exercising for one block of time. Get up and move around at least every couple of hours, Dr Sheridan says.

There are many options: the executive who rides an exercise bike in the privacy of his office, the medical registrar who runs up hospital stairs, the researcher who does isometric exercises while sitting at her desk.

Just say no. Learn to delegate, advises Dr Sheridan. If too many obligations or commitments are wearing you out, learn to say, 'No, thank you.'

Lose weight. If you are obese, losing weight will be a great help, says William Fink. Follow a sensible diet combined with exercise. Losing more than one kilo a week isn't healthy and will wear you down.

Get less sleep. You can have too much of a good thing, even sleep. 'If you oversleep, you tend to be groggy all day,' Fink says. 'Six to eight hours sleep a night is enough for most people.'

Blow out the candle. Burning the candle at both ends – not going to bed until 2am and getting up at 5am, for example – will leave you feeling burned out.

Have 40 winks. Naps don't suit everybody, but they can help to recharge older people who aren't sleeping as soundly as they used to, and parents with young children who wake in the night. Young people with hectic schedules and short nights might consider taking naps, Dr Ricer says. If you decide to take naps, try taking them at the same time each day and for no more than an hour.

WHEN TO CONSULT A DOCTOR

Fatigue may be just a signal that you need to manage your life better or that a cold or the flu is coming on.

But it also can be a warning sign of serious illness. Chronic conditions, such as diabetes, lung disease or anaemia cause fatigue, says Dr Ricer.

Fatigue is also a symptom of many other illnesses including hepatitis, mononucleosis, thyroid disease, depression and cancer. So if your tiredness persists, don't try to diagnose yourself; see your doctor.

Breathe deeply. It's one of the best ways to relax and energize at the same time, according to doctors and athletes.

Have just one drink. Alcohol is a depressant and will calm you down, not rev you up. Limit your alcohol intake to one drink, Dr Ricer suggests, or don't drink at all.

Eat a light lunch. Some doctors advise a light lunch to help prevent that post-lunch droopy-eyed need to sleep. If you are too often tired after lunch, this advice is worth trying. Soup, salad and a piece of fruit is a light, nutritious meal.

Or make lunch your main meal. If a light lunch doesn't satisfy you, Dr Young suggests eating your largest meal of the day at lunchtime and following it with a 20-minute walk. Eating most of your calories early in the day gives you the fuel you need to keep going. But you have to be selective in the type of fuel you choose. Carbohydrate, for example, is a fast burner. Fat, on the other hand, burns slowly, so it will slow you down.

Take a holiday. In many cases, what's needed is a holiday, says Dr Ricer. 'If you haven't had a break for a long time, it can be the perfect energy booster.' That's *really* good advice.

Divert your energy. Strong emotion is not only mentally draining, it can also be physically draining, says Dr Young. Try and redirect strong emotions such as anger, and apply that pent up energy to your job or a workout.

Colour your world. If you live in a dark gloomy house, you're going to feel low, Dr Ricer says. He suggests bringing in a little sunshine – literally or metaphorically. Several studies have shown that lots of colour and variety are important in keeping energy levels high. Red, for example, is good for short-term, high-energy stimulation, while green is good at eliminating distractions and maintaining focus for long periods of time.

Tune in. Music can light your fire, Dr Ricer says. Listen to U2, Vivaldi, Coldplay, Kylie Minogue – whatever and whoever peps you up.

Set yourself a target. Some people simply need deadlines to keep moving forwards, Dr Sheridan says. If you're like that, set yourself both short and long-term deadlines – so neither becomes too routine.

Take a shower. When fatigue starts to affect one New York stockbroker, he doesn't buy or sell. He stops to splash his face with cold water.

But if he were at home, a cool shower would be even more invigorating. Cascading water emits negative ions into the air, which then surround the body. Negative ions are thought to make people feel happier and more energetic.

Drink up. Dehydration can cause fatigue. Drink at least eight 250ml glasses of water each day, even more when you're active. If you know you're going to have a really active day, drink up the day before, and continue to do so throughout the busy day. Drummond King, an over-50s triathlete, has learnt from experience that it's best to drink lots of fluids the day before his body is going to need them. 'The major problem is dehydration and the fatigue that goes with it,' he says. 'Now I spend the day before a competition with a water bottle in my hand.'

Rethink your medications. Do you really need to take all those prescription and over-the-counter medicines? You may be shocked at what eliminating or reducing dosages of certain medications may do for you.

Sleeping pills, for example, are notorious for their next-day hangover effects. Other culprits, according to doctors, are drugs for treating high blood pressure and cough and cold remedies.

If you suspect a medication exhausts you, discuss it with your doctor. Maybe you can try a new prescription or, better still, stop the medicine altogether. But never stop taking a prescription drug without your doctor's approval.

If it feels good, do it. There's no denying the pleasure of a massage, jacuzzi or sauna. It's hard to say scientifically whether or not they lessen fatigue, says Fink. 'But many people swear by them. I'm convinced, too – if people feel better, they perform better.'

But don't let drugs fool you. Many so-called 'recreational' drugs are

Think positive

Where your mind goes, your body follows. It is now generally accepted that the mind influences the body. Here are some attitudes that can boost your energy levels.

Think positive. Championship athletes do it, successful chief executives do it – and so should you.

'It's important to think positively,' says Mary Trafton, an avid hiker and marathon runner. 'If I step in a huge puddle while hiking, I don't think, Oh dear, I'm going to be cold and tired. I think about the woolly socks I am wearing for protection and warmth.'

Be motivated. When you think about it, it's pretty hard to do much of anything if you're not motivated. But it's almost impossible to accomplish tasks that require mega-energy if your heart just isn't in it.

Take Drummond King, a veteran triathlete. He says that when he's too far behind to win a race, he finishes at walking pace instead of running. But when there's a chance of winning, or a bet on how long it will take him, he somehow finds the energy reserves to keep running.

Be confident. The chances are, if you feel you can do it, you will have the energy to do it. And once you've proved that you have the energy, you'll become even more confident.

---

taken for their supposed energizing, feel-good properties. Seventy-two million 'pep pills' – amphetamines – were handed out to soldiers in World War Two to keep them awake longer (Hitler himself used them daily). The jumpiness, aggression, loss of appetite, nausea and panic that these can cause were ignored or even welcomed, and the profound fatigue as the amphetamines wore off was simply treated with ... more amphetamines.

It was only in the 1970s that the addictiveness and health dangers of amphetamines led to their strict control for medical use. 'I shall never forget a young, long-distance lorry driver patient of mine,' says family doctor, Stephen Amiel. 'He used amphetamines so he could drive across Europe without stopping. His heart muscle was destroyed by them: he spent a year fighting for breath and died aged 38 waiting for a heart transplant.'

Ecstasy (a related drug) and cocaine are also energizing at first, but fatigue on comedown is just one – and probably the least serious – of the many downsides of using these drugs, warns Dr Amiel.

Change your routine. Sometimes fatigue can be caused by being in a rut. Even the simplest of changes, says Dr Ricer, can make a difference. If you always start your day by reading the paper, try reading something inspirational instead. If you always eat fish for supper on Mondays, cook chicken next Monday. If you run every day, try alternating your runs with cycle rides.

Curb your caffeine. One or two cups of coffee can kick you into gear in the morning, but the benefits usually end there. Too much caffeine is as bad for you as too much of anything. Drinking coffee throughout the day for energy can actually backfire says Dr Ricer. Caffeine is a magician. 'It makes you feel as though you have more energy, but you don't really.'

FEVER

12 cooling tactics

Think of fever not so much as a threat, but as your body's early-warning system. It's the way your body protects itself against infection and injury – and a tool it uses to enhance its natural defence mechanisms. Before antibiotics, doctors would deliberately infect patients with malaria, in the hope that the high fevers would cure syphilis.

The mechanics are quite simple. Your brain tells your body to move blood from the surface of your skin to the interior of the body. The white blood cells and antibodies in your blood can then get to the source of the infection and get to work eliminating it. With blood so far away from the skin, the body surface loses less heat and your temperature rises. But before you take steps to cool it down, listen to what the doctors say.

Make sure you have a fever. Although 37°C (98.6°F) is considered the norm, that number is not etched in stone. 'Normal' temperature varies from person to person and fluctuates widely throughout the day. Food, excess clothing, emotional excitement and vigorous exercise can all raise your temperature, says Thomas Gossel, a professor of pharmacology. 'In fact, vigorous exercise can raise body temperature to as high as 39.5°C (103°F). Furthermore, children tend to have higher temperatures than adults and greater daily variations. So here's a general rule: if your temperature is 37.5–38°C (99–100°F), it may suggest a fever. If it is over 38°C (100°F), it is a fever,' he says.

Dr Gossel adds that often someone's appearance is a better indicator of their condition than hard-and-fast numbers. Someone with a raised

WHEN TO CONSULT A DOCTOR

See a doctor when:

- a fever is associated with a stiff neck. If there's a non-fading rash (see *Rashes*, page 464) as well, seek medical attention **immediately**;
- a fever above 38.5°C (101°F) lasts for more than three days or fails to respond at least partly to treatment;
- a fever rises above 39.5°C (103°F) under any conditions.

Babies and frail elderly people, or anyone with chronic illnesses, such as diabetes, heart or respiratory disease, may not be able to tolerate prolonged high fevers.

temperature who looks ill needs attention more quickly than one who looks and seems well.

Don't fight it. If you have a fever, remember this: a fever is not an illness – it's a symptom of one. When your body senses a bacterial or viral invasion, it releases substances that tell your brain to raise your internal temperature, causing a fever. An elevated body temperature makes it harder for bacteria and viruses to reproduce and spread. So, in essence, your body's natural defences can actually shorten an illness with its quick response and increase the power of antibiotics. These factors should be weighed against the discomfort involved in letting a slight fever run its course, says public-health expert Stephen Rosenberg.

But if you feel the need for relief, try the following steps.

Drink lots. When you're hot, your body sweats to cool you down. But if you lose too much water – as you might with a high fever – your body turns off its sweat ducts to prevent further water loss. That makes it more difficult for you to cope with your fever. The answer is to drink lots. As well as plain water, doctors recommend the following:

Fruit and vegetable juices. They're high in vitamins and minerals, says nutritionist Eleonore Blaurock-Busch, and that's exactly what you need to build up your strength. She particularly favours nutrient-dense beetroot juice and carrot juice.

One doctor's botanical tea. Although any tea will provide fluid, several are particularly suitable for fever, says Dr Blaurock-Busch. One mixture she likes combines equal parts dried thyme, linden flowers

Thermometer ins and outs

Mothers are famous for being able to gauge temperatures just by feeling their children's foreheads.

If you didn't inherit the knack, you'll need to rely on thermometer readings. Here's how to get the safest, most accurate results.

• There are many types of thermometer available, including digital, ear and glass galinstan thermometers, which contain a safe alternative to mercury.

• All of these are good alternatives to old-fashioned mercury thermometers, which can cause neurological problems if the glass breaks and the mercury vapour is inhaled.

• Wait at least 15 minutes after eating or drinking anything hot or cold or after smoking before taking an oral reading. These activities alter mouth temperature and will cause inaccurate readings.

• Hot baths also affect readings.

• Before using a glass thermometer, hold it by the top (not the bulb) and shake it with a quick snap of the wrist until the coloured dye drops below 35°C (96°F). If you are worried about dropping and breaking it, shake the thermometer over a bed.

• Place the thermometer under the tongue in one of the 'pockets' located on either side of your mouth rather than in front. These pockets are closer to blood vessels that reflect the body's core temperature.

• Hold the thermometer in place with your lips, not your teeth. Breathe through your nose rather than your mouth so that the room temperature doesn't affect the reading. Leave a glass thermometer in place for at least three minutes.

• After use, wash a glass thermometer in cool, soapy water. Never use hot water or store near a heat source.

and chamomile flowers. Thyme has antiseptic properties, chamomile reduces inflammation and linden promotes sweating, she says. Steep a teaspoon of the mixture in a cup of boiling water for five minutes. Strain and drink warm several times a day. Herb tea-bags and loose herbs are sold in health food stores.

Linden tea. This tea by itself is also good, she says, and can prompt sweating to bring out a fever. Use a tablespoon of the flowers in a cup of boiling water. Prepare as above and drink hot often.

Willow bark. This bark is rich in salicylates (aspirin-related compounds) and is considered nature's fever medication, says Dr Blaurock-Busch. Brew into a tea and drink in small doses.

Ice. If you're too nauseated to drink, you can suck on ice. For variety, freeze fruit juice in an ice-cube tray.

Use warm or cool compresses. Wet compresses – a squeezed-out flannel works well – help to reduce the body's temperature output, says Dr Blaurock-Busch. Ironically, she says, warm moist compresses can do the job. But if you start to feel uncomfortably hot, apply cool flannels to the forehead, wrists and calves. Keep the rest of the body covered.

But if the temperature rises above 39.5°C (103°F) don't use warm compresses at all. Instead, apply cool flannels to stop the fever from getting any higher. Change them as they warm to body temperature and continue until the fever drops.

Note: Don't use cold compresses: cold causes the skin's blood vessels to shut down, shunting the blood inwards and raising your core temperature further.

Try a tepid sponge. Evaporation has a cooling effect on body temperature. Community nurse Mary Ann Pane recommends tepid tap water to help the skin dissipate excess heat. Rather than sponging the whole body, pay particular attention to spots where heat is greatest, such as the armpits and groin area.

Wring out a sponge and wipe one section at a time, keeping the rest of the body covered. Body heat will evaporate the moisture, so you don't need to towel dry.

The low-down on painkillers. If you're very uncomfortable, take an over-the-counter pain reliever. For adults, Dr Gossel recommends aspirin, paracetamol or ibuprofen taken according to package directions.

So which one should you take? All are effective, but some work better for particular ailments. For example, aspirin and ibuprofen are non-steroidal anti-inflammatory drugs (NSAIDs), so they're effective at reducing muscle pain and inflammation.

Paracetamol is recommended if you have a sensitive digestive system or are allergic to aspirin. It doesn't work as well as NSAIDs for inflammation and muscle aches, but it's a safer drug and has minimal side-effects.

Paracetamol and NSAIDs are different types of drug and can be used together. If your fever does not respond to one type alone, you can use full daily doses of both for a few days.

A combination of paracetamol and ibuprofen is safe for children in appropriate doses too, but **children under 16 should not be given aspirin-containing drugs,** as there is a small risk of a fatal condition called Reye's syndrome.

Dress comfortably. Use common sense with clothing and blankets, says Nurse Pane. If you're very hot, take off extra covers and clothes so that body heat can evaporate into the air. But if you feel chilled, wrap up until you're just comfortable.

Don't sweat it out. Resist the temptation to sweat a fever out by co-cooning yourself in extra blankets. You'll feel worse for longer and increase your risk of dehydration

Keep babies cool. Babies can be left in a vest and nappy if they're feverish, provided the room is at a reasonable temperature.

Create a healing atmosphere. Do your best to make the sickroom conducive to healing, says Dr Blaurock-Busch. Don't overheat it – German doctors generally recommend that room temperature does not exceed 18°C (65°F), she says.

Soft light, fresh air. Let in just enough fresh air to promote recuperation but not to create a draft. And keep the lighting subdued so that it's properly relaxing. Keep cool air circulating with a gently oscillating fan if you have one.

Eat – if you want to. Don't fret over whether you should feed a fever or starve one. Some doctors, like Dr Blaurock-Busch, recommend a juice fast until the fever is reduced nearly to normal.

Others think that you should eat during a fever because the body's increased heat uses up calories. Ultimately, of course, the choice is yours and depends on your appetite. Just remember to keep up your fluid intake.

FLATULENCE
11 wind-reducing ideas

It's hard to be serious about flatulence – even the scientists who study the subject poke fun at their own research, writing of failed experiments that ended 'without even a whiff of success'. Consider Michael Levitt, one of the top researchers in the field. His peers know him as 'the man who brought status to flatus and class to gas'. In his own words, Dr Levitt describes his work as 'an attempt to pump some data into the field filled largely with hot air'. He's found that the average person passes downwind 10 times a day: over a litre of gas for most men, and about 800ml for most women.

Hot air and a colourful history, too. Hippocrates investigated flatulence extensively, and ancient physicians who specialized in it became known as 'pneumatists.' In early American history, such great men as Benjamin Franklin taxed their minds seeking a cure for 'escaped wind'. Here, we try and take flatulence seriously.

Lay off the lactose. People who are lactose intolerant (see *Lactose Intolerance* page 375) can have flatulence problems from eating dairy foods, says nutritionist Dennis Savaiano. Lactose-intolerant people have a low intestinal level of the enzyme lactase, which is needed to digest lactose, a type of sugar found in many dairy foods.

But you don't necessarily need to be diagnosed as lactose intolerant to have an unwanted reaction. Some people can handle only certain amounts or kinds of milk products. If you or your doctor suspect that your favourite dairy food is causing your problem, try eating it in smaller servings or along with a meal for a day or two until you notice where wind begins to be a problem.

Keep off the carbonated drinks? Fizzy drinks are notorious for causing upwind – belching. The carbon dioxide that gives them their fizz is absorbed by the time it reaches the intestine, and so this in itself cannot cause flatulence. Many carbonated drinks contain fructose, though, and

KITCHEN CURES

Sugar-coated fennel seeds are served after meals in India, observes Dr Andrew Weil, just as we might serve after-dinner mints. Fennel is known as a carminative – a substance that can disperse gas from the intestinal tract, he says. The seeds can also be brewed as tea.

some people's intestines handle this sugar poorly, giving rise to downwind flatulence, explains family doctor Stephen Amiel.

Avoid gas-promoting foods. The primary cause of flatulence is the digestive system's inability to absorb certain carbohydrates, says nutritionist Samuel Klein. You probably know that beans are flatus producers, but many people don't realize that cabbage, broccoli, Brussels sprouts, onions, cauliflower, wholemeal flour, radishes, bananas, apricots and many more foods can also produce a lot of wind.

Eat less air. Every schoolboy, of the grown up variety too, knows that if you deliberately gulp down some air, you can produce a belch to impress (?) your friends. Excess swallowed air can also find its way downwards too and reappear as flatulence, says Dr Amiel. Some people who suffer from anxiety gulp air as a nervous tic (aerophagy – 'eating air'); other causes are excessive chewing of gum, eating too quickly, or over-enthusiastic slurping of drinks.

Fight off fibre-induced flatus. Although we encourage dietary fibre for digestive health, some high-fibre foods increase gas,' says gastroenterologist Richard McCallum.

If you are adding fibre to your diet for health reasons, start with small amounts so that the bowel gets used to it. That lessens the increase of flatus, and doctors have found that most people's wind production returns to normal within a few weeks of adding fibre.

Take a digestif herb. Wind is often caused by slow digestion. Food simply sits in the gut for too long, ferments and gives off gas. Speedy digestion prevents this, and, says clinical herbalist Douglas Schar, there are several remedies that will get things moving. Herbs have long been used in after-dinner digestif liqueurs like Chartreuse and Kümmel. Angelica, mint, fennel, caraway, dill and gentian are good examples. The best way to take any of these herbs is in tincture form, available from health food stores. Take the recommended dose after every meal to get your digestion moving and reduce wind production.

Use charcoal to absorb gas. Studies have found that activated charcoal – available as tablets or biscuits – is effective in eliminating excessive gas. 'Charcoal absorbs gases and may be useful for flatulence,' says Dr Klein. 'It's probably the best available treatment – after appropriate dietary changes have been made and other gastroenterological diseases have been treated or ruled out.' Try Bragg's charcoal tablets or biscuits or Lanes charcoal tablets.

Note: Check with your doctor if you are taking any medication, because charcoal can soak up medicine as well as gas.

Look under the sofa. A surefire (no pun intended) way to get rid of trapped gas is to kneel on the floor with your head on the ground and your bottom in the air, like you are trying to find something under the sofa, says Dr Amiel. Rest your forehead on your forearm, relax and wait. Within a minute or two, the trapped gas will exit relatively noiselessly and inoffensively. If someone comes in unexpectedly, just say you're looking for something under the sofa. (Tip: for this excuse to work, you need a sofa!)

Get quick relief from popular antacids. While many doctors

Bean cuisine – reduce the wind

If you love beans and pulses but hate living with the consequences, there is a solution.

Clearly, these foods cause flatulence, although the longer they're cooked for, the less the problem. Beans seem to lose a lot of their gas-producing properties in water. Studies show that soaking beans for 12 hours or germinating them on damp paper towels for 24 hours can significantly reduce the amount of gas-producing compounds in beans.

The most effective gas-cutting solution is a good soak followed by cooking in a pressure cooker.

recommend activated charcoal for relief of intestinal gas, pharmacists say that dimethicone-containing products, such as Asilone, are still the most popular with consumers. Unlike activated charcoal's absorbent action, dimethicone's defoaming action relieves flatulence by dispersing and preventing the formation of mucus-surrounded gas pockets in the stomach and intestines.

FLU
21 remedies to beat the bug

Flu is a viral infection, so antibiotics are powerless against it. The best defence against flu is avoidance (see *Resist the flu virus* on page 238). But if avoidance didn't work and you have flu, take these steps to help ease your symptoms.

Stay at home. Flu is a very infectious disease that spreads like wildfire, says pharmacologist Thomas Gossel. So don't be a workaholic or a martyr. Stay at home until at least one day after your temperature returns to normal. And keep your children away from school until they have fully recovered.

Get some rest. You shouldn't have much trouble following this advice, as you're probably too sick to do much else. Bed rest is essential, says Dr Gossel, because it lets your body put its energy into combating the infection. Being active while you're still quite ill weakens your defences and leaves you open to complications.

Drink up. Liquids are especially important to prevent dehydration if you have a fever. In addition, fluids can provide vital nutrients when you're too ill to eat. Thin soups are good, as are fruit and vegetable juices. Nutritionist Eleonore Blaurock-Busch advises drinking juices that are rich in vitamins and minerals.

Family doctor Jay Swedberg recommends diluting fruit juice with water. 'A little sugar provides necessary glucose, but too much can cause diarrhoea when you're ill,' he says. 'Also, dilute ginger ale and other sugar-sweetened soft drinks. And allow them to go flat before drinking, because their bubbles can create gas in the stomach and make you feel sick.'

Cool down. Real flu is associated with a high temperature, says family

WHEN TO CONSULT A DOCTOR

Influenza can be as deadly today as it was in 1918, when Spanish flu killed more than 20 million people worldwide. Family doctor Stephen Amiel warns that flu can lead to secondary bacterial infections, causing bronchitis and pneumonia; encephalitis; or the worsening of asthma, diabetes, heart failure, AIDS and many other chronic illnesses. So call a doctor if:

• you develop pains in your chest;

• you have difficulty breathing;

• your phlegm changes to yellow, green or bloody;

• confusion or drowsiness develops;

• you're not sure if what you have is flu (for example you have a rash, urinary symptoms, severe vomiting or diarrhoea);

• your acute symptoms are not subsiding after a week or so;

• you or your child are in a high risk group (see above).

If there is known to be influenza in the community (the virus is monitored by public health laboratories), and if you are in a high risk group, your doctor may be able to prescribe an antiviral drug like zanamovir (Relenza). This is effective in shortening the duration of a flu attack, but only if you can start the treatment within 48 hours of the onset of symptoms, says Dr Amiel. Doctors are recommended not to prescribe these drugs if you are otherwise healthy.

People often underestimate flu. 'A bout of real flu can leave you feeling debilitated and depressed for many weeks,' says Dr Amiel. 'So don't expect to back on your feet and firing on all cylinders within days.' See your doctor though if you think you are not recovering normally, both physically and mentally.

---

doctor Stephen Amiel. This makes your headache worse, increases dehydration, can leave you wringing wet and makes you feel even more wretched. There are a number of ways to cool your body down – for a list of suggestions see *Fever*, page 228.

Take painkillers. Aspirin, paracetamol or ibuprofen can reduce the fever, headache and body aches that accompany flu. Follow label instructions. Because symptoms are often more pronounced in the afternoon and evening, take painkillers regularly during this period, says Dr Gossel.

Paracetamol is a different class of drug from aspirin and ibuprofen

Resist the flu virus

Individual immunity and the particular strain of flu virus circulating in a given year play a large role in determining who will submit to flu. But there are steps you can take to reduce your susceptibility.

Have a flu jab. Every year, scientists develop a vaccine against the most recently circulating strain of the virus. So the best thing you can do to protect yourself against flu is to be vaccinated, says family doctor Stephen Amiel.

Influenza vaccination is usually available at your doctor's surgery from late September/early October, and you should make every effort to have yours as soon as possible. The jab is virtually painless: you may have an ache in your arm for a day or so, and some people get a very mild feverish illness for a day or two. The vaccine cannot cause flu.

Some people are at higher risk from the complications of flu and flu vaccination for them should be considered essential, says Dr Amiel. Have a flu jab every year if:

- you are 65 years old or over;
- whatever your age, you have a chronic heart or chest complaint, including asthma; chronic kidney disease; diabetes; lowered immunity due to a disease or treatment such as steroid medication or cancer treatment; any other serious medical condition – check with your doctor if you are unsure;
- you live in the same household as a high-risk person;
- you live in an old people's home or a nursing home.

In cases where the jab doesn't prevent flu, it considerably lessens the disease's severity. Don't wait

(which are both anti-inflammatory NSAIDs), so the two types of drug can be used in combination, says Dr Amiel. If your symptoms do not respond to one type alone, you can use full daily doses of both for a few days. A combination of paracetamol and aspirin or ibuprofen is safe for adults. Children can be given a combination of paracetamol and ibuprofen in appropriate doses too.

Note: Do not give aspirin to children under 16.

Think twice about what you take. Over-the-counter cold cure medicines may give you temporary relief of symptoms, says Dr Gossel. Those with antihistamines, for instance, can dry up a runny nose.

But be careful – these drugs may suppress your symptoms to the point where you feel better. Prematurely resuming your normal activities

until the virus is rampant before acting, as the vaccine takes about two weeks to work. And don't have the flu jab if you're allergic to eggs – the vaccine is made from them – or if you are pregnant.

Flu vaccination is extremely effective against the influenza virus itself, says Dr Amiel but there are other flu-like illnesses which are around throughout the year. So don't assume that you're immune to flu and don't need a vaccination as winter comes on.

Don't rubbish the vaccination if you still get colds or a flu-like illness, says Dr Amiel. It can be a life-saver.

Avoid crowds. Because the virus spreads easily, stay away from cinemas, theatres, shopping centres and other crowded places during an epidemic. And keep your distance from sneezing or coughing people,

even if it means getting out of a lift or giving up your seat on the bus.

Come in from the cold. Prolonged exposure to wet and cold weather lowers your resistance and increases your risk of infection.

Give up bad habits. Smoking and alcohol can also impair your resistance to illness.

Smoking, in particular, harms the respiratory tract and makes you more susceptible to flu.

Kiss at your own risk. Kissing is an efficient way for flu to spread, says Dr Gossel. Just sleeping in the same room as a sick partner is asking for trouble. So, if possible, move to a spare room.

Keep your strength up. Don't get tired or run-down. Paint the sitting room or clean the attic some other time, not during the flu season.

can bring on a relapse or trigger serious complications.

Suck something sweet. Sucking on boiled sweets or lozenges keeps your throat moist so it feels better, says community nurse Mary Ann Pane. If you're worried about calories, look for sugar-free brands. They're just as effective.

Humidify the air. Raising the humidity in your bedroom helps to reduce the discomfort of a cough, sore throat and dry nasal passages. A humidifier may also be helpful if you have chest congestion or a blocked nose, says Calvin Thrash, a health-education specialist.

Pamper your nose. If you've been blowing your nose a lot, it is

Is it really flu?

People often complain of having flu when all they have is a nasty cold. Although similarities exist between the two illnesses – and their treatment – they are caused by entirely different viruses. The worst part of a cold might last longer, but flu generally causes more discomfort. Here is a comparison of common symptoms.

Fever. Prominent with flu, coming on suddenly; rare with a cold.

Headache. Prominent with flu; rare with a cold.

General aches. Prominent, often severe with flu; slight with a cold.

Fatigue. Extreme with flu, lasting two to three weeks; mild with a cold.

Runny nose. Occasional with flu; common with a cold.

Sore throat. Occasional with flu; common with a cold.

Cough. Common and possibly severe with flu; mild to moderate hacking cough with a cold.

---

probably pretty sore. So lubricate your nostrils frequently to decrease irritation, says Nurse Pane. A lubricant such as K-Y Jelly is preferable to petroleum jelly, which dries out quickly.

Soothe aching muscles. One characteristic of flu is sore muscles. Warm them and ease their pain with a warm bath or a heating pad, says Nurse Pane.

Warm your feet. Soaking your feet in hot water may help if you have a headache or nasal congestion. The warm water helps to widen blood vessels, thereby diverting bloodflow from your head to your feet, which relieves congestion.

Breathe fresh air. Make sure your sickroom has a good supply of fresh air, says Dr Thrash. But avoid a draft. Prevent chills with snug bedclothes.

KITCHEN CURES

A sore or scratchy throat often accompanies flu.

Get some relief – and wash out any secretions collecting in your throat – by gargling with a saltwater solution, says community nurse Mary Ann Pane. Dissolve a teaspoon of salt in 500ml of warm water. This concentration mimicks the pH level of body tissues and is very soothing, she says. Use as often as you like, but make sure you do not swallow the liquid.

Ask for a massage. A back rub may help to activate your immune system to fight flu, says Dr Thrash. And it's very comforting.

Eat lightly and wisely. During the worst phase of flu, you probably won't have an appetite at all. But when you're ready to make the transition from liquids to more substantial fare, put the emphasis on bland, starchy foods, says Dr Swedberg. 'Dry toast is fine. So are bananas, stewed apples, boiled rice, rice pudding, porridge and baked potatoes, which can be topped with yoghurt.' For a refreshing dessert, peel and freeze very ripe bananas, then purée them in a food processor.

FOOD POISONING

33 ways to prevent it, or deal with it

Raw or undercooked meat or poultry, improperly washed fruit and vegetables, sun-warmed pizza, moussaka or potato salad and a host of other foods can harbour microscopic organisms capable of triggering potentially life-threatening cases of food poisoning.

According to the UK's Food Standards Agency, around 5.5 million people in Britain suffer from food poisoning each year and, of these, 4.2 million believe that their illness was caused by food eaten outside the home. Infectious intestinal disease (or IID) was responsible for 590 deaths in the UK in 2000 – and, says the FSA, many of these deaths will have been due to food poisoning. Even non-life-threatening cases of food poisoning can make you feel miserable, resulting in dizziness, queasiness, diarrhoea, vomiting, abdominal cramps, headache and fever.

Toxic bacteria get into food in a variety of ways, generally as a result of inadequate cooking or processing. Once inside you, these bugs attack your intestines. For a day or so, you feel wretched as your body tries to battle back. Here's what the experts say to do to help your body fight food poisoning.

Fill up on fluids. The bacteria irritate your intestinal tract and trigger a great deal of fluid loss from diarrhoea, vomiting or both. Drink lots of fluids to prevent dehydration. Water is fine if that's all you can tolerate at first, but this should be followed as soon as possible by other clear liquids such as apple juice, or chicken or vegetable stock.

Soft drinks are okay, too, if you drink them flat, says microbiologist

Don't let it happen again

You can't always blame the bistro or the sandwich bar down the road for stomach upsets. The truth is, says Daniel Rodrigue, an expert on infectious diseases, many cases of food poisoning probably come from carelessness in your own home.

Follow these commonsense rules to significantly decrease your chances of poisoning yourself or your family.

- Wash your hands with warm water and soap for at least 20 seconds before and after preparing food to avoid passing on bacteria such as staphylococcus. This is especially important before and after handling raw meat and eggs.

- If you have an infection or a cut on your hands, wear plastic or rubber gloves. Be sure to wash your gloved hands just as often as you would wash your bare hands.

- Heat or chill raw food. Bacteria can't multiply above 66°C (150°F) or below 5°C (40°F).

- Don't leave food at room temperature for more than two hours, and avoid eating anything that you suspect may have been unrefrigerated for that long. Bacteria thrive in warm protein food made with meat or eggs, cream-filled pastries, dips, potato salad and so forth.

- Raw food can harbour bacteria.

Don't eat raw protein food like fish, poultry, meat or eggs. Consider avoiding sushi, oysters and Caesar salad or mayonnaise made with raw eggs.

- Don't use eggs if they have hairline cracks – they could harbour salmonella bacteria. Don't sample raw cake mix made with eggs. This advice is particularly important if you're pregnant.

- Don't buy cooked seafood, such as prawns, if it's displayed in the same cabinet as raw fish.

- Buy fresh seafood only from reputable fishmongers or supermarkets where the products are kept properly refrigerated or on ice.

- Cook meat – especially pork, beefburgers and sausages – until the pink disappears, chicken until there is no redness visible in the joints and the juices run clear, and fish until it flakes easily. Complete cooking is the only way to ensure that all harmful bacteria have been killed.

- Don't taste-test foods before they're cooked, especially pork, fish and eggs.

- Don't let raw meat juice drip onto other food. It can taint otherwise harmless food.

- Use a separate chopping board and utensils when handling raw meat, and wash them with hot, soapy water after use to prevent cross-contamination.

- Scrub fruit and vegetables thoroughly. Remove the outer leaves of leafy vegetables.

- Scrub can openers and worktops and clean out crevices to prevent bacteria from hiding there.
  For all areas that come in contact with food, use hot water and detergent, and then a bleach solution.

- Replace sponges and dishcloths often and use kitchen paper to wipe worktops.

- Thaw meat in the refrigerator. Or thaw it in the microwave and cook it immediately it's thawed. Bacteria can multiply on food surfaces while the centre is still frozen.

- When using the microwave to defrost, follow the instructions and leave at least 5cm of space around the item to allow air to circulate.

- Refrigerate leftovers within a maximum of two hours. After cooking, place food in shallow containers, so it cools more quickly.

- When you re-heat leftovers, they need to be heated and stirred until they are piping hot all the way through. Sauces, soups and stews should be brought to a full boil.

- Don't reheat food more than once.

- Avoid reheating takeaways unless you are certain the food has been recently cooked and not reheated already.

- Avoid takeaways altogether if you have lowered immunity.

- Do not refreeze thawed raw meat, fish or cooked food. Thawed raw meat and fish can be refrozen if it's cooked first.

- Storage times for properly refrigerated foods vary, but generally use leftovers within three to five days.

- Never pick and eat wild mushrooms unless you have adequate training in the identification of edible species. Some contain toxins that attack the nervous system and can be deadly.

- Use common sense and don't taste any food that doesn't smell or look right.

- Avoid cracked jars or swollen, dented cans or lids, clear liquids that have turned milky, or cans or jars that spurt or smell 'off' when opened. They could contain dangerous bacteria.
  Make sure you discard the contents carefully so that pets can't eat them.

WHEN TO CONSULT A DOCTOR

With a normal case of food poisoning, the symptoms – stomach cramps, nausea, vomiting, diarrhoea and dizziness – disappear in a day or two. But for the very young, the elderly or someone with a chronic health condition or immune disorder, food poisoning can be very serious. Those people should contact a doctor at the first signs of food poisoning.

Even if you don't fall into one of those categories, call a doctor immediately if your symptoms are also accompanied by:

- difficulty in swallowing, speaking or breathing; changes in vision; muscle weakness or paralysis, particularly if this occurs after eating mushrooms, canned food or shellfish;
- fever over 38°C (100°F);
- severe vomiting – meaning you can't even hold down any liquids for a continuous period of 12 hours or more;
- severe diarrhoea for more than a few days;
- persistent, localized abdominal pain;
- dehydration – you have extreme thirst, a dry mouth or decreased urination, and when you pinch the back of your hand, the skin stays pinched;
- bloody diarrhoea.

Food poisoning is a public health concern. If you think you have food poisoning, especially if you think the source is outside your home, you should contact your doctor, who can arrange for appropriate tests, and inform the relevant public health authorities.

If you work with sick people, in a nursery, school, residential home, or in any food handling occupation, you must contact your doctor if you think you have food poisoning. You will need to have the all-clear from public health officials before you can return to work.

Vincent Garagusi. Otherwise, the carbonation can further irritate your stomach. Defizzed Coca-Cola, for reasons yet to be determined, has the added bonus of settling your stomach.

Sip little, sip often, sip slowly. Trying to gulp down too much at once may trigger more vomiting, says Dr Garagusi.

Replenish electrolytes. Vomiting and diarrhoea can flush out important electrolytes – potassium, sodium and glucose. Experts suggest that you replace them by sipping commercially prepared electrolyte products like Dioralyte or Rehidrat. Or try this rehydration recipe: mix fruit juice (for potassium) with ½ teaspoon of honey (for glucose) and a pinch of salt (for sodium). De-fizzed cola, lemonade or Lucozade will have a reasonable balance of glucose and electrolytes too (stir to get rid of the bubbles). This may be your best option if you're dealing with a miserable child who's reluctant to drink otherwise.

Milk is best avoided for a few days, as your intestine will often be temporarily intolerant of the lactose in it and you could make matters worse. Breast milk is an exception: if your baby has vomiting and diarrhoea, you should continue to breastfeed, although you may need to supplement with clear fluids: ask your health visitor or doctor.

Save antacids for heartburn. They can reduce the acids in your stomach and weaken your defence against bacteria. If you take an antacid, it's possible that the bacteria could multiply in greater numbers and more rapidly.

Don't interfere with progress. Your body is trying to flush the toxic organism out, explains Daniel Rodrigue, a specialist in infectious diseases. In some cases, taking antidiarrhoeal products (like Imodium, Kaopectate or Lomotil) may interfere with your body's ability to fight the infection. So stay away from them and let nature take its course. If you feel you need to take something, talk to your doctor first.

Reintroduce bland foods. Usually within a few hours to a day after the diarrhoea and vomiting have subsided, you'll be ready for some 'real' food. But take it easy. Experts suggest starting with easily digestible foods. Try breakfast cereal, rice pudding, crackers or clear broth. Avoid high-fibre, spicy, acidic, greasy, sugary or dairy foods that could further irritate the stomach. Do this for a day or two. After that, your stomach will be ready to get back to its routine.

FOOT ACHES
12 ways to relieve sore feet

Our feet look after us every day, taking us through all kinds of activity, whatever the weather. Each foot is a complex piece of engineering, containing 26 bones, 33 joints, 107 ligaments, 19 muscles and many tendons that hold it together and help it to move in various directions. The average person takes 8000 to 10,000 steps a day. However, we tend to ignore our feet and take them for granted, that is, until they cause us problems.

Amazingly, it's not really the daily workout that batters our feet. It's more often a combination of badly fitting shoes and neglect. But much can be done to ease foot pain. Here's what our experts recommend.

Put your feet up. The best thing you can do for your feet when you get home is to sit down, put your feet up and exercise your toes to get the circulation going again, says Gilbert Wright, orthopaedic surgeon and foot specialist. Elevate your feet at a 45-degree angle to your body and relax for 20 minutes.

Soak them in salts. A tried-and-tested foot revitalizer is to soak your feet in a basin of warm water containing one to two tablespoons of Epsom salts, says podiatrist Mark Sussman. Rinse with cool, clean water, then pat your feet dry and massage with a moisturizing gel or cream.

Run hot and cold. Dr Sussman recommends this spa treatment: sit on the edge of the bath and hold your feet under running water for several minutes. Alternate one minute of comfortably hot water with one minute of cold, repeating several times and ending with the cold. The contrasting bath will invigorate your whole system.

Note: If you have diabetes or impaired circulation, don't expose your feet to extremes of temperature.

Massage away your aches. It's really nice to have your feet massaged with baby oil, says Dr Sussman. If you can't find a willing partner, then either before or during a soak give yourself a foot massage, says aromatherapist Judith Jackson.

WHEN TO CONSULT A DOCTOR

Foot specialist Mark Sussman says you should definitely see a doctor if:

• you have pain in your feet that continually worsens during the day;

• your feet get to the point where you can't keep your shoes on;

• you have trouble walking first thing in the morning.

Painful burning in the feet can be a sign of poor circulation, athlete's foot, a pinched nerve, diabetes, anaemia, thyroid disease, alcoholism or other problems, and always warrants a visit to your doctor.

Work over the whole foot, squeezing the toes gently, then pressing in a circular motion over the bottom of your foot. One really effective movement is to slide your thumb as hard as you can in the arch of the foot.

Get relief with ice. Another way to refresh tired feet is to wrap a few ice cubes in a wet flannel, then rub it over your feet and ankles for a few minutes.

Ice acts to relieve inflammation, and it also acts as a mild anaesthetic, says podiatrist Neal Kramer. Then dry your feet and wipe them with witch hazel, cologne, alcohol or vinegar for a cooling and drying effect.

KITCHEN CURES

Soaking your feet in tea can be very soothing.

Aromatherapist Judith Jackson suggests brewing a strong peppermint or chamomile tea. Steep four tea bags in two cups of boiling water. Add the brew to a large basin of warm water. Soak your feet for five minutes. Slosh your feet in the water and let the tea's warm scent relax you. Then drain the water and pour some cold water over your feet. Follow that with warm water from the tap and then more cold.

Exercise. Many doctors recommend that you exercise your feet and leg muscles throughout the day to ward off aches and keep the circulation going. Try these ideas.

- If your feet feel tense and cramped during the day, give them a good shake, as you would your hands if they felt cramped. Do one foot at a time, then relax and flex your toes up and down.

- If you have to stand for long periods of time, walk on the spot whenever you can. Keep changing your stance, and try to rest one foot on a stool or step occasionally. If possible, stand on carpeting or a spongy rubber mat.

- To relieve stiffness, remove your shoes, sit in a chair and stretch your feet out in front of you. Circle both feet from the ankles 10 times in one direction, then 10 times in the other. Point your toes down as far as possible, then flex them up as high as you can. Repeat 10 times. Now grasp your toes and gently pull them back and forth.

- For a mini-massage, take off your shoes and roll each foot over a golf ball, tennis ball or rolling pin for a minute or two.

Choose thick soles. Try wearing shoes with thick, shock-absorbing soles to shield your feet from rough surfaces and hard pavements. Don't let your soles become too thin or worn, because they won't do the job they're supposed to do. Women's thin-soled, pointy-toed high heels are classic villains, says Dr Wright. If you have to dress up for work, ease foot strain by wearing walking shoes or trainers to and from work and changing into heels at the office.

Change heel heights. Wearing high heels tightens the calf muscles, which leads to foot fatigue, says foot surgeon John Waller. So changing heel heights from high to low during the day is a good idea.

Wear insoles. High heels have the added disadvantage of causing your foot to pitch forward as you walk, putting painful pressure on the ball of your foot, says Dr Waller. To prevent this discomfort, wear a half-insole to help keep your foot in place. And be sure to take the insoles with you to the shoe shop to ensure that they'll fit comfortably into your new shoes.

Buy shoes in the afternoon. As your feet expand during the day, you should buy shoes with enough space to accommodate the slight swelling. Measure your feet while standing up, and always try on both shoes. If one foot is a bit larger than the other, buy the pair that feels best on the bigger foot.

Stretch your shoes. When you add insoles to shoes that you already have, make sure they don't cramp your toes, says Dr Sussman. If they do feel tight, you may be able to stretch the shoes to accommodate the insoles. Fill a sock with sand, stuff it into the toe of the shoe and wrap the shoe in a wet towel. Let it dry out over the next 24 hours. Repeat once or twice, if necessary.

FOOT ODOUR
11 ways to stop the smell

Any parent who has chaperoned a trip to the sports centre recognizes it instantly. Twenty-five little boys and girls take off their shoes to expose socks that should have been changed days ago. It's the ripe pong of 50 sweaty little feet.

Doctors don't have to look far for the cause of foot odour. Bacteria feed on the dead skin beneath our socks producing the characteristic smell. Exercising, wearing shoes that don't breathe – anything that makes

WHEN TO CONSULT A DOCTOR

Your foot odour may be due partly to athlete's foot (see *Athlete's Foot*, page 56), a fungal infection, which usually starts between the toes. Eradicating this may help your foot odour. See your doctor if you can't get rid of athlete's foot yourself.

Eczema of the feet may become infected and smelly, requiring steroid creams and antibiotics.

If you have any ulcers or sores on your feet that won't heal, see your doctor whether they smell or not, especially if you know you have diabetes or circulation problems.

the feet moist – can make the smell worse. The key to eliminating foot odour is good foot hygiene.

Wash – often. Keep your feet scrupulously clean. Use warm, soapy water and wash your feet as often as needed – several times a day if you sweat a lot or notice a smell. Scrub gently with a soft brush, even between your toes, and dry your feet thoroughly.

Powder your toes. After washing, apply foot powder, talc or an antifungal spray. Another good method for keeping feet cool and dry is to treat your shoes – sprinkle the insides with talcum powder, says podiatrist Suzanne Levine.

Use an antiperspirant. Control odour with either an antiperspirant or a deodorant. You can buy foot deodorants or simply use your underarm brand. Remember that deodorants eliminate odour, but they don't stop perspiration. Antiperspirants take care of both problems. Dr Levine recommends products that contain aluminium chloride hexahydrate such as Driclor (available from pharmacies).

Note: Don't use aluminium chloride on cracked or raw skin – it will sting like mad.

Use shoe sense. 'Closed shoes aggravate sweaty feet and set up a perfect environment for bacteria to grow, leading to more odour and more sweat,' says Dr Levine. Wear sandals and open-toed shoes when you can, but stay away from rubber and plastic shoes, which don't allow feet to breathe easily. And never wear the same shoes two days in a row. It takes at least 24 hours for shoes to dry out thoroughly.

Change your socks – often. The answer to sweaty, smelly feet is to change socks as frequently as possible – even three or four times a day, says podiatrist Glenn Copeland. Wear socks made of natural fibres like cotton, which are far more absorbent than socks made from synthetic materials.

Take frequent soaks. Various soaking agents can help to keep the feet dry, which may also control odour.

Tea. Tannin, found in tea, is a drying agent. Boil three or four tea bags in a litre of water for about 10 minutes, then add enough cold water to make a comfortable soak, suggests dermatologist Diana Bihova.

Soak your feet for 20 to 30 minutes, then dry them and apply foot powder. Do this twice a day until you get the problem under control. After that, repeat it twice a week to keep foot odour from recurring.

Bicarbonate of soda. This makes the foot surface more alkaline, thereby cutting down on the amount of odour produced, says Dr Levine. Dissolve a tablespoon of baking soda in a litre of water. Soak twice a week for about 15 minutes a time. You can also sprinkle baking soda in your shoes.

Vinegar. A acidic footbath may also help. Dr Levine recommends half a cup of vinegar in a litre of water. Soak for 15 minutes twice a week.

Potassium permanganate. Soak your feet daily in a solution of potassium permanganate. This is especially good for foot odour associated with athlete's foot or infected eczema. You can obtain tablets at the pharmacy (Permitabs): dissolve one tablet in four litres of water. The solution stains clothes and will stain your skin brown temporarily.

Hot and cold water. Alternate hot and cold footbaths, says Dr Levine. This procedure constricts the bloodflow to your feet, reducing perspiration.

KITCHEN CURES

Try radishes. Liquidize about two dozen radishes, add a quarter teaspoon of glycerine, put in a spray-top container and use daily to reduce foot odour.

This brew can also be used as an underarm deodorant.

Do your feet work harder than you do?

Sometimes feet sweat a lot because they simply work harder than they should, says podiatrist Neal Kramer. You may have a structural defect (such as flat feet) or a job that keeps you on your toes all day. Either would increase the activity of your foot muscles. And the harder your feet work, the more they sweat. Although feet that sweat don't necessarily smell bad, the wetness provides a good environment for odour-producing bacteria.

'If you correct the underlying problem with an arch support or some other orthotic shoe insert,' says Dr Kramer, 'you can cut down the amount of sweat produced. If muscles don't have to work as hard, they don't produce as much heat.'

Then make yourself a third footbath of ice cubes and lemon juice. Finally, rub your feet with alcohol to cool and dry them. In hot weather, when your feet sweat a lot, you could probably do this every day.

Note: People with diabetes and those with poor circulation should not use this treatment.

Sprinkle sweet-scented sage. Try sprinkling the fragrant herb sage into your shoes to control odour, says Dr Levine.

Try insoles. Some shoe insoles, such as Odor-Eaters, contain activated charcoal, which absorbs moisture and helps to control odour.

Keep your cool. The sweat glands in your feet, similar to those in your armpits and palms, respond to emotions, says dermatologist Richard Dobson. Stress can trigger excessive sweating. That, in turn, can increase bacterial activity in your shoes, leading to extra odour. So try not to get frazzled.

Watch what you eat. As bizarre as it may sound, says Dr Levine, when you eat spicy or pungent foods, such as onions, peppers or garlic, their essential oils can be excreted through the sweat glands in your feet. Which means your feet can end up smelling like your lunch.

FROSTBITE

13 safeguards against a winter chiller

Frostbite occurs when your extremities (fingers, cheeks, ears, nose and toes) get so cold that their temperature drops below freezing. It often affects mountaineers and people on skiing holidays. If frost damage is caught quickly, it is fully reversible (frostnip); if not, the result may be the loss of tissue (frostbite). Less extreme forms of injury include chapped lips and skin. Symptoms include an uncomfortable coldness which then becomes painful and, finally, numb. Yet less severe forms of frostbite can occur quickly in very cold weather when you're simply shovelling snow or changing a tyre. Here's what you need to know about this menace.

Know the signs. Frostnip is the least severe form of frostbite and usually leaves skin somewhat numb and white. The cheeks, tip of the nose, and ears are most likely sites for frostnip, says surgeon Bruce Paton. Peeling and blistering are also possible after the affected area is warmed.

Peeling and blistering after warming are more likely with superficial frostbite, a more serious condition. Frostbite is an injury in which the tissues of the body freeze. The skin is also frozen harder than with frostnip, but not so deeply that all resiliency is lost.

'Frostbite is the body's way of trying to preserve heat by shutting down circulation to an extremity,' says A&E surgeon Ruth Uphold. 'Unfortunately, as you develop frostbite, you might not even know that you have it because of the numbness.'

Look out for each other. If you are out on the ski slopes, make a deal to watch a friend's face – specifically the ears, nose and cheeks – for any noticeable change in colour, and get him to do the same for you.

Hide from the wind. Obviously, getting out of the elements into a warm place is a good idea. But if that's impossible, at least get out of the wind – windchill factors contribute significantly to frostbite.

Think before warming. Don't use dry, radiant heat, such as a heat lamp or campfire, Dr Paton says, if your skin appears to be frostbitten. Frostbitten skin is easily burned.

Use yourself. If you can't get indoors, take advantage of your own body heat. To warm fingers and hands, for example, tuck them in your armpits. 'Rolling yourself into a ball also makes you more energy efficient,' says Tom Schimelpfenig, an expert in mountain rescue.

WHEN TO CONSULT A DOCTOR

Frostbite demands professional medical attention. Tissue is dying which could lead to infection, the loss of fingers or toes and, in extreme cases, the loss of an arm or leg.

With deep frostbite, the skin is cold, hard, white and numb. When rewarmed, the skin may turn blue or purple. It may also swell and blisters might form. The idea, of course, is to treat frostbite quickly and effectively so none of that happens. Here's what you should do while you wait for medical attention.

Do not allow a frostbitten part to refreeze. Water crystals are bigger when the part refreezes, which causes even more tissue damage.

Use your head. It's best not to walk on frozen feet, but it's better than allowing a frozen foot to thaw and refreeze. If you think walking may be your only route to survival, leave your shoe or boot on the frostbitten foot, says surgeon Bruce Paton. 'The foot could blister and swell if you took a boot off, and you wouldn't be able to get it back on.'

Don't rub it with snow. That just creates friction with the skin, says Dr Uphold, and you also lose more heat when you get wet.

Wear mittens. Wear mittens instead of gloves – mittens are warmer – and pull on a fleece hat that protects your ears, advises A&E doctor James Sturm.

Avoid booze. 'You only think alcohol is warming you from the inside out. Alcohol actually causes more heat loss,' says Dr Uphold.

Don't smoke. Smoking decreases peripheral circulation and makes the extremities more vulnerable to frostbite, Dr Uphold says.

Hang loose. To protect circulation, wear loose clothing and don't wear any rings on your fingers, says Schimelpfenig.

Don't get wet. Heat loss is greatly accelerated by contact with water.

Don't delay. As soon as you feel your hands or feet are getting excessively cold, get indoors and get warm, advises Schimelpfenig.

Avoid contact with metal. Just a few moments with your bare hand on a metal wrench can lead to frostbite in severe cold.

GENITAL HERPES

15 managing strategies

Most people in the UK carry herpes simplex – 70 per cent facially (see *Cold Sores*, page 132) and 10 per cent genitally. One in four will be diagnosed because their symptoms are obvious or uncomfortable. The rest of us either have no symptoms, or such mild ones that they are never diagnosed.

There are two types of herpes simplex virus: Type 1 causes most oral herpes infections and up to half the cases of genital herpes; Type 2 almost always causes genital herpes only, but, with the growing popularity of oral sex, there is an increasing overlap.

Genital herpes is most often acquired during sexual contact, says family doctor Stephen Amiel, but a person with an active facial cold sore can transfer the virus to their own genitals – or other parts of the body, including the eye. The herpes virus does not survive off the body for long, so infection is very unlikely from household surfaces.

Genital herpes sounds dire and, until HIV/AIDS came along, was the sexual infection people dreaded most. There are treatments that help, though, and its long-term dangers have been overstated in the past, says Dr Amiel.

Your first attack of herpes may start with a flu-like illness, with tingling or irritation in the genital area. Typically, a small red, swollen area on the genitals or nearby then develops clusters of small blisters or vesicles, which burst to form shallow, painful ulcers. Occasionally, there may be only a small, painless ulcer. The lymph nodes in your groin may become swollen and tender and you may have a discharge. Passing urine may be extremely painful.

Once the initial attack of herpes comes and goes (usually in two to three weeks), the virus lies dormant for most of the time. But if the immune system is disrupted or put under pressure, through stress, illness or even menstruation, the virus can reactivate. Subsequent attacks are usually infrequent and rarely as severe as the first one. Although herpes is one of the most common sexually transmitted diseases (STDs), the blisters only recur in about one per cent of infected people. To limit outbreaks, try these steps.

Boost your immune system. Experts don't know exactly what causes the herpes virus to lie dormant for long periods and then abruptly awake to wreak havoc. But many think that a weakened immune system allows the virus to recur. To help prevent this from happening, it's a good idea to keep your immune system fit and robust with a balanced diet, lots of rest and relaxation and regular exercise.

WHEN TO CONSULT A DOCTOR

Early treatment with an oral antiviral drug during a first or recurrent attack of genital herpes is likely to reduce the duration of your symptoms, the extent of your sores and the number of days you continue to be infectious to others, says family doctor Stephen Amiel. Treatment in a first attack does not reduce the likelihood of further attacks, but if you have a high rate of recurrence, your doctor might put you on a low daily dose for some months. Antiviral creams like Zovirax are not particularly effective in genital herpes, and are not recommended.

If you are pregnant, make sure you tell your doctor that you have herpes, since the virus can infect newborns. You may be given oral antiviral treatment in late pregnancy if you had a first attack earlier in the pregnancy, but you will hopefully still be able to have a vaginal delivery. If you have a first attack in late pregnancy, though, you will probably be advised to have a Caesarean section, says Dr Amiel. A recurrent attack, even at the time of delivery, is less serious, and will not necessarily mean a Caesarean.

If your general immunity is low, either because you are on drugs like steroids or chemotherapeutic agents for cancer, or because of something like HIV/AIDS, the herpes virus can spread rapidly and cause a life-threatening infection, says Dr Amiel. Seek medical help urgently if you are in an at-risk group and you develop a herpes infection. Rarely, the herpes virus can cause meningitis or encephalitis even in otherwise well people. Symptoms can include fever, fits, headaches, personality change or coma.

If you suffer from severe eczema, you are also more at risk of a herpes infection spreading rapidly and should seek medical advice as soon as possible.

A strong link was once suspected between genital herpes and cervical cancer. That link is not as strong as once thought: women with herpes should have smears at normal three-yearly intervals, unless there are other indications for more frequent ones, such as a previous abnormal smear, or deep pain during, or bleeding after, intercourse.

Try a herbal strategy. Herpes is a viral condition and, once you have it, you have it forever. The immune system is responsible for keeping herpes in remission, and you need to work with your immune system to keep it that way, says clinical herbalist Douglas Schar.

Herbal immune stimulants with antiviral activity, such as echinacea, astragalus, maitake and burdock can all be used to prevent herpes episodes. Stress impairs the immune system, so if you know you are heading into a storm, use any of these herbs to boost your immune system and prevent an outbreak. If you are ill or run down, the herbs can give you a boost and prevent an attack. And if you feel an attack coming on, take a herbal remedy to stop it in its tracks.

The most effective strategy is to plan ahead. This simply means keeping herbal immune stimulants in the house so that they are there, ready to take immediately, as soon as you need them.

Use soap and water. You may be inclined to bombard your newly discovered sores with everything in your medicine cabinet. As with any sore, you do need to be concerned about developing a secondary (bacterial) infection, but soap and water is all you need or want to keep the area sufficiently germ-free, says Will Whittington, a medical researcher who specializes in STDs. Use a pH-neutral or dermatological soap to avoid stinging.

Add salt. Half-a-cup to a cup of household salt added to the bath water will soothe and promote healing of the ulcers, says Dr Amiel.

Steer clear of ointments. Genital sores need lots of air to heal. Petroleum jelly and antibiotic ointments can block this air and slow down the healing process, says Stephen Sacks, an expert on herpes viruses. Never use a cortisone cream, which can inhibit your immune system and actually encourage the virus to grow, he says.

Warm the discomfort away. During your primary attack or bad secondary attacks, taking a bath or shower to get warm water over the genital area three or four times a day may provide soothing relief. When you get out of the shower or bath, blow the genital area dry with a hair dryer, set on low or cool so as not to burn yourself. The air from the dryer is also soothing and may speed up the healing process by helping sores to dry out, says Dr Sacks.

Wear loose-fitting cotton undies. Since air is essential for healing, wear pants that let your skin breathe – that is, cotton, not synthetics, says nurse Judith Hurst, medical adviser to a herpes support group.

Around the house, you may feel more comfortable wearing a skirt or loose shorts and no pants at all, adds Dr Amiel. If you wear nylon tights, make sure the gusset is made of cotton. If you want to wear a lycra swimming costume, cut the cotton crotch out of a pair of knickers and sew it into the swimsuit.

Ease a painful pee. Urination during a first herpes outbreak can bring intense pain as acidic urine passes over open sores. This is particularly true for women. Try keeping the urine stream away from your sores with some rolled-up toilet paper, suggests Dr Sacks.

Occasionally, a first attack can be so painful that you are unable to pass urine at all, says Dr Amiel. Don't panic: take some painkillers, get into a bath as hot as you can comfortably cope with and allow yourself to urinate in the bath. Don't be tempted to stop drinking, warns Dr Amiel. Drinking extra fluids will dilute the urine, so that it stings less.

Don't touch. Although the disease is called *genital* herpes, it is possible, though not very common, to spread the virus to other parts of the body by touching an open sore and then bringing your fingers into contact with, say, your mouth or eyes. For this reason, it's important to wash your hands if you touch a sore, says Mitch Herndon, who runs a herpes

The mind and body connection

Why do some people carry the herpes virus for years without an attack, while others carrying the virus experience regular attacks?

The answer is largely in the mind, says clinical psychologist Christopher Stout. 'People who are more tense and depressed, carry more hostility, and are more easily aroused to anger, seem to suffer more frequent outbreaks,' says Dr Stout. 'These kinds of attitudes are thought to suppress the body's immune system.'

Nurse Judith Hurst agrees: 'I don't care how much research is done over the next 1000 years, I'm convinced that stress will always be the number one factor,' she says.

But if you weren't subject to stress before you learned you had herpes, you're probably feeling stress now.

This can create a situation in which your stress contributes to outbreaks, which contributes to stress, causing a vicious cycle.

The question is, how do you get off this roller coaster?

Learn all that you can. Read about herpes, talk with your doctor, try to make as much sense out of, and gain as much control over, your situation as you can, says Dr Stout.

Join a support group. See the tip 'Call for help' for details of a website and helpline. Support groups offer camaraderie, emotional support and a place to talk confidentially and share information, says Hurst.

Learn relaxation techniques. Find one that works for you, such as meditation or yoga, says Dr Stout.

telephone helpline. If you think you might scratch at night, cover sores with a gauze dressing, he says.

Consider these supplements. American studies suggest that the amino acid lysine helps to heal sores and prevent their recurrence. Amino acids may not be suitable if you have liver or kidney problems, if you are pregnant or breastfeeding. As with all such supplements, there is no official guarantee of safety, purity or effectiveness. Good dietary sources of lysine include fish, chicken, cheeses, potatoes, milk, brewer's yeast and beans.

Other supplements that may fight off herpes attacks include zinc, in ointment form or capsules, or the food additive butylated hydroxytoluene (BHT), taken as a supplement. But studies are small and have had mixed results: these are unproven remedies.

Note: High doses of zinc and BHT may be dangerous and should be taken only under a doctor's supervision.

Call for help. If you have any questions regarding your condition, help is available. The Herpes Viruses Association (HVA) has a helpline: 020 7607 9661, and a website (www.herpes.org.uk) that provides useful information and a list of patient support groups.

Don't do unto others. Remember how you got herpes? You now have a responsibility to protect others. When you have sores, you are highly contagious – so avoid sex. When you have no sores, you are unlikely to pass on the virus, but there is no guarantee, says Dr Amiel, so you may wish to use a condom for further protection and peace of mind.

GINGIVITIS
21 ways to stop gum disease

Fewer than half of British adults have frequent dental check-ups, and only 62 per cent of children are registered with NHS dentists, despite treatment being free. The British Dental Association says that, while overall dental health is far better than it was two decades ago, the number of adults having regular check-ups is falling. This explains, at least in part, why 19 out of 20 of us will suffer from gum disease at some point in our lives.

Most adults have gingivitis to some degree. The condition is the first sign of periodontal disease and the main reason that adults lose their teeth. Gingivitis is simply inflammation of the gums. The normally pale pink gums turn bluish red. They become tender and swollen between the teeth and bleed easily, especially when brushing.

Gingivitis is caused by plaque and tartar both above and below the gumline. If left untreated, it can lead to periodontitis, in which pus collects in deep pockets of the gum, teeth become sensitive to pressure, loosen and fall out. Here are some ways recommended by dentists to stop this from happening.

Brush properly. If you want to get rid of gingivitis, you have to take time to floss and brush correctly. Take three to five minutes two or three times a day for good oral hygiene, says dentist Robert Schallhorn.

Brush at the gumline. The plaque-catching area around the gumline is where gingivitis starts, and is the most neglected area when we brush, says dentist Vincent Cali. Use your brush at a 45-degree angle to your teeth so that half of your brush cleans your gums while the other half cleans your teeth.

Have two toothbrushes. Alternate between them, advises Dr Cali. Allow one to dry while using the other.

Consider electric. Studies show that using an electric toothbrush improves oral health, though manual toothbrushes are just as effective as long as you're brushing properly. Electric toothbrushes are especially useful for people with limited manual dexterity as the rotating head can clean hard-to-reach areas.

Build up bone. Gingivitis is the beginning of what Dr Cali calls periodontal osteoporosis. Just as the bones in the rest of your skeleton can shrink and become brittle, so, too, can your jawbone. Bolster your bones with plenty of calcium (found in dairy products, salmon, almonds and dark green leafy vegetables such as kale and broccoli), exercise and a no-smoking policy.

Try a gum massage. Grip your gums between your thumb and index finger (index on the outside) and rub, suggests dentist Richard Shepard. This increases healthy blood circulation to your gums.

Use a gum stimulator. A specially designed triangular gum stimulator, available from some dentists and pharmacies, is better than a toothpick for massaging the gums, says Dr Cali. It also cleans the surfaces between the teeth. Place the rubber point so that it rests between two teeth. Point the tip in the direction of the biting surface until the stimulator is at a 45-degree angle to the gumline. Apply in a circular motion for 10 seconds, then move on to the next tooth. Some electric toothbrushes come with a gum stimulator attachment.

Stock up on vitamin C. Vitamin C won't cure gingivitis, but it can help to prevent bleeding gums, according to an American study. The suggested daily intake is 100 to 500mg. Fresh fruit and vegetables are the best dietary sources of vitamin C, but keep the cooking of them to a minimum to preserve their full vitamin content.

Brandish an interdental brush. An interdental brush is a specially designed brush (available at most pharmacies) shaped like a tiny bottle brush. It slides between your teeth or under your crown or bridge to get at those hard-to-reach places, says dentist Roger Levin.

Use a mouthwash. An antibacterial mouthwash may help gingivitis. Look out for those listing cetylpridinium chloride or domiphen bromide on the label. Research shows that these are the active ingredients in mouthwash that reduce dental plaque.

Examine your lifestyle. Too much stress? Too little relaxation? Do you work with toxic chemicals? Any of these factors can adversely affect your gums. Look at every aspect of your lifestyle to see what you can change to make your life more healthy, advises Dr Cali.

Cut down on drinking and smoking. Excessive smoking and drinking drains your body of vitamins and minerals vital to a healthy mouth.

Scrape your tongue. Remove the bacteria and toxins hiding there. It doesn't matter what you use to scrape with, as long as it isn't sharp, says Dr Cali. He recommends a small spoon, a wooden ice lolly stick, a tongue depressor or your toothbrush. Scrape from back to front 10 to 15 times.

Vary the routine. Don't try to perform all these oral ablutions in one day. Massage your gums one day, and scrape your tongue the next. If you do something different after you brush and floss, you won't bore yourself to death.

Zap bacteria with H_2O_2. Buy a three per cent solution of hydrogen peroxide, mix it half-and-half with water, and swish it around your mouth for 30 seconds. Don't swallow. Use three times a week to inhibit bacteria, says Dr Cali.

Try folic acid. There is some research evidence that a 0.1 per cent solution of folic acid used as a mouth rinse (5ml twice a day for 30 to 60

WHEN TO CONSULT A DOCTOR

If your gums still bleed when you brush your teeth and remain sore and swollen despite your efforts at good oral hygiene, see your dentist. You risk more serious periodontal disease and the possible loss of your teeth if you ignore sore, bleeding gums. Serious warning signs that should send you straight to your dentist are:

• bad breath that doesn't go away within 24 hours;

• your teeth looking longer – a result of the gums shrinking away from your teeth;

• your mouth feeling out of alignment when you shut it because your teeth meet differently;

• your partial dentures fitting differently;

• pus pockets forming between your teeth and gums;

• teeth becoming loose or falling out.

Swollen, bleeding gums are a common side-effect of phenytoin, a drug used for epilepsy. This may be helped by folic acid mouthwash (see facing page), but if badly affected, you should talk to your doctor about alternatives.

Painless, bleeding gums may signify a clotting disorder of the blood, or overtreatment with anticoagulants like warfarin. See your doctor as soon as possible, especially if you have bruising, or unexplained or excessive bleeding elsewhere, too.

days) reduces gum inflammation and bleeding in people with gingivitis. The folic acid solution is rinsed around the mouth for one to five minutes and then spat out. The evidence for benefit from folic acid tablets is less convincing.

Herbs may help. Echinacea, chamomile and myrrh have been found by herbalists to have anti-inflammatory and antimicrobial actions which can help in gingivitis. They can be found made up as a mouthwash or toothpaste.

Wash with a water jet. Use an oral irrigation device to flush water around your teeth and gums, says Dr Cali. To use it correctly, direct the water jet between your teeth like dental floss, not down into your gums.

Eat a raw vegetable a day. Crunching on carrots and celery sticks will keep gingivitis away, says Dr Cali. Hard and fibrous foods clean and stimulate teeth and gums.

Try baking soda. Mix a teaspoonful of baking soda into a paste with a little water and apply it with your fingers along the gumline. Then brush. You'll clean, polish, neutralize acidic bacterial wastes and deodorize in one fell swoop, says Dr Cali.

Free dentistry for mums-to-be. Pregnant women should take special care of their gums. Pregnancy hormones increase the sensitivity of gum tissue to plaque bacteria, increasing the likelihood of gum disease. Dental care is free for all women during pregnancy and for a year after delivery, so take advantage of this and see your dentist regularly.

GOUT
15 coping ideas

Gout is an extremely painful joint condition – so painful that most patients can't even bear the weight of a sheet on the tender joint. The throbbing pain often hits at night, turning the skin red-hot and leaving the affected joint swollen and tender for five to 10 days.

Once considered the domain of royalty, gout is actually a fairly common disorder, affecting 16 men in every 1000, but only three women in every 1000. Contrary to popular belief, people don't get gout from drinking too much port, but because there is something wrong with the chemical processes of their body.

We all have a substance called urate in our blood, and in a gout sufferer, this substance can build up and form needle-shaped crystals in the joints, making them intensely painful. Gout may be caused by an inherited enzyme deficiency but there are a number of other things that can precipitate it too, including certain foods, alcohol, drugs and other diseases.

Often the big toe is affected, but gout can cause pain in almost any joint. One small bit of good news is that gout usually affects only one joint at a time. In older people, though, attacks are more likely to affect several joints at once, often the fingers, and women become more susceptible than men.

The typical gout victim is a middle-aged man, who may be overweight and have a family history of the disease. If you're a current – or potential – sufferer, take some advice from the experts.

WHEN TO CONSULT A DOCTOR

If you experience sudden and intense pain in a joint, call your doctor. Even if the pain goes away in a day or two, it is important to see your doctor, because gout left untreated can lead to more pain and joint damage.

If this is your first attack, your doctor will want to:

- establish the diagnosis, usually by blood tests, but occasionally by taking a little fluid from an inflamed joint;

- rule out other causes of an acutely inflamed joint, like a septic arthritis or psoriasis;

- establish the cause of your gout: excess alcohol, perhaps, or medications for high blood pressure, low dose aspirin for heart disease and some cancer drugs; associated illnesses such as kidney disease, bone marrow disorders, obesity and raised blood triglycerides;

- prescribe NSAIDs or colchicines, an anti-gout medicine used for thousands of years, derived from the autumn crocus plant. Occasionally, your doctor might prescribe a short course of prednisolone (an oral steroid), or give you a steroid injection.

If you have more than three gout attacks, or suffer from complications such as uric acid kidney stones or gouty arthritis, your doctor may want you to take allopurinol once an attack has passed. This reduces uric acid formation and must be continued long-term. You will need to continue with NSAIDs or colchicines too for a while, usually three months or so, as allupurinol can make acute gout worse at first.

Get some rest. During an acute attack, rest and elevate the affected joint, says pathologist Agatha Thrash. You'll probably have little trouble following this advice because the pain will be so intense.

Take ibuprofen. It is the tremendous inflammation around the affected joint that causes the pain. So when you need a painkiller, make sure it's one that can reduce inflammation – namely ibuprofen, says arthritis specialist Jeffrey Lisse. If the recommended dose doesn't provide relief, consult your doctor before increasing it. You may be told to increase to a maximum of 2.4g a day.

Other nonsteroidal anti-inflammatory drugs (NSAIDs), with the exception of aspirin, probably work just as well, but ibuprofen has fewer side-effects. If you're unable to take or tolerate NSAIDs, your doctor may be able to give you alternative pain relief.

Avoid aspirin. All pain relievers are not created equal. Aspirin can actually make gout worse by inhibiting the excretion of uric acid, says Dr Lisse. Paracetamol doesn't have anti-inflammatory properties and isn't therefore as effective in acute gout as NSAIDs, but you can add paracetamol and codeine-type analgesics to your NSAIDs for extra pain relief.

Use herbs to clean up. Gout is caused by the deposition of waste in joints. This happens when the body does not excrete waste properly, but instead stores it in the joints of the extremities, says clinical herbalist Douglas Schar. The solution, he says, is to increase waste excretion.

Diuretic and laxative herbs get the body's waste excretion systems pumping so that toxins go where they should go – out of the body. 'My favourites are dandelion leaf, chicory root and burdock root,' says Schar. 'All can be bought at health food stores and are best taken in tea form. Three cups a day, brewed according to label instructions, will go a long way towards relieving an active case of gout, and will help to prevent a relapse once the condition has cleared up.'

Apply ice. If the affected joint is not too tender to touch, try applying a crushed-ice pack, says rheumatologist John Abruzzo. The ice has a soothing, numbing effect. Place the pack on the painful joint for about 10 minutes. Cushion it with a towel or sponge. Reapply as needed.

Drink lots of water. Large amounts of fluid can help to flush excess uric acid from your system before it can do any harm. Physiologist Robert Davis recommends plain water. 'Most people just don't drink enough water,' he says. 'For best results, drink five or six glasses a day.'

As a bonus, lots of water may also help to discourage the kidney stones that also affect people with gout.

Avoid high-purine foods. 'Foods that are high in substances called purines contribute to higher levels of uric acid,' says professor of medicine, Robert Wortmann. Avoiding such foods is wise.

Those foods most likely to *induce* gout include high-protein animal products. Those highest in purines are anchovies, sardines, herring, offal, game, meat extracts and shellfish.

Limit other purine-containing foods. Foods that may contribute to gout contain a moderate amount of purines. These foods include asparagus, dried beans and pulses, cauliflower, mushrooms, oatmeal, spinach, wholegrain cereals and breads, and yeast. Also included here are all fish, meat and poultry (apart from the high-purine ones listed above). Limit these foods to one small serving five days a week.

Skip the beer. Avoid alcohol if you have a history of gout, says pharmacist Gary Stoehr. Alcohol seems to increase uric acid production and inhibit its secretion, which can lead to gout attacks in some people. Beer may be particularly harmful because it has a higher purine content than wine and other spirits, says nutrition expert Eleonore Blaurock-Busch.

If you do have the odd tipple, minimize your risk of a reaction by drinking slowly and buffering wine with easily absorbed carbohydrates such as bread and fruit, suggests Felix Kolb, a professor of medicine.

Control your blood pressure. If you have high blood pressure as well as gout, you have double trouble. That's because certain drugs prescribed to lower blood pressure, such as diuretics, actually raise uric acid levels, says pharmacist Branton Lachman. So taking steps to lower your blood pressure naturally is wise. Try decreasing your salt intake, losing excess weight and exercising. But never discontinue any prescribed medication without consulting your doctor.

Beware of fad diets. If you're overweight, slimming is imperative. Heavier people tend to have high uric acid levels. But stay away from fad diets, which are notorious for triggering gout attacks, says Dr Lisse. Such diets – including fasting – cause cells to break down and release uric acid. So work with your doctor or health visitor to devise a gradual weight-loss programme.

Make a charcoal poultice. Charcoal draws toxins from the body, notes Dr Thrash. She recommends mixing a tablespoon of activated charcoal powder BPC (which you can order from chemists) with three tablespoons of flaxseeds (also known as linseed) ground to a fine powder in a blender, and enough very warm water to make a paste. Apply to the affected joint. Cover with a cloth or cling film to hold it in place. Change every four hours or leave on overnight.

If you prefer a warm soak instead of a poultice, make a charcoal-and-water paste and then gradually add enough hot water until you can comfortably

KITCHEN CURES

Cherries have long been a folk remedy for gout. Although there is no hard scientific evidence that cherries help to relieve gout, many people find them beneficial. It doesn't seem to matter whether they are sweet or sour, canned or fresh. Recommended amounts vary from a handful (about 10 cherries) a day up to 250g. People have also reported success taking one tablespoon of cherry concentrate a day, says pathologist Agatha Thrash.

submerge your foot in the mixture. Soak for 30 to 60 minutes. Make sure you use an old basin, and don't get any charcoal on clothes or bed linen because it stains.

Taken by mouth, activated charcoal can help to reduce uric acid levels in the blood, says Dr Thrash. Try Bragg's charcoal tablets or biscuits or Lanes charcoal tablets four times a day: on getting up, mid-morning, mid-afternoon and at bedtime.

Note: Charcoal inhibits the absorption of many other drugs, so check with a pharmacist or your GP before taking it.

Watch those vitamins. Be careful when taking vitamins, because too much of certain nutrients can make gout worse, says Dr Blaurock-Busch. Excess niacin and vitamin A, in particular, may bring on an attack. It's best to talk to your doctor before increasing your vitamin intake.

Don't hurt yourself. For some unknown reason, gout often strikes a joint that's been previously bruised, so try not to stub your toe, says Dr Abruzzo. It's a good idea to avoid wearing tight shoes, which can also damage your joints.

GREASY SKIN
6 ideas for a shine-free face

Nobody dies from greasy skin, so researchers aren't exactly racing to find a cure. Indeed, the best advice most experts have to offer is to keep your skin clean. No magic there, then.

Greasy skin has many more causes than solutions. Heredity plays a big part, as do hormones. For instance, pregnant women sometimes notice an increase in skin oil as hormonal activity changes. Women taking certain types of contraceptive pills often do as well. Stress can cause our oil glands to kick into overdrive. And the wrong cosmetics can easily aggravate an otherwise mild case of greasy skin.

But there is one big advantage to having greasy skin: in the long run, oily skin tends to age better and wrinkle less than dry or normal skin. Meanwhile, here are some tips for a cleaner, drier face.

Try a mud pack. Clay masks cleanse the skin of surface greasiness and tone it – for a while anyway, says dermatologist Howard Donsky. But their effects are only temporary.

WHEN TO CONSULT A DOCTOR

If you think your contraceptive pill is making your skin more greasy, talk to your doctor or family planning clinic nurse about changing to a more oestrogen-dominant type. Don't stop taking your current pill in mid-packet: it's better to continue with them until you see your doctor, or use alternative methods such as condoms until a suitable alternative is found.

Use soap and hot water. 'Hot water is a good solvent,' says dermatologist Hillard Pearlstein. Washing greasy skin with very warm water and plenty of soap dissolves skin oil better than cold water and soap.

Buy medicated soaps. Finding a drying soap is not a problem. (Finding one that *won't* dry the skin is actually more of a challenge.) Many dermatologists recommend specialized degreasing soaps such as Neutrogena, or Boots ACT wash bar, formulated for spots. But you don't need to spend lots of money, says dermatologist Kenneth Neldner. Most ordinary soaps are pretty drying – the key is to use lots of soap and really scrub the skin, he says.

Follow with an astringent. Astringents containing alcohol are your best bet; try Neutrogena Clear Pore Lotion or Clearasil Pore Cleansing Lotion.

For an effective, inexpensive astringent, try witch hazel, which contains some alcohol and works well. Alcohol-free astringents contain mostly water and are not as effective as those with alcohol, but they may help if you have sensitive skin.

Dermatologists say that rather than washing your face several times a day, which can leave it dry and irritated, you're better off carrying astringent pads with you and using them to cleanse your face.

Use herbal teas. Any of the herbal astringents will help to dry out oily skin, says clinical herbalist Douglas Schar. Popular astringents include China tea, oak bark, geranium bark and geum. Make a weak tea using any one these herbs, let it cool, strain and apply to greasy areas with a cotton wool ball.

Another simple remedy, says Schar, is to dab oily areas with a used tea bag several times a week. This tip doesn't even require a visit to the health food shop.

Forget any food connection

Although some beauty writers recommend special diets for reducing oily skin problems (usually cutting out fried and fatty foods), our experts dismiss such things as pure fantasy.

There's no relationship between diet and oily skin, says dermatologist Hillard Pearlstein.

The condition is genetic – you either have it or you don't. You can't turn off your oil glands with diet.

Dermatologist Kenneth Neldner agrees. 'I don't think diet has any effect. If it does, the medical community knows nothing about it.'

Choose cosmetics with care. Make-up comes in two major categories: oil-based and water-based. If you have oily skin, use only water-based products, says Dr Neldner. Many cosmetics are specially formulated for oily skin. They soak up and cover oiliness so that the skin doesn't look as greasy. But no cosmetic has any magical ingredient to slow down or stop oil production.

HAEMORRHOIDS
16 tips to ease the discomfort

Haemorrhoids may have changed the course of history. It is said that Napoleon was so distracted by the pain and discomfort of haemorrhoids that this contributed to his defeat at Waterloo. But haemorrhoids, or piles, are a common ailment this side of the Channel too, affecting about half the UK's population by the age of 50.

Haemorrhoids are areas of congested tissue, full of blood vessels, in the anal canal and lower rectum. Increased pressure over long periods causes these normal areas to become more engorged and swollen. They become painful when, under the pressure of straining, they protrude through the anus and their blood supply is cut off by the tight anal sphincter. The haemorrhoids become more congested; they get bigger and then are more likely to come down the next time. If the blood supply is cut off for long enough, the haemorrhoid strangulates – it thromboses, dies and shrivels, but the process can be excruciatingly painful.

More commonly, haemorrhoids cause bleeding from the anus during or after straining, usually bright red blood which may be noticed on wiping, or which may coat the stool or drip into the pan. Over time, haemorrhoidal bleeding may be persistent or severe enough to make you anaemic. The bleeding is usually painless: pain is a feature only of more severe piles, and may well indicate some other condition. Haemorrhoids may also cause a mucus discharge and itching (see *Anal Fissures and Itching,* page 38). A prolapsed pile may be seen or felt at the anus as a smooth, grape-like, bluish, tender lump and sometimes you may have a sense of fullness or discomfort in the rectum.

Heredity and age make some people more vulnerable to haemorrhoids, but they can also be caused by – and remedied by – such things as diet and toilet habits. Here's what our experts suggest to relieve the pain and discomfort of this common problem.

Aim for soft, easy bowel movements. Straining on the toilet provides just the kind of pressure needed to engorge and swell the veins in your rectum. Hard stools then make matters worse by scraping the already troubled area. The solution is to drink lots of fluids, eat plenty of fibre and observe the following remedies.

Ease the passage of stools. Once you've increased the fibre and fluids in your diet, your stool should become softer and pass with less effort. You may help your bowels move even more smoothly by lubricating your anus with a little petroleum jelly, says colorectal surgeon Edmund Leff. Use a cotton bud or finger to apply the jelly about 1cm into the rectum.

Clean yourself gently. After moving your bowels it's extremely important to clean yourself properly and gently, says family doctor John Lawder. Toilet paper can be scratchy, and some types contain chemical irritants. Buy only unscented white toilet paper, and dampen it under the tap before you wipe.

Use premoistened wipes. Most chemists and supermarkets now sell moist toilet wipes that are soft on your bot and safe to flush.

Don't scratch. Haemorrhoids can itch, and scratching can make them feel better. But *don't* give in to the urge to scratch. You can damage the walls of the delicate veins and make matters worse, says Dr Lawder.

Don't lift heavy objects. Lifting heavy objects and strenuous exercise can act much like straining on the toilet, says Dr Leff. If you're prone to haemorrhoids, get a friend to help or pay someone to move that piano or dresser.

WHEN TO CONSULT A DOCTOR

If you've never had haemorrhoids, but all of a sudden you experience discomfort, it may well be due to something else. If discomfort is accompanied by itching and you've recently returned from a trip abroad, for example, you might have worms. You will need treatment to get rid of them. A lump at the anus may be due to an abscess, skin tags or anal warts.

'Never assume that rectal bleeding is due to haemorrhoids,' warns family doctor Stephen Amiel. 'Other causes need to be ruled out, including colitis, diverticular disease, polyps, anal fissures and cancer.' Even if haemorrhoids have been previously diagnosed, your doctor should have the opportunity to reassess your symptoms and diagnosis, in case something else is going on instead of, or as well as your haemorrhoids.

At other times, an enlarged vein in your anus can clot, creating a swollen hard area that's very painful, says family doctor John Lawder. In most cases, the clot can be removed with minor surgery.

Haemorrhoids that don't heal may require medical intervention to halt blood flow to the tissue or to remove it. Options include laser and traditional surgery and sclerotherapy (in which a chemical solution is injected to shrink the vessel).

Increasingly, specialists and some GPs, too, tie off moderate haemorrhoids with rubber bands: they then shrivel away as their blood supply is cut off. This procedure can be done in minutes, says Dr Amiel.

Soak in the bath. Sitting with your knees raised in 8–10cm of warm water in a bath is a remedy that still tops most experts' lists as a way to deal with haemorrhoids, says Byron Gathright, a colorectal surgeon. The warm water helps to kill the pain and also increases the flow of blood to the area, which can help to shrink the swollen veins.

Reach for the ice. If prolapsed haemorrhoids are particularly painful, use an icepack to anaesthetize and shrink them, suggests family doctor Stephen Amiel. Wrap some crushed ice in a plastic bag (a pack of frozen peas or coffee beans works very well too) and then a small cloth or flannel. Take some painkillers – avoiding constipating codeine-containing ones – and lie down with your bottom on a slight incline to get the help of gravity. Apply the icepack for no more than 20 minutes at a time, and no more than three times a day. Severe anal itching from haemorrhoids also responds well to this remedy.

Apply a haemorrhoid cream. There are many haemorrhoid creams and suppositories on the market, and while they generally will not make your problem disappear (contrary to what the ads may say), most work as local painkillers to relieve some of the discomfort, says Dr Gathright.

Creams are best. Choose a haemorrhoid cream over a suppository, says Dr Leff. Suppositories are useless for external haemorrhoids. Even for internal haemorrhoids, they tend to float too far up into the rectum to do much good.

Creams containing local anaesthetic may cause local sensitization if used for long periods, and those containing steroids should not be used if there might be local infection present. Some people find creams containing heparinoids, like Lasonil, helpful. These are said to act by dissolving congealed blood and reducing swelling.

Try herbal tannins. Tannins, found in plants, were once used to tan animal hides to make them into leather. They worked because they are astringent, which means that they shrink and tighten tissues. And that is just as true for a haemorrhoid as it is for a hide, says clinical herbalist Douglas Schar.

The three most effective tannin-rich herbs – long used to reduce the swelling and discomfort of haemorrhoids – are witch hazel, oak bark and geranium root. Buy them in tincture form from a health food store and apply with a cotton wool ball three times a day. The advantage of tannins, says Schar, is that they take care of immediate symptoms and, used regularly, will prevent a relapse.

Watch your weight. Because they have more pressure on their lower extremities, overweight people tend to have more problems with haemorrhoids, just as they do with varicose veins, says Dr Lawder.

Control your salt intake. Excess salt can make haemorrhoids worse. Salt retains fluids in the circulatory system that can cause veins in the anus and elsewhere to bulge, says Dr Lawder.

Avoid certain foods and drinks. While specific foods don't make haemorrhoids worse, they can contribute to your anal discomfort by creating further itching as they pass through the bowels. Watch out for excessive coffee, strong spices, beer and cola, says Dr Leff.

Lie on your left side if you're pregnant. Pregnant women are particularly prone to haemorrhoids, in part because the uterus sits directly on the blood vessels that drain the haemorrhoidal veins, says obstetrician Lewis Townsend. A good haemorrhoid remedy if you are pregnant is to lie on your left side for about 20 minutes every four to six hours, he says. This helps to decrease pressure on the main vein draining the lower half of the body.

Constipation, common in pregnancy, also makes haemorrhoids more likely. See *Constipation*, page 144 for some ways to avoid this. Straining during labour can make haemorrhoids temporarily worse, but the good news is that they usually disappear after delivery.

Give it a little push. Sometimes the word 'haemorrhoid' refers not to a swollen vein but to a downward displacement of the anal canal lining. If you have such a protruding haemorrhoid, try gently pushing it back into the anal canal, says Dr Townsend. Haemorrhoids left hanging can develop into painful clots.

HAIR PROBLEMS
27 treatments for hair on head and body

While the average human head has 150,000 hairs, some people think they have too few and others think they have too many, if not on their head then elsewhere on their bodies – faces, bikini area, underarms or legs.

Although a really bad hair day can *feel* like the end of the world, most hair problems are merely cosmetic and easily dealt with. Here's what our experts have to say about unwanted hair, dry hair and greasy hair. (For tips and remedies for excessive hair loss, see *Alopecia*, page 34.)

Too Much Hair

Visible hair in places where you'd rather look smooth can be embarrassing. There are numerous ways to eliminate unwanted hair, with the best method dependent on the type and location of hair you're trying to get rid of, says dermatologist Victor Newcomer.

Shave it. Simple and quick, shaving works fine for hair in places where next-day stubble is okay, such as your legs. Contrary to what you may have heard, shaving doesn't make hair grow back faster or coarser, says Dr Newcomer.

Bleach it. Hiding the hair rather than removing it is a painless option for light, fuzzy hair above the lip, but it doesn't work as well on thick or dark growth.

Wax it. Waxing is best for light fuzz, Dr Newcomer believes. He says that the least painful waxing methods are prewaxed plastic strips and kits for sugaring, a process that coats hairs with a mixture of sugar and wax, then removes the hair when it is pulled off.

Note: Don't use wax if you're taking oral isotretinoin (Roaccutane) for acne, or for six months after you stop taking it, as this medication makes skin more sensitive. Similarly, don't wax areas if you're using tretinoin creams (Retin-A, for example) on them, or for three months after you stop. These medications make skin more sensitive. Sunburnt or broken skin should never be waxed.

Depilate it. Chemical hair removers like Immac work by dissolving the hair, so they are too harsh to use on sensitive, sunburned or broken skin.

Interestingly, a drug called eflornithine, used to cure sleeping sickness in Africa, seems to be effective in inhibiting hair regrowth after removal when used in a cream (Vaniqa). Long-term studies on its effectiveness and safety are awaited, and it is not yet generally available in the UK.

If your skin becomes irritated after using a depilatory, soothe it with aloe.

Greasy Hair

Blondes may have more fun, but they also have greasier hair. And those with silky, baby-fine hair tend to have the worst problems with greasiness.

Oil is particularly conspicuous on fine, straight hair, and much less so on thick or wiry hair. Heat and humidity can accelerate oil production, as can hormonal changes. The male hormone androgen, for example, can activate the oil-producing sebaceous glands. Stress raises levels of androgen in the bloodstream of women as well as in men. Because they have more androgen than

KITCHEN CURES

If you have greasy hair, you may find some helpers in the kitchen cupboards.

Try a cider vinegar rinse. Put a teaspoon of cider vinegar in a pint of water and use as your final rinse. This solution removes soap residue that can weigh down oily hair. And don't worry about smelling like a salad; the vinegar's smell evaporates quickly.

Freshen up with lemon. Squeeze the juice of two lemons into a litre of water – ideally distilled water, says hairstylist David Daines, and use as a final rinse.

Switch to beer. 'Mousse dries the hair and clogs the pores,' says Daines. He recommends using fresh beer as a setting lotion for greasy hair.

WHEN TO CONSULT A DOCTOR

Excessive hair and hair texture problems can signal hormonal imbalances, illness, nutritional deficiencies or stress. See a doctor if you notice a sudden change in your hair, just to rule out any serious underlying cause.

Even if your problem is cosmetic, doctors can offer a number of solutions that aren't available over the counter.

women, men tend to have greasier hair. Anyway, if your problem is greasy hair, here's what our experts advise.

Get the right cut. Ask your hairdresser to cut some body into your hair. Layers are the key, says hairstylist David Daines. If you wear your hair long and one length, the weight pulls it down, making it lie flat on your head.

Shampoo often. The most important thing you can do to combat an excessively oily scalp is to shampoo every day, particularly if you live in a city. When summer heat and humidity stimulate your scalp's oil glands, you may want to shampoo twice a day, says dermatologist Lowell Goldsmith.

Choose a clear shampoo. 'Clear, see-through shampoos tend to have less goo in them,' says dermatologist Thomas Goodman. They clean oil away better, without leaving a residue behind.

Give yourself a scalp massage. This should be done just before a shampoo, never between washes, says hair care specialist Philip Kingsley.

Double bubble. People with especially greasy hair or scalps, should shampoo twice, advises Dr Goldsmith. Leave the shampoo on the scalp for five minutes each time. This won't harm your hair or scalp.

Forget conditioner. If you have greasy hair that tends to flatten out as the day goes on, the last thing you want to do is coat it with more oil. Try doing without conditioner, suggests Dr Goodman.

Just aim for the ends. If you find you do need a conditioner, look for a product that contains the least amount of oil or one that is largely oil-free. Then, just condition the ends and leave the roots.

Apply astringent. You can help to slow down oil secretion by applying a homemade astringent directly to your scalp. Kingsley suggests applying a mixture of equal parts witch hazel and mouthwash, with cotton wool balls, to the scalp only. The witch hazel acts as an astringent, and the mouthwash has antiseptic properties, he says. If your scalp is very oily, use this before each shampoo.

Don't overbrush. 'People with oily hair have to be careful not to be too vigorous with brushing,' says Dr Goldsmith. Brushing from the roots carries oil from your scalp to the ends of your hair.

Learn to relax. When you're under stress, your body produces more androgens, and androgens boost oil production. Relax, says Kingsley. Experiment with different relaxation techniques, such as meditation, tai chi or yoga, and practise the one that works best for you.

Consider your birth control pill. Oral contraceptives affect a woman's hormone balance. That, in turn, affects oil production. Dr Goodman suggests that you mention excessively oily hair to your doctor when discussing the Pill.

Dry Hair

Dry, flyaway hair can be unattractive and unmanageable. Ironic as it may sound, too much water may be responsible for the hair's parched condition, particularly water of the salty, chlorinated or soapy variety.

Swimming and overshampooing are two common causes of arid, flyaway locks, says hairstylist Jack Myers. Other culprits, he says, include colourings, perms, curling tongs, excessive blow-drying and overexposure to wind and sun.

Here are some ways to rescue dried-out hair.

Shampoo with care. Shampooing doesn't only wash away dirt, it also washes out the hair's protective oils, says Dr Goodman. If your hair is dry from too much lather, give it a break by washing less often. Use only a mild shampoo, one labelled 'for dry or damaged hair'.

Use a conditioner. When hair becomes dry, the outer layers, or cuticles, peel off the central shaft. Conditioners glue the cuticles back to the shaft, lubricate the hair and prevent static electricity (which creates frizz). Find a conditioner that works well for you and use it after every shampoo, says Dr Goodman.

Snip off those split ends. Dry hair tends to suffer most at the ends. The answer is to snip them off, says Finnish hairstylist Anja Vaisanen. Have

KITCHEN CURES

Try these salon-approved kitchen cures for dry hair.

Slap on some mayonnaise. 'Mayonnaise makes an excellent conditioner,' says Steven Docherty, former senior art director at the Vidal Sassoon Salon. He recommends leaving the dressing in your hair for between five minutes and an hour before washing it out.

Try a fizzy solution. 'Beer is a wonderful setting lotion. It gives a crisp, healthy, shiny look, even to dry hair,' says Docherty. Spray it onto your hair using a pump bottle after you've shampooed and towel-dried, but before you blow-dry or style. Don't worry about smelling like a pub – the smell of the beer quickly disappears.

Go for natural nutrients. Hairdresser Joanne Harris makes a nutrient-rich conditioner in her kitchen. 'I take blackened bananas and mash them with mushy avocados,' she says. Leave the tropical purée in your hair for 15 minutes, and then wash it out over the kitchen sink.

a trim every six weeks or so to keep split ends under control.

Chill out. Hot curling tongs and heated rollers can both contribute to dry hair, says hairdresser Joanne Harris. She suggests that you rediscover those unheated, plastic cylinder rollers from years gone by.

For straightening, wrap slightly moist hair under and around rollers (like a pageboy hairdo) for about 10 minutes.

For curling or adding wave, try using sponge rollers overnight or sleeping in damp plaits.

Protect your hair from the elements. 'Whipping wind can fray your hair just like a piece of fabric,' says Steven Docherty, formerly of the Vidal Sassoon Salon. The sun, too, takes a great toll on our hair.

Docherty recommends wearing a hat on breezy, balmy summer days and blustery, frosty winter days.

Wear a bathing cap. Chlorine is very destructive, says Docherty. Wear a fitted rubber swimming cap whenever you visit the swimming pool. For extra protection, first rub a little olive oil into your hair.

HANGOVERS

19 ways to deal with the day after

The best and only foolproof cure for a hangover is 24 hours. In the meantime, many of the symptoms – the headache, nausea and fatigue – can be alleviated. Here's how.

Get some pain relief. A headache is invariably part of the package that goes with a hangover, says family doctor Stephen Amiel. Aspirin or ibuprofen will help, but these can irritate and occasionally cause bleeding from a stomach that may already be inflamed from too much alcohol. Avoid them if you have a history of persistent indigestion or ulcers, or are on warfarin, or you have a known sensitivity to these anti-inflammatory drugs.

Paracetamol is toxic to the liver in large doses, and can be dangerous if your liver is already damaged by alcohol but, says Dr Amiel, most experts agree that a full daily dose of paracetamol (4 grams in 24 hours), will not do a social drinker any harm as a hangover cure.

A herbal alternative. Willow bark is a natural pain reliever, according to pharmacologist Kenneth Blum. 'It contains a natural form of salicylate, the active ingredient in aspirin,' he says. He recommends taking it in capsule form.

Replenish your water supply. 'Alcohol causes dehydration of your

---

The CAGE questionnaire

To find out whether or not you might have a drink problem, take this simple questionnaire test. If you answer 'yes' to two or more of the following questions, it is highly likely (more than 90 per cent) that you have an alcohol dependency problem and should seek professional help, says family doctor Stephen Amiel.

C Have you ever thought that you should CUT DOWN on your drinking?

A Have you ever felt ANNOYED by others' criticism of your drinking?

G Have you ever felt GUILTY about your drinking?

E Do you have a morning EYE OPENER?

How to avoid a hangover

Once you've had a hangover you never want another. But it doesn't mean that you have to give up alcohol altogether.

'There's evidence emerging that the chief cause of hangover is acute withdrawal from alcohol,' says Mack Mitchell, who runs a research organization that investigates the effects of alcohol. 'Your brain cells physically change in response to the alcohol's presence, and when the alcohol's gone – when your body's burned it up – you go through withdrawal until those cells get used to doing without the alcohol.'

Couple that with the effects alcohol has on the blood vessels in your head (they can swell significantly depending on the amount you drink), and you end up living through a day after that you'd rather forget. So how do you avoid it?

Drink less. Sounds obvious, but it can be surprisingly difficult to say no. Your safe weekly maximum (14 units for a woman, 21 for a man) should be spread out over the week, not consumed in one or two sessions. One unit (10g of alcohol) is equivalent to a small glass of wine, a single pub measure of spirits or a half pint of standard strength beer. Be honest with yourself, and firm with others, says family doctor Stephen Amiel. Don't be sucked into feeling obliged to drink more when someone buys a round of drinks; opt for low alcohol or non-alcoholic drinks between alcoholic ones; don't be afraid to say 'No thanks, I'm driving,' or 'No thanks, I'm seeing what it's like to cut down a bit.'

Drink slowly. The slower you drink, the less alcohol actually reaches the brain – even though you may actually drink more in the long run. The reason, according to Dr Mitchell, is simple maths: your body burns alcohol at a fixed rate.

body cells,' says John Brick, a specialist in the effects of alcohol on the body. 'Drinking plenty of water before you go to bed and again when you get up the morning after may help to relieve the discomfort and headache caused by dehydration.'

Take B-complex vitamins. Drinking drains the body of these valuable vitamins. Research shows that your system turns to B vitamins when it is under stress – and overtaxing the body with too much booze definitely qualifies as stress, says Dr Blum. Replenishing your body with a B-complex vitamin can help to shorten the duration of your hangover.

Give it more time to burn that alcohol, and less will reach your blood and brain.

Drink on a full stomach. This is probably the best thing you can do, besides drinking less, to reduce the severity of a hangover, says Dr Mitchell. 'Food slows down the absorption of alcohol, and the slower you absorb it, the less alcohol reaches the brain.' What food you eat doesn't matter much.

Drink the right drinks. What you drink can play a major role in what your head feels like the next morning, according to pharmacologist Kenneth Blum.

The main villains are known as congeners, substances found in all alcoholic drinks. How they work isn't known, but they're closely related to the amount of pain you experience after drinking.

The least risky drink for congeners – and hangovers – is vodka. The worst are cognacs, brandies, whiskies and all sparkling wines.

Red wine is also bad, but for a different reason. It contains tyramine, a histamine-like substance that produces a killer headache.

Avoid bubbly. That doesn't just mean champagne. Anything with bubbles in it – gin and tonic is just as bad as champagne – is risky. The bubbles move the booze into your bloodstream much more quickly. Your liver tries to keep up but it can't, and the overflow of alcohol pours into your bloodstream.

Don't mix your drinks. The old rule of not mixing grape (wine and cognac) with grain (beer and whisky) seems to help.

Be size sensitive. With few exceptions, there's no way a lightweight can keep up with a heavyweight drinker and wake up the winner. So if you are have a slight build, scale down your drinking.

Take amino acids. Amino acids are the building blocks of protein. Like vitamins and minerals, they can also be depleted by alcohol. Replenishing amino acids will help to repair the ravages of a hangover, says Dr Blum. Eat a small amount of starch, too, to help get amino acids back into the bloodstream. Amino acids are sold in capsule form at health food stores.

Eat a good meal. If you can tolerate it, that is. A balanced meal will replace the loss of essential nutrients, explains Dr Blum. But keep the meal light – not a hearty fried breakfast.

Drink fruit juice. 'Fruit juice contains a form of sugar called fructose,

WHEN TO CONSULT A DOCTOR

There are few of us, doctors included, that haven't had the occasional hangover, says family doctor Stephen Amiel. It's miserable at the time, and may give a laugh to our friends and colleagues, and that's it. But if a hangover is a regular occurrence, some serious questions need to be asked about your alcohol intake.

Alcohol dependency affects one in 20 adults in the UK: men aged 20–24 are most at risk, but it can creep up on anyone. Alcohol is implicated in one in seven road deaths, 40 per cent of domestic violence cases and many cases of child abuse. Physical health problems include cirrhosis of the liver, pancreatitis, heart failure, gastro-intestinal haemorrhages, injuries from accidents or fights, gout and impotence. Mental health problems include depression, panic disorder, memory loss, dementia and psychosis. You should seek professional help and/or support from self-help organizations if:

- you score more than two 'yes' answers on the CAGE questionnaire (see page 277);
- you have health problems you think may be alcohol-related;
- you are neglecting your work or family because of alcohol;
- you have been in trouble with the law because of alcohol;
- you have been violent or abusive towards your partner or child when you've been drinking;
- you are worried about a member of your household's drinking.

which helps the body to burn alcohol faster,' explains Seymour Diamond, a headache specialist. A large glass of orange juice or tomato juice will help to accelerate removal of the alcohol still in your system the morning after.

Try toast and honey. Honey is a concentrated source of fructose, and eating a little the morning after is another way to help your body flush out remaining alcohol, says Dr Diamond. The toast is just the delivery system for the honey.

Drink some broth. A clear broth made from stock cubes or any home-made stock will help to replace the salt and potassium that your body loses when you drink, says Dr Diamond.

Two cups of coffee. Coffee is a vasoconstrictor, which means that it reduces the swelling of blood vessels that causes headache, says Dr Diamond. 'Two cups can do a great deal to relieve the headaches associated with hangovers.' But don't drink too much. You don't need coffee jitters on top of the alcohol jitters.

Leave the hair on the dog. The 'hair of the dog that bit you' treatment – a morning alcoholic drink to reverse the effects of alcohol withdrawal, merely postpones the inevitable hangover, says Dr Amiel. Needing a so-called 'eye-opener' is a danger sign that your drinking is out of control: you may well be on the way to alcohol dependency.

Let time heal. Treat your symptoms as best you can. Get a good night's sleep, and the next day, hopefully, all will be forgotten. But hopefully not forgotten to the extent that you go off and do the same thing the next night!

Drinking affects next-day performance

After a night of drinking, feeling fine doesn't mean you are fine, according to a study on US Navy pilots. Using simulators, the pilots' flying skills were assessed when stone-cold sober and 14 hours after drinking enough to get drunk.

'Pilots who said they felt absolutely fine and in whom we couldn't find even a trace of alcohol still couldn't fly as well as they did during times they were off alcohol completely,' says Von Lierer, a cognitive psychologist.

What does that mean for the rest of us? 'If you have an important business meeting the next day, a key presentation you have to give – any situation where you need peak performance – I

wouldn't drink the night before,' says Dr Lierer.

Drivers suffer the same deterioration in performance as pilots, according to a Swedish study published in *JAMA* (the *Journal of the American Medical Association*).

Researchers tested 22 volunteers driving Volvos (what else!) through a coned test route. At surprise intervals, they received a signal that meant they were to swerve the car right and left around the cones.

Braking time and the number of cones hit were used as measures of driving ability. Nineteen of the 22 volunteers scored significantly worse while hungover.

HEADACHE AND MIGRAINE

38 hints to head off the pain

An estimated eight million people in the UK suffer from regular severe headaches. About 90 per cent of headaches are classified as muscle contraction, or more commonly, 'tension headaches'. These headaches hit hardest with the onslaught of bills, work and arguments. The pain is all over the head. You may feel a dull ache or a sense of tightness and perhaps experience a sense of not being clearheaded, says headache expert Fred Sheftell. People often describe it as feeling like a tight band around their head.

There is hardly anyone who doesn't have a headache now and then. For most of us it is an occasional nuisance swiftly solved with a couple of painkillers. But for others, headache is a chronic problem which can ruin their career and their relationships. 'Some people are born with biology that makes them headache prone,' explains headache expert Joel Saper. Other people suffer from a particularly debilitating form of headache – migraine.

'Migraines can be crippling,' says neuroscientist Patricia Solbach. Migraine affects about 10 per cent of the UK population. Most sufferers are women, and half of them relate their migraine attacks to their menstrual cycle. The symptoms vary but migraine is usually a moderate to severe one-sided headache which pulsates or throbs. It gets noticeably worse with activity and there are other symptoms, too, including nausea and vomiting, diarrhoea and an increased sensitivity to noise, light or smells. Some people experience an aura (symptoms like flashing or zig-zagging lights) before the onset of the headache.

Whatever type of headache you suffer from, you are in the best position to recognize what triggers your headaches. It's up to you to do everything within your control to prevent or treat them. If you get frequent headaches, start by keeping a headache diary. This will help you to identify trigger factors, and also to monitor your response to treatment.

Home Headache Prevention

People who get headaches know that an ounce of prevention is worth a pound of cure. Since many headaches are caused by tension, lots of these preventative measures focus on stress relief.

Breathe deeply. Deep breathing is a great tension reliever. 'If your stomach is moving more than your chest then you're doing it properly,' says Dr Sheftell.

Cluster headaches

Cluster headaches – which almost always affect men – cause severe pain, often around or behind an eye. Unfortunately, cluster headaches tend to come back, even after long periods of remission. Cluster attacks may occur every day for weeks, or even months. The cause is unknown, but it's probably either hormonal or genetic, says neurologist Seymour Solomon. The male hormone testosterone is currently being studied for possible connections to cluster headaches. But doctors have noticed one common factor: men who have cluster headaches are often heavy smokers. So give up smoking, or at least cut back. And don't take naps, advises neurologist Joel Saper.

Do the body scan. Dr Sheftell suggests mentally checking yourself for signs that you are tensing up and precipitating a headache. Watch out for clenched teeth, clenched fists or hunched shoulders.

Go with the flow. Maybe older people are better at this – headaches are more common in younger individuals, says headache expert Seymour Diamond. 'And younger people are under more stress – trying to make a living, supporting a family. But it's important to not overdo it.' Decreasing your expectations, both of yourself and others, wouldn't hurt.

Relax with imagery. 'Imagine that the muscle fibres in your neck and head are all scrunched up,' says Dr Sheftell. 'Then begin to smooth them out in your mind.'

Have a sense of humour. People who take life too seriously tend to walk around with their faces all scrunched up, says Dr Sheftell. And they are probably wondering why they have another headache.

Sleep comfortably. Sleeping in an awkward position, or even on your stomach, can cause the muscles in your neck to contract and trigger a headache. Dr Diamond advises sleeping on your back.

Don't oversleep. Sleeping in may feel relaxing, but it's not a good idea. So no matter how tempting, avoid having a lie-in at weekends, advises Ninan Mathew, who runs a headache clinic. You're more likely to wake up with a headache. The same goes for napping.

Exercise to prevent. Exercise is a useful preventative measure, says headache expert Seymour Solomon. Moving your body is a great way to release stress.

Avoid wearing perfume. 'Strong perfume can trigger migraine,' warns Dr Solbach.

Stand tall, sit straight. Slouching can cause the muscles in your neck to contract and trigger head pain. And avoid leaning or pushing your head in one direction, says Dr Diamond.

Be gentle. Believe it or not, even if you're headache-free and 'in the mood', you might develop a headache during sex. 'It's considered an exertion headache,' says neurologist Robert Kunkel, 'and it's more common in people with migraines than in those who have tension headaches.'

Seek quiet. Excessive noise is a common trigger for tension headaches.

Protect your eyes. Bright light – be it from the sun, fluorescent lighting, the television or a computer screen – can lead to screwing up your eyes, eye strain and, finally, headache. Sunglasses are a good idea if you're going to be outside. If you're working indoors, take regular breaks from the computer screen and try wearing tinted glasses, suggests Dr Diamond.

Watch your caffeine intake. If you drink coffee regularly, and don't get your daily dose of caffeine, your blood vessels will dilate, possibly giving you a headache, says Dr Solbach. Too much caffeine will also give you a headache, so try to limit yourself to two cups (or a mug) of coffee a day.

Don't chew gum. The repetitive chewing motion can tighten muscles and bring on a tension headache, says Dr Sheftell.

Go easy on the salt. High salt intake can trigger migraines in some people.

Try prevention with feverfew. No one really understands why migraines or cluster headaches occur, and no one is entirely sure why feverfew takes them away. But, according to clinical herbalist Douglas Schar, long-term use of feverfew helps most sufferers.

Research suggests that the herb interferes in some way with the inflammatory processes that cause these headaches. Herbal practitioners know from experience that a dose of feverfew, taken every morning, reduces their incidence. 'But don't expect instant relief,' says Schar. 'You'll need to persevere for several months before you can judge this remedy.' Buy feverfew at the health food store and follow label instructions.

Eat on time. Skipping or delaying meals can cause headaches in two ways. A missed meal can cause muscle tension and, when blood sugar drops from lack of food, the blood vessels of the brain tighten. When you eat again, they expand, leading to a headache. Try eating several small meals rather than infrequent large ones.

Know your danger foods. For some headache sufferers, milk is a trigger. And there are other headache foods. Cut out cured meats like frankfurters, luncheon meat, peperoni and salami as these contain nitrates. And nitrates dilate blood vessels, which can mean serious head pain, says Dr Mathew.

Read the labels. Some people's headaches are triggered by monosodium glutamate (MSG). Many foods are loaded with it, so read labels carefully for additives like hydrolysed protein, glutamate or caseinate – all MSG in disguise.

Reactions to MSG have been reported after exposure to anything from soya sauce to soaps and shampoos.

Go organic. Some wines, beers and champagnes contain metabisulphites as preservatives. In sensitive individuals, these can trigger wheezing, flushing, sneezing and headache. Look for low sulphite wines and beers – organically produced ones are likely to be relatively safe for you.

Say no to chocolate, cheese and nuts. They all contain tyramine, a major culprit in causing headaches. The good news is that many young people outgrow this chemical reaction. The body seems to build up a tolerance, says Dr Diamond.

Don't smoke and drive. You shouldn't smoke, anyway. But smoking with the car windows open when you're driving in heavy traffic gives you a double hit of carbon monoxide. This gas appears to adversely affect brain mechanisms that can spark a killer headache, warns Dr Saper.

Curtail the cocktails. One alcoholic drink probably won't hurt, but don't drink too much. Also, some drinks – especially red wine – contain tyramine.

Eat ice cream slowly. You can probably remember more than one occasion when you've taken a mouthful of ice cream and seconds later felt

Give your face a workout

All you need is your face and a mirror, and you're ready to do some exercises devised by Dr Harry Ehrmantraut, author of *Headaches – The Drugless Way to Lasting Relief*. The exercises are designed to relax the muscles of the face and scalp and teach you conscious control over these muscles so that you can take action at the first sign of a headache.

- Eyebrows up and return: lift both eyebrows up quickly, then relax and let them drop down.

- Right eyebrow up and return: this is difficult, so hold the other eyebrow in place and then move the right eyebrow up, as before.

- Left eyebrow up and return.

- Squeeze both eyes tight shut and release: do this quickly, hold briefly, then relax.

- Squeeze right eye tight shut and release: squeeze the right side of your face hard enough to raise the corner of your mouth.

- Do the same with the left eye.

- Frown deeply and release: squeeze eyebrows down and in towards the bridge of your nose.

- Yawn wide and close: slowly open your mouth by lowering your jaw gradually to a wide position. Then close slowly.

- Open jaw, move right and left: open mouth slightly and slide jaw from right to left, then from left to right.

- Wrinkle nose: squeeze nose upwards, as if smelling a nasty smell.

- Make funny faces: ad-lib this one, stretching your mouth into weird shapes, like children do.

an intense rush of pain to your head. Eat ice cream slowly, Dr Saper advises. This lets your palate cool gradually instead of receiving a shock of cold.

Consider riboflavin. Fifty-two litres of chocolate syrup. Nine hundred bowls of cornflakes. These might prevent a headache – if they weren't guaranteed to give you a stomach-ache first. They add up to a super-high dose of riboflavin, or vitamin B_2, the dose which research suggests may be necessary to ward off headaches.

'I wouldn't use riboflavin as my first line of attack,' says Dr Solomon. 'But it might be worthwhile exploring riboflavin with patients who haven't responded well to other treatments.'

Home Headache Relief

If, despite your best efforts at prevention, your head is throbbing, here are some expert-recommended ways to get rid of the pain.

Don't over-rely on painkillers. For that once or twice a month tension headache, ibuprofen – an over-the-counter anti-inflammatory – may work well.

Codeine-containing analgesics may be useful in aborting a severe headache but with regular use you run the risk of making your headaches worse. As the codeine wears off, you get mild withdrawal symptoms – mainly a headache! If you take more pills for the headache, the spiral continues. A similar analgesic-overuse headache cycle is occasionally seen with paracetamol and ibuprofen.

Caffeine is added to many compound over-the-counter painkillers. This gives you a boost and may make you feel better more quickly, but caffeine overuse can also cause headache in its own right.

Don't delay. If you do decide to take a painkiller for a headache, take it right away – at the beginning of the headache, advises Dr Solbach. Otherwise, it may not do you much good.

Herbs and solitude. It's hard to be a nice person or stop and smell the roses when you feel as if your head is about to explode, says Douglas Schar. Tension headaches are best treated with seclusion therapy – time alone – and a dose of cramp bark. Cramp bark (*Viburnum opulus*) relaxes the blood vessels that serve the brain, which in turn relaxes the headache. Usually a 5ml dose of cramp bark tincture 1:5, and some time in a darkened quiet room, will do the trick.

To exercise or not. If a headache isn't too severe, exercise can help to make it better, says Dr Solbach. A slight tension headache can often be relieved if you exercise. Don't exercise if it's severe. You'll just make your head hurt more, especially if you're experiencing a migraine.

Go hot or cold. Some people like the feeling of cold against their foreheads or necks and find that it eases the pain, says Dr Solbach. But others prefer hot showers or putting heat on their necks.

Use your hands. Both self-massage and acupressure can help, according to Dr Sheftell. Two key points for reducing pain with acupressure are the web between your forefinger and thumb (squeeze there until you feel pain) and under the bony ridges at the back of the neck (use both thumbs to apply pressure there).

WHEN TO CONSULT A DOCTOR

Most headaches are straightforward tension headaches. But occasionally headaches are warning symptoms for serious conditions. These signs are red flags alerting you to see your doctor.

- The headache is your first or worst, especially if it came on suddenly.
- You are over 40 and have not had recurrent headaches before.
- The headaches are worse in the morning or wake you from sleep.
- A headache is constant and progressively worsening over a period of days.
- The headaches are worse on bending forwards.
- The headache follows recent head injury.
- The headache is associated with a rash, intolerance of light, unexplained vomiting or fever.
- The headaches have changed locations.
- The headaches are getting stronger.
- The headaches are coming more frequently.
- The headaches do not fit a recognizable pattern; that is, there seems to be nothing in particular that triggers them.
- Headaches have begun to disrupt your life; you've missed work on several occasions.
- The headaches are accompanied by neurological symptoms, such as numbness, dizziness, blurred vision or memory loss.
- The headaches coincide with other medical problems or pain.

Or use someone else's. An upper body massage, focusing on the neck and shoulders, face and scalp, can work wonders for tension headaches.

Some experts maintain that increasing bloodflow to knotted muscles disperses lactic acid more quickly, relieving muscle pain, but the evidence for this is scanty. Others believe that massage increases serotonin and endorphin levels, making you feel good and moderating your response to pain.

Pretend it's a flower. 'Put a pencil between your teeth, but don't bite,' says Dr Sheftell. 'You *have* to relax to do that.' The relaxation – and distraction – could help to ease the headache.

Wear a headband. The old wives' remedy of tying a tight cloth around the head has some merit to it, says Dr Solomon. It decreases bloodflow to the scalp and lessens the throbbing and pounding of a migraine.

Herbs for hormone headaches. The hormone headache begins at puberty and can play a role in a woman's life till the last hot flush of menopause, says Schar. In this case, chasteberry, known botanically as *Vitex agnus-castus*, is the solution. 'If your headaches are linked to your periods,' says Schar, 'I recommend taking a daily dose of chasteberry. It must be taken every morning, just like the contraceptive pill, and should be taken for several months before you can decide whether or not it is making a difference.' Buy capsules at a health food store and use according to label instructions.

Sleep. A lot of people simply sleep off a headache, says Dr Mathew.

HEART PALPITATIONS
11 ways to calm a rapid heartbeat

An adult's heart normally beats between 60 and 80 times a minute. Any disturbance of the normal rhythm of the heart is known as arrhythmia. The heart rate may become abnormally fast or slow and it may or may not be irregular. Arrhythmias are very common and can happen naturally, or be due to heart disease or other causes, such as a reaction to a drug.

Lots of people have arrhythmias and know nothing about it, because they have no symptoms. Sometimes, though, arrhythmias may lead to palpitations, which people describe as an unpleasant sensation of their heartbeat 'thumping' in the chest. The palpitations may be occasional and irregular, commonly occurring at rest. Called ventricular extrasystoles or ectopic beats, this type of palpitation feels like the heart is 'missing a beat'. Extrasystoles are caused by an abnormal electrical discharge triggering off a contraction of the heart muscle, and are generally harmless. Unlike other palpitations, they usually disappear during exercise. Common causes of fast, but regular, palpitations include exercise, fever, stress, caffeine and alcohol. Here's how to slow them down.

Slow yourself down. Think of your speeding heart as a flashing red light saying, stop what you're doing; calm down; rest. Rest is, in fact, the best way to stop an attack, says cardiologist Dennis Miura.

WHEN TO CONSULT A DOCTOR

There are many causes and many different types of palpitations, says family doctor Stephen Amiel. Whilst many are easily explained and can be managed by using home remedies, there are some which signify potentially serious heart problems; others which accompany conditions like an overactive thyroid, anxiety states or depression; some which may be explained by natural phenomena like the hormonal changes of pregnancy or menopause; and still others which may be due to medications, like asthma-relieving pumps, ephedrine and some antihistamines.

Even after taking a careful history and examination, doctors may well find it difficult to diagnose the cause of your palpitations without further tests: blood tests for thyroid disease, anaemia or electrolyte disturbances; an electrocardiogram, and sometimes a 24-hour heart monitor arranged in conjunction with your local cardiology department.

For these reasons, says Dr Amiel, if you have anything other than mild, occasional, short-lived palpitations that are easily explainable by stress, emotion or over-indulgence, you should see your doctor, especially if you are already known to have heart disease or other health problems. If you get shortness of breath, chest pains, light-headedness or fainting with your palpitations, you should seek medical help urgently.

Try the vagal manoeuvre. How fast your heart beats and how strongly it contracts are regulated by sympathetic nerves and parasympathetic nerves (or vagal nerves). When your heart pounds, the sympathetic network is dominant. (That's the system that basically tells your body to speed up.)

What you want to do is switch control to the mellower parasympathetic network. If you stimulate your vagal nerve, you initiate a chemical process that affects your heart in the same way that a gentle foot on the brake slows down your car. One way to do this is to take a deep breath and bear down, as if you were having a bowel movement, says family doctor John Lawder.

Rely on the diving reflex. When sea mammals dive into the coldest regions of the water, their heart rates automatically slow down. That is nature's way of preserving their brains and hearts, says Dr Miura. You can trigger your own diving reflex by filling a basin with icy water and plunging your face into it for a second or two.

Or break the ice an easier way. Just as effective, and sometimes easier when you're out and about, says family doctor Stephen Amiel, is an ice-cold drink. Fill a glass with ice cubes and sip slowly as the ice melts.

Break the coffee habit. Ditto for cola, tea, chocolate, diet pills, ecstasy, cocaine, amphetamines or stimulants of any form. Overuse of stimulants increases your risk of palpitations, says Dr Miura.

Cut out cigarettes and alcohol. Far from calming your heart down, nicotine and alcohol can both contribute to heart irregularities and palpitations, says Dr Amiel.

Look after your hypothalamus. What goes on in your head – your midbrain specifically – rules your heart, says vascular specialist James Frackelton. That's why you must give your hypothalamus the support it needs – through diet, exercise and a positive attitude – to maintain stability and control over your autonomic nervous system.

Stress, poor diet and pollutants can cause your hypothalamus to lose its grip on the autonomic nervous system, allowing the system to slip into high gear or what Dr Frackelton terms 'sympathetic overload'.

Here's how to help your hypothalamus retain control.

Eat healthy, regular meals. If you skip meals and then fill your stomach with sweets or soft drinks, you'll get a sugar 'hit' but that is quickly followed by a fall in blood sugar levels. Your body then releases adrenaline to mobilize the glycogen (sugar) stored in your liver to correct the low blood sugar levels. It's this adrenaline rush that stimulates a sudden increase in heart rate and the feeling of panic.

Tailor your meals to suit your metabolism. People who have a fast metabolism should eat more protein foods, says Dr Lawder. Proteins take longer to digest and help to prevent your blood sugar from falling too low. When your blood sugar drops, it triggers the process discussed above.

Learn to let go. Dr Lawder says he's noticed a relationship between perfectionist, upwardly mobile, success-orientated individuals and palpitations. You need to learn progressive relaxation, or to visualize serenity, tranquillity, calmness and peace, says Dr Lawder.

Eat foods rich in magnesium. In the muscle cells of the heart, magnesium helps to balance the effects of calcium, which stimulates muscular contractions within the cell itself. Magnesium creates rhythmic contraction and relaxation, helping the enzymes in the cells pump calcium out, and making the heart less likely to get irritable, says Dr Frackelton. Magnesium is found in soya beans, nuts, beans and bran.

Note: Do not take magnesium supplements without checking with your doctor, as an excess can itself cause heart problems, says Dr Amiel.

Make sure you get enough fruit. Potassium is another mineral that helps to slow down heart action and reduce irritability of the muscle fibres, says Dr Lawder. The mineral is found in fruit and vegetables (bananas and oranges are especially good sources), so getting enough shouldn't be difficult. But you can deplete it if your diet is high in salt or if you use diuretics or overuse laxatives.

Note: As with magnesium, do not take potassium supplements without checking with your doctor, as an excess can itself cause heart problems.

Exercise. You can do a lot by getting fit, says Dr Frackelton. 'When you do the kinds of exercise that raise the heart rate, it tends to reset at a lower level. People who don't exercise usually have a heart rate of around 80. When they begin to do a little bit of jogging, their heart rates go up to 160 or 170. But with regular exercise, they can bring their resting heart rate down to 60 or 65.

Exercise also gets rid of aggression in a healthy way because you're using up excess adrenaline, he says.

Turn to herbs. There are two excellent treatments for heart palpitations, says clinical herbalist, Douglas Schar. These are motherwort and hawthorn. Motherwort's scientific name, *Leonorus cardiaca*, suggests the plant's use. This herb is primarily used to slow down a rapid heartbeat and to improve cardiac activity. Herbalists prescribe it for nervous palpitations that are likely to occur when someone is under pressure or strain.

The second plant grows in most hedgerows – the common hawthorn (*Crataegus*). This plant quells unpleasant palpitations and has extra benefits. When taken long term, it strengthens the heart muscle and improves blood circulation.

Both herbs are available from health food stores and should be used according to label instructions. Motherwort is recommended for use when an attack is under way or when you might expect an attack. Hawthorn, on the other hand, works best when taken on a daily basis.

Note: Always consult your doctor first before commencing herbal remedies for palpitations or other heart problems.

HEARTBURN
25 ways to put out the fire

Heartburn is caused by a number of things, but in most cases it's acid reflux. That is, some of the digestive juices normally found in the stomach find their way up into the oesophagus, the pipe between the stomach and mouth.

The stomach has a protective lining that shields it from acid, but the oesophagus has no such lining. That's why stomach acid burns it, sometimes so badly that people think they're having a heart attack. Of course, heartburn is nothing to do with the heart at all, but the burning pain of heartburn, which can rise from the upper abdomen right up towards the neck, can easily be confused with angina. The overlap of symptoms can be confusing for doctors too, particularly as heart pain can sometimes be felt in the stomach area. 'When I was a medical student,' says family doctor Stephen Amiel, 'we were taught, "When a young man complains of his heart, look at his stomach, but when an old man complains of his stomach, look at his heart".'

Heartburn due to acid reflux, though, is often associated with other symptoms: an acid taste in the mouth, worsening of the pain on bending forwards or lying down, nausea, wind, burning on swallowing hot drinks, hoarseness and a night-time cough.

Overeating is the most common cause of heartburn. But it's not the only one. You can get heartburn without over-indulging. Try these soothing tips.

Don't overdo it. Stomach acids can be forced up into the oesophagus when there's too much food in your stomach. Fill your stomach more and you'll force up more acid. There can be many reasons for heartburn, but for the occasional sufferer it's usually eating too much food too fast, says nutritionist Samuel Klein.

Give that burger to the dog. Greasy, fried and fatty foods tend to sit in the stomach for a long time and promote surplus acid production. You can discourage future attacks if you avoid fatty meats and dairy products, says Larry Good, an expert in digestive problems.

Don't blame spices. Chilli peppers and their spicy cousins may seem like the most likely heartburn culprits, but they're not. Many people with heartburn can eat spicy foods without added pain, says Dr Klein. Then again, some can't.

Antacids do help

Over-the-counter digestive aids are generally effective and safe. The antacids most highly rated by our experts are those which are a mixture of magnesium hydroxide and aluminium hydroxide. (One constipates and the other tends to cause diarrhoea; combined, they counter each other's side-effects.)

Although the mix may be relatively free of side-effects, it is not a good idea to stay on these antacids for more than a month or two, says gastroenterologist Francis Kleckner. They are so effective that they could mask a serious problem that requires expert care.

Our consultants agree that liquid antacids, although not as convenient as tablets, are generally more effective.

Acid production inhibitors, like ranitidine and cimetidine, are also available over-the-counter in low dose preparations. They, too, can work almost too well in masking underlying problems: if you find you need them on frequent occasions or for long periods, you must consult your doctor.

Oranges and lemons. Citrus fruits might seem like trouble, but the acid they contain is kids' stuff compared to what your stomach produces, says gastroenterologist Francis Kleckner. He says let your tummy decide.

Take an antacid. Over-the-counter antacids generally bring fast relief from occasional heartburn, says Dr Klein. These products help to neutralize the acid in your stomach, while acid blockers can decrease the production of acid in the stomach for several hours. You can take these before a meal as well as afterwards.

Milk can make it worse. 'Some people recommend milk for heartburn – but there's a problem with it,' says Dr Klein. 'It feels good going down, but it stimulates acid secretion in the stomach.' Milk contains fats, proteins and calcium, all of which can stimulate the stomach to secrete acid.

Leave the mints in the saucer. Mints are one of several foods that tend to relax your lower oesophageal sphincter, the little valve that keeps acid in your stomach – and the little lid that can often protect you even when you do over-indulge.

Other foods that can relax your sphincter include beer, wine, other alcoholic drinks and tomatoes. This may be especially noticeable if you're pregnant. Not only does the baby increase the pressure in your abdomen, but your oesophageal sphincter is also relaxed by pregnancy hormones.

Go easy on caffeine. Caffeinated drinks such as coffee, tea and cola may irritate an already inflamed oesophagus. Caffeine also relaxes the sphincter.

Let your drinks cool down. Very hot drinks can aggravate an already sensitive and inflamed oesophagus, says Dr Amiel. Take your time and, if you do have the odd tea or coffee, drink them lukewarm.

Don't eat chocolate. The number one food to avoid when you're experiencing heartburn is chocolate. It's double trouble for those with heartburn: it is nearly all fat *and* it contains caffeine.

Avoid fizzy drinks. All those little bubbles can expand your stomach, having the same effect on the sphincter as overeating, says Dr Good.

Clear the air. 'It doesn't matter whether it's yours or someone else's tobacco smoke – avoid it,' says Dr Kleckner. It will relax your sphincter and increase acid production.

Watch that spare tyre. The stomach can be compared to a tube of toothpaste, says Dr Kleckner. If you squeeze the tube in the middle something's going to come out of the top. A roll of fat around the gut squeezes the stomach much as a hand would squeeze a tube of toothpaste. But what you get is stomach acid.

Loosen your belt. Think again of the toothpaste analogy, says Dr Kleckner. You can obtain relief from heartburn simply by wearing braces instead of a belt.

Tight skirts, and especially body-shaping, tummy-controlling underwear can also cause big trouble for heartburn sufferers.

Bend at the knees to lift. If you bend at the stomach, you'll be compressing it, forcing acid upwards. Bend your knees instead. It not only protects you from acid – it's also better for your back.

KITCHEN CURES

A popular remedy for heartburn is a teaspoon of cider vinegar in half a glass of water sipped during a meal. 'I've used it many times – it definitely works,' says home-remedy expert Betty Shaver. It may sound bizarre to ingest an acid when you have an acid problem, she admits, but there are good acids and bad acids.

Check your medicines. The source of your heartburn could be a medication. Several prescription drugs, including certain antidepressants, sedatives, antibiotics, heart and high blood pressure tablets, anti-inflammatory painkillers and steroids can all aggravate heartburn. If you have heartburn and are on any prescription drugs, discuss them with your doctor, advises Dr Kleckner.

Little and often. 'Little and often' should be the watchwords for all your meals, says Dr Amiel. And don't drink too much fluid at the same time as you eat. Food and stomach acids float upwards on the liquid and are more likely to enter the oesophagus.

'Never eat within two-and-a-half hours of bedtime,' adds Dr Kleckner. A full stomach and gravity working together are likely to force stomach acid upwards into the oesophagus.

Don't lie flat. If you lie flat, you'll have gravity working against you. Stay upright and the acid in your stomach is more likely to stay in your stomach. 'Water doesn't travel uphill, and acid doesn't either,' observes Dr Kleckner.

Herbal heartburn helpers

Go into your health food store, and the chances are you'll find a number of herbs reputed to fight heartburn. Herb researcher Daniel Mowrey has studied the evidence carefully and concludes that some herbal remedies do relieve and prevent heartburn.

Ginger. This, says Mowrey, is the most helpful. 'I've seen it work often enough to be convinced,' he says. 'We're not sure how it works, but it seems to absorb the acid and have the secondary effect of calming the nerves.' Take it in capsule form just after you eat. Start with two capsules and increase the dosage as needed. You know you've taken enough when you start to taste ginger in your throat.

Bitters. A class of herbs called bitters, used for many years in parts of Europe, is also helpful. Examples of common bitters are gentian root and goldenseal. 'I can vouch that they work,' Mowrey says. Bitters can be taken in capsule form or as a liquid extract, just before you eat.

Aromatics. Aromatic herbs like catnip and fennel are also said to be good for heartburn, but the evidence is inconclusive.

WHEN TO CONSULT A DOCTOR

Heartburn is especially common between the ages of 35 and 64. But anyone, especially over the age of 45, developing heartburn or indigestion frequently or constantly (two or three times a week for more than a few weeks) should see their GP, advises family doctor Stephen Amiel. Although heartburn caused by simple acid reflux is likely, it could also be the sign of an ulcer, or possibly something worse.

Longstanding heartburn may be due to a hiatus hernia, where part of the stomach slips up through the diaphragm. This condition, whilst not life-threatening, may require long-term medication to suppress stomach acid production, or occasionally surgery. Chronic acid reflux into the oesophagus may cause scarring and narrowing of the oesophagus, and may increase the risk of cancer of the oesophagus. That's why it's particularly important to see your doctor if your symptoms are chronic, or if they change (especially if you start to have difficulty swallowing your food). She may want you to be investigated, usually by having an endoscopy, where a camera is passed down the oesophagus.

Whatever your age, says Dr Amiel, see your doctor as soon as possible if your heartburn is accompanied by weight loss, difficulty in swallowing, vomiting or proven anaemia.

You should seek **immediate** medical attention if:

• you vomit fresh blood or fluid containing what look like coffee grounds;

• you pass a bloody or tarry black stool;

• you have chest or upper abdominal pain associated with shortness of breath, dizziness or lightheadedness, especially if the pain is pressing or crushing in nature, and/or radiates to your neck, jaw, shoulder or arm (these symptoms may indicate a heart attack).

Raise the bedhead. Elevate the head of your bed by 10–15cm. You can do this by putting blocks under the legs of the bed or by putting a wedge under the mattress at the head of the bed. A sloping bed will discourage heartburn – but don't expect extra pillows to do the trick. Too many pillows will crease you up in your midriff area, says Dr Amiel. This will increase the pressure on your stomach contents and force the acid upwards.

Take life a little easier. 'Stress can cause an increase in acid production in the stomach,' says Dr Klein. Relaxation techniques could help to reduce tension levels and allow your body chemistry to rebalance itself.

HEAT EXHAUSTION
17 tactics to stave off trouble

Each summer, with everything from garden hoes to golf clubs in hand, those of us cautious enough to carry umbrellas when rain is forecast push ourselves beyond safe limits in the sun. This can result in heat exhaustion, a condition in which an excessive loss of body fluid causes a rise in body temperature.

It's important to understand that no one is immune from heat exhaustion, not even the fittest athlete, says A&E doctor Richard Keller. That's because the hotter we get, the more we perspire, and if we sweat too much we start to run low on water. Heat exhaustion is generally caused by dehydration or, in rare cases, salt depletion (we lose salt along with our sweat).

Thirst is likely to be the first symptom, followed by loss of appetite, headache, pallor, dizziness and a general flu-like feeling that may include nausea and even vomiting. In extreme cases, the heart may race and concentration become difficult. Hopefully, you won't find yourself in that situation. Here's how to avoid it and, if necessary, how to cope with it.

Get out of the sun. This is as critical as it is obvious, especially for someone already experiencing heat exhaustion. Otherwise, body temperature could continue to rise, even if you're resting and drinking water. Going back into the sun, even hours later, could cause a relapse.

Drink water. It's still the best drink to turn to for hydration, says Dr Keller. It should be taken a little at a time, not gulped down. 'Ideally, you should have stoked up on water before going out in the sun,' he adds.

Eat fruit and vegetables. 'They have a fairly high water content and good salt balance,' says Dr Keller.

Drink isotonics. Liquid Power, Isostar and Lucozade Sport are known as isotonic drinks. They have a similar carbohydrate electrolyte concentration to the body's own fluids and are widely used by athletes and sports men and women who can lose a lot of potassium and sodium when they sweat heavily – especially when training in summer.

Avoid salt tablets. Once routinely handed out to athletes and anyone else who wanted them, most doctors now consider these pills bad medicine. 'They do the opposite of what they're supposed to do,' says physiologist Larry Kenney. 'The increased salt in the stomach keeps fluids there

Careful when you're clubbing

Heat exhaustion can happen at night too. Dancing for hours in a crowded, badly ventilated nightclub, especially if you're drinking alcohol, can result in significant dehydration.

The use of drugs like ecstasy and amphetamines adds a far more dangerous dimension: the initial energizing and mood-enhancing effect of these drugs can make you oblivious to time and keep you dancing far longer than your body can cope with. Ecstasy can also disrupt your body's heat regulation mechanisms, leading to hyperthermia and liver damage.

Periods of rest and steady fluid replacement are vital, but don't overdo the water. Clubbers who've drunk huge amounts of water (14 litres in one case) whilst under the influence of drugs have died of fluid overload.

longer, which leaves less fluid available for necessary sweat production.'

Avoid alcohol and caffeine. Both speed up dehydration and can make you sweat more than normal, says Dr Keller.

Don't smoke. Smoking constricts blood vessels, Dr Keller says, and can impair your ability to acclimatize to heat.

Go slower. Whatever you're doing outdoors, you should do it more slowly than usual when it's hot, Dr Keller advises.

Pour a cold one – on yourself. Dousing your head and neck with cold water will help if it's hot and dry, says Dr Kenney, because the water evaporates and cools you off. It won't help much in humid conditions, though. Don't make it too icy, though: very cold water constricts the blood vessels in the skin, increasing your core temperature as blood is diverted inwards.

Improvise a fan. Use a newspaper, a sunhat or a baseball cap – whatever you have to hand – to create your own cool breeze.

Give the weather forecaster some credit. They aren't always right, but if they say it is going to be a scorcher, don't make that the day you begin painting the outside of your house.

WHEN TO CONSULT A DOCTOR

If it's not treated, heat exhaustion can progress to heatstroke, which can be deadly. But it is sometimes difficult to distinguish between heat exhaustion and heatstroke. For this reason, a person who does not respond within 30 minutes to self-help measures for heat exhaustion should be taken to a doctor. It's important to get emergency care quickly, otherwise complications such as shock and kidney failure could develop.

Heatstroke is a major malfunction of the body's thermo-regulatory system – internal temperature is allowed to rise dangerously high. Symptoms can be similar to those of heat exhaustion – dizziness and nausea, for example. In addition, the person may become very disorientated and even agitated. When the body stops regulating temperature, a heatstroke victim tends to stop sweating – but not always.

Although fainting may or may not signal heatstroke, it warrants immediate medical care. If the person revives quickly – in 2 to 5 minutes – it's more likely to be heat exhaustion. With heatstroke, fits or a coma are additional possibilities. And unless heatstroke strikes in a hospital car park, you'll need to give some fast first aid. Here are recommendations on how to treat heatstroke until you can get the victim to a doctor.

Cool with water. Splash the person with water instead of immersing him or her in cool water, if possible. The water will evaporate from the skin more quickly and have a cooling effect.

Apply cool, damp towels. Again, this is a better option than immersing the person in ice-cold water.

Take advantage of technology. If possible, move the person into an air-conditioned area.

Give fluids to drink. Give water, as long as the person is conscious.

Take charge. Sometimes, an afflicted person lets pride get in the way of treatment. If you think someone is severely affected by heat, bully them into the shade.

Cheat the sun. You can't beat the sun, so do what you have to do outdoors early and late in the day. 'On hot days, we start work at daybreak,' says roofing safety director David Tanner. 'Then we knock off about 2 or 3 o'clock in the afternoon.'

Don't bare your chest. 'You pick up more radiant heat exposure with your shirt off,' says physical education expert Lanny Nalder. 'Once you start perspiring, a shirt can cool you when the wind blows through it.'

Wear a hat. Choose a well-ventilated hat that shades your neck. A wide-brimmed hat with tiny holes around the brim is a good choice. 'The blood vessels in your head and neck are very close to the skin surface, so you tend to gain or lose heat there very quickly,' says Dr Kenney.

Wear cotton/polyester blends. Surprisingly, cotton/polyester blends breathe better than shirts that are 100 per cent cotton.

Wear light colours. They reflect the heat, while dark colours absorb it.

HICCUPS
18 home-tested cures

Pregnant women know a secret many of the rest of us don't. Before they're born, babies hiccup in the womb. A pregnant woman can feel the little spasms and see her tummy move, too. Most of us hiccupped before we were born and keep on doing it every now and then for the rest of our lives. Nobody is really sure why. Some scientists believe hiccupping is the last vestige of a primitive reflex that at one time served a useful purpose, now long forgotten. They have a better idea, though, about what causes hiccups – eating too fast and swallowing too much air.

Foods that are too hot or spicy, water or air that is too cold, fumes, nervousness, intense emotion, sudden laughter or fizzy drinks may all trigger the sudden contraction of your diaphragm. The involuntary sharp intake of air in turn triggers a part of your throat (your glottis) to snap shut, giving rise to the tell-tale 'hic'. Hiccups usually stop spontaneously after several seconds or minutes; rarely, a bout can last much longer.

Hiccup cures date from antiquity and there are hundreds. But the general goal of all hiccup cures is either to increase carbon dioxide levels in the blood or to disrupt or overwhelm the nerve impulses causing the hiccups: that may be a fancy way of saying that if you divert the brain enough by trying to do something difficult or silly enough, your hiccups will just go away. Note, these are home-tested, not scientific cures. Maybe one of these treatments will be your cure.

Try a little bribery. 'My brother has a hiccup cure that he swears works every time,' says family doctor Stephen Amiel, 'though I've never dared try it myself.' Dangle a £20 note in front of someone who's hiccupping and say it's theirs if they hiccup again. Try as they might to hiccup again, they're stopped dead in their tracks.

Nine weird hiccup stoppers

Try running through this list of favourite treatments until you find one that works for you.

- Yank forcefully on your tongue.
- Gargle with water.
- Tickle the roof of your mouth with a cotton bud at the point where the hard palate meets the soft palate.
- Put an ice pack on the abdomen just beneath your ribcage.
- Chew and swallow dry bread.
- Suck a lemon wedge soaked with Angostura bitters.
- Compress the chest by pulling the knees up or leaning forward.
- Hold your breath.
- Suck crushed ice.

Drink water upside-down. Try curing hiccups by filling a glass of water, bending over forwards, and drinking the water upside-down from the wrong side of the glass, says gastroenterologist Richard McCallum. 'That always works, and I firmly recommend it for my healthy patients.'

Blow slow. A researcher for a publishing company, Christine Dreisbach Murray often works through lunch and sometimes suffers the consequences – a bad case of hiccups. 'I used to try holding my breath, but lately, I've been blowing air out in a slow, steady stream. Simple, but it works.'

KITCHEN CURES

'One cure I find effective is a teaspoon of sugar, swallowed dry,' says gastroenterologist André Dubois. 'That often stops hiccups in minutes.
The sugar probably acts in the mouth to modify the nervous impulses that would otherwise be telling the muscles in the diaphragm to contract spasmodically.'

Swallow the hiccup. 'When you're eating, just be quiet and eat,' says home-remedy expert Betty Shaver. 'Then you won't get hiccups.' If you've already got hiccups, hold your breath for as long as possible and swallow every time you feel a hiccup sensation coming. Do that two or three times, then take a deep breath and repeat.

Acrobatic hiccup cure. Here's a tip recommended by researcher Dawn Horvath. Fill a paper cup with water and put it on a worktop. Put your index fingers in your ears, and bend over at the waist to pick up the cup using the little finger and thumb of each hand. Then, while holding your breath, drink the water down in one or two gulps.

The tot tickle. When you have a roomful of active children running around giggling and laughing at a day nursery, you can be sure some will end up with hiccups. 'I tickle them while they hold their breath, and they try hard not to laugh,' says childcare expert Ronnie Fern. 'It works. I suppose it makes you gasp for breath and your diaphragm goes back to doing what it's supposed to do.'

A herbal helper. Hiccups are an unpleasant combination of muscles and nerves backfiring, and when they occur for more than a few minutes, they can be very uncomfortable. One of the best herbal nerve/muscle relaxants is valerian, says clinical herbalist Douglas Schar. It soothes all kinds of spasms. Try taking 5ml of 1:5 tincture to relieve hiccups.

The paper bag trick. We were going to leave out the tip of breathing into a brown paper bag: everybody probably knew it already and – worse still – it never works very well, anyway. But then we heard about postal clerk Pat Leayman. She's cured numerous hiccupping colleagues using nothing more sophisticated than a brown paper bag.

'You have to blow in and out exactly 10 times, and you have to do it really hard until you're red in the face,' says Leayman. 'You also have to do it fast, and you have to form a good seal around your mouth with the bag so that no air can get in. If you follow these directions exactly, the bag will work every time.'

WHEN TO CONSULT A DOCTOR

Hiccups can be embarrassing and uncomfortable, says family doctor Stephen Amiel, but they're not harmful in themselves: an American pig farmer had continual hiccups for 65 years without suffering unduly, although the same could not be said for his family.

Hiccups are rarely the first sign of serious illness but, occasionally, they can be a symptom associated with other conditions, including pneumonia, liver or kidney problems, excessive alcohol consumption, asthma, stroke or brain tumour. They can also follow abdominal surgery, or be associated with certain medications, such as muscle relaxants.

If you're badly affected by hiccups, your doctor may be able to give you a tranquillizer like chlorpromazine or haloperidol to help.

HIGH BLOOD PRESSURE
20 pressure-lowering strategies

High blood pressure, or hypertension, has been called a 'silent' disease because it causes no symptoms for years or even decades. In the UK, 41 per cent of men and 33 per cent of women have high blood pressure. Over 65, the chances of your having high blood pressure are even higher: more than half of all people over this age in the UK are estimated to have a blood pressure at or above 160/95 millimetres of mercury (mmHg), when the upper acceptable limit is no more than 140/90, and in some cases 140/85mmHg. Certain ethnic groups, such as those of South Asian, African and Caribbean origin, are particularly likely to have high blood pressure.

Without treatment, hypertension can cause heart disease, stroke and kidney disease. It is estimated that hypertension directly causes several thousand deaths a year, but it is a major contributory factor, too, in many of the 50,000 deaths from stroke and 100,000 deaths from coronary heart disease annually. Yet half of all people with hypertension don't even know they've got it. 'When I started out in practice,' says family doctor Stephen Amiel, 'we learned about the "rule of halves": half the people with hypertension don't know they have it; of those that do know, half are not on any treatment for it, and only about half of those on treatment are controlled adequately. We're getting better at controlling hypertension we know about, but there are still huge numbers of people out there with a blood pressure time bomb ticking away.'

Smoking, obesity and a sedentary lifestyle all contribute to high blood pressure, but in many cases doctors are not sure what causes it. Studies have shown, however, that most people with high blood pressure can control or even eliminate it with some basic lifestyle changes.

Know your BP. Because high blood pressure causes no symptoms at first, there's no way to know you have it without being tested. 'People often think of their blood pressure only when they get a symptom associated with hypertension, like a nose bleed or headaches,' Dr Amiel says. 'Usually though, these symptoms are nothing to do with high blood pressure. You can't rely on your body warning you that you have hypertension.'

Doctors are encouraged to check an adult's blood pressure every few years when they get the chance – over 90 per cent of the adult population will see their GP for some reason at least once in three years. 'But it's up to everyone to make sure their blood pressure is known,' says Dr Amiel. 'Ask your doctor or practice nurse to check it when you see them. Or you can, for a small fee, get a pharmacist to check it.'

Blood pressure DIY? Some people buy their own blood pressure monitors. Studies show that people who check their blood pressures at home several times a month may keep it under better control. It's also a good way to rule out 'white-coat hypertension', in which blood pressure goes up at the doctor's surgery but is normal the rest of the time.

'Some of these machines are wildly inaccurate, though,' says Dr Amiel, 'and people can become obsessed with checking their pressure to the point where it seriously undermines their health rather than benefits it.' Even if you have your own machine, you should still have your blood pressure checked by a nurse, pharmacist or doctor on a regular basis.

Lose weight if you need to. It's the most important thing you can do to manage high blood pressure, says nutrition expert Nilo Cater. If you're overweight, you're between two and six times more likely to develop high blood pressure. The heavier you are, the worse your blood pressure is likely to be.

That's because the more you weigh, the more blood circulates through your arteries, causing an increase in pressure. As a result, both the heart and circulatory system are under increased strain.

You don't necessarily have to lose a lot of weight to improve your blood pressure readings. In fact, research suggests that losing between just three and nine per cent of your weight may be enough to lower your blood pressure to a healthier range.

Despite the plethora of weight-loss plans around, the basic approach is pretty simple: eat fewer calories than you burn, reduce your consumption of high-fat (and high-calorie) foods and exercise regularly.

Get some exercise every day. Regular exercise can lower blood pressure by 5 to 10 per cent, says David Capuzzi, an expert in heart disease prevention. That may not sound like much, but it's often enough to stop high blood pressure developing. Research suggests that you'll get the most benefit by exercising five hours a week. Jogging, cycling and weightlifting are all excellent, but everyday aerobic activities like walking or brisk gardening can also make a difference.

Give up cigarettes. If you're a smoker, this is probably the last advice that you want to hear, but it makes a real difference. Every time you smoke, your blood pressure shoots upwards, staying high for an hour or more. Put another way, even if you smoke only 10 cigarettes a day, your blood pressure may be constantly in the danger zone.

There is no direct evidence that stopping smoking reduces blood pressure overall in people with hypertension, says Dr Amiel. 'BUT – and it's a very big but – there's a huge amount of evidence that smoking is itself one of the biggest risk factors for heart disease and stroke (as well as

WHEN TO CONSULT A DOCTOR

Your blood pressure readings ideally should be below 140/85 millimetres of mercury (mmHg). If either of these numbers is raised, it's time to make the necessary changes to bring BP down.

Lifestyle changes may lower blood pressure to a healthy range, but many people also require medication. 'I find this the most difficult thing to persuade my patients of,' says Dr Stephen Amiel. 'They come in with a bad finger but feeling perfectly well; I check their blood pressure, it's high even when I re-check it and, within months, they may be on tablets which they hate. But persistent hypertension is such a killer, it's worth the effort for me and, I believe, all the downsides for my patients. Age isn't important – there's lots of evidence that – although the side-effects of medication need to be watched especially carefully – the older you are, the more you stand to gain from having a lower blood pressure.'

The main classes of blood-pressure-lowering drugs include diuretics, which reduce fluid in the body; beta-blockers, which slow heart rate; and ACE inhibitors, which cause blood vessels to dilate. These drugs are quite safe, but they can cause a variety of side-effects, including dizziness or dehydration. They can also cause blood pressure to drop too low in some cases.

Report any side-effects to your doctor straight away. With so many drugs available, he or she shouldn't have any trouble in finding one that provides the benefits without the discomfort. Often, a combination of several different types will be necessary, says Dr Amiel. Different drugs can increase each other's effectiveness, and low doses of each keeps side-effects to a minimum.

many other diseases). So if you've got hypertension, why take more risks than you need to?'

Smoking is probably the hardest habit to break. Some people succeed by going cold turkey, but you're more likely to be successful if you get some help by attending stop-smoking workshops, for example, or using nicotine patches or other medications to break tobacco's grip. (See *Addiction*, page 21.)

Learn about it. Check out the website Blood-Pressure-Treatments.co.uk for detailed information about tackling high blood pressure.

Cut down on salt. Salt has been pinpointed as a major dietary cause of hypertension. The average western diet contains much more salt than our bodies actually need. Nearly everyone could benefit from eating less salt. Sodium attracts water, so too much dramatically increases your blood volume (much of which is water to begin with). This, in turn, raises blood pressure. Look out for low-sodium or sodium-free processed foods, and avoid crisps, pickles, salted meat or fish and other salty foods.

Add salt at the table, not in the kitchen. Foods absorb a lot of salt when they cook, which reduces the intensity of the flavour. That means you need to sprinkle on yet more salt to get the taste you want. So add salt at the table to get the most flavour from the least salt.

Read food labels. Sodium hides in some unexpected places. Even a healthy wholegrain breakfast cereal may contain 100mg (or more) of sodium per serving. Checking labels is the best way to keep within healthy limits.

Get enough potassium. Think of potassium and sodium as being at opposite ends of a see-saw. As your levels of potassium increase, sodium levels decline, leading to a reduction in blood pressure. The recommended daily intake for potassium is 3500mg, but people who are using some diuretics – medications to control high blood pressure – may need a little more, says heart expert Howard Weitz. The richest sources of potassium are fruit – especially bananas – and vegetables.

To achieve a modest drop in blood pressure, says Dr Amiel, people with hypertension need about two grams of extra potassium a day (the equivalent of five bananas). You can also buy potassium supplements, and salt-lovers can buy a potassium-containing salt alternative (LoSalt). Even if you can't face five bananas a day, a low fat, high fruit and vegetable diet has been shown to be beneficial in lowering blood pressure, as well as having many other health benefits.

Get enough calcium and magnesium. These minerals aren't a treatment for high blood pressure, but your blood pressure may rise if you don't get enough calcium and magnesium in your diet, says nutritionist Kristine Napier.

The current UK recommendation is 700mg of calcium a day (though in America the advice is to have 1000–1200mg per day). Some of the best sources of calcium are semi-skimmed or skimmed milk, fortified soya milk and fortified orange juice.

For magnesium, eat plenty of leafy green vegetables, whole grains, beans and pulses. Lean meats and poultry also contain good amounts of magnesium. The recommended daily amount of magnesium is 300mg for men and 270mg for women.

Put fish on the menu. It contains omega-3 fatty acids, which can help to lower blood pressure, can reduce the risk of blood clots in the arteries, and have been shown to reduce death rates in people who have already had a heart attack, says Dr Cater. All fish contain omega-3s, but the best sources are oily fish such as salmon, mackerel and fresh (not tinned) tuna. Tinned sardines are also a good source of omega-3s.

Season with garlic? The evidence that garlic can reduce blood pressure is patchy, says Dr Amiel, though there are plenty of claims that not only blood pressure, but also cholesterol and sugar levels can be beneficially reduced by eating a clove of raw garlic a day. There is some evidence that garlic, rather like aspirin, reduces the tendency of blood to clot too quickly and this may reduce the risk of heart disease and stroke in people with hypertension.

Supplement with coenzyme Q_{10}. This powerful antioxidant is found in meat and fish and many health benefits have been claimed for it, says Dr Amiel. Coenzyme Q_{10} improves energy supplies to heart muscle cells, helping them to pump more efficiently with less effort. That, in turn, helps to lower blood pressure. Blood levels of coenzyme Q_{10} may decline with age and in certain conditions such as heart failure. Experts recommend taking about 100mg per day, but if you already have heart failure, you should consult your doctor beforehand.

Try hawthorn. This herb has a long tradition as a remedy for heart ailments. European and Chinese doctors use it to lower blood pressure. Take 400 to 600mg a day.

Drink in moderation. Small amounts of alcohol don't affect blood pressure and may even be good for the heart. Too much alcohol, on the other hand, causes blood pressure to rise. For men, two drinks a day are the upper limit; women should have no more than one drink a day.

'We don't advise people who don't drink to start,' Dr Weitz stresses. The benefits of alcohol for cardio-protection are modest at best, but the potential risks from alcohol are significant.

Manage stress. Emotional stress doesn't cause long-term increases in blood pressure, but it can cause the numbers to rise temporarily. Stress can also trigger heart attacks in those with underlying cardiovascular problems, says Dr Weitz. Allow yourself time to slow down and relax – with meditation, deep breathing or other stress-reduction techniques.

Take snoring seriously. Frequent snoring may be a symptom of sleep apnoea, a condition in which breathing intermittently stops during sleep.

This can raise blood pressure and cause heart irregularities known as arrhythmias, says Dr Weitz.

Apart from snoring, symptoms of sleep apnoea include morning headaches or feeling tired when you get up. If you think you may be suffering from sleep apnoea, see your doctor (see *Snoring*, page 505).

Keep an eye on cholesterol. High cholesterol doesn't cause high blood pressure, but it can make the arteries narrower, less flexible and less likely to dilate during exercise or at other times when the heart needs more blood, says Dr Weitz.

Raised cholesterol also results in fatty deposits, or plaque, on artery walls. Continued high blood pressure can cause the deposits to rupture, increasing the risk of dangerous clots. 'Eighty per cent or more of heart attacks are caused by the rupture of plaque,' he says.

KITCHEN CURES

The omega-3 fatty acids in fish may lower blood pressure slightly and reduce the risk of blood clots in the arteries. But what if you don't like fish? Try flaxseed (linseed). It has a pleasant, nutty taste, and it's loaded with omega-3s along with cholesterol-lowering fibre.

Sprinkle ground seeds onto breakfast cereals or mix them into soups, stews or other cooked dishes.

When you shop for flax seeds, buy them ground, or buy whole seeds and grind them at home. Don't eat the whole seeds, because they'll pass through your digestive tract without being absorbed.

As part of your overall treatment plan for high blood pressure, you'll probably be advised to keep your total cholesterol no higher than 5.2 millimoles per litre of blood (5.2mmol/L) – the maximum safe upper limit – but lower is better, especially if you already have established heart disease or diabetes (see *High Cholesterol*, page 310).

Dietary changes, such as eating more fibre and reducing your intake of saturated fat, can cause cholesterol to drop significantly. Getting regular exercise, losing weight, and, if necessary, taking medications are also important parts of long-term cholesterol control.

HIGH CHOLESTEROL

30 steps to take control

Your heart beats an average of 100,000 times a day. With every beat, it sends 60–90mls of blood whooshing through your vascular system – some 60,000 miles of arteries, veins and capillaries.

The heart is an impressive organ, but its efforts won't do much good unless the vascular highway is free from obstructions. But build-ups of cholesterol and other fatty substances in the arteries restrict the flow of blood and promote the development of blood clots. Over time, this can lead to heart attacks, strokes and other cardiovascular diseases.

Cholesterol itself isn't harmful. In fact, the body produces this waxy substance daily to manufacture cell membranes, bile acids, vitamin D and a variety of sex hormones. Problems only occur when cholesterol levels in the blood rise to unhealthy levels. It's estimated that almost half the 100,000 deaths a year from heart disease in the UK are attributable at least partly to high cholesterol. And nearly 70 per cent of us have cholesterol levels above the recommended maximum.

Research conducted for the British Cardiac Patients Association (BCPA) found that 85 per cent of British adults do not know their cholesterol level. And only one in three of those surveyed knew that their cholesterol level should be under 5.2 millimols per litre (mmol/l).

We often talk about cholesterol as though it's a single substance, but there are two main types:

- Low-density lipoprotein (LDL) is the harmful form. High levels of LDL promote the development of a dense, fatty layer called plaque on artery walls. As the plaque layer gets thicker over the years, it's harder for blood to squeeze by. Plaque also promotes the development of blood clots that can impede or stop the flow of blood.

- High-density lipoprotein (HDL) is beneficial. Its job is to remove excess LDL from the blood and carry it to the liver for disposal.

This complicates things when it comes to working out numbers, and knowing what your cholesterol level should be, says family doctor Stephen Amiel. The headline figure for maximum total cholesterol is 5.2mmol/l, and below 5.0mmol/l if you already have heart disease or diabetes. But your total cholesterol can be higher, and still be OK, if your HDL is high, he explains. So increasingly, doctors are calculating the relative contribution of HDL and LDL to your total cholesterol and basing risk on this. This is normally expressed as a TC:HDL ratio, obtained by dividing your total cholesterol (TC) by your HDL. The higher your HDL, the lower –

and better – will be your ratio. A ratio of less than 3.5 is ideal.

Medication is sometimes required to bring cholesterol into a healthy range, but many people can control it by making simple changes to their diets and lifestyles.

Cut right back on saturated fats. Found in meats, butter and a variety of processed foods, saturated fat is converted by the liver into cholesterol. If your cholesterol is already hitting the danger zone, cut right down on saturated fat, says nutritionist Kristine Napier.

'Don't eat red meat more than once or possibly twice a week, and limit servings to about the size of a pack of cards,' she advises.

Eat more fibre. Found in plant foods, dietary fibre – especially the soluble fibre in oats, beans, barley and asparagus – can lower your cholesterol by between two and five per cent. Unfortunately, the average British diet is low in fibre. Unfortunate because fibre lowers cholesterol in several ways, Napier explains. It absorbs water and swells in the stomach, increasing your feeling of fullness. In addition, soluble fibre dissolves and forms a gel in the intestine. The gel traps cholesterol molecules before they get into the blood.

Everyone should eat at least one food rich in soluble fibre a day, advises Napier. More is better: research shows that people who eat 7g of soluble fibre a day have lower blood cholesterol levels.

Cook with olive oil. It's the favourite oil throughout the Mediterranean and the benefits are clear. People in Greece, Spain, Italy and other Mediterranean countries are about half as likely as Britons to die of heart disease, even when their total cholesterol levels are fairly high.

The Mediterranean diet, which we're increasingly being encouraged to emulate, comprises more bread, more fruit and vegetables and more fish. It also means eating less meat and less cream, and choosing margarine –

Do just *one* thing

Try a cholesterol-lowering margarine. Traditional margarine is made with hydrogenated fats, which can raise cholesterol as much as saturated fat does. Some new margarines like Benecol contain plant sterols – compounds that help to prevent cholesterol from getting into the blood.

One large study found that people who used Benecol for a year had a drop in total cholesterol of 10 per cent and a decrease in LDL of 14 per cent.

Even people who are on medication can see an additional 15 per cent reduction in LDL by having two servings (one tablespoon counts as a serving) per day.

made from rapeseed, sunflower or olive oil – rather than butter.

Olive oil – along with grapeseed, sunflower and other oils high in mono-unsaturated fats – lowers levels of harmful LDL without lowering HDL at the same time. Olive oil, especially cold-pressed extra-virgin, is also rich in phytochemicals that help to prevent cholesterol from sticking to artery walls.

Olive oil isn't medicine, of course. It's still 100 per cent fat, which means it can add a lot of calories to your diet. The idea is to use it instead of butter or other fats in the diet, not in addition to them.

Make your meals meatless. Most of the saturated fat in our diet comes from meat, which is why anyone with high cholesterol should consider eating a vegetarian diet, at least on most days of the week. A mostly vegetarian diet not only can lower cholesterol levels, for some people it can also help to stabilize arterial deposits that have already formed, says David Capuzzi, a specialist in cardiovascular disease prevention.

Boost fibre with psyllium. One tablespoon of this crushed seed – also known as ispaghula – available in most health food stores and pharmacies, provides as much fibre as a serving of bran cereal. If you sometimes find it difficult to get enough fibre-rich foods in your diet, you may want to take a tablespoon or two of psyllium daily. You can mix it in water and drink it or sprinkle it on cereals, into smoothies or on other foods.

'Psyllium is a good source of soluble fibre,' says nutrition expert Nilo Cater. Adding 3g of soluble fibre to the diet can result in a 5 per cent reduction in LDL within a month or two.

Fill up on oats. This cereal grain has had a lot of attention for its cholesterol-lowering properties for good reason: the soluble fibre in oatmeal and oat bran help to prevent cholesterol from getting into the bloodstream.

Studies find that eating a bowl of cooked porridge every day for breakfast has a noticeable cholesterol-lowering effect. But don't use instant oats – most of the beneficial soluble fibre has been stripped out.

Put fish on the menu. It contains omega-3 fatty acids, healthy fats that lower LDL and triglycerides – harmful blood fats that have been linked to heart disease – while raising HDL at the same time. Fatty fish such as salmon, mackerel and fresh tuna (not tinned) contain the most omega-3s, Napier says.

Eat flaxseed. A nutty-tasting grain seed, flaxseed (or linseed) is loaded with cholesterol-lowering omega-3s. It's also rich in soluble fibre and phytoestrogens, which help with cholesterol control, Napier says.

'Don't use flaxseed oil,' she adds. 'You'll be missing out on the fibre as well as some of the phytoestrogens.' Also, the oil contains many more calories than the seeds, so using too much can lead to weight gain, and you can even raise your cholesterol levels as a result.

Health food stores sell whole or ground flaxseed. If you buy whole seeds, grind them at home; the whole seeds aren't broken down during digestion, Napier says, and will pass straight through you.

Follow the 'rule of five'. Some breakfast cereals, especially the sugary kind, are fibre lightweights; others provide a real fibre kick. Check the labels and buy only cereals that provide at least 5g of fibre per serving. Shredded Wheat, for example, contains 5.2g of fibre in a 45g serving, and Bran Flakes has 6.75g in a 45g serving.

Enjoy whole grains. Forget 'white' anything – white rice, white bread or white flour. Most of the fibre has been stripped away during processing. Whole grains, on the other hand, are loaded with it. A slice of wholemeal bread, for example, has about 2g of fibre, three times more than a slice of white bread. 'You can fool the kids (or your partner) by buying high-fibre white-coloured bread in most supermarkets,' says Dr Amiel. 'They won't notice the difference!'

Switch to brown rice. It takes longer to cook than the white varieties, but it's higher in fibre and contains more rice oil, which is thought to have cholesterol-lowering effects, Napier says. And it's delicious.

Eat more grapefruit. It contains a type of fibre called pectin, which blocks the absorption of cholesterol and other fats into the blood. Red grapefruit is better than white because it's richer in the carotenoid called lycopene, an antioxidant that helps to prevent LDL from sticking to artery walls.

Snack on nuts. Even though they're almost dripping with fat, studies find that people who eat nuts are less likely to develop heart disease. Most nuts are high in mono-unsaturated and polyunsaturated fats. Replacing saturated fat in the diet with these 'good' fats can cause a significant drop in LDL, says Dr Cater.

Include milk in your diet. While full-fat milk, cheese and other dairy foods are extremely high in saturated fat, fat-free and low-fat dairy foods have negligible amounts. Plus, studies suggest that low-fat dairy foods can help to combat high blood pressure, Napier says.

Add mushrooms to recipes. Studies show that shiitake mushrooms can

WHEN TO CONSULT A DOCTOR

If you have had your cholesterol levels checked by a pharmacist and the figure is not as good as it should be, see your doctor. He or she may prescribe cholesterol-lowering drugs. These are very effective but are usually recommended only when dietary and lifestyle changes haven't worked.

Your doctor will look at more than just cholesterol numbers when considering drugs. Even quite a high cholesterol level or TC:HDL ratio may increase your risk of heart disease and stroke only slightly, if you have no other risk factors, says family doctor Stephen Amiel. The factors your doctor will take into account when determining whether to recommend medication may include:

• your age and gender (risks are higher if you're older and if you're male);

• whether you smoke;

• if you have a strong family history of heart disease or raised cholesterol;

• whether you're diabetic;

• whether you have high blood pressure;

• whether you've already had heart problems, a stroke or circulatory problems.

Quite sophisticated formulae are now available for this risk assessment. Although they only give a guide as to the statistical probability of a heart attack or stroke, they can help your doctor and you to decide whether it is desirable and necessary for you to embark on what will probably need to be lifelong medication.

lower cholesterol and triglyceride levels. Supermarkets often sell fresh shiitake mushrooms. Try sautéing them for delicious and healthy additions to soups, stews, sauces, omelettes and stir-fried meals.

Crunch into an apple. Apples are rich in the soluble fibre pectin. Experts have found that pectin mops up excess cholesterol in your intestine, like a sponge soaks up spills, before it can enter your blood and clog up your arteries. Then the pectin is excreted, taking fat and cholesterol along with it.

Eat vitamin C-rich foods. This vitamin is an antioxidant that helps to prevent cholesterol from sticking to artery walls and blocking the flow of blood. You can get a lot of vitamin C in your diet by eating plenty of fruits and vegetables, especially green and red peppers, spinach, tomatoes, and oranges or other citrus fruits.

Drink green tea. It's rich in polyphenols, antioxidants that keep LDL from sticking to artery walls. Black tea contains some of the protective compounds, but green tea, which undergoes less processing, is a better source.

Add soya to your diet. It's a staple in Asian cuisine, which may be one reason heart disease is much less common in Asian countries than in the West. Soya foods such as tofu, tempeh and soya milk contain chemical compounds called isoflavones, which appear to reduce the amount of cholesterol that the liver produces. People who eat about 30g of soya protein a day can have drops in total cholesterol of about 10 per cent. 'Soya is most effective in people with very high cholesterol levels,' says Dr Cater. To incorporate more soya in your diet:

- Eat whole soya beans. They contain more of the beneficial compounds than processed soya foods. Soak the dried beans overnight, drain the water, and then cook them in a covered container for two to three hours.

- Add tofu to recipes. It has little flavour of its own, but it absorbs the flavours of other ingredients. Tofu can be used in stews, casseroles or stir-fries in place of cheese or meat.

- Try tempeh. Along with miso, it's a fermented soya bean product with a slightly smoky taste – and it's exceptionally high in isoflavones.

- Make a soya smoothie. A delicious way to get more soya in your diet is to blend 30–90g of tofu with a variety of fresh fruits and a cup of soya milk.

Toast your health with red wine. Dozens of studies suggest that drinking moderate amounts of red wine can reduce the risk of heart attack – possibly by 30 to 50 per cent, in some cases. Wine raises levels of HDL and helps to prevent blood clots from forming in the arteries. It also contains antioxidant compounds that reduce cholesterol build-up in the arteries.

'Red wine tends to get most of the attention, but research suggests that any form of alcohol may help,' says Dr Cater.

More isn't better, however. The risks of drinking too much alcohol vastly outweigh the cholesterol-controlling benefits.

Add more onions to recipes. They contain a powerful antioxidant called quercetin, which helps to prevent LDL from accumulating in the arteries. In addition, the sulphur compounds in onions raise levels of beneficial HDL. All onions are helpful, but red onions contain the highest levels of other antioxidants called flavonoids.

Shop for colour. The next time you're in the produce department at the supermarket, look at all the colours: fruits and vegetables with red, orange and yellow hues are all rich in carotenoids, plant pigments that make cholesterol less likely to stick to artery walls, Napier says.

Carotenoid-rich foods include tomatoes, red peppers, sweet potatoes and carrots. Research shows that those who eat the most fruits and vegetables – and get the most carotenoids – are less likely to develop heart disease than those who get smaller amounts.

Ask your doctor about niacin. Also known as vitamin B_3, niacin can raise levels of beneficial HDL and lower LDL, says Dr Cater. Unfortunately, it takes very high doses of niacin to have these effects. And unpleasant side-effects are common. 'At the amounts needed to obtain any beneficial effects, niacin is a drug, not a vitamin,' says Dr Cater. 'It should only be taken under the supervision of a doctor.'

Be a glutton for garlic. Clinical herbalist Douglas Schar is convinced that garlic is the answer. 'While working in north Spain, I became perplexed,' he says. 'People ate a diet terribly rich in animal fat and yet did not appear to have the heart disease I see in Britain or the USA. One day at an open-air market, I got a clue as to why this was the case. The housewives were all buying carrier bags full of garlic. And they weren't buying for the month – they were buying for the week!'

It's difficult to be sure how much of a contribution the garlic itself plays, as opposed to the overall Mediterranean diet discussed earlier. The evidence is contradictory, says Dr Amiel. One review of various trials in 1992

KITCHEN CURES

When you're trying to lower cholesterol, beans are among the best foods you can eat. They're very high in soluble fibre, which traps cholesterol in the intestine and helps to keep it out of the bloodstream.

All beans are high in fibre, but some varieties really stand out. Black beans, for example, have 7.5g of fibre in a serving. Butter and kidney beans have about 6.5g and black-eyed peas contain about 5.5g.

The drawback with beans is that they take forever to cook. Make life easy and use tinned beans. They're as good at lowering cholesterol as dried ones.

suggested a 10 per cent reduction in cholesterol levels was possible with garlic; but more recent reviews (1998) showed that garlic powders and oils had no effect on cholesterol levels.

Perhaps, though, it's worth a try. 'But for it really to have an effect,' says Schar, 'you need to include large amounts of garlic in your cooking on a regular basis.' The effort may well be worthwhile. Not only may garlic lessen your risk of heart attack, there is also some evidence that it stimulates your immune system, boosting your resistance to other illness.

Maintain a healthy weight. If you're overweight, your metabolism undergoes changes that can cause cholesterol levels to rise. 'Losing even 5 to 10 per cent of your weight if you're overweight can lower LDL,' says Dr Cater. If you adapt your diet – by eating less fat and more fibre, for example – in order to lose weight, LDL levels will drop even more.

Get regular exercise. Walking, swimming, jogging and even lifting weights can raise levels of beneficial HDL, says Dr Cater. And because people who exercise also may lose weight, this can cause a corresponding drop in harmful LDL cholesterol.

Any exercise is beneficial, but you'll gain the most benefit if you do it regularly – say, for 20 to 30 minutes each day, five or six days a week.

Try to quit smoking. Smoking lowers levels of HDL and increases LDL. It also damages LDL molecules in the blood, making them more likely to stick to artery walls.

HIVES

8 hints to stop the itching

This common skin condition goes by several names: hives, nettle rash or, more scientifically, urticaria ('urtica' is Latin for nettle). Hives are usually reddish or white, itchy, raised bumps in the skin that can join together to form patches called weals. As anyone who's been stung by nettles will remember, the sensation of hives is unbearable; a cross between itching and a burning pain. Sometimes you feel you could scratch them to pieces; sometimes you can't bear them to be touched. Either way, when you have hives, you can hardly think of anything else.

Hives tend to occur when you're exposed to certain foods, drugs, insect bites, plants, metals or other allergens. This exposure causes special cells in your body to start releasing histamine, making blood vessels leak fluid into the deepest layers of your skin.

But allergic reactions aren't the only cause of hives. Emotional stress, cold weather, even sunshine can trigger them. The weals may disappear in minutes or hours, but usually within a couple of days. While you wait for them to disappear, follow these tips to relieve the itching and swelling.

Send antihistamines to the rescue. Over-the-counter antihistamines – often found in cold and hay fever medications – are just about the best thing you can do without a prescription, says allergy specialist Leonard Grayson. Your pharmacist can advise you on what to take.

Antihistamine creams are not generally recommended. 'They are not as effective as oral antihistamines,' says family doctor Stephen Amiel. 'They are awkward to apply if your rash is extensive and, most importantly, they can cause local sensitization of the skin.'

Note: Most antihistamines make you drowsy, and they should *never* be mixed with alcohol.

Cool down. Applying cold compresses, sitting in cool baths or rubbing an ice cube over the hives are the best topical treatment for hives, Dr Grayson says. The cold shrinks the blood vessels and keeps them from opening, swelling and allowing too much histamine to be released.

A touch of the natural

Here are a few alternative treatments for hives.

Take herb tea. If you suspect emotions cause your hives and if you want to stay away from drugs like antihistamines, try a nerve-calming herb tea, suggests herbalist Thomas Squier. He recommends peppermint or passionflower. Or try chamomile, valerian or catnip.

Make a poultice or paste. Herbal manuals often suggest a poultice of crushed chickweed leaves as a remedy for itchy skin.

Some people make a paste of water and cream of tartar and apply it to hives, replacing it when the paste dries and crumbles.

Put on pressure. Natural medicine expert Michael Blate gets rid of hives with acupressure. Deeply massage the point on your trapezius (the muscle that runs between your neck and shoulder) found midway along the muscle and just a couple of centimetres over the back of the ridge. 'If it doesn't hurt, you haven't found exactly the right spot,' he says.

WHEN TO CONSULT A DOCTOR

Hives can kill by blocking breathing passages. If you get hives in your mouth or throat, dial 999 immediately. If you know that you're subject to this kind of reaction, you should have a readily available kit to deal with it.

This kit consists of a pre-filled syringe of adrenaline which, when injected into the muscle of the leg by yourself or someone with you, reverses the effects of histamine. Adrenaline kits are available on prescription from your doctor.

This life-threatening allergic reaction, called anaphylactic shock, causes several symptoms, usually immediately or within two hours of exposure to the offending substance. So if you know you're vulnerable to anaphylactic shock, carry an adrenaline kit with you at all times, make sure it is not date expired, and make sure you, and preferably those with you, know how to use it. Even if you respond quickly to the injection, you should still seek immediate medical attention as a precaution.

Symptoms of anaphylaxis include hives; a sense of uneasiness; agitation; tingling, itchy, and flushed skin; swelling of the fingers, lips or tongue; coughing; sneezing; and difficulty breathing as the windpipe swells and closes off. Your heart may malfunction and beat erratically. You may also go into shock.

Anyone with long-term hives or severe acute hives should also see a doctor.

For bigger areas, make an icepack with several ice cubes or crushed ice, a pack of frozen peas or frozen coffee beans, wrap them in a small towel and leave in place for no more than twenty minutes at a time, says Dr Amiel.

'But the relief is only temporary,' says Dr Grayson. 'And if you get hives from cold weather or water, you're out of luck.' Note that hot water will make the itching worse.

Use calamine lotion. This astringent may help temporarily to soothe the itch of hives. Because astringents reduce discharge, they may stop the blood vessels from leaking fluid and histamine. Other astringents that may help hives include witch hazel and zinc oxide.

Try the alkaline answer. 'Anything that's alkaline usually helps to relieve the itching,' says Dr Grayson. So try dabbing milk of magnesia on your hives. 'It's thinner than calamine, and I think it works better,' he says.

Prevention, prevention. 'There are myriad causes of hives,' says dermatologist Jerome Litt. 'You have to be a detective to find out what causes them.' Some of the more common causes are drugs, foods, cold, insect bites, plants and emotions.

Once you find out the cause, of course try and avoid exposure. And if you know you're likely to get hives for whatever reason, he suggests, take an antihistamine beforehand. It may prevent them.

HOSTILITY

12 ways to dissipate the anger

Fits of rage and hostility are so common these days that terms like 'going ape' or 'losing your rag' have become part of everyday language. Left unchecked, however, hostility is serious business. It can kill the lucrative deal at work, sabotage your efforts as a parent and ruin relationships.

People who think it's okay to let tempers explode, reasoning that it's good to get it out, are probably harming themselves more than they think, says psychologist Paul Hauck. 'Inappropriately expressed or repressed anger can overshadow all the good things a person does,' he says. 'Anger can ruin you if you let it.'

It doesn't take a degree in nuclear physics to know that explosive anger eventually takes its toll on a person. Numerous studies have shown that angry people face heart disease in record numbers compared to their calmer counterparts.

Uncontrolled anger has also been linked to other conditions, including white-blood-cell-count abnormalities, asthma, diabetes and anorexia nervosa, as well as to everyday complaints such as backaches.

As if the toll on your body weren't enough, consider how it affects the quality of your everyday life. 'Anger, if not expressed appropriately or if repressed, can be the dynamite that explodes an important relationship or gets you fired from a job,' says Dr Hauck.

No one is suggesting that you never get angry. How you handle that charged energy, though, is what makes the difference.

Anger Avoidance

The real secret to controlling your rage is never to let yourself reach exploding point. Here's what our experts suggest to keep your anger from building up.

Exercise at lunchtime. Anger and tension tend to build up as the day progresses. By swimming or walking at lunchtime, you'll diffuse some of the hostility and tension that have built up in the first half of the working day. 'Find a form of exercise that you enjoy and that helps to relieve the everyday stresses, and you'll be less susceptible to letting rage take over,' says psychotherapist Aaron Kipnis.

Take an extra 10 minutes. Once a week, treat yourself to a 70-minute lunch break – without your mobile phone – and don't rush to get back to the grind. The chances are you're working 50-plus hours a week, and that extra 600 seconds without any communiqués from your boss, colleagues or family won't get you sacked and will do you wonders, says anger-management expert John Lee.

Break the chain. Plan ahead to avoid a build-up of minor everyday things that could make you blow your top. For example, if you're flying, take a book or a crossword with you, because you'll probably encounter delays, says Lee.

Brainstorm. Make mental notes of things that have upset you in the past

---

Why are we so angry?

There are numerous theories as to why we're so hostile nowadays. But experts have identified some concrete reasons for our tempers.

We're overworked. 'The average adult works more hours than ever before,' says Karyn Buxman, an expert in stress management. With technological advances like pagers and mobile phones, we're always on call. Pressures build up over time and make us pretty angry.

We're more accepting. In our fathers' day, a man was the voice of reason, staying ever calm, cool and collected. Today, we are more laissez-faire about behaviour, says psychologist Paul Hauck. 'We feel it's okay to blow up at our boss or swear at someone on a train.'

We're programmed that way. Combine the reasons above with the fact that we're genetically made to react decisively when faced with a crisis. It's a fight-or-flight survival mechanism that dates back to the stone age, says psychotherapist Aaron Kipnis. But instead of burning off all that aggressive energy by hunting a mammoth, it builds up and has nowhere to go.

As a result, that charged energy sometimes gets taken out on your boss, the driver who cuts you up, or your partner.

and think of other ways to respond in the future, says clinical psychologist Marilyn Sorensen. If you don't incorporate new ways of behaving or thinking into your repertoire, you will continue to act in the same way, she says.

Ask yourself if this is really the behaviour and image you want to project. If not, think of other ways to see the situation and consider what you could do or say differently.

Prepare for hecklers. Stand-up comedians have a repertoire of responses to deal with hecklers. You should, too, suggests stress management expert Karyn Buxman. 'We all work with certain people who push our buttons,' she says. Think ahead and develop a humorous and kind response or two to keep them off balance. Humour is a great tool for diffusing tense situations.

Is it really anger? Many people, especially men, have a limited repertoire of emotions, says family doctor Stephen Amiel. 'I recognize this in myself,' he says. 'I know I respond with anger when I'm actually feeling sad, guilty or afraid.'

Be more honest with yourself, and with others, about what exactly is churning you up and, instead of an inappropriate angry outburst (which will usually make you feel even more sad, guilty or fearful), express your genuine feelings.

Anger Diffusion

Despite our best efforts, we all get angry sometimes. Here's how to keep your flash of fury from turning into an ugly incident.

Postpone the discussion. If you find yourself coming to the boil, remove yourself from the situation to clear your head, suggests Dr Sorensen. Tell a loved one or colleague that you're too angry at the moment and suggest a later time to re-address the problem.

Give time travel a try. Take a page from Michael J. Fox in *Back to the Future* and transport yourself 10 months or 10 years into the future. 'Will what's making you angry right now really matter in 10 years, 10 months – or even 10 minutes?' asks Buxman.

'For 99 out of 100 things, probably not.' And if you're about to do something impulsive, think about the repercussions of your action.

Keep physically busy. When anger strikes, do something constructive with your hands, legs, feet, face and jaw – anything that will release the tension in your muscles and distract you. For instance, if you're at home, take a bath towel in both hands and twist it as tightly as you can, sug-

WHEN TO CONSULT A DOCTOR

Inwardly directed or repressed anger and hostility can be damaging to your physical and mental health, says family doctor Stephen Amiel. As well as contributing to a number of physical illnesses like heart disease, it can lead to physical self-harm with alcohol, drugs, or more direct self-injury, like cutting; and it can contribute to depression and even suicide.

Inappropriate anger and aggression can sometimes be a symptom of underlying physical or mental illness, as well as, of course, an outcome of alcohol or 'recreational' drug misuse. Temporal lobe epilepsy, brain tumours and certain hormonal imbalances can occasionally manifest themselves in this way; and low sugar levels in people with diabetes can cause irrational aggression – an early warning sign of a hypoglycaemic attack. Depression, bipolar disorder and schizophrenia are all serious mental illnesses in which aggression may be a symptom. Certain medications are also linked to aggression: testosterone, oral steroids, anabolic steroids used illicitly by athletes, and possibly some of the newer SSRI antidepressants.

Finally, outwardly directed hostility can have devastating consequences for you or those around you, says Dr Amiel. Picking fights, driving dangerously, and shouting at or hitting your partner or children are red flag warning signs that you need help, and quickly.

See your doctor if you think aggression is a symptom or a cause of any of the above. Apart from excluding and treating physical or mental health problems, you may need a review of your medication, a referral for anger management help, drug or alcohol misuse treatment, stress counselling or other forms of therapy.

gests Lee. As you twist it, sigh, groan or grunt. After 10 to 15 minutes, imagine that the knots that used to be in you are now in the towel.

If rage affects you at work, grab a toy. Everyone should keep things to amuse them in their desks, says Buxman, whether it's wind-up toys or squishy balls.

Divert your attention. If, for example, the person in front of you in the '10 items or less' supermarket queue has 36 items and you're furious about it, Buxman recommends distracting yourself until the numerically challenged shopper has gone through.

Look at one of the magazines at the checkout, or talk to the more law-abiding person in the queue behind you.

Are you about to explode?

Lynne McClure, an expert in anger management, says that the signs leading up to full-blown rage are easy to spot. Beware of these:

Palpitations. Your heart feels as if it's about to pound its way out of your chest, and your breathing becomes quite shallow.

Overheating. Your temperature rises and you start to sweat. 'That,' says Dr McClure 'is where the saying, "hot under the collar" comes from'.

Fixation. You're consumed with whatever is making you angry. 'If you're in a meeting with 14 people and find that you're completely riveted by the one person that made you angry two weeks ago, then you have a problem,' she says.

Overreacting. You let everyday things, such as lack of toner in the photocopier, set you off. 'When little things enrage you, it's often a sign of unresolved anger,' says Dr McClure.

Don't drink alone. When you're angry, a can – or 12 – of beer may seem like your best friend. But drowning your anger with alcohol, especially alone, only makes the problem worse. It's when you're drunk that you're most likely to leave your boss a threatening voicemail.

Instead, call your best friends and invite them out for a gripe session/happy hour. Enjoy a few drinks, and use the time to vent your anger and get it out of your system. Before you know it, you'll be laughing and will have forgotten what got you steamed up in the first place.

Scream blue murder. If you've had a bad day at work, Lee suggests pulling into the nearest car park and, with the windows closed, screaming as loud as you possibly can. Swear. Name names.

If you're at home, take a pillow and yell into it. The pillow will muffle the noise so that the neighbours can't hear you. How long should you scream for? 'As long as you have the energy to yell,' says Lee. 'It might seem simple, but you're releasing that anger straight away.'

Hot Flushes
16 ways to put out the fire

Perhaps the most common complaints women have about the menopause revolve around the dreaded hot flushes – waves of heat that start in the chest and spread to the neck and head, leaving them sweaty, hot, flushed, irritable and uncomfortable. According to gynaecologist Mary Jane Minkin, about 75 per cent of women experience hot flushes. A single hot flush can last from 30 seconds to 30 minutes, but two to three minutes is the norm. Women usually experience them for three to five years.

Hot flushes are even more annoying at night. A night sweat wakes you from deep sleep, soaked in sweat. Because night sweats disrupt sleep, they can be even harder to deal with than daytime hot flushes. They can leave you exhausted and desperate for a good night's sleep.

Hot flushes and night sweats are the result of the drop in oestrogen that women experience during perimenopause (the two to eight years before menopause) and menopause, which actually occurs after 12 months with no periods. This oestrogen deficiency, as well as other hormonal changes, interferes with the way your body regulates heat.

Millions of women have turned, over the years, to hormone replacement therapy (HRT) to relieve the misery of hot flushes, as well as some other symptoms of the menopause like dry skin and vaginal dryness. Millions more have turned to HRT as a way of preventing osteoporosis, heart disease, stroke, Alzheimer's disease, and some cancers. Still others have hoped that HRT would prove to be the elusive elixir of youth, keeping body and mind forever young.

But in recent years, evidence has begun to mount that some of these great claims for HRT cannot be sustained. HRT can certainly work wonders for flushes and dryness; it improves sleep disrupted by flushes, and this may improve mood and quality of life; it will certainly help in preventing osteoporosis and some bowel cancers; and it may slow down the development or progression of Alzheimer's. But it won't protect against heart disease or stroke, and in some cases, it may increase the risk slightly; and it does slightly increase your risk of breast cancer and thrombosis.

So nowadays, the decision to go onto HRT is a more complex one, depending among other things on the severity of your menopausal symptoms and your risk of developing osteoporosis. HRT is contra-indicated in some women, and more women are choosing not to take long-term HRT, or to discontinue it. For these women, if the heat is too much to bear, the tips below will help you to handle both daytime and night time hot flushes.

WHEN TO CONSULT A DOCTOR

Hot flushes and night sweats are rarely serious enough to demand medical attention. But if you are feeling lousy, or you haven't slept well for weeks, you shouldn't put up with them.

Hormone replacement therapy (HRT) may be the answer for you, even if you only choose to take it for a few months. Otherwise, there are also other medications you may be offered for your flushes, such as clonidine. Occasionally another condition may be responsible for your flushes or night sweats. Your doctor may want to do a blood test to confirm that you are indeed menopausal, and if not, he or she may need to rule out thyroid disease, severe anxiety, or possibly TB or cancer.

Finally, given the confusion and uncertainty about longer term HRT, it may be worth a discussion with your doctor, to look together at the risks and benefits for you as an individual of starting HRT, or continuing it.

Banish binge drinking. Dr Minkin says that drinking a glass of wine a day is fine. If you're drinking a *bottle* a day, however, it might be a problem. Along with its other health risks, excessive alcohol is definitely a strong aggravator of hot flushes. Alcohol causes blood vessels to dilate. More blood goes to the surface of the skin and produces a hot flush.

Forego hot coffee. Hot caffeinated beverages are another common hot flush trigger. 'You can drink cola or hot herbal tea if you like,' says Dr Minkin. 'It's not the heat or the caffeine alone that seems to cause hot flushes. But the combination of the two really seems to bring them on.'

Rely on exercise. Not only does it give strength to your heart and bones, regular exercise also reduces the occurrence of hot flushes and night sweats. Exercise reduces menopausal symptoms, helps you to sleep, keeps bones strong and maintains a healthy heart, says Dr Minkin. Exercise three to five times a week for 30 to 45 minutes at a time.

Find a low-sweat form of exercise. There's just one problem with recommending exercise for menopausal women. 'When women have hormonal problems, the last thing they want to do is sweat,' points out gynaecologist Larrian Gillespie. She recommends a low-sweat form of exercise such as swimming, yoga or Pilates – which improves flexibility and strength without building bulk.

Give hormone replacement therapy a try. There's a myth that it's dangerous to go on and off hormone replacement therapy (HRT), says Dr Minkin. The truth is, HRT is very flexible. So if hot flushes and night sweats make your days and nights miserable, Dr Minkin recommends at least trying HRT for a couple of months. If you don't like it, you can stop the medicine whenever you like. If you decide you want to go back on it again, you can do that, too.

Consult your calendar. 'One thing I do encourage women to do if they're going to stop oestrogen is to stop it in a cool month,' says Dr Minkin. If you stop in July, you'll discover that a sweltering summer afternoon is a really bad time to have a hot flush.

Try some black cohosh. 'Black cohosh is mysterious,' says Dr Minkin. The herb is not a plant-like oestrogen, like the phytoestrogens found in soya and flax, and nobody is really sure why it works. Still, says Dr Minkin, dozens of studies and her own patients have convinced her that black cohosh is a legitimate herb for relieving hot flushes. The herb is sold in health food stores and online. Follow directions on the label.

Discover red clover. Another herb that might be effective against hot flushes is red clover. A natural phytoestrogen, this herb has proved useful in clinical studies. Red clover is sold in health food stores and online. Follow directions on the label.

Give soya a try. Incorporating more soya foods into your diet may be quite helpful for overcoming hot flushes and other menopausal symptoms. The advantage of soya – bursting with phytoestrogens – is its wide availability. Aim for one to two servings a day (the amount found in a typical Asian diet). You can buy a wide array of soya foods at supermarkets.

Or try these foods. Soya products aren't the only foods that can give you a good dose of hot flush-relieving phytoestrogens. Other foods to incorporate into your daily diet include chickpeas, lentils and almost any kind of bean.

Try abdominal breathing. For some women, abdominal

KITCHEN CURES

Brew a cup of sage tea. This common kitchen herb is often the herbalists' choice for reducing or eliminating night sweats. To make a cup of sage tea, place four heaped tablespoons of dried sage in a jar with a cup of hot water. Seal tightly and steep for four hours. When you need it, strain the brew, warm it up and drink.

breathing alone can help to reduce the severity of a hot flush. To give it a try, lie on your back with your hands on your tummy. Imagine that your abdomen is a balloon that you fill with air as you inhale and deflate as you exhale. Repeat this six to eight times a minute whenever you have a hot flush.

Try old-fashioned sleep aids. If night sweats keep you up at night, try these tips from Dr Minkin: drink a glass of warm milk, take a warm bath or simply blank out the day's events.

Wear cotton. If night sweats are a problem, pure cotton sheets and pillowcases will 'breathe' and wick moisture away from your skin. Avoid flannel, satin or cotton/polyester blends, which trap wetness around your body. It may also help to keep a light cotton quilt at the foot of your bed. If you get the chills following a nocturnal flush, pull this over you for comfort. Other cottony items to have on hand while fighting night sweats include a cotton, short-sleeved, knee-length nightgown, cotton underwear and a small cotton towel to wipe up the sweat. Avoid full-length nightgowns and synthetic blends of underwear. They'll trap heat and make you feel uncomfortable.

Keep a fan by the bed. It can cool you down at night during those heat waves. Or install a ceiling fan over your bed. To keep cool and exercise at the same time, Dr Gillespie walks on a treadmill under a ceiling fan.

HYPOTHERMIA
17 safeguards against a winter menace

A staggering 30,000 deaths a year in the UK are thought to be the result of exposure to cold. The causes not only include increased susceptibility to viruses like flu, but also hypothermia – one of the deadliest cold-induced conditions. The charity Age Concern estimates that an extra

8000 elderly people in the UK will die with each one degree Celsius drop in temperature below the winter average. What's particularly shocking about these statistics is that, with the right approach to dealing with the cold, these deaths are largely preventable.

In parts of Scandinavia and in Germany, which are much colder in winter than the UK, there is very little excess mortality in the winter months at all (seven per cent in Norway and Sweden, and four per cent in Germany, compared with 19 per cent in England and Wales). The reasons for this do not do us credit. In much of the rest of Europe, houses are better maintained, drier and better insulated; older people are less likely to be too poor to heat their homes adequately; more resources are available to keep older people well nourished and mobile; and people are more aware of the dangers of the cold, how to avoid those dangers, and who needs extra care and support during a cold spell.

Hypothermia occurs when exposure to cold reduces the body's core temperature – and it can occur even at relatively mild outdoor temperatures if exposure is prolonged. If not caught and treated early on, hypothermia leads to a rapid fall in the body's ability to function normally. Those most at risk are the elderly and babies under one year old.

Someone with hypothermia may show the following signs: drowsiness, lethargy or confusion; slurred speech and unsteady movement; pale and puffy hands and face; and skin cold to the touch. You may think that they are drunk or have had a stroke. If you find someone suffering from hypothermia, contact the emergency services straight away, as extreme hypothermia requires urgent medical attention. Even with apparently milder cases, you should always call a doctor. In the meantime, the aim is to rewarm the person and the room slowly. Follow these steps:

Remove cold wet clothes. Replace all cold, wet clothing with warm, dry clothing or blankets as quickly as possible to prevent further heat loss, but don't pile on too many heavy blankets.

Keep heat at bay. Rapid rewarming with hot water or massaging cold hands and feet should be avoided as, if not done properly, it could lead to serious tissue damage. Rely instead on gradual rewarming with blankets and slow reheating of the room. In an emergency, if dry clothes or blankets are not available, use your own body heat to warm the victim, but don't risk hypothermia yourself in the process.

Don't offer a warming brandy Do not give alcohol or cigarettes to someone suffering from hypothermia. Offer warm, nourishing drinks or soup, as long as the person is conscious enough to swallow them safely.

Prevention is better than cure. Avoid getting chilled in the first place

How do you help a hypothermia victim?

The human body was designed to work at an internal temperature of 37°C. Just a 3.5°C drop could be enough to kill. Below 33.5°C, cardiac arrest can occur, says A&E doctor James Sturm.

Hypothermia, simply defined as low body temperature, begins in its mildest stage at about 35.5°c. Symptoms include shivering, slow pulse, lethargy and a general decrease in alertness. If body temperature drops low enough, muscles turn rigid, and the person may lose consciousness.

Falling into an icy pond would bring on hypothermia in less than an hour, but most cases result from prolonged exposure to cold temperatures. Elderly people are at greater risk of hypothermia because their bodies regulate temperature less effectively.

If hypothermia occurs, follow these tips and get the victim to a doctor as soon as possible.

• Move the person to a warmer place.

• Wrap him or her in blankets.

• Give the victim warm liquids. But don't give any alcohol. Alcohol gives an artificial feeling of warmth but actually causes more heat loss.

by wearing lots of layers of clothing, drinking warm drinks and eating well.

Keep moving. The best way to keep your circulation going is to keep moving, whether this means doing light housework or going for a walk – well wrapped-up, of course. Even if your mobility is severely impaired, small frequent movements of your arms and legs whilst sitting in your chair can generate a little warmth and increase your circulation.

Just one room. It can be expensive to keep a house warm in winter – prohibitively so if you are trying to make ends meet on a pension. The charity Age Concern suggests keeping just one room really cosy and warm in winter.

Watch the temperature. Age Concern provides a free easy-to-read room thermometer. Try to keep the room you spend most of your time in at 21°C (70°F).

Improve insulation. If possible, insulate your home as well as yourself against the cold. Grants may be available from councils for loft insulation and minor repairs, broken window panes should be replaced, badly-fitting windows should be repaired or replaced with double glazing. Otherwise, you can temporarily stop draughts through windows or under doors with cloth, polythene or newspaper. Clingfilm can be stretched across windows to provide temporary secondary glazing: some DIY shops sell kits for the purpose. Heavy curtains, when drawn, will also keep heat in.

Reduce damp. If your windows and doors are too airtight, you run the risk of damp if you leave wet washing around, let pots boil for too long, or run the bath without having at least a little ventilation. Some heating fuels like paraffin and butane can also generate a lot of water vapour. You may be able to get financial help with installing an extractor fan or dehumidifier.

Check your heating. If you're elderly or disabled, you should qualify for a free gas or electricity safety check once a year under the Priority Service Register scheme, but you should also make sure your heating system is serviced on a regular basis. Be especially careful that they check for blocked flues and chimneys to prevent carbon monoxide build-up. And make sure that there aren't trailing flexes from electric fires. Keep gas and electric fires away from curtains and blankets.

Make sure of your benefits. Fuel poverty is a major factor in hypothermia. Severe weather fuel benefits are available to all elderly people if the temperature falls sufficiently. You may qualify for attendance allowance if you need extra care, and there are grants available for the installation of central heating if you are over 60 and on income-related benefits already.

WHEN TO CONSULT A DOCTOR

You should call for medical attention immediately if you find someone suffering from hypothermia, says family doctor Stephen Amiel. But your doctor can also help you or your relative to avoid hypothermia, by:

- reviewing medical conditions that impair mobility, such as heart disease, arthritis or chest problems;
- checking for conditions that slow down your metabolism, like an underactive thyroid;
- checking your medication, and perhaps changing drugs that make you drowsy or make falls more likely;
- referring you for physiotherapy to help with mobility problems and to teach you how to get up safely if you fall;
- accessing occupational therapy and social services to help make your home safer and warmer;
- referring you to a specialist falls clinic for further investigation if you have frequent falls.

Use a hottie. A hot water bottle or electric blanket will help to keep you warm in bed. Never use both together though. Wear socks in bed. And don't forget: you lose a good deal of heat from your head, so wear a woolly nightcap. You can also get heated pads for your chair.

Use a lifeline. Illness or a fall can be deadly to an elderly or disabled person if they can't summon help. 'Almost every winter,' says family doctor Stephen Amiel, 'I get called out by a neighbour or home help who's gone into a house and found someone marooned on the floor. They've had a fall or become unwell and been unable to get to the phone.

'Sometimes,' he says, 'they've been there overnight or even longer: hypothermia and dehydration have often done more harm than the fall.'

This scenario can be avoided. Keep a cordless or mobile phone nearby. Better still, alarm pendants, like the Piper Lifeline system, can be worn round the neck. Pressing the button can summon help 24 hours a day via your telephone. 'But you **must** wear it at all times,' says Dr Amiel. 'Too often I visit a patient and there's their pendant, hanging on a hook on the other side of the room.' Many councils provide alarms free to vulnerable people on low incomes, and you can also get financial help with telephone installation and standing charges.

Love thy neighbour. Age Concern runs a 'Be a Good Neighbour' scheme in winter. It asks us to be aware of elderly people living nearby and to help them with small jobs like shopping, or keeping paths free of snow and ice.

Babies get hypothermia too. Babies are also vulnerable to the cold, especially in the first year of life. A hypothermic baby may look normal, says Dr Amiel, but is likely to be drowsy, limp and reluctant to feed. Skin to skin contact is the best way to warm a baby up: cuddle him against your chest, with both of you wrapped up in a warm bed. Prevent cold rooms in the same way as you would for an elderly person, but don't be tempted to overheat a baby's bedroom: 16–20°C (61–68°F) is the recommended range if the baby is adequately clothed. A vest and winter babygro are adequate for all but the coldest nights, even if you're worried that the baby will kick his bedclothes off. Again, don't forget a hat.

Walk home with friends. Hypothermia can strike anyone. When it's freezing outside and you're out on the razzle, get a taxi or make sure someone walks you home, says Dr Amiel. If you're drunk, and you fall or slip on the ice, or just fall asleep in someone's front garden, hypothermia can kill you before you're found.

Stay in your car. If you get stranded in your car on a subfreezing night, stay put. If you try to walk for help you risk hypothermia, and death.

IMPOTENCE

15 ways to overcome it

Improved treatments for impotence are gradually shedding light on this once hushed-up condition. It's now so out in the open that, following prostate cancer surgery, US senator Bob Dole even appeared in television commercials for the impotence wonder drug, Viagra.

Doctors define impotence, or erectile dysfunction as it is correctly known, as the consistent inability to sustain an erection sufficient for sexual intercourse. It is estimated that one in ten UK men over the age of 21 suffer from impotence at some point in their lives. And even more men have an occasional problem achieving an erection. However, evidence suggests that most sufferers do not seek medical help.

'If men are honest, every one of them will tell you they've experienced impotence at least once in their lives,' says urologist Neil Baum. 'It can be devastating when it occurs,' he says. 'A man's whole concept of his masculinity may be undermined.'

Until the early 1970s, experts thought that underlying psychological problems caused most erection difficulties. Today, the medical community recognizes that most long-term impotence (about 75 per cent) is caused by a disease, an injury or as the side-effect of a drug. The most common disease predisposing to impotence is diabetes – more than a third of men with diabetes will have erectile dysfunction, and sometimes this may be the first sign that diabetes has developed. Narrowing of the arteries, hypertension, neurological conditions like multiple sclerosis, pelvic injury and prostate surgery may all cause impotence too, but hormonal problems like low testosterone account for only three per cent of cases. Here's what our experts advise to overcome impotence.

Give yourself time. 'As a man gets older, it may take a longer period of genital stimulation to get an erection,' says Dr Baum. 'For men aged 18 to 20, an erection may take a few seconds. In your thirties and forties, maybe a minute or two. But if a 60-year-old doesn't get an erection after a minute or two, that doesn't mean he's impotent. It just takes longer.'

The time period between ejaculation and your next erection also tends to increase with age. In men aged 60 to 70, it can take a whole day or longer to regain an erection. This is a normal consequence of ageing.

Look at your medicines. Prescription drugs might be at the root of the problem. Or it might be over-the-counter antihistamines, diuretics or sedatives – not every individual reacts to drugs in the same way.

Drug-induced impotence is most common in men over 50, says Dr Baum, with almost 100 drugs cited as potential causes of impotence. If

WHEN TO CONSULT A DOCTOR

Men of any age can be treated for impotence. When home remedies fail to help, your doctor may want to review your medication, rule out causes like diabetes or refer you to a urologist for assessment. Available treatments, depending on the cause and extent of the problem, include:

- drug therapy, including testosterone replacement therapy and drugs that allow more bloodflow into the penis, such as Viagra;
- vacuum devices that draw blood into the penis and hold it there for an erection;
- surgically implanted devices that can be mechanically expanded when an erection is desired;
- surgery to correct bloodflow problems to the penis;
- intracavernosal injections or transurethal therapy;
- psychotherapy.

you suspect your medication, consult your doctor or pharmacist and ask about changing the dose or switching to a different drug. But do not attempt to do this on your own.

Beware of 'recreational' drugs. Other troublemakers include cocaine, marijuana, opiates, heroin, morphine, amphetamines and barbiturates.

Go easy on the alcohol. Shakespeare was right when he said in *Macbeth* that alcohol provokes desire but takes away the performance. That happens because alcohol is a nervous-system depressant. It inhibits your reflexes, creating a state that's the opposite of arousal, says urologist Richard Berger. Even two drinks before dinner can affect performance.

And over time, too much alcohol can upset hormones. 'Chronic alcohol abuse can cause nerve and liver damage,' says Dr Baum. Liver damage results in excessive levels of female hormones in men. Without the right proportion of testosterone to other hormones, you won't achieve normal erections.

Try saw palmetto for stress-related impotence. Stress turns off testosterone production and this can result in loss of libido and poor sexual performance. 'Working with hard-working men has made me realize how common this problem is,' says clinical herbalist Douglas Schar. 'Men who work too hard often end up playing little if at all!'

Saw palmetto, often prescribed by herbalists for prostate problems, really makes a difference to stress-related loss of libido, says Schar. Buy it from a health food store and follow label instructions. You'll need to take the remedy for two or three weeks before you notice a difference.

Use herbs to boost bloodflow. As we age, poor circulation can become a problem, says Schar. Feet and hands are not the only parts of the body affected. If poor circulation is causing erection problems, herbal circulatory stimulants may help. Gingko, ginger and red pepper are favourites amongst herbalists. All are sold in health food stores and should be taken according to label instructions. Take one of these a few hours before you want blood circulating to the relevant parts, says Schar.

What's good for the arteries is good for the penis. The penis is a vascular organ, says urologist Irwin Goldstein. The same things that clog your arteries – dietary cholesterol and saturated fat – also affect bloodflow to the penis. In fact, he says, all men over the age of 38 have some narrowing of the arteries to the penis. High cholesterol (see *High Cholesterol,* page 310) is a major cause of impotence – so watch what you eat.

Don't smoke. Studies show that smoking affects the circulatory system, impairing the efficient bloodflow in the blood vessels – including those in the penis. Around 40 per cent of men with impotence are smokers, says Dr Baum, compared to 30 per cent of men in general.

Feel good about your body. If you've been thinking about losing weight, learning karate or starting a weight-training programme, do it. The better you feel about your body, the better you'll feel going into the event, says James Goldberg, who runs an impotence clinic.

But don't overdo exercise. Excessive exercise stimulates the body's natural opiates, the endorphins. 'We're not sure how they work, but they tend to lessen sensation,' says Dr Goldberg. Exercise is good for you, but you can have too much of a good thing.

Forget sex if you're in pain. Your body also produces its own opiates when you're in pain, says Dr Goldberg. These opiates can turn off any sexual stimuli. There's not much you can do, he says, except wait until you feel better.

Relax. Being in a relaxed frame of mind is crucial to maintaining an erection. This is why. Your nervous system operates in two modes. When the sympathetic nerve network is dominant, your body is literally 'on alert'. Adrenal hormones prepare you to fight or take flight. Your blood moves away from your digestive system and penis and into your muscles.

You can turn on your sympathetic nervous system just by being too anxious, says Dr Baum. For some men, the fear of failure is so overwhelming that it floods the body with adrenaline. That's the opposite of what you need to achieve an erection. The key is to relax and let your parasympathetic nervous system take over. Signals that travel along this network will direct the arteries and sinuses of the penis to expand and let more blood flow in.

Avoid whole-body stimulants. That means caffeine and certain substances sold as potency enhancers. As stated above, it's important to be relaxed during sex, says Dr Goldberg. Stimulants tend to constrict the smooth muscle that must dilate before an erection occurs.

Refocus your attention. One way to relax is to focus with your partner on the more sensual aspects of intimacy. Play with and enjoy each other without worrying about an erection. 'The skin is the largest sexual organ in the body,' says Dr Goldberg, 'not the penis.'

Plan ahead. Decide in advance what you'll do if you don't get an erection, suggests Dr Berger. If you're not so focused on the erection itself, it makes it easier for erection to occur.

Talk to your partner. Don't risk increasing the tension in the bedroom by maintaining a miserable silence. Together, try and work out what's going on. Pressure at work? Worry over a child's illness? A sensitive, unresolved issue? 'If you understand some of the things that can cause impotence, you can explain it without attributing it to something that's not there,' says Dr Berger. 'And you should talk about what your alternatives are. Will you continue your lovemaking in a different way? Don't let an erection, or lack of it, interfere with your intimacy.'

INCONTINENCE
22 ways to gain control

Urinary incontinence is a symptom, not a disease. But the consequences of involuntary loss of urine can be debilitating to a person's self-esteem, social life, and job. That's why urologist Robert Schlesinger describes incontinence as a social disease. 'People will go to almost any extent to adjust their lives to it. I had one patient who didn't leave her house for three years because she was so ashamed.'

One in 10 people in the UK are affected by urinary incontinence. A common myth is that incontinence only affects the elderly. In fact, many younger people are also affected, though they are embarrassed to talk about it. Among 15–64 year-olds, about 5 per cent of men and up to 25 per cent of women suffer from incontinence. The condition affects more than a third of women over 60.

No one should be stigmatized by incontinence, says Katherine Jeter, founder of an organization that supports people with the problem. 'Nearly everybody can be made better or cured.' That's saying something, when you consider that more than three million adult Britons are incontinent.

There are two types of incontinence: stress and urge incontinence. If coughing, laughing, exercising or sneezing cause you to leak small amounts of urine, you may have stress incontinence, which is the most common form in women and is treatable. Physical changes resulting from pregnancy, childbirth and the menopause are the common culprits behind stress incontinence.

Urge incontinence happens when you cannot 'hold on'. It seems to strike for no apparent reason, and more women than men are affected. Urge incontinence is often caused by illness and is common in older people. But it is not a normal part of ageing, says geriatrician Neil Resnick. 'It's not inevitable, and it's not irreversible.' Sometimes, minimal effort can reduce or even prevent the problem.

Keep a bladder diary. For a week, write down everything you eat, drink, when you go to the loo and when you leak urine, Dr Jeter suggests. The diary will help you and your doctor to track down the cause.

Go easy on fluids. Your bladder diary may reveal that you've been downing gallons of water a day, Dr Jeter says. 'If you drink a little less, your incontinence problem should ease up.'

Note timing, too. It's better to sip water throughout the day rather than pouring it down all at once. And it's especially important to stop drinking water within three or four hours of going to bed, especially if you get up during the night to pee, adds Joseph Montella, a urologist and gynaecologist.

But not too easy. Cutting your fluid intake to below-normal levels can lead to dehydration, worsening urinary problems and, possibly, serious illness. Doctors usually advise people to drink eight glasses of water a day to prevent dehydration.

Avoid alcohol. Booze is a great stimulant for trotting to the loo.

WHEN TO CONSULT A DOCTOR

The vast majority of people with mild to moderate symptoms do not have to rush off to see a doctor. Give yourself three months to see if lifestyle changes help, says gynaecologist Abraham Morse.

Other symptoms – such as painful urination, incontinence along with painful intercourse, or cloudy or blood-tinged urine – are signs that you should see your doctor. Urinary tract infections and tumours can cause the bladder to go into overdrive. An increase in the amount of urine you're passing, accompanied by increased thirst, may indicate the onset of diabetes: this is something your doctor can easily check for.

You should also call a doctor if you're having large 'accidents' rather than small leaks. Or if accidents are accompanied by numbness or weakness in your arms or legs, vision changes or a change in bowel habits. These symptoms could indicate nerve damage or other neurological problems, such as Parkinson's disease.

Avoid caffeine. Caffeine is another well-known diuretic. It also irritates the bladder and stimulates muscle contractions, which can aggravate the symptoms of urge incontinence, explains Abraham Morse, a urologist and gynaecologist.

Caffeine is found in drinks, but also in foods such as chocolate and in medicines including several painkillers and cold-cure remedies. Limit caffeine intake to no more than 200mg a day, about the amount in two cups (or one mug) of coffee. Your diary will help you see if you're having too much. Switching to decaffeinated coffee or tea will help, but it may not eliminate the problem, Dr Morse adds. Other substances in coffee and tea also act as bladder irritants.

Avoid grapefruit juice. Grapefruit juice is a famous diuretic, which is why it formed the basis of the once-popular grapefruit diet.

Drink cranberry juice. It's good for bladder health because it helps to prevent urinary tract infections, a common problem for people who live with many forms of incontinence. Cranberry juice also helps to deodorize the urinary tract, making accidents a little less noticeable.

Drink still water. The carbon dioxide bubbles in fizzy water and soft drinks make urine more acidic, which can trigger the urge to urinate.

Stay loose. Constipation can contribute to incontinence. So eat a high-fibre diet and be sure to drink adequate amounts of fluid. One incontinence clinic's prescription is to eat popcorn every day.

Don't smoke. Nicotine and other chemicals in tobacco smoke can irritate the bladder, says Dr Montella. And if you have stress incontinence, coughing can trigger leaking.

Lose excess weight. People who lose even a few pounds can reduce their incidents of incontinence.

Go twice. When you urinate, stay on the toilet until you feel your bladder is empty. Then, stand up and sit down again, lean forwards slightly and try again.

Know when to go. It's a good idea to empty your bladder on a regular basis, Dr Jeter says. For example, don't sit at the dinner table and hold it until dinner's over. Holding on too long may lead to bladder infection and an overstretched bladder. Also, if you have an over-full bladder and a weak sphincter muscle, you're likely to leak when you cough, sneeze or laugh. Your best bet is to empty your bladder before and after meals, and at bedtime.

Do just *one* thing

Bladder drill training is one of the best treatments for certain types of incontinence. The idea is simple. Rather than going to the toilet every time you need to pee, only go at specific times – every hour on the hour, for example, whether you feel the urge or not.

Do this for five to seven days, then increase the interval between bathroom visits to 90 minutes, advises urologist and gynaecologist Abraham Morse. Do this for another five to seven days, then increase the interval to two hours. Keep increasing the time intervals until you reach four hours.

Hold your urine as best you can between toilet visits. You might experience leaks, but that's okay. As long as you stick to the clock, you'll eventually gain more control. 'Research shows that about 50 per cent of people see a significant improvement with bladder training,' says Dr Morse.

Do pelvic floor exercises. Pelvic floor exercises were developed in the late 1940s by Dr Arnold Kegel to help women with stress incontinence during and after pregnancy. The experts say that these exercises reduce and may even prevent some forms of incontinence in both sexes and at all ages. Here's how to do them.

i) Without tensing the muscles of your legs, buttocks or abdomen, imagine that you're trying to hold back a bowel movement by tightening the ring of muscles (the sphincter) around the anus. This exercise identifies the back part of the pelvic muscles.

ii) When you're urinating, try to stop the flow and then restart it. This identifies the front part of the pelvic muscles.

iii) You're now ready for the complete exercise. Working from back to front, tighten the muscles while counting to four slowly, then release. Do this for two minutes at least three times a day – that's 100 repetitions.

Anticipate accidents. If you know you're going to sneeze, cough, lift or bounce up and down, squeeze that sphincter first to ward off an accident.

Don't panic if you have no warning. If you have urge incontinence, you have almost no warning of the need to go. Don't panic. Instead, at first notice, relax. The same muscles you use to clench your buttocks can also be used to short-circuit those 'got to go' sensations. Clench the muscles as tightly as you can and hold the tension for a few seconds. Doing this several times in a row often makes the urge to urinate disappear. 'It's like biting your lip when you want to sneeze,' says Dr Morse. When the urge passes, walk slowly, without panicking, to the nearest toilet.

Quieten your mind. Another strategy for sudden urges is to 'breathe deeply, calm yourself down, and be confident that you're not going to make a mess,' says Dr Morse. If you can calm yourself for 30 to 60 seconds, there's a good chance that the urge will go away.

The idea is to gain control over your bladder, rather than panicking, adds Dr Montella. Wait until you're calm, then go to the loo.

Be ready for emergencies. If incontinence at night is a problem, keep a bedpan or commode within reach of your bed.

Compensate for your age. As you age, it takes longer to get anywhere – including the toilet. So make sure you always know where the nearest lavatory is, and position yourself as close as possible to it, says Dr Jeter.

Buy special supplies. There are several brands of absorbent pants, pads and shields. The products absorb 50 to 500 times their weight in water, neutralize odour and congeal fluid to prevent leakage. The kind you need depends on your anatomy and the kind and degree of incontinence you have. It's understandable if you're embarrassed to buy them. Find an understanding pharmacist and ask to have your package waiting for you when you arrive, or buy online and have them delivered to your door.

Reduce tension. 'Whenever you're anxious or depressed, your body sensations are magnified in a negative way,' says Dr Morse. 'If you're anxious to begin with, feeling as though you have to rush to the toilet is one more thing that can push you over the edge.'

Take a hint from your bladder and unwind. Give yourself an hour each day to do something just for you, like taking a walk, watching some television, wandering round a museum or going to the cinema.

Infant Colic

14 ideas to quieten the cries

Any parent who has tried to soothe an inconsolable infant at the witching hour just before supper will tell you that it's the hardest thing in the world to cope with a baby convulsed by the unstoppable screams caused by colic. First time parents especially can find their baby's colic devastating and terrifying, says family doctor Stephen Amiel. Just when you think you're getting the hang of this new baby business, colic can come along and shake you out of your just-about established routine and sense of achievement. Is he ill? Am I feeding him enough, or too much? Why can't he tell me what's wrong? Why am I such a hopeless parent?

Ancient scholars first described infantile colic in the 6th century. Modern parents have no trouble describing it today. The baby cries wrenching sobs, pulls his knees up to his abdomen, and appears to be in great pain. He may produce some wind, then go quiet, then scream again.

Nothing much seems to have changed over the centuries, and nothing much seems to help. Colicky babies cannot generally be quietened with feed or a nappy change, and episodes may last for several hours. Colic tends to be most severe at four to six weeks of age and gradually subsides by three to four months. While none of the remedies offered below will cure colic, most have brought some relief to suffering parents, so you may want to give them a try. And remember that this will pass. Colic disappears as mysteriously as it begins.

Don't beat yourself up. There is no convincing evidence that babies get colic because their parents are stressed or anxious, says Dr Amiel. Your baby's colic will naturally cause some tension and anxiety, rather than the other way round. But babies are sensitive to their parents' mood and household tensions do affect their behaviour. So, exclude other causes of excessive crying, such as hunger, cold or itching, and satisfy yourself that your baby is not ill. Then everyone, including the baby, will benefit if you do your best to relax and see colic as a misery that is no one's fault, and above all, one that will eventually go away.

Try the colic carry. 'I'm a big believer in the colic carry,' says childcare expert Anne Price. Extend your forearm with your palm up, then put the baby on your arm chest down, with her head in your hand and her legs on either side of your elbow. Support the baby with your other hand and walk around the house with her in this position. 'It definitely helps.'

Excessive handling of your baby is actually not helpful, though, says Dr Amiel. There is no harm in leaving her to cry for a little, if you are happy all she has is colic.

Burp that babe. 'My experience is that at least some colicky babies do have more abdominal wind than the norm and may be more difficult to burp,' says paediatric nurse practitioner Linda Jonides.

Her recommendation is to watch the position of the baby when feeding (upright is all right) and burp frequently. When bottle-feeding, burp after every ounce, and try a variety of teats. The teat hole size should not be too big or too small, or your baby will gulp too much air as she fights to control the flow or to get enough milk. Turn the bottle upside down: single drops of milk should form steadily if the hole size is right. Some parents swear by the Playtex disposable nurser – which is probably the closest in shape and action to breastfeeding – but it is not widely available in the UK.

Stop drinking milk. Some childcare specialists believe that colic is caused when cow's milk is transmitted from mother to infant through breast milk. Though some research casts doubt on this connection, experts agree that a maternal diet free of cow's milk may be worth a try, especially in families with a strong history of allergies. Start by eliminating all dairy products from your diet for one week and see what happens, says Dr Amiel.

If you bottle-feed your baby, talk to your health visitor about changing to a hypo-allergenic formula for a trial period of one week. Soya milk has not proved to be particularly beneficial in controlling colic.

Check the diet connection. 'Occasionally, some foods set a baby off,' says paediatrician Morris Green. He suggests that breastfeeding mothers try and see if there's any correlation between what they eat and bouts of colic. Potential troublemakers include caffeine-containing drinks, chocolate, bananas, oranges, strawberries, grapes and highly spiced foods.

Drink a soothing tea, mum. Many nursing mothers report that colic can be remedied by the consumption of fennel or chamomile tea, says clinical herbalist Douglas Schar. The theory is that the soothing tea makes its way into breastmilk and settles the baby's sore tummy. In the old days, says Schar, mothers sweetened chamomile tea and spoonfed the baby

WHEN TO CONSULT A DOCTOR

If you think your baby has colic, your health visitor is the best person to speak to first, says family doctor Stephen Amiel. She'll be able to check the baby's weight, go through feeding and winding techniques with you, and generally reassure and support you. If your baby is failing to thrive despite adequate milk being available, your health visitor will advise you to see your doctor who will want to rule out infection or other causes.

Medicine and milk. Medication for infantile colic is generally disappointing, but your doctor may prescribe dimethicone, which a few small studies have shown sometimes to be beneficial. You can also get one hypo-allergenic milk, Nutramigen, on prescription, if you are giving this route a try. Gripe water can be bought over the counter, but it is not prescribed, as there is little evidence it makes any difference to colic.

Urgent attention. Sudden onset of apparent pain in a baby, if associated with projectile vomiting and reluctance to feed, or continuous crying without the squirming and drawing up of the knees characteristic of colic, should always be checked by a doctor at the earliest opportunity, says Dr Amiel. Your baby may have a serious infection or possibly a bowel blockage from, for example, a strangulated hernia.

Help for mum. You should also see your doctor or health visitor if you feel you are not coping with your colicky baby's demands, says Dr Amiel. The early months of parenthood can be a difficult and lonely time for anyone, especially for single parents. But 10 to 15 per cent of mothers suffer symptoms of postnatal depression, a sometimes serious condition which requires treatment.

Warning signs include losing your temper with the baby, even to the point of wanting to harm him, or blaming him irrationally for other things too, like having a dirty nappy; getting excessively irritable with your partner or other children; becoming tearful, sad or withdrawn; becoming excessively anxious or panicky; losing your appetite and sleeping badly, even when the baby is quiet; or having thoughts of self-harm.

with it to ease the problem. 'However, this remedy has not been verified by contemporary clinical trials,' warns Schar, 'and giving babies remedies before they have been cleared scientifically, is always questionable.'

Try swaddling the baby. 'I recommend swaddling a colicky baby,' Jonides says. For some reason, wrapping a baby snugly in a blanket has a calming effect. She also suggests using a baby-carrier to hold the baby so that your arms are free to get on with other things.

Use a vacuum cleaner instead of a lullaby. Colicky babies seem to love the noise made by a vacuum cleaner. Science has failed to explain this mystery. 'The noise of a vacuum cleaner running does seem to calm a colicky baby,' says Dr Green. Some parents tape-record the sound of a vacuum cleaner and play it back when baby starts fussing. Others simply start vacuuming the carpet and hope the child outgrows colic while there's still some pile left.

Price suggests a two-pronged attack: 'If you wear the baby on your front in a baby-carrier and vacuum at the same time, it's a double whammy. That colicky baby goes out like a light.'

Try the spin dryer trick. 'Put the baby in an infant seat and rest it against the side of a running spin-dryer so the baby gets that buzzing sound and vibration through the seat,' suggests paediatric nurse Helen Neville. 'There's something about the vibration that really soothes a colicky baby.' Sounds weird? Wait until the baby cries for another three hours or so – you'll try anything.

Take the baby for a spin. If you and the spin dryer can't take any more, bundle the baby in her infant seat into the car and go for a drive. 'Twice around London's North Circular was my second daughter's record,' says Dr Amiel, 'but twenty minutes was usually more than enough. It gave my wife – and the neighbours – a break and, with the radio full on, everyone was happy.'

Give yourself a break. If you're lucky enough to have parents, in-laws or friends who can look after the baby for an hour or two, grab the opportunity with both hands to go out for a walk or a meal, says Dr Amiel. The baby will be fine (and probably good as gold), and you'll get a bit of peace and perspective back.

Warm that tummy. 'A hot-water bottle or heating pad set on low and placed on the baby's tummy sometimes helps,' Jonides says. (Put a towel between the baby and the hot-water bottle to make sure the tummy doesn't get burned.)

Keep a diary. It's a really good idea to keep a log of when the baby cries, Neville says. Often, it may seem that the baby was miserable for two solid hours, when it was really only 45 minutes. A log will show how long the baby cries for, and – more importantly – what might be bringing it on.'

Buy or borrow a mechanical swing. A regular swinging motion seems to be good for colic. 'Many babies will be quiet at least for long enough to let you get through supper when they're swinging.' says Jonides.

INFERTILITY

21 ways to get a baby on board

Few experiences can compare to the joy of bringing a child into the world – and virtually nothing is as distressing as trying for a baby, and failing.

Infertility is defined as the inability to conceive a child within one year. A variety of factors contributes to infertility, including genetics, health and lifestyle. And while infertility may be traced to a single cause in either you or your partner, it can also be caused by a combination of factors, from infection to stress to medication.

If you and your partner have been unable to get pregnant, you're far from alone. Infertility affects one in seven couples in the UK. Of these couples, the problem occurs in a man's reproductive system 30 to 50 per cent of the time and in a woman's reproductive system – which has more tasks to perform in the baby-making process – 50 to 70 per cent of the time. But take heart, especially if you're an older wanna-be parent. While you and your partner will want to see a doctor to determine the exact cause of your infertility, there's a lot that you can do on your own to increase your odds of conceiving a child. Try any or all of these expert-recommended tips.

Remedies for Women

Plan ahead if you can. Unfair as it is, it's a biological fact: a woman's age has a dramatic impact on her fertility, says obstetrician Robert Stillman. Population studies indicate that more than 90 per cent of women under the age of 24 are able to conceive successfully. That figure drops sharply with age; by the time women are between the ages of 35 and 44, the odds are a little better than 1 in 3.

That's *not* to say that if you're in your twenties or early thirties, you should have children if you're not emotionally or financially prepared, says Dr Stillman. But knowing ahead of time that your odds of conceiving dwindle with age can help you to make an informed decision about when to get pregnant.

Practise think-ahead birth control. Some hormonal methods of birth control can linger in the body for some time after you stop them. Depo-Provera (a three-monthly injection), for example, can delay a return to normal fertility for anything up to a year or more, so you need to factor this in to your plans, especially if you are over 35. If you prefer a hormonal method of birth control (rather than, say, condoms or diaphragms), use the Pill, recommends Dr Stillman. 'When you're ready to conceive, there will be less chance of a long delay.'

Achieve a 'fertile weight'. Twelve per cent of all infertility cases stem from weighing too much or too little. If you're overweight, losing just five to 10 per cent of your weight can dramatically improve your chances of ovulating and conceiving. If you're drastically underweight, do your best to gain. 'Women need a certain amount of body fat to carry and bear a child,' says Dr Stillman.

Keep up with your workouts. It's a myth that women should stop exercising while they're trying to conceive, says reproductive expert John Jarrett. In fact, regular exercise can help you to cope with the emotional stress that you might be feeling as you try to get pregnant.

Time your ovulation. Women usually ovulate – release an egg from an ovary – 14 days before they menstruate. To find out when you ovulate, use an ovulation detection kit, recommends fertility expert Linda Giudice. These kits, which you can buy over the counter, measure your levels of urinary luteinizing hormone (LH), a hormone that stimulates egg maturation and release. Use the test between 8am and 10am when LH levels surge, she says.

Get ahead of your hormones. The ovulation detection test reads positive 24 hours before you actually ovulate. When you get that positive result, have intercourse that night (or day), the next day or both.

Or throw timing out of the window. If a woman has a reliable 28-day cycle, she ovulates around day 14, says Dr Jarrett. Having sex on days 10, 12, 14, 16 and 18 will pretty much cover your fertile period. If your cycle is longer or shorter, but still reliable, count back 14 days from the expected first day of your period to calculate when you ovulate.

Lie still. Lying still for five to 10 minutes after intercourse may improve your chances of conceiving, as it helps keep your partner's semen where it needs to be, says Dr Stillman. But you don't need to do anything drastic – like hanging upside down in gravity boots – to keep semen inside you.

WHEN TO CONSULT A DOCTOR

If you're under 35, and you and your partner have not been able to conceive after a year of unprotected sex, see your doctor. If you're 35 or older, see your doctor if you haven't conceived after six months.

Avoid soya-based foods. Women who are trying to conceive should avoid soya foods, such as tofu and soya milk, advises Dr Stillman. 'They contain plant oestrogens, called phytoestrogens, that compete with a woman's natural oestrogen, and they can disrupt a woman's ovulation cycle,' he says.

Choose chasteberry. Also known as *Vitex agnus-castus*, chasteberry stimulates the pituitary gland to increase the production of LH, explains Serafina Corsello, an expert in alternative medicine. This results in higher levels of progesterone during the second phase of a woman's menstrual cycle, called the luteal phase. Progesterone is important for fertility because it helps to develop a thick, blood-rich uterine lining into which a fertilized egg can implant.

Many women between 30 and 45 have a drop-off in progesterone, which leads to shortened cycles and the inability to implant an egg. You should use chasteberry (available in health food stores) for several months before trying to get pregnant. Follow instructions on the label.

Boost fertility with black cohosh. As we age, our fertility decreases. This does not help the increasing numbers of people who are trying for a family later in life. Black cohosh, usually thought of as a menopause herb, can be used to help older women conceive.

According to clinical herbalist Douglas Schar, black cohosh plays two roles in age-related infertility. 'I tell patients who are putting off childbearing to think about using black cohosh to keep their reproductive tract in good health – so it's ready when they are ready. And older women whose periods are becoming erratic can use the herb to stabilize their cycle and thereby increase their chances of

KITCHEN CURES

Men who want to be dads should consider filling their plates with fresh fruit and vegetables. The nutrients they contain may help to grow healthy sperm.

Research suggests that abnormally high levels of free radicals may cause infertility in some men. Free radicals are 'crippled' oxygen molecules that are generated naturally by our body processes. They damage healthy cells – and possibly sperm.

It seems that the antioxidant vitamins found in fresh produce, like beta-carotene, vitamin C and vitamin E, may benefit the sperm of men under high oxidative stress – for example, smokers and keen exercisers – because these vitamins help to neutralize free radicals.

Do just *one* thing

Quit smoking. 'No question – smoking is a major factor in infertility,' says reproductive specialist John Jarrett. 'If both partners smoke, their chances of successful conception drop by as much as 50 per cent.'

In men, the heavy metals in cigarette smoke get inside the head of the sperm and poison the mechanism by which the sperm penetrates the egg. In women, heavy metals prevent cell division from occurring, which leads to miscarriage.

Women over 35 who are planning to have children have another good reason to quit. Smoking makes you infertile by bringing on the menopause an average of two years earlier.

pregnancy.' Black cohosh is available from health food stores; follow label directions.

Start preparing for success. If you're trying to conceive, make sure that your body is in good shape for a pregnancy, advises family doctor Stephen Amiel. Start to take folic acid supplements to help prevent birth defects like spina bifida. A 400 microgram tablet a day is enough: tablets can be bought over the counter or on prescription from your doctor.

Other vitamin supplements or iron are rarely necessary if you have a balanced diet with plenty of fruit and vegetables, and you should avoid extra vitamin A, which can be harmful in pregnancy. Get your rubella (German measles) status checked by having a blood test, avoid people with chickenpox unless you are sure you are immune, and avoid foods that might carry dangerous bacteria – blue cheeses, patés, unpasteurized milk, raw eggs and cook-chill meals.

Stop smoking, cut down your alcohol and check with your doctor before taking prescription or over-the-counter medications.

Relax? This is common advice to people who are trying to conceive, says Dr Amiel, but there is little consistent evidence that stress itself is a cause of infertility. Of course it can be tense and a bit of a passion-killer time planning your lovemaking around ovulation, and the disappointment of yet another period starting can be acute, taking its toll on a relationship. So make a special effort to support each other, and make time for each other right through the month.

Remedies for Men
Stay out of hot water. A hot bath can lower a man's fertility because the heat can kill the sperm in his testes, says Dr Stillman.

Wear baggy pants. It really is true: it's better to wear loose underwear that allows your testicles to 'breathe,' says Dr Giudice. 'Tight pants raise the temperature of a man's testicles, which can kill sperm or decrease the ability of sperm to fertilize an egg.'

Treat supplements with caution. Supplements containing the amino acids carnitine and acetyl-L-carnitine, known to play a part in sperm development, are available via the internet. 'They are expensive,' says Dr Amiel. 'A six-month supply will cost several hundred pounds, and the evidence for their success is pretty patchy.'

Remedies for Men and Women

Use condoms. If you're not currently in a monogamous relationship but want to have children one day, use a condom – every time. Sexually transmitted diseases such as chlamydia and gonorrhoea, which often cause no symptoms, can cause infertility in both men and women.

Don't overdo it. Having sex until you're ready to drop will not increase your chances of conceiving, says Dr Stillman. 'In fact, having sex four or five times a day is counterproductive.' That's because a man's sperm count drops dramatically after ejaculation and takes about 48 hours to reach pre-ejaculation levels.

Drink lightly or not at all. Research shows that women who drink as few as five drinks a week may hinder conception. Men who consume large amounts of alcohol can impair their fertility, too. A heavy drinker may end up with a damaged liver. Oestrogen levels rise in men with liver damage, which can often cause impaired sperm production.

INGROWING HAIRS
10 ideas for a clean shave

An ingrowing hair lives up to its name, for instead of growing outwards, it grows back into the skin. When the tip of the hair punctures the skin, it can cause inflammation and pain. Naturally curly hairs, especially beard hairs, often grow inwards.

If inflammation is a problem, many experts recommend letting the hair grow into a beard if at all feasible. When hairs are longer, they don't twist around and puncture the skin.

Dermatologists say that tweezers are the only way to get rid of an ingrowing hair, but there are other ways of making sure that ingrowing hairs don't return. Follow these tips to ease your discomfort.

Use tweezers. If you can see an ingrowing hair beneath the skin, apply a warm flannel for a couple of minutes to soften the skin, advises dermatologist Rodney Basler. Then sterilize a needle or tweezers and pluck the hair. Finally, wipe the area with an antiseptic such as surgical spirit.

Bring it to the surface. If you can't see the ingrowing hair, don't fish for it, Dr Basler warns, because it might not be an ingrowing hair at all. Instead, treat it with a warm compress until you can see a hair lurking there. Then use a sterilized needle or tweezers, followed by an antiseptic.

Think about growing a beard. 'The curlier your hair is, the more likely you are to get ingrowing hairs,' says Dr Basler. If it's a real problem, seriously consider growing a beard.

Soften your bristles. If you cannot consider growing a beard, then properly preparing your bristles for shaving helps to prevent ingrowing hairs. Wash your face thoroughly with soap and water for two minutes, recommends dermatologist Jerome Litt. That softens the hair. Rinse well, apply shaving cream or gel and leave it on for two minutes before shaving to further soften the hair.

Hide behind your shadow. Reconcile yourself to having a permanent five o'clock shadow, Dr Basler says. Don't shave too close. The best way to do this is to use an electric razor.

Don't use a twin blade. Twin-bladed razors are double trouble. The first blade cuts and sharpens the hair; the second blade cuts below skin level, Dr Litt says. The result is that the sharpened hair curls around and slips back into the skin. Instead, use a single-bladed razor and settle for a shave that isn't as close.

Train your bristles. Does your beard grow in several directions? Dr Litt advises you to train it to grow out straight. Do this by shaving in two directions: down on the face, and up on the neck (to prevent neck nicks). Don't shave in all different directions or back and forth. You won't get as clean a shave to begin with, but if you keep shaving down your face and up your neck, your beard should start growing out straight in a matter of months.

Try the aftershave special. Put a damp towel on your face for a few minutes after shaving. It softens the bristles so they're less able to repenetrate the skin, says Dr Basler. And use a creamy aftershave balm, not the normal alcohol-based aftershave splash. It's soothing and keeps the hair moisturized.

Fight infection. If a bristle burrows under your skin despite your best efforts, you can cut down on the amount of bacteria it takes with it.

A 10 per cent benzoyl peroxide solution has some antiseptic effect, Dr Basler says, and could help if used as an aftershave. Most aftershaves contain lots of alcohol which also helps to decrease the bacteria on the skin.

Ladies, shave down instead of up. Women tend to shave their legs from ankle to knee, says Dr Litt. This is against the grain and can cause ingrowing hairs. Instead, shave downwards, from knee to ankle.

Ingrowing Toenails
7 ways to look after your feet

The pain of an ingrowing toenail can make a monster of even the most placid person. Ingrowing toenails usually start when a toenail – usually one of the big toenails – grows or is pushed into the soft, tender tissue next to it. People whose toenails are noticeably curved are more susceptible, but anyone can be affected. The result is red, painful, tender toes. The long-term goal is to prevent future ingrowing toenails, but the immediate aim for most people is to ease the pain. Here's how to do both.

Try an over-the-counter product. There are one or two over-the-counter products that may soften the toenail and the skin around it, thus relieving pain, says podiatrist Suzanne Levine. Scholl Toenail Softening Solution or Pickles Toenail Softener are two that might help. Make sure you follow directions carefully. Don't use these products if you have diabetes or poor circulation.

Get a wisp of relief. You want to help the embedded toenail to grow out over the adjacent skin fold. Start by soaking your foot in warm water to soften the toenail, says family doctor Frederick Hass. Dry carefully, then gently slide a wisp (not a wad) of sterile cotton beneath the burrowing edge of the toenail. The cotton will slightly lift the toenail so that it can grow past the tissue it is digging into. Apply an antiseptic as a safeguard against infection. Change the cotton insert each day until the toenail has grown past the trouble spot.

Protect toes from accidents

While ingrowing toenails are usually caused by improper cutting, they can also result from accidents, says GP Frederick Hass. Stubbing your toe is one cause. Dropping a heavy object on your foot is another.

Wear sturdy, comfortable shoes for housework, he says. And if your job involves handling heavy objects, then buy work shoes with steel toecaps. They will protect your toes in all but the most serious accidents.

Don't cut a V. Don't try the old wives' remedy of cutting a V-shaped wedge out of the centre of the toenail, warns podiatrist Glenn Copeland. This will not cause the sides to grow towards the centre and away from the ingrowing edge: toenails only grow from the cuticle upwards.

Let your toes breathe. Badly fitting shoes can cause an ingrowing toenail, especially if your toenails tend to curve. Avoid pointed or tight shoes that press on your toenails, says Dr Levine. Instead, wear sandals when you can, or broad-toed shoes. And avoid tight socks and tights.

Cut toenails straight across. Never cut your toenails too short, says Dr Hass. Soften them first in warm water to reduce possible splitting,

WHEN TO CONSULT A DOCTOR

If your toe becomes infected, see a doctor, says foot specialist Suzanne Levine. Signs of infection include swelling, redness and pain or warmth when touched. Pus-filled blisters may also form.

'If you let an ingrowing toenail become seriously infected, you can end up in big trouble,' she warns. 'Several patients have come to me only after their toes became red and swollen with pus. If your circulation is poor, you run the risk of gangrene.'

If you have diabetes or poor arterial circulation to your feet, ask your doctor to refer you to a podiatrist (chiropodist) for advice on how best to cut your toenails and care for your feet. If you have problems cutting your own nails because of poor eyesight, thickened toenails or disability, the podiatrist can cut them for you regularly. If you are housebound, ask for a home visit from the podiatry service.

then cut straight across with a substantial, sharp, straight-edged clipper. Never cut a toenail in an oval shape so that the edges curve down into the skin at the sides. Always leave the outside edges parallel to the skin. And don't trim the toenail any shorter than the tip of your toe; you want the nail to be long enough to protect the toe from pressure and friction.

Repair mistakes. If you accidentally cut or break a toenail too short, carefully smooth it at the edges with an emery board or nail file so that no sharp points are left to penetrate the skin, says Dr Hass.

INSOMNIA
22 steps to a good night's sleep

Insomnia ranks just behind the common cold, stomach upsets and headaches as the reasons people go to their doctors. In a Gallup poll of more than 1000 adults, one-third said that they woke in the middle of the night and couldn't get back to sleep.

At one time, doctors might automatically have prescribed a sedative to help you get some sleep, but that isn't always the case today. Researchers and doctors are learning more about sleep each year, broadening their knowledge of how to deal with its related problems.

Indeed, there are quite a few commonsense approaches that you can use to try and correct the problem yourself. It may take just one therapy; it may take a combination. In any case, the key to success is discipline. As psychologist Michael Stevenson, says: 'sleep is a natural physiological phenomenon, but it's also a learned behaviour'.

Set a rigid sleep routine – seven days a week. Sleep medicine experts insist on people trying to be as regular with their habits as possible, says Merrill Mitler, a psychiatrist who specializes in sleep problems.

The key is to get enough sleep so that you can make it through your day without feeling drowsy. To achieve that goal, try to get to bed at the same time each night, which will help to set your system's circadian rhythm, the so-called body clock that regulates most internal functions. Just as important is getting up at the same time each morning.

Set a sleeping time of, say, 1am to 6am. If you manage to sleep soundly through that five-hour period, add 15 minutes each week until you find yourself waking in the middle of the night. Work on getting through that waking period before adding another 15 minutes. You'll know when you reach the point where you've had enough sleep – you'll wake up refreshed, energetic and ready to take on the day.

If you wake up during the night and can't get back to sleep within 15 minutes, don't fight it, says Dr Mitler. Stay in bed and listen to the radio until you're drowsy again.

Again, be sure to wake up at your normal routine time in the morning – don't lie in trying to make up for 'lost' sleep. That applies to weekends as well. So don't lie in on Saturday and Sunday mornings. If you do, you may have trouble falling asleep on Sunday night, which can leave you feeling washed out on Monday morning.

Don't waste your time in bed. As you grow older, your body needs less sleep. Most newborn babies sleep for up to 18 hours a day. By the time he or she reaches the age of ten, a child's need for sleep has usually dropped to about ten hours.

Experts agree that there is no 'normal' amount of sleep for an adult. The average is seven to eight hours, but some people operate well on as few as five hours, while others need up to ten. The key is to become what experts call an efficient sleeper.

Go to bed only when you're sleepy, advises Edward Stepanski, who runs a sleep research centre. If you can't fall asleep in 15 minutes or so, get up and do something pleasantly monotonous. Read a magazine article, not a book that may engross you. Knit, watch television or do a puzzle. Don't play computer games that excite you or begin jobs you feel you need to finish, such as the washing. When you feel drowsy, go back to bed. If you still can't fall asleep, repeat the procedure until you can. But remember: always get up at the same time in the morning.

Have some quiet time before bed. 'Some people are so busy that when they lie down to go to sleep, it's the first time that they've had a chance to think about what's happened during the day,' says psychiatrist David Neubauer.

An hour or two before going to bed, sit down for at least 10 minutes. Think about the day's events and try to put them into some sort of perspective. Try and work out solutions to any problems. Plan what you'll do tomorrow. This exercise will help to clear your mind of the niggles that can keep you awake once you're under the duvet.

Keep your bedroom sacred. 'If you want to go to bed, be prepared to sleep,' says Magdi Soliman, a pharmacologist who specializes in nervous disorders. 'If there's something else to do, you won't be able to concentrate on sleeping.' So don't watch TV, talk on the phone, argue with your partner, read, eat or perform mundane tasks in bed. Use your bedroom only for sleep and sex.

Light therapy

A dose of bright light in the morning can help chronically poor sleepers to set their circadian rhythms, or body clocks, to a more regular pattern.

According to Jean Joseph-Vanderpool, a sleep researcher, many people find that they just can't get going in the morning.

He conducted an experiment in which, when subjects woke up at around 8am, they were placed in front of high-intensity, full-spectrum fluorescent lights for two hours. This strong light resembles daylight on a bright summer morning. Those lights 'told' the body it was morning and time to get moving. Then, in the evening, the subjects donned dark glasses so that their bodies knew it was time to begin to wind down.

After several weeks of the therapy, the volunteers reported more alertness in the morning and better sleep at night. At home, says Dr Joseph-Vanderpool, you can achieve the same effect by going for a walk, sitting in the sun or doing some gardening as soon as you get up. In winter, talk to your doctor about the best type of artificial light to use.

See SAD (Seasonal Affective Disorder), page 480 for more information on daylight-mimicking artificial lights.

Get off the vicious cycle. One of the commonest causes of insomnia is worry that you're not going to sleep and worry that you'll be too tired to function the next day. Short-term insomnia is common and harmless. Fatigue does affect performance but, mostly, people function perfectly well enough on no sleep – ask any new mum!

Avoid stimulants after twilight. Coffee, colas and even chocolate contain caffeine, a powerful stimulant that can keep you up, so try not to consume them after 4pm, says Dr Mitler. Don't smoke either; nicotine is also a stimulant. Stimulant 'recreational' drugs like ecstasy, cocaine and amphetamines will, of course, also disrupt your sleep.

Say no to a nightcap. Avoid alcohol at dinner and throughout the rest of the evening, suggests Dr Stevenson. And don't make a so-called nightcap to relax you before bed. Alcohol depresses the central nervous system, but it also disrupts sleep. In a few hours, usually during the middle of the night, its effects wear off, your body slides into withdrawal, and you'll wake up.

Look at your medicines. Certain drugs can disrupt sleep. If you take prescription medicine routinely, ask your doctor about its side-effects. If a drug could be interfering with your sleep, your doctor may be able to alter the prescription or adjust the time of day that you take it.

Drugs to look out for include diuretics, some antidepressants, steroids, beta-blockers, painkillers containing caffeine, slimming tablets, asthma reliever inhalers and some pseudoephedrine-containing cold remedies.

One of the reasons doctors are reluctant to prescribe sleeping tablets is that stopping them after regular use can cause 'rebound' insomnia.

Look at your work pattern. Research shows that people who work shifts that regularly swing between day and night have problems sleeping, says Mortimer Mamelak, who runs a sleep clinic. The stress of such a disruptive pattern can make you feel jet-lagged all the time, and sleep mechanisms can break down altogether. The solution is to try and get a regular shift – even if it's at night.

Eat a light snack before bedtime. Bread and fruit will do nicely an hour or two before you hit the sack, says psychologist Sonia Ancoli-Israel. So will a glass of warm milk. Avoid sugary snacks that can excite your system or heavy meals that can put a strain on your body.

And use common sense. If you're older, don't drink lots of fluids before going to bed, or you might need the loo in the middle of the night.

Create a comfortable sleep setting. 'Insomnia is often caused by stress,' says Dr Stevenson. 'You get into bed, you're nervous and anxious, and that impairs your ability to sleep. Before long, the bedroom becomes associated with sleeplessness, and that triggers a phobic response.'

You can change that by making the bedroom as comfortable a setting as possible. Redecorate the room in your favourite colours. Soundproof the room and use black-out curtain linings or blinds to keep out the light.

Buy a comfortable bed. It doesn't matter whether it's a sprung mattress, a waterbed, a futon or a mat on the floor. If it feels good, use it. Choose loose-fitting cotton night clothes. Make sure the bedroom's temperature is just right – not too hot, not too cold. Make sure there's no clock within view to distract you during the night.

Turn off your mind. Stop yourself from reliving a stressful day by focusing your thoughts on something peaceful and non-threatening, says Dr Stevenson. Play some soft, soothing music as you drift off, or some environmental noise such as the sound of a waterfall, waves crashing on a beach or the sound of rain in a jungle. The only rule is that it's not intrusive or distracting.

A herbal approach

Insomnia is nothing new. Since the beginning of time, people have reached for herbal medicines when sleep is a problem. There are various different types of insomnia, and the important thing is to find the best herbal remedy for your particular problem, says clinical herbalist Douglas Schar. The following herbs are all sold at health food stores. Choose one that most closely matches your sleep problem.

Chamomile. A bright, daisy-like flower, chamomile has an age-old reputation for calming nerves and gently aiding sleep. Probably the first stop for a person looking for a herbal remedy for sleep, it's an excellent herb for an insomniac to try. 'When I think of chamomile,' says Schar, 'I think of someone a little highly strung and inclined to nervousness. Drinking one or two cups of tea before bed will help to soothe such a person into a relaxing sleep.'

Valerian. This is the best-studied herbal sleep aid. Research shows that the herb not only helps you to fall asleep faster but

also improves sleep quality. Valerian, says Schar, is perfect for those with tension and stress-related sleep problems. For people who bring their work home, and then into bed, nothing could be better. Try taking a valerian capsule 30 to 45 minutes before bedtime, according to label directions.

Anemone pulsatilla. Also known as pasqueflower, this herb is specifically recommended for people who become anxious or fearful when they should be winding down for a good night's sleep, says Schar. 'If your thoughts pick up speed when they should be slowing down, and they tend to be on the negative side, anemone may be the herb for you. Take it half-an-hour before bedtime, and relax into sleep.'

Californian poppy. This, according to Schar, is the herbal equivalent of knock-out drops – almost everyone succumbs to its effects. Probably the strongest of the herbal sleep remedies, Californian poppy should be used with caution: avoid operating machinery or driving a car.

Use mechanical aids. Earplugs can help to block out unwanted noise, especially if you live on a busy street or near an airport, says Dr Ancoli-Israel. An eyemask will screen out unwanted light. An electric blanket warms you, especially if you're someone who always feels chilly.

Try relaxation techniques. The harder you try to sleep, the greater the chances you'll end up gnashing your teeth all night. That's why it's

WHEN TO CONSULT A DOCTOR

Serious sleep problems can sometimes result in what experts call chronic insomnia. Your doctor will want to see if there's an underlying physical or mental cause. Physical causes may include: breathing problems from chronic airways disease, nocturnal asthma or heart failure; pain from arthritis; neurological problems causing involuntary leg movements or spasms; indigestion or reflux; itching from dermatitis; bladder problems or diabetes causing frequency of urination; or hot flushes from the menopause.

Mental causes can include: chronic anxiety; alcohol or drug dependence; depression or bipolar disorder. If you cannot easily fall asleep or stay asleep all night for a month or so, you may need your doctor's help.

If you are given sleeping tablets to get you over a short-term crisis or bad patch of insomnia, try not to use them for long periods. You are also less likely to become dependent on them if you use them on alternate nights rather than every night. Sometimes just having one on your bedside table can reassure and relax you enough to get a good night's sleep.

important to relax once you're in bed. The problem with insomnia is that people often try too hard to sleep, says Dr Stevenson. The key is to stop worrying and avoid getting worked up. Try deep breathing, muscle stretches or yoga. CDs or cassettes are available that can teach you how to progressively relax your muscles. Here are two techniques that doctors have found particularly successful.

- Slow down your breathing and imagine the air moving slowly in and out of your body while you breathe from your diaphragm. Practise this during the day so that it's easy to do before you go to bed.

- Programme yourself to turn off unpleasant thoughts as they creep into your mind. To do that, think about enjoyable experiences you've had. Reminisce about good times, fantasize or play some mental games. Try counting sheep or counting backwards from 1000 in sevens.

Have a warm bath. Normal body temperatures are at their highest point during the day and lowest when we are asleep. One theory suggests, therefore, that the body begins to get drowsy as its temperature drops. So try taking a warm bath four or five hours before bedtime. This will raise your temperature. Then, as your temperature begins to fall, you'll feel more tired, which will make it easier to fall asleep.

Go for a walk. Get some exercise late in the afternoon or early in the evening, suggest Drs Neubauer and Soliman. It shouldn't be too strenuous – a short walk is fine. Not only will it tire your muscles, but it will also raise your body temperature and may help to induce sleepiness as a warm bath would. Exercise may also help to trigger the deep, nourishing sleep that your body craves most for replenishment.

Try sex before bedtime. They say the only sleep that's sounder than the sleep of the just is the sleep of the just after. For many, sex is a pleasurable and mentally and physically relaxing way to unwind before settling down to sleep. Researchers have found that hormonal mechanisms triggered during sexual activity help to enhance sleep. But it depends on the person, according to sleep expert James Walsh. 'If sex causes anxiety and creates problems, it's not such a good idea. But if you find it enjoyable, it can do a lot for you.'

IRRITABLE BOWEL SYNDROME
21 coping suggestions

Many people with irritable bowel syndrome, or IBS, develop a sixth sense about public toilets – they know where to find one in a hurry, and they're used to leaving a table of friends at dinner to dash to the loo.

Doctors aren't sure what causes IBS, but many believe it's a muscle contraction or 'motility' disturbance. The walls of the intestines are lined with layers of muscles that contract and relax as they move food from the stomach through the intestinal tract. In people who don't have IBS, the muscles contract and relax in regular rhythm. In people with IBS, it seems that the contractions are stronger – and they last longer.

Another theory blames an overgrowth of intestinal bacteria, says Mark Pimentel, a gastroenterologist and expert on IBS. Research suggests that some IBS sufferers have a condition known as 'small intestine bacterial overgrowth', in which the bacteria that normally live in the colon somehow find their way into the relatively sterile small intestine. The small intestine responds with an increase in gas and bloating after meals, as well as noticeable changes in usual bowel habits. There is some controversy about this theory, however.

Whatever the cause, coping with IBS means identifying the food, drinks or stressful events that trigger alternating bouts of diarrhoea, constipation and abdominal pain. Sometimes, people with IBS get all three at the same time. A sense of bloating or fullness and mucus in the stool are other symptoms.

But there's some reassuring news: firstly, IBS does not appear to raise your risk of colorectal cancer, and secondly, IBS doesn't trigger changes in bowel tissue or cause inflammation. If you've been diagnosed as having IBS, try these tips to ease symptoms and discomfort.

Take stress in your stride. There's a strong link between stress and an irritable bowel, says gastroenterologist Douglas Drossman. What you don't want to do is become stressed because you have an irritable bowel.

During flare-ups of abdominal pain, take a deep breath. 'Think about what's happening. Recognize that it's happened before and it will pass. You're not going to die, because people don't die from an irritable bowel,' he says.

Become more relaxed. Anything you can do to help yourself unwind should help to alleviate your symptoms, says Dr Drossman. You may benefit from relaxation techniques like meditation or yoga.

If the stress in your life is particularly hard to deal with, consider psychological counselling. The key is to find what works for you.

Keep a stress diary. People with an irritable bowel have an intestinal system that overreacts to food, stress and hormonal changes. 'Think of your irritable bowel as a built-in barometer, and use it to help you determine what things in your life are most stressful,' says Dr Drossman.

If, for instance, you have stomach pain every time you talk to your boss, see this as a sign that you need to work on that relationship (perhaps by talking it over with your boss, a friend, a family member or a therapist). Keep a record of your symptoms for a week or two, taking note of what was happening just before their onset to see if any patterns emerge.

Log in your food and drink intake, too. Certain foods and drinks can activate an irritable bowel, so it's also helpful to record in your diary the foods and drinks that give you the most trouble, says Dr Drossman.

Add fibre to your diet. Many people with IBS do much better simply by adding fibre to their diets, says gastroenterologist James Rhodes. Fibre tends to be most effective for people who tend towards constipation and small, hard stools, but it may also help you if you're experiencing diarrhoea. The best fibre to add to your diet is the insoluble type – found in bran, whole grains, fruit and vegetables.

Psyllium seed to the rescue. An easy way to increase your fibre intake is with crushed psyllium seed, also known as ispaghula, says Dr Drossman. It's a natural laxative sold in pharmacies and health food stores. Unlike the chemical laxatives often found on the same shelf, psyllium-based laxatives such as Metamucil are non-addictive and generally safe, even when taken over long periods.

Drink lots of fluid. To keep your bowels moving smoothly, you not only need fibre but also fluids. You need to drink more on a summer day when you play tennis than on a winter day at home, but as a general rule you should drink between six and eight glasses of fluid a day, says Dr Rhodes.

Reconsider dairy products. One fluid you may be better off without is milk. Many people who say they have IBS are in fact lactose intolerant (see *Lactose Intolerance*, page 375), says William Snape, a specialist in bowel disorders. It means that your body has difficulty absorbing lactose, an enzyme found in milk. Your doctor can test you for lactose intolerance, or you can give up dairy products for a couple of days and see how you do. Either way, you may find that this one dietary change clears up all your problems.

Put out that cigarette. Smoking often makes matters worse for people with IBS, says Dr Snape. The most likely culprit is nicotine, so if you're trying to give up with the help of nicotine gum, you may not see any improvement in your tummy problems until you've weaned yourself off the gum, too.

WHEN TO CONSULT A DOCTOR

A change in bowel habit, or alternating constipation and diarrhoea, especially when accompanied by abdominal pain triggered by stressful situations and relieved by passing stools, are classic signs of IBS. It is rare though to develop true IBS over the age of 40. So if you develop the classic symptoms of IBS for the first time, and you're over 40, see your doctor in case there is another cause. Other symptoms may indicate a more serious condition. See your doctor if you have:

- blood in your stool;
- unexplained weight loss;
- diarrhoea that causes you to wake up at night;
- constipation, diarrhoea, abdominal pain or any combination of the three so severe that you can't work or lead life normally for several days.

Imagine yourself pain-free

It's normal to panic during an attack of abdominal pain. But ironically, stress makes the pain worse by tensing the bowel. How can you break this nasty cycle? With visualization, says Donna Copeland, a specialist in behavioural medicine. It's an effective tool for dealing with pain and anxiety.

If you feel pain, stop what you're doing, find a comfortable place to sit or lie down, close your eyes and – instead of focusing on your pain – imagine yourself:

- diving into the warm ocean surf off a beautiful, white, sandy tropical island beach;
- standing on top of a tall, snow-capped mountain, breathing the cool air and listening to the crunch of snow beneath your feet;
- walking through a lush garden in a far-off, exotic land.

Don't chew gum. Nicotine gum is not the only kind of gum that can give you trouble. Gums and sweets artificially sweetened with sorbitol are not easily digested and can worsen IBS, says Dr Drossman. While the amount of sorbitol found in a stick of gum isn't likely to affect you much, if you chew 10 or more pieces a day, it's time to cut back.

Cut out fat. Here's another good reason to eat a low-fat diet. Fat stimulates colonic contractions, says Dr Snape. In other words, it can worsen your IBS. A good start is to cut out rich sauces, fried foods and oily or creamy salad dressings.

Say no to wind. Some people with IBS are particularly sensitive to wind-producing foods, says Dr Rhodes. If you fall into this group, you may find relief by avoiding such flatulence promoters as cooked dried beans, cabbage, Brussels sprouts, broccoli, cauliflower and onions.

Add bran slowly. If you're adding fibre such as bran to your diet, add it gradually to give your body time to adjust. Too much fibre, too fast, can produce gas, says Dr Rhodes.

Beware of spicy foods. Some people with IBS are sensitive to foods flavoured with chillis and other spices, says Dr Rhodes. Try eating lots of spicy foods for a week and then bland foods the next week, and see whether your condition changes.

Cut coffee. Coffee is a major cause of discomfort for people with IBS, says Dr Snape. To some extent, the culprit may be caffeine, but it may also be the resins in the coffee bean itself. Try switching to decaffeinated coffee. If that doesn't help, try cutting out coffee altogether.

Change your tipple. Alcoholic beverages can exacerbate your problems, but it's probably not the alcohol itself, says Dr Snape. Instead, it's the complex carbohydrates in beer and the tannins in red wine that appear to cause the most grief. People with IBS should avoid these two drinks.

Soothe with herbal medicine. 'Based on my experience as a clinical herbalist,' says Douglas Schar, 'people who suffer from an irritable bowel always suffer from tension.' Not surprisingly, herbal remedies that ease tension are a great help in relieving irritable bowel.

Two classics, says Schar, are valerian and crampbark. Both remedies diminish the effects of stress on the body and this has a knock-on effect on the irritable bowel. Buy either in tincture form (tincture 1:5) and take 5ml three times a day. You should notice an improvement within a week of using either one of these remedies.

Eat small, regular meals. It's not only *what* you eat, but how you eat that can vex an irritable bowel, says Dr Snape. Digesting a lot of food eaten all at once overstimulates the digestive system. That is why it's much better to eat frequent small meals than infrequent large ones.

Go for a jog. 'Good body tone, good bowel tone,' says Dr Rhodes. Exercise strengthens the entire body, including the bowel. It helps to relieve stress, and it releases endorphins that help you to control pain. All in all, regular exercise will almost certainly calm an irritable bowel. But be careful not to overdo it: too much exercise can lead to diarrhoea.

Hot-water bottle to the rescue. If you experience abdominal pain, the best thing to do is to sit or lie down, take a deep breath, and try to relax. Putting a hot-water bottle on your tummy is very comforting and can also help, says Dr Snape.

Jaw Pain and TMJ Problems
17 ideas to ease the discomfort

If your teeth don't meet properly you can have problems not only in your teeth themselves, but also in your gums, in the temporo-mandibular joint (TMJ), where your lower jaw articulates with your skull, or in the muscles that move your jaw. Signs of TMJ problems include clicking or popping noises when you open or close your mouth, difficulty opening your mouth or chewing, locking of the jaws open or closed, grinding or pain in your jaw joints and pain, ringing or buzzing in your ears. You may feel a dull ache around the ear, radiating into your face, neck, the back of your head and even down into your shoulders.

The temporo-mandibular joint needs equal support from both sides of both jaws. If you have missing teeth, they may need to be replaced either with a partial denture or bridgework.

Many experts believe that most cases of TMJ pain have several causes. Trauma, stress, misaligned teeth, orthodontic treatment and arthritis are just some of the factors associated with TMJ problems. Sometimes it can be triggered by opening the mouth too wide, especially when sideways pressure is applied. 'I've seen patients in terrible trouble with their TMJs after taking too big a bite out of an apple, after a long session in the dentist's chair, or after an overenthusiastic kissing session with their girlfriend,' says family doctor Stephen Amiel. According to the British Dental Health Foundation, up to one in four people in the UK may have some symptoms. Men and women are affected equally, but women tend to seek treatment more often than men. In most cases, jaw pain is temporary and can usually be relieved with simple measures.

Apply heat or cold. In other words, do whatever you can to increase bloodflow to the area. Heat is better for recurrent or prolonged conditions, but cold is more effective for relieving acute pain and reducing the swelling that goes along with it, says dentist Sheldon Gross. Don't alternate the two or use cold therapy for a prolonged period, as this could damage the tissues. For cold treatment, wrap an ice pack or a bag of frozen peas in a teatowel. Apply to the affected area for five to 10 minutes, or until it feels a little numb. Do not exceed 20 minutes. Repeat every two hours for up to two days, or until the pain is relieved. Apply heat therapy, using a warm compress, for the same length of time.

You can also try gently stretching and massaging the jaw as long as the muscles don't cramp. If you get blood flowing in the area, you are likely to alleviate some of your symptoms, says Dr Gross. This will help to increase your range of motion and strengthen the joint.

Take an anti-inflammatory and massage the jaw. 'Aspirin is a marvellous drug for any muscle or joint problem,' says orthodontist Harold Perry. He suggests following a dose of aspirin with a self-massage of the jaw several minutes later. You could also try ibuprofen, another anti-inflammatory, to relieve pain and reduce swelling.

Check your body position. If you work at a desk, check your body position regularly throughout the day. Make sure that you, and especially your chin, are not leaning over the desk, says Owen Rogal, a dentist who specializes in facial pain. Your back should be supported. As a general guideline for sitting or standing, your cheekbone should be over your collarbone and your ears should not be too far in front of your shoulders.

Don't rest your head on a pillow. Instead, tuck yourself in with a pillow under your knees. You could also use wedge-shaped pillows that are designed for reclining. Sleeping in this position – on your back throughout the night with your head, neck, shoulders and upper back in alignment and less pressure on your lower back – can be very relaxing for

WHEN TO CONSULT A DOCTOR

The most common signs of temporo-mandibular joint problems – facial and jaw joint pain or swelling; headaches; toothaches; aching neck, shoulders or back; and a clicking, grating or popping noise or pain when opening or closing your mouth – are usually nothing more than minor to moderate annoyances that will go away once the condition is treated. Few people develop significant long-term effects.

Some symptoms, however, are more serious and should be investigated. If you cannot open your mouth, cannot brush your teeth and are having sharp headaches, then see your doctor. Sudden onset of pain in the ear or around the TMJ should also be checked out.

Anti-inflammatory drugs may be prescribed for you if you have recent onset TMJ problems, but for more chronic cases, drugs such as amitriptyline, trimipramine or fluoxetine work well. These drugs, which are used also as antidepressants, are increasingly being used for the management of chronic pain of various sorts, even in people who are not depressed.

Your dentist or doctor may also be able to refer to a dental or facial pain specialist in particularly stubborn cases.

Seven habits to break

Don't:

- sleep on your front with your head turned to one side;
- lie on your back with your head propped up at a sharp angle to read or watch television;
- cradle the telephone between your shoulder and chin;
- prop your chin on one or both hands for too long;
- carry a heavy shoulder bag with the strap on the same shoulder for any length of time;
- look upwards for long periods of time – so don't paint ceilings or sit in the front row at the cinema;
- grind or clench your teeth.

your jaws, says Dr Rogal. If you usually sleep on your side, put a beanbag on either side of your head to stop you from rolling over.

Limit your jaw movement. If you feel a yawn coming on, restrict it by holding a fist under your chin, says Andrew Kaplan, a dentist who runs a clinic for TMJ and facial pain. Yawning can strain the jaw.

Don't chew gum. Repetitive chewing can stress the jaw. Control other similar habits, such as biting your lips or fingernails – and use your pencil for writing, not chewing, advises Dr Gross.

Stop grinding your teeth. Gnashing teeth, referred to by doctors as bruxism, is often associated with TMJ pain and may exacerbate existing symptoms, says Dr Kaplan. If you find that you're clenching your teeth during the day, invariably as a result of stress, take some deep breaths, try some relaxation exercises (see *Stress*, page 518) and loosen up your TMJs by rapidly making small opening and closing movements of your mouth 20 times or so. You look and sound like a rather manic goldfish, says Dr Amiel, but in the privacy of your car or office, who cares?

Use a mouthguard. Buy the kind of mouthguard sold in sports shops that you soften in hot water and then bite down on to form a fit in your mouth. It shouldn't feel loose or uncomfortable. Wearing one during the day can help to reduce grinding and clenching, says Dr Gross. If your symptoms seem worse in the morning, wear your mouthguard at night. You may be grinding your teeth in your sleep.

Consider acupressure. To find the point that will ease TMJ pain on the left-hand side of your face, rest your left forearm on a table with your palm flat down, says pain specialist Albert Forgione. Put the fingers of your right hand on your left forearm so that your index finger is in the fold of your elbow and the rest of your fingers lie next to each other. Wiggle your left middle finger and feel the corresponding ligament move at the edge of your right index fingertip. Press moderately hard on this point for 15 seconds (the point will feel sensitive and even hurt when you find the right spot). Do this three times in a row, pausing briefly in between. Switch sides to relieve pain on the right-hand side of your face.

Avoid hard, crunchy food. If you have a lot of pain in and around your mouth, eat soft and liquid foods for a while, suggests Dr Perry.

JET LAG
13 hints for arriving alert

When you fly across several time zones, your body has to adjust to a new time and a new place. It takes a while for the internal body clock to reset itself to the new day or night cycle, which is why you get jet lag. And the more time zones you cross, the more you suffer. No matter which way you're going, each time zone crossed requires about one day of adjustment, says Charles Ehret, a researcher into the effects of time changes on animals and people. The inner body clock is really a whole set of clocks controlled by a master clock, he says. 'Every cell in the body is a clock, and they're all brought together by a special pacemaker in the brain.'

Jet lag causes fatigue, lethargy, inability to sleep, trouble concentrating and making decisions, irritability, perhaps even diarrhoea and a loss of appetite. Though you can't make time stand still, there's a lot you can do to take some of the sting out of jet lag.

Adopt a routine. Weeks, or at least days, before you leave, maintain a sensible routine. 'People who have no order in their lives – who stay up late to watch a film and start doing the washing at 2am – have more trouble with jet lag,' says Dr Ehret.

Get enough sleep. If you get too little sleep before your trip, your jet lag will be worse, says Dr Ehret. 'Give yourself about 15 extra minutes of sleep on each of the last few nights before you travel.'

Fly by day, arrive at night. The best way to combat time changes is to arrive at your destination mid-evening, have a light meal and go to bed by 11pm local time,' says psychiatrist Timothy Monk. This will give your body the best chance of adjusting to the change in time zones.

Drink plenty of fluids during the flight. Aeroplane cabins are notoriously dry, says Dr Monk, and fluids help to combat the dehydration that induces fatigue. Dehydration obviously won't help you beat jet lag.

Avoid alcohol. Alcohol is a diuretic and further dehydrates you. Ask for juice or water instead.

When in Rome... When you arrive, start adapting to your environment as quickly as possible. Get involved, notice the street names and listen to the language or local accents, says Dr Ehret. This will help you to adjust.

Socialize. This is especially important if your body craves sleep but it's only mid-afternoon local time. When we socialize, our bodies assume it's daytime because we are, by nature, daytime creatures, says researcher Marijo Readey.

Don't nap. Or if you do, limit the nap to an hour. Napping, Dr Monk says, just delays your adjustment to the new time zone.

Soak up some sunshine. Get out in the sun at your destination as much as possible, says Dr Monk. This exposure helps to keep your biological clock in the stimulated and awake state during daylight hours.

When light strikes the eye, neurotransmitters are released that send a signal to specific regions of the brain, explains Dr Ehret. In turn, these brain regions tell the rest of the body that your awake-and-active phase is about to begin. Look after your skin though, warns family doctor Stephen Amiel. Protecting yourself against sunburn, sunstroke and skin cancer takes precedence over avoiding jet lag (see *Sunburn*, page 524).

Make a date with the sun. Some experts believe that the time of day you get out in the sunshine is also important. Light earlier in the day appears to shift the body's clock to an earlier hour, while light later in the day seems to shift the body's clock to a later hour, according to psychiatrist Al Lewy.

So if you've travelled east, Dr Lewy suggests getting outdoor light in the morning. And if you've travelled west, try getting outside light in the afternoon. This only works if you've crossed six time zones or less.

Exercise. Exercise, especially outdoor exercise, gets your body pumped up, helps alertness and gets you out in the sunlight.

Think before you react. Put off any important decision-making for 24 hours or at least until you feel well-rested, advises Dr Ehret. You won't think your clearest after a long trip. People often make bad business decisions soon after arrival, and only realize later that jet lag was the reason.

Get ready to go home. If possible, use these tips to prepare for your return journey home, too. Jet lag is a two-way flight.

KNEE PAIN
22 ways to make it better

The knee is the strongest joint in the human body, absorbing a force equivalent to four and a half times your body weight just when you walk downstairs. Yet despite its power, the knee is also the joint that causes the most suffering.

Sports-related knee injuries are becoming increasingly common. But you don't have to be an athlete to experience knee pain. Car accidents commonly involve knee injuries. So do falls. Some knee pain stems from overuse or age-related wear and tear on the joint.

Knee pain often affects older people, largely due to osteoarthritis, a degenerative wearing down of the cartilage cushions in the joint, causing bones to scrape painfully against each other.

Part of the problem is design, or rather the inability of knee design to change whenever human beings place new demands on it. The knee is ill-suited to the jobs we ask it to do, says knee surgeon James Fox. It wasn't designed for football, car accidents, or plumbing or carpet laying all day long. If your knees ache because of overuse or abuse, here are some ways to make them feel better.

Lose weight. Body weight is a major contributor to knee problems, says Dr Fox. Every kilo of excess weight is multiplied by about six in terms of the stress placed on the knee area. So if you're five kilos overweight, that's an extra 30kg your knee has to carry around. As Dr Fox observes, you don't put Mini tyres on a juggernaut.

Don't rely on knee supports. Knee supports are sold in most sports shops, but the experts say to leave them on the shelf. They shouldn't be used for anything more than to remind you that you have a bad knee, says Dr Fox. And some can do more harm than good, says athletics trainer Marjorie Albohm, by pushing your kneecap into the joint.

Take a painkiller. Ibuprofen, which reduces inflammation and provides pain relief, is recommended by our experts. It also causes fewer stomach problems than aspirin. Paracetamol is fine as a painkiller, but it does little to reduce inflammation. Studies have shown that ibuprofen can significantly improve joint mobility in people with acute knee ligament damage.

You can take paracetamol and ibuprofen together, in full daily doses, for added pain relief, says family doctor Stephen Amiel, as they have different modes of action. If you have stomach problems or you're on warfarin though, stick to paracetamol or consult your doctor first, as nonsteroidal anti-inflammatory drugs (NSAIDs) like ibuprofen can cause bleeding from the gut, especially in the elderly. Your doctor may be able to give you medication to protect your stomach while you're taking anti-inflammatories.

NSAID-containing creams can bring some relief, with fewer side-effects than tablets, although there is conflicting evidence about their comparative effectiveness.

Ask for a prescription. A newer class of anti-inflammatory pain relievers, COX-2 inhibitors, offers the same benefits as ibuprofen while being even easier on the stomach. Many doctors now recommend celecoxib (Celebrex) or rofecoxib (Vioxx) for people with severe pain and a history of gastrointestinal problems.

Try a supplement. Glucosamine and chondroitin have been gaining in popularity in the treatment of osteoarthritis. Although controlled studies of these compounds have produced mixed results, they appear to have an impact on pain. So far, their effect seems to be slightly less robust than nonsteroidal anti-inflammatory drugs (NSAIDs) such as ibuprofen, and their full effect is not seen for four to six weeks. Larger trials are underway.

Take your vitamins. Certain vitamins can help to rebuild cartilage and tendons and reduce joint pain. Some experts recommend taking daily doses of vitamins A, B_6, C, E and niacin.

Use a liniment. As old-fashioned as it may sound, some menthol rubbing lotions produce heat, which can relieve symptoms and make you feel more comfortable, says Dr Fox.

Reach for arnica. Knee joints are often injured through accidents or strain-related damage. The first thing an unhappy knee does is to swell up, says clinical herbalist Douglas Schar. When you take an awkward step or lift something too heavy, and one of your knees objects, Schar suggests you try witch hazel or arnica cream – both available from health food stores. Apply three times a day to speed up repair of the injury and greatly reduce the pain.

Another soother is a daily soak in Epsom salts, says Schar. Buy from a pharmacy and mix according to package instructions.

Ask your GP about chilli cream. Knees are subject to wear and tear injuries because we use them day in and day out. When a knee problem becomes an ongoing part of life, ask your doctor about toning down the pain with a cream containing capsaicin, an extract from chilli peppers, suggests Schar. This substance appears to block the transmission of pain from the knee to the brain. The problem is still there, but you don't feel it to the same degree. Two capsaicin creams are available in the UK – Axsain and Zacin – but both are prescription-only.

Reduce inflammation with essential fatty acids. Chronic knee problems involve inflammation. Essential fatty acids, found in cod liver oil, evening primrose oil, borage seed oil, hemp seed oil and blackcurrant seed oil, can be used to reduce this inflammation and make the knee much less painful, says Schar. Choose one and take it as a daily supplement, but don't expect to feel the effects for a few weeks.

Try black or white. Black cohosh, commonly prescribed for menopausal problems, was originally used to treat chronic joint complaints. White willow, another traditional joint pain remedy, has long been used to make a creaky joint swing smoothly and with less pain. Buy either remedy at the health food store and use according to label instructions. Schar says you should notice an improvement within two weeks.

Update your shoes. If your shoes don't absorb shock anymore, says Gary Gordon, a foot surgeon who specializes in sports injuries, that shock has to go somewhere. So it goes through your foot, up your shin, and into your knee. Sometimes it keeps going, up to your hip and back.

If you run 25 miles a week or more, you need new shoes every two to three months, Dr Gordon says. If you run less than that, you need new shoes every four to six months. Aerobic dancers and netball and tennis players who practise twice a week can probably get away with new shoes every four to six months. But if you exercise four times or more each week, you also need new shoes every two months. Most people don't really want to hear this – except perhaps the shoe manufacturers.

Strengthen with exercise. The only things holding the knee together are the muscles and ligaments, says Dr Fox. Building up the muscles is critical, because the muscles are the real supporting structures. If they don't have their power or endurance, you'll have trouble with your knees.

Stronger muscles provide you with a stronger joint, one that's better able to withstand the considerable strain that even walking or climbing stairs places on the knees. The goal of these exercises is to strengthen your quadriceps, the muscles in front of your legs, and your hamstring muscles, in the back of your thighs. These two muscles must be in balance, says Dr Fox. If only one or the other is developed, it causes stress on the knee joint. The following exercises are not hard to do, and they hurt a lot less than aching knees.

Note: If an exercise causes increasing discomfort or pain, stop. You must listen to your body. Don't try and work through the pain.

Isometric knee builder. Sit on the floor with your sore knee straight out in front of you. Place a rolled towel under the small of the knee, then tighten the muscles in your leg without moving the knee. Hold that contraction and work up to where you can keep the muscles taut for at least 30 seconds, then relax. Repeat this tightening and relaxing process up to 25 times. You can do isometric exercises at other times too: tighten and relax your thigh muscles in the same way while you're waiting at a bus stop or doing the washing up.

Sitting leg lifts. Sit with your back against a wall and place a pillow in the small of your back. (Sitting against a wall ensures that the leg muscles do the lifting. This type of leg lift won't aggravate back pain.) Once you're in that position, do the isometric contraction described above for a count of five, then raise your leg a few inches and hold it to a count of five, then lower it and relax for a count of five. Work up to doing three sets of 10 lifts each, always using the five-count for pacing.

Hamstring helper. Lie on your stomach with your chin to the floor. With an ankle weight (or a sock filled with coins and draped over your ankle) and your knee bent, slowly lift the lower leg 20 to 30cm off the floor, then slowly lower it back down, stopping before you touch the floor. Repeat the movement again, always working slowly and steadily through each repetition. Work up to three sets of as many of these as you can comfortably do (largely determined by the amount of weight you use).

Change your sport. Athletes with chronic knee problems have to alter their levels of training or their activity, says Albohm. But that doesn't mean giving up. If you like squash and you have a chronic knee condition that squash has gradually made worse, you're probably going to have to stop playing.

So what are your options? You could try swimming, cycling or rowing – all activities that are good for your health without placing great strain on the knees. The key phrase is 'non-weight-bearing' activity. In fact, by helping to strengthen thigh muscles, non-weight-bearing exercises such as cycling and rowing can give you better knees without sacrificing aerobic capacity or how many calories you burn.

Whatever you do, don't give up a healthy lifestyle because of knee pain. No one should have to stop being active, says Albohm. Simply avoid anything that hurts your knee.

Change to a softer running surface. 'When you run a mile, your foot strikes the ground between 600 and 800 times,' says Dr Fox. A lot of runners' pain is caused by tendinitis that results from poor training habits, especially running on hard surfaces. The problem can often be minimized by a change in running surface.

Choose grass as a running surface in preference to tarmac and tarmac before concrete. Concrete is the hardest surface of all and should be avoided as much as possible.

Don't make a habit of jogging on pavements. Try to find a golf course to run on once the golfers have left.

Try RICE. Following any activity that causes knee pain, Albohm says, immediately rest the knee and apply ice, compression and raise your leg for 20 to 30 minutes. That advice is nicknamed RICE: rest, ice, compression and elevation. 'Don't underestimate the power of ice,' says Albohm. Ice is a tremendous anti-inflammatory and will really help the condition.

Keep the routine simple: when you return from exercising, just prop the leg up, wrap an elastic bandage around it and apply an ice pack for 20 to 30 minutes. That should always be the first thing you try for relieving pain.

Use heat with caution. When there is no swelling present, using a heating pad before an activity may enable you to exercise with less pain. But, Albohm warns, if there's any swelling, don't use heat.

Furthermore, don't use heat after an activity, she warns. Assuming that the area is irritated by activity, then applying heat is going to increase the irritation.

Exercise in water. The buoyancy of water makes it the perfect place to gently exercise a sore knee joint. Try your regular knee exercises underwater. Swimming and water walking will keep you in shape without straining your knees.

WHEN TO CONSULT A DOCTOR

Abrupt twisting motions (such as in golf or skiing) or an impact to the side of the knee (perhaps from a car accident or football tackle) may cause an injury to the cruciate ligament or the medial or lateral collateral ligaments of the knee. These injuries may or may not involve pain when they occur, but you may hear a buckle sound or pop.

Tendinitis and ruptured tendons can occur with overuse or when you attempt to break a fall. A forcible twist to a flexed knee can result in a torn cartilage (meniscus). The knee usually swells and may lock. These injuries may settle with time but locking or giving way of the knee unexpectedly may persist long after the injury, indicating that there is loose cartilage requiring surgical removal.

Knee injuries may be followed by swelling, tenderness, radiating pain and perhaps some discoloration and loss of mobility. They should be treated with ice packs, and require medical care as soon as possible.

Get into low gear. Many experts recommend cycling, either on an exercise bike or the open road, as an alternative to running, which is renowned for causing knee strain and pain. But cyclists can also damage their knees, usually by thinking that the harder it is to pedal, the more exercise you get. Harder pedalling puts more strain on the knees. In general, a lower gear, which makes it easier to pedal, is a better gear, says Albohm.

Find the trigger point for pain. There's a trigger point on the inside of the thigh that contributes to 'weak knee syndrome', says sports physiotherapist and masseur Rich Phaigh. That trigger point is responsible for a lot of generalized pain on the inside of the knee, too.

To get rid of that pain, move your hand straight up from the kneecap along the front of the thigh for about 8cm, then move it inwards for another 5–10cm. With the tip of your thumb, press in firmly and hold until you feel the muscle release its tension – anywhere from 30 to 90 seconds – and then release.

First and finally, stretch. Many of fitness consultant Lisa Dobloug's clients are older. Her emphasis is on the quality, not quantity, of exercise and the importance of stretching.

It's very important to warm up and cool down properly, she says. Take about 10 minutes and do very light stretching before you begin exercising. You could go through the motions of whatever exercise you'll be doing without really extending it. Then do a little aerobics – jogging on the spot or walking around.

After you've finished exercising, stretch for flexibility and to counteract the pounding that the exercise has given your knees. Dobloug recommends this stretch to combat stiffness. Lie on your back and pull your knees into your chest, then start to straighten one leg, she says. Act as if you're trying to press your heel towards the ceiling. Hold the stretch for a count of 10 while breathing slowly, then relax. Repeat with the other leg.

LACTOSE INTOLERANCE
9 soothing ideas

Even though low-fat dairy products are regarded as healthy foods, not everyone can digest them. Indeed, some four to five million people in the UK are lactose-intolerant, all suffering varying degrees of abdominal pain, nausea, cramps, bloating, gas and diarrhoea. Just how many dairy foods a lactose-intolerant person can eat without causing symptoms varies from one person to another.

Lactose intolerance occurs when the small intestine doesn't produce enough lactase, an enzyme required for the digestion of lactose, the natural sugar found in dairy products.

Premature babies are often lactose intolerant, but otherwise it's un-common in children before the age of three. Asian, African and Afro-Caribbean people are much more likely to be lactose intolerant, and it can also affect people temporarily after a bout of gastroenteritis.

Most people develop some degree of lactose intolerance by the time they're 20, and, while it can be a nuisance, lactose intolerance is not a serious medical problem.

But you may be able to have your ice cream and eat it, too. Here are some useful suggestions.

Take the tolerance test. Since everyone's degree of tolerance is dif-ferent, find out how much of a good thing you can have before you stop enjoying it, says Theodore Bayless, who runs a clinic for digestive disor-ders. The obvious thing to do is decrease the amount of milk and dairy products you eat until your symptoms go away. Even a few sips of milk can bother some people, he says.

Don't forget your calcium. Dairy products are a major source of calcium, Dr Bayless says. Most people should get the calcium equivalent of two glasses of milk a day. If milk is your main source of calcium and you cut back on it, then you should boost your calcium intake by eating calcium-rich foods like sardines with bones, spinach, broccoli, calcium-fortified breakfast cereals and perhaps calcium supplements.

Don't drink milk on its own. Some people find that their symptoms disappear if they take dairy produce as part of a meal, Dr Bayless says.

Inoculate yourself. It may be worth trying to take just a small amount of milk each day, gradually increasing the dose to build up your tolerance, Dr Bayless suggests. Cut back again if your symptoms reappear.

Eat yoghurt. The fermentation process that produces yoghurt depends on organisms that also produce lactase, the enzyme in short supply in lactose-intolerant people, says gastroenterologist Naresh Jain. The bacteria themselves also probably break down the lactose in the milk. Most otherwise healthy lactose-intolerant people should be able to tolerate yoghurt.

Choose fat free yoghurt and try to eat it every day. Yoghurt with fat in it sits in the stomach for longer, which means stomach acids have more of a chance to kill the beneficial organisms in the yoghurt. Since lactose digestion takes place in the small intestine, you want your organisms to get there as soon as possible.

Add your own lactase. You can buy lactase enzyme from pharmacies in liquid form. A few drops of lactase liquid, or a capsule added to a litre of milk, renders the milk flatulence-free with a slightly sweeter taste. Try Lifeplan lactase enzyme capsules and Biocare lacatse enzyme liquid.

Try buttermilk. Buttermilk, available in some supermarkets, is fairly well tolerated, Dr Jain says. That's because it contains less lactose per serving than wholemilk, semi-skimmed or skimmed milk. And despite its name, buttermilk is very low in fat and cholesterol.

Eat cheese. Cheese contains less lactose than milk. Choose hard cheeses as they are the longest fermented. Swiss cheeses and mature Cheddars contain only a trace of lactose and are least likely to cause digestive upset, says gastroenterologist Seymour Sabesin.

Beware of bulking agents. Lactose is widely used in pills and nutritional supplements. Some pills contain enough lactose to trigger symptoms of lactose intolerance. Read labels and ask your pharmacist if your medication contains lactose.

LARYNGITIS

17 ways to find your voice

The most noticeable symptom of laryngitis is loss of voice or hoarseness. The throat may also feel raw or tickly, and people with laryngitis often feel a need to clear their throats. Straightforward laryngitis is a rather gratifying illness to get as, apart from the hoarseness, there are few other symptoms. You get lots of sympathy for sounding so awful, yet you rarely feel ill.

The common cold and other viral infections of the upper airways are the most common causes of laryngitis. Laryngitis may also accompany flu, bronchitis, pneumonia, measles, whooping cough or any infection of the upper airways. As any singer will tell you, excessive use of the voice, exposure to tobacco smoke, even allergic reactions, can bring it on, too.

In order for you to sound like you, the air you exhale through your larynx, or voice box, as you speak has to vibrate through your vocal cords in just the right way. When the cords are scarred or swollen, they don't create the right shaped 'container' for that air.

Even a slight change in the vocal cords can render a person's voice un-recognizable. The vocal cords contain a central muscle bundle, various layers of connective tissue and a skin-like covering called the mucosa. 'An alteration in any one of these layers can disrupt the optimal vibration through the tissue,' says throat specialist Scott Kessler. So if you sound as husky as Lauren Bacall, follow our experts' tips to recover your true voice.

Don't talk. No matter what triggered the laryngitis, the most important thing you can do for your voice is to give it a rest, says Laurence Levine, an ear, nose and throat specialist. Try to spend a day or two without talking.

Don't even whisper. If you have to communicate, pass notes. Whispering makes the vocal cords bang together as hard as shouting, explains throat specialist George Simpson.

Don't take aspirin. If you've lost your voice through shouting too loudly, you've probably ruptured a capillary, says Dr Levine. So stay away from aspirin. Aspirin increases clotting time, which can impede healing. Use paracetamol instead to control fever, aches and pains.

Use a humidifier. The mucosa that blanket your vocal cords need to be kept moist. When they're not, mucus can become sticky, a virtual flypaper for irritants. Fight back with a humidifier, says Dr Kessler.

Steam it away. Steaming can also restore moisture. Robert Feder, throat specialist and singing coach, suggests leaning over a bowl of steaming water for five minutes twice a day. Set the bowl on a steady surface and your face about a forearm's length away from the water, and breathe. Create a steam tent with a towel over your head and the bowl.

A safer and more convenient alternative can be bought at the pharmacy: a device like a baby's feeding mug with an attached mask that fits over your nose and mouth. Half fill with steaming water and inhale.

Drink plenty of fluids. Dr Simpson recommends eight to ten glasses a day, preferably water. Dr Feder suggests fruit juice and tea with honey or lemon.

Don't chill drinks. Warm fluids are best, says Dr Feder. Cold drinks can aggravate the problem.

Breathe through your nose. Breathing through your nose humidifies

WHEN TO CONSULT A DOCTOR

Straightforward laryngitis is almost always caused by a virus and it will go away on its own within a few days without antibiotics. There are a number of other causes of hoarseness though, including: sinus infection; acid reflux where stomach acid comes up the oesophagus and irritates the throat; an underactive thyroid gland; injury or paralysis of the vocal cords; smoking; long-term alcohol misuse; nodules on the vocal cords caused by chronic misuse of the voice; and cancer of the larynx. Many of these conditions are associated with other symptoms too, and your doctor should be able to help your hoarseness by treating the underlying cause.

Cancer of the larynx is obviously the condition that must not be missed: if your hoarseness persists, despite resting your voice, for more than three weeks, you must see your doctor for further investigation, however well you feel otherwise. Most of the time, nothing serious will be found, but you will need to be investigated urgently to make sure you don't have a tumour.

Consult your doctor immediately if your hoarseness is accompanied by throat pain so severe that you cannot swallow your own saliva: you may have an abscess on the tonsil (quinsy), requiring urgent treatment.

the air, says Dr Kessler. Breathing through your mouth exposes the voice to dry, cold air.

Quit cigarettes. Smoking is a prime cause of throat dryness.

Go easy on the alcohol. Alcohol is a chemical irritant to the larynx. It can aggravate laryngitis, and long term alcohol excess can cause permanent change to your larynx and increase your risk of throat cancer.

Choose lozenges carefully. Avoid mint and mentholated products, says Dr Feder. They can temporarily paralyse your throat muscles and slow down the recovery process. Stick to honey or fruity soft lozenges.

Suck liquorice. In ancient Greece and Rome singers and orators used liquorice to keep their vocal apparatus in fine form. To this day, singers in the know use the herb to keep their voices working properly.

Clinical herbalist Douglas Schar says that singers who have to work in smoke-filled environments swear by liquorice for keeping their voices smooth. Liquorice works for chronic and acute laryngitis by soothing the inflammation at the root of the problem. Buy liquorice lozenges at the health food store and suck five or six during the course of the day.

Beware of aeroplane air. Talking on a flight can sabotage your voice because the pressurized air inside the cabin is so dry. To keep your vocal cords moist, breathe through your nose, says Dr Kessler. Chew gum or suck boiled sweets so that you have to keep your mouth closed.

Check your drugs. Some prescription drugs can be very drying, our experts say. Check with your doctor if you're uncertain. Likely culprits include blood pressure and thyroid tablets, and antihistamines.

Use a microphone. If your job requires you to raise your voice to be heard, use an amplifier to make yourself louder. This will help to protect your voice, says Dr Levine.

Respect your voice. If you have a presentation to do and you wake up hoarse, it's better to postpone or cancel rather than risk doing long-term damage to your voice, says Dr Kessler.

Consider voice training. If your job involves speaking a lot – teaching, for example – consider having voice training. In a non-trained voice, the muscles that suspend the larynx strain against each other, says Dr Levine. Training the voice can get those muscles to work together as a team.

LEG PAIN

7 tips to alleviate the aching

A variety of problems can lead to aching legs, including back problems, muscle spasms, infections and nerve damage. Overuse or injury also can cause leg pain. Most commonly, leg pain stems from trouble with the arteries or veins. (See also *Phlebitis*, page 443 and *Varicose Veins*, page 552.)

If you experience a cramp-like pain in the calf when you walk, which disappears quickly when you rest, then you are probably suffering from a condition known as intermittent claudication. It is caused by narrowed arteries in the leg reducing blood supply to leg muscles. Conditions such as diabetes, high blood pressure or raised cholesterol levels can cause narrowing of the arteries, as can smoking.

Just as plaque-clogged blood vessels in the heart lead to angina (chest pains), intermittent claudication is a sign of restricted bloodflow in the the areas furthest from the heart – the periphery. Intermittent claudication should not be taken lightly. If you've been diagnosed as having this condition, you should see your doctor regularly to monitor the underlying vascular disease. The pain, after all, is only a symptom. The disease can be a killer. Fortunately, there are several things that you can do at home to rid yourself of the pain of claudication and slow down the progression of peripheral vascular disease.

Stop smoking. 'The number one thing on everyone's list with this affliction should be to stop smoking,' says vascular specialist Jess Young. Between 75 and 90 per cent of all people with intermittent claudication are smokers.

Stopping smoking is so important, in fact, that our experts say you must quit before any other remedy listed below will work. And if you are not convinced, then consider the following: cigarette smoking increases the damage the disease can do by substituting carbon monoxide for oxygen in the already oxygen-starved muscles of your legs. Nicotine also causes constriction of the arteries, which further restricts bloodflow, possibly damaging the arteries themselves and leading to blood clots. In extreme cases, these clots can result in gangrene and may necessitate amputation of a limb.

Start walking. Exercise is the most important thing you can do after stopping smoking, says Dr Young. The type of exercise our experts overwhelmingly recommend is the simplest of all – walking. Though the pain in your legs can be uncomfortable, and can make it difficult to walk, it is

WHEN TO CONSULT A DOCTOR

Leg pain is a symptom of many conditions, some very serious. If your pain is severe, worsens rapidly or lasts for more than a week, see your doctor as soon as possible.

Intermittent claudication is made worse by walking. If you only get pains in your legs when you are in bed, you probably have muscle cramps. These are usually harmless and may respond to gentle stretching of the calves before you go to bed, a prescription of quinine bisulphate tablets, or a review of your existing medication. **But**, leg pain in bed when you already have intermittent claudication may be a danger sign that the narrowing in your arteries has become critical, and you should tell your doctor immediately.

Chronic foot problems that get infected are a leading cause of amputation in people who have intermittent claudication. If you have a cut, graze, blister or other foot problem that becomes red, swollen, hot and painful with infection, see your doctor.

See your doctor, too, if you need help to stop smoking.

important to take gentle exercise as this encourages the growth of new blood vessels.

'Get out every day for at least an hour of walking,' says Dr Young. 'You have to bring on the discomfort of intermittent claudication in order for walking to do any good.' Walk until you feel the pain, he says, but don't stop at the first sign of pain. 'Wait until it gets moderately severe. Stop and rest for a minute or two until it goes away, then start walking again.' Repeat that pain/walk cycle as often as you can during your daily hour of walking.

Improvement won't happen overnight, however. It will take two or three months before you see results, so don't be discouraged.

Exercise, whatever the weather. Walking may be the best exercise, but cycling on an exercise bike can also help if it works the calves, says circulation expert Robert Ginsburg. 'In fact, any indoor exercise that works the calves enough to bring on the pain of claudication can help.' Try climbing stairs, running on the spot, skipping and dancing – but check with your doctor before trying these more strenuous exercises.

Lose weight. Obesity is a major problem for people with claudication, not only because of the strain it places on circulation but also because of the damage it inflicts on the feet.

Avoid heating pads. Because of the restricted bloodflow in the legs, people who have intermittent claudication often experience cold feet. But regardless of how cold your feet may be, never warm them with a heating pad or a hot-water bottle. Because bloodflow is restricted, the heat can't be dissipated and could actually burn your feet. Try wearing loose woolly bed socks instead.

Good news on alcohol. Modest amounts of alcohol may help prevent intermittent claudication. This protective effect is seen with wine and beer rather than spirits, and is lost if you drink more than the recommended maximum of three standard drinks a day for men, and two for women. A standard drink (unit) is half a pint of normal strength beer, a small glass (85ml) of wine or a single pub measure of spirits.

Have your blood pressure and cholesterol checked. If you have intermittent claudication, your blood pressure and cholesterol levels should be monitored, says Dr Young. 'These are important risk factors that can markedly increase the severity of the underlying disease.'

MEMORY PROBLEMS
21 ways to forget less

If you spend any time with older adults, then you'll probably hear wry comments about getting senile – usually when someone forgets an appointment, or can't remember a word or name on the tip of their tongue.

Despite the jokes about memory loss, one of the greatest fears people have is of losing their memory or mental faculties as they age. It's worth remembering that there's a huge difference between occasional memory lapses and conditions like dementia or Alzheimer's disease, which are caused by underlying disease.

High blood pressure, for example, can contribute to declines in memory. So can depression, fatigue, high cholesterol, stroke, alcohol abuse, drug side-effects and a variety of nutritional deficiencies. It's essential to see a doctor if your memory is suddenly worse than it used to be, or if it seems to be going downhill.

Patchy forgetfulness is rarely a sign of disease, however. Nor is it something you necessarily have to live with. With a combination of mental exercises and lifestyle changes, there's a good chance that you can improve your memory and keep it strong for years to come.

Give your mind a workout. The brain is like any other part of the body. The more it's exercised and challenged, the stronger it gets, says neurologist Gunnar Gouras. People who are mentally active form additional neural connections, Dr Gouras explains. In other words, they have a larger 'reserve' of brain circuits, so they're more likely to stay mentally sharp. A study of 678 nuns, for example, found that those with the most education and language abilities were least likely to develop Alzheimer's later in life.

So keep your mind busy. Do crossword puzzles. Read challenging books. Play Scrabble or go to the cinema. Virtually any activity that keeps the mind active could help to reduce the risk of age-related memory loss.

Break information into bite-sized pieces. It's easy to forget – or fail to learn – information that comes in large chunks. It's much easier to remember things when you break them down into smaller bits, says psychiatrist Cynthia Green. Phone numbers are a good example. They're usually divided into two or three sections – the area code, the first three numbers and the final four numbers. They're not too hard to remember because they're broken into small, manageable pieces of information.

Make mental connections. When you were at school, you probably learnt to spell 'together' by thinking of three words: to get her. It was a way of linking new information with something you already knew.

'At a conference I met a woman called Celia,' says Dr Green. 'As soon as she said her name, I connected it to a friend of mine who's also called Celia, which made the name easier to remember.'

You can form connections with almost anything. Suppose your pin number is 1418. Link it to something that you already know, like the dates of World War One, or you could give each number its corresponding letter of the alphabet and make the letters into a sentence. Or perhaps your locker number at the public swimming pool is 27: you might think, that's the age I was when I got married.

Try the sentence technique. Another way to remember names or other information is to weave them into little sentences, says Dr Green. If you meet someone named Frank Hill, for example, you might think something like, 'Frankly, he's over the hill.'

Write it down. Diaries, calendars and notebooks are invaluable memory aids. Apart from the fact that you can write things down and look them up later, the act of writing can make them easier to remember, says Dr Green.

One theory about memory loss is that it's caused by unstable oxygen molecules in the body, called free radicals, damaging cells and blood vessels in the brain. You can't rid yourself of free radicals, but you can counteract some of their harmful effects by eating fresh fruit and vegetables.

Fruit and vegetables are rich in antioxidants, and they are believed to protect us from several age-related diseases of the brain. Next time you're pushing your trolley through the fresh produce aisle, go for the fruits and vegetables with the brightest colours – yellow peppers, red tomatoes, blackcurrants, oranges – as they're the ones with the highest concentration of antioxidants.

Create 'forget-me-not' spots. Some things are always getting lost – car keys and reading glasses, for example. One of the best memory aids is simply to put these and other commonly mislaid items in the same places all the time.

As soon as you walk through the door, put your keys on the hall table, Dr Green suggests. Always keep your reading glasses next to the sofa or bed. As long as you're consistent, you'll never have to worry about losing these or other things again.

Make sleep a priority. The brain needs sleep to perform properly, says psychiatrist and sleep expert Allan Hobson. When you're asleep, the brain works on information gathered during the day. Aim for at least eight hours sleep a night. If you're less alert than you'd like to be, take a look at how much sleep you're getting, and sleep more if you need to, suggests Dr Hobson.

Check your B_{12}. The B vitamins, especially vitamin B_{12}, play a key role in memory and mental functions. 'As people get older, it becomes harder to absorb B vitamins from food,' says Dr Green. 'A vitamin B_{12} deficiency can cause significant memory loss.'

There is no evidence that taking B vitamin supplements helps memory if your B_{12} levels are normal to start with, says family doctor Stephen Amiel, and in many cases of established B_{12} deficiency, only regular B_{12} injections will help. A blood test can easily establish if you're B_{12} deficient.

Get extra vitamin E? There are claims that vitamin E can help the memory loss of Alzheimer's disease. It's an antioxidant nutrient that helps to block the harmful effects of free radicals, unstable oxygen molecules in the blood. It can reduce build-ups of cholesterol and other fatty substances in blood vessels in the brain, as elsewhere, and it also appears to reduce inflammation. The evidence is controversial though, says Dr Amiel, and more trials are needed before the benefits of vitamin E can be established one way or another. There are also concerns that high doses may do more harm than good, with a number of side-effects being reported, including worsening of angina and diabetes.

Give ginkgo a try. Researchers at the University of Surrey found that people aged between 50 and 59 who took 120mg of ginkgo three times a day experienced improvements in memory, concentration and alertness. A herbal remedy, ginkgo appears to improve circulation and helps brain cells to get all the nutrients they need in order to stay healthy.

According to clinical herbalist Douglas Schar, gingko can be used to prevent age-related senility in those with a family history of the condition, to increase memory in those that have lost some of theirs – and even to help those with normal memories get a little more! Recent research has shown that gingko improves the memory capacity of healthy people, says Schar. So if you're thinking about going back to college as a mature student, then gingko may help you to get through those exams.

Consider Siberian ginseng. Many people suffer from memory problems when they are mentally and physically exhausted. By the time the day is over, the mind has processed as much information as it can process and goes into

Do just *one* thing

Pay attention. If your memory isn't as good as you'd like it to be, make a special effort to focus your attention on the things you want to remember.

The main reason we forget things is that we weren't paying attention in the first place, says psychiatrist Cynthia Green.

One way the brain sorts information is by routing it to short-term or long-term memory. Long-term memories tend to stay with us, while short-term memories tend to be fleeting. If you don't focus your attention on remembering new things, they'll never make the transition into long-term memory.

'My favourite technique for remembering names is repetition, in which I say the name back to the person,' says Dr Green. You can use the same technique for anything. When you put the car keys down, for example, simply repeat to yourself where you're putting them. When you meet someone new, repeat their name in your head a few times. Making the effort to remember things will help to ensure that you do.

shut-down mode. If poor memory is a symptom of being worn out, herbal medicines known as adaptogens may help. These raise resistance to exhaustion and this has a knock-on effect on memory. Try Siberian ginseng, Chinese ginseng or oat straw. All three are available in capsule and tincture form at health food stores and should be taken according to label instructions. Expect it to take a week or two before you notice an effect.

Rosemary for remembrance. So the saying goes. Herbalist Brigitte Mars believes it. 'When my daughter was revising for her chemistry finals, I told her to dab some essential oil of rosemary in her hair,' she says. 'She also applied the oil just before taking the exam. Smelling the scent during the test helped to remind her of the material she'd studied.'

Note: Don't take rosemary oil by mouth – it's toxic, and never apply it undiluted to your skin because it will cause irritation.

Exercise regularly. Walking, cycling and other forms of exercise are among the best ways to increase bloodflow throughout the body, including in the brain. Regular aerobic exercise also protects from illnesses such as stroke, diabetes and high blood pressure, all of which can cause memory problems, says Dr Green.

WHEN TO CONSULT A DOCTOR

Because declining memory can be caused by many physical problems – such as depression, thyroid disorders, alcohol-related problems, nutritional deficiencies or even urinary tract infections – it's important to see a doctor as soon as you notice any changes, says psychiatrist Cynthia Green. Ask yourself if your memory has got significantly worse in the last six months. Are the changes affecting your ability to lead a normal life? Are your friends or family worried? The answers to these questions will give you an idea of the seriousness of the changes.

Another thing to consider is whether you're taking a new medication. Many drugs, including antihistamines and drugs for heartburn, anxiety and high blood pressure, can have memory impairment as a side-effect. Often, switching to a new drug or changing the dose may be all that is needed to reverse the problem.

Some cases of mild to moderate memory loss due to Alzheimer's respond to medication. Drugs like donepezil, galantamine and rivastigmine are showing promising results in improving memory and general functioning in older people. These drugs can only be initiated by hospital specialists, so would involve a referral from your doctor.

Treat your brain gently. Your skull provides an amazing degree of protection to your brain, one of the body's most delicate organs, but a blow to the head will still cause the brain, which has the consistency of porridge, to bounce around inside the skull. A severe blow can cause concussion or haemorrhage, but the impact on memory of repeated minor trauma to the head can be devastating, says Dr Amiel. Studies on boxers have shown significant memory problems in most professional ex-boxers, even when there are no outward signs of being 'punch drunk'. Amateur boxers are at risk too, despite the protective headgear that should always be worn. And, says Dr Amiel, if you or your child cycle, make sure protective headgear is worn at all times.

Keep stress at manageable levels. People who are frequently tense or anxious tend to have high levels of stress hormones. Over time, high levels of these hormones can affect the area of the brain that controls memory.

Stress and anxiety also affect memory indirectly. If you're tense all the time, you're more likely to have sleep problems – and the resulting fatigue can make it harder to remember things. 'You can't avoid stress entirely,' says Dr Green, 'but you can balance it with activities that help you to relax. It might be making time to do some colouring with your children, to take a lazy bath or to have a massage.' Anything that shifts your attention away from what's causing your stress can be helpful.

Keep cholesterol low. Research suggests that adults who take prescription drugs to lower cholesterol have a significantly lower risk of developing Alzheimer's disease. More research is needed to show conclusively that reducing cholesterol – either with drugs or through dietary changes – will protect against Alzheimer's disease or memory loss, says Dr Gouras. But because lowering cholesterol has so many other benefits, such as reducing the risk of stroke or heart disease, it's worth making the effort.

Drink more water. About 85 per cent of the brain consists of water. If you don't drink enough, you can get dehydrated, which leads to fatigue and makes it harder to remember things. Aim for at least eight 250ml glasses of water a day.

And less alcohol. The news on alcohol and memory is all bad, says Dr Amiel. Even small amounts of alcohol impair our memory, by inhibiting the transfer and consolidation of information into our long-term memory bank. You're less likely to remember things you've learned if you then go out for a few drinks, and a heavy drinking session can impair your memory, concentration and ability to learn for up to 72 hours afterwards.

'Alcohol often makes people do things that they remember all too well afterwards, but wish they could forget,' says Dr Amiel. 'But more serious binges can result in "blackouts": these are really memory wipe-outs rather than any loss of consciousness and are a real danger sign of alcohol dependence,' he warns.

Alcohol also disrupts sleep patterns, leading to fatigue and further impact on your memory. Long-term alcohol abuse can cause permanent damage to the connections between nerve cells in your brain, leading to irreversible memory problems, personality changes and dementia, and alcohol abuse during pregnancy can cause permanent brain damage to the unborn child.

Fight depression. It makes it hard to concentrate, and it also makes people feel tired and sluggish. Among elderly adults, in fact, depression is often mistaken for Alzheimer's disease or other forms of dementia, says Dr Gouras.

MENOPAUSE
17 ways to cope with the change

Menopause is not a disease. It does not have to be a horrendous life-altering change. Many women sail through their menopause with few symptoms, and many of the symptoms women do have to deal with can be controlled naturally.

Doctors define menopause one full year after a woman's last period. This can occur in a woman's forties or her sixties, but most commonly, the change takes place when a woman is in her early fifties.

Symptoms of the menopause vary widely. They may not affect a woman at all, or they may hit like a force 10 gale. As women age, their oestrogen levels drop, which triggers menopausal symptoms and also increases their risk of cardiovascular disease and osteoporosis. The most common symptoms are weight gain, vaginal changes (including dryness and loss of elasticity), sleep disturbances, emotional changes and hot flushes (see *Hot Flushes*, page 325).

It may sound awful, but it doesn't have to be. Eat properly, exercise and talk to your doctor about hormone replacement therapy (HRT), other medications or herbal remedies. They can all help to smooth your transition, enabling you to enjoy the benefits of menopause: no more pre-menstrual tension, no more periods and no more pregnancy worries.

Give up smoking. Your chances of developing heart disease and osteoporosis jump during menopause. Smoking makes those odds rise even higher. And smokers hit the menopause two years earlier on average than non-smokers, says gynaecologist Mary Jane Minkin.

Refrain from binge drinking. Too much booze is bad for both bone and heart health as you move into the menopause. 'A glass of wine a day is fine,' says Dr Minkin. But a bottle a day is definitely not good for your heart or your bones. Worse still, alcohol brings on hot flushes (see *Hot Flushes*, page 325), one of the greatest banes of the menopause.

Get enough calcium. You can get a healthy dose of 1000mg of calcium a day from dairy products. But most women don't drink a lot of milk or eat a lot of cheese because they're worried about saturated fat and calorie intake, says Dr Minkin. To ensure adequate calcium intake, she recommends taking 1000mg of supplementary calcium a day.

And get it now. Don't wait until your forties and fifties to up your calcium intake, says family doctor Stephen Amiel. 'The time to start is in your teens and twenties: 50 per cent of your adult bone mass is laid down during adolescence. Plenty of calcium in your diet then can be an insurance policy when you reach menopause.' Low fat dairy products are the best source of dietary calcium, but look out also for fortified juices, cereals and even white bread.

Do just *one* thing

Exercise regularly. 'Exercise reduces menopausal symptoms, helps you to sleep, helps your bones and helps your heart,' says gynaecologist Mary Jane Minkin.

But find a variety of activities you really enjoy. Saying you're going to exercise is one thing, but, as gynaecologist Larrian Gillespie points out, most women only stick with it for about six weeks.

To counteract the loss of flexibility women face as they grow older, Dr Gillespie recommends a type of exercise called Pilates that focuses on flexibility and strength for the whole body without building muscles. It also has the advantage of being a low-sweat form of exercise, as are swimming and yoga.

Strengthen your bones by brisk walking for 20 to 30 minutes three times a week at least, by using a step machine or by gentle jogging. 'You need some impact for new bone to be laid down,' says family doctor Stephen Amiel. 'Evidence suggests that just walking can give your bones at least a third of the benefit that HRT does.'

Don't forget vitamin D. This is the other nutrient that Dr Minkin pinpoints as crucial to good menopausal health. Most dietary vitamin D comes from fortified foods such as milk and other dairy products. Your skin also synthesizes vitamin D when exposed to sunlight. If your diet is poor, you are elderly or you have an Asian diet, you are more likely to be deficient in vitamin D, and you should consider a dietary supplement. You can kill two birds with one stone by taking a combined calcium and vitamin D tablet to give you the 10mcg of vitamin D you need a day.

The truth about HRT. A myth exists that it's dangerous to go on and off HRT. 'It's not,' says Dr Minkin. In fact, she says, women should feel free to experiment with HRT until they find the combination that works best for them – or decide that they don't need it at all.

Taking HRT longer term does need some thought, as recent evidence suggests that the risks and benefits are more evenly balanced than was once thought. See *Hot Flushes*, page 325, for more information on this.

Eat smaller, more frequent meals. Women metabolize foods differently from men, says gynaecologist and diet expert Larrian Gillespie. Men use carbohydrates for energy, and women store carbohydrates as fat to allow them to procreate in the face of starvation. Changes in oestrogen levels make these differences even more pronounced as we grow older. Dr Gillespie recommends eating five or six smaller meals during the day rather than three large ones. And include plenty of fresh fruit and vegetables, beans and pulses.

Use a lubricant. A classic complaint of menopause, decreased sexual desire, is sometimes caused by physical changes in the vagina. If a lack of interest in sex is, in part, due to sheer discomfort, then buy an over-the-counter lubricant such as KY Jelly. But if there are emotional issues involved, you and your partner need to work on your relationship.

Try old-fashioned sleep aids. If sleep is a problem, Dr Minkin advises some of old-fashioned remedies. You'll sleep more restfully if you drink a mug of warm milk, take a warm bath and try not to focus on the day's events.

Share your troubles. Much of the stress of the menopause for women results from other life changes that are happening at the same time. Children may be leaving home, parents are ageing and developing health problems, husbands are going through their mid-life crises – or second childhoods. Friendships can help you to overcome these emotional land-

WHEN TO CONSULT A DOCTOR

If your periods are becoming fewer and lighter as you reach your fifties, you are getting no disabling symptoms, and you are not at increased risk of osteoporosis, then there is no need to consult your doctor.

Remember though that you will need to continue to use contraception for a year after your last period if you are over 50, and for two years if you are over 40. 'I've seen at least five patients over the years who came to tell me they were menopausal because their periods had stopped, and they were several months pregnant!' says family doctor Stephen Amiel.

You **should** see your doctor in the following circumstances:

• you have irregular bleeding, your periods are becoming heavier or more frequent, or you bleed after sex;

• you are at increased risk of osteoporosis (your menopause is starting earlier than 45; you've had a hysterectomy before 50, even if your ovaries were not removed; you have had few menstrual periods in your life because of low body weight, over-exercising or anorexia; you have been on long-term steroids; you have a strong family history of osteoporosis; you are a heavy smoker or drinker; you have reduced mobility);

• your symptoms of menopause are affecting you physically, emotionally or socially despite home remedies;

• you have not been called for your routine breast screening (mammography) and you are 51 or over;

• you need your regular cervical smear test. New guidelines suggest that over the age of 50, you only need smears five yearly if they have been normal previously, and you no longer need a smear over the age of 65, provided your last smear was normal and you have no symptoms of abnormal bleeding.

Any vaginal bleeding occurring after the menopause requires urgent medical attention. Although there are many innocent causes, 10–20 per cent of cases will be due to cancer.

mines. 'Volunteer to give some time to a charity, or join a menopause support group,' says Dr Minkin. 'These are great ways to meet friends, share life's stresses or just get together.'

The Amarant Trust is a UK charity for women going through the menopause. For help and support ring their Helpline on 01293 413000. All calls are answered personally by menopause nurse specialists, and lines are open from 11am to 6pm every weekday. Or visit their website at www.amarant-menopausetrust.org.uk.

Get your partner to read all about it. You might understand what's happening to you, but your partner may be totally oblivious to, or bemused by the changes going on in your body and won't understand how hard things are for you from time to time. Ask your partner to read about it, says Dr Minkin. Once he understands the changes you are going through, he'll hopefully react with patience and encouragement.

Chase it away with chasteberry. Menopause is a natural phenomenon, says clinical herbalist Douglas Schar, not an illness. What is true is that you can experience chaotic hormone levels during the menopause, which can make this natural transition most unpleasant.

Chasteberry (*Vitex agnus-castus*) has been used for centuries to balance hormones. Research suggests that it does this by working on the pituitary gland. The remedy is available from healthfood stores in capsule or tincture form. Follow label instructions.

You'll need to use the remedy for a month or more before judging its effects, says Schar, but more often than not, it makes the menopause much more manageable.

Buy black cohosh. 'This is my favourite herb for menopausal symptoms. It really makes a big difference,' says family doctor Connie Catellani. Studies show that black cohosh alleviates symptoms of hot flushes, night sweats, vaginal dryness, sleep disturbances, nervousness, irritability and depression. Scientists don't know exactly how black cohosh works, but it appears to help balance oestrogen levels.

Some doctors advise against using it for more than six months at a time as its long-term effects have not been studied. So far, there have been no reported adverse effects from its continued use, and Dr Catellani has patients who have taken it for three or four years with no problems.

KITCHEN CURES

Try soya-based foods. As a natural phytoestrogen, soya has proved useful for helping women overcome the symptoms of the menopause. Phytoestrogens are thought to provide a substitute for the body's own oestrogen, helping to relieve symptoms like hot flushes and dry skin. The phytoestrogens in soya are called isoflavones.

A variety of soya products are available from supermarkets, including tofu and soya milk.

Dry sweats with sage. Sage (*Salvia officinalis*) has long been used to dry up abnormal sweating, says Schar. It was prescribed for the very severe sweating of malaria as well as the disturbing night sweats and hot flushes of menopause. Buy sage tincture 1:5, and take 2.5ml, or half-a-teaspoon, three times a day. The remedy will work within a day or two.

Seek out St John's wort. If the menopause is causing hormone-related depression, Dr Catellani suggests trying St John's wort (hypericum). The herb, long recognized for its ability to fight melancholy, has been shown to be as effective as some prescription antidepressants for mild to moderate depression. It's also less likely than prescription drugs to cause side-effects such as fatigue or loss of sexual interest. You may need to take the herb for two or three weeks before you notice an effect. But don't suffer in silence: if symptoms persist, see your doctor as soon as possible.

MORNING SICKNESS
12 ways to counteract queasiness

Morning sickness is a term used to describe the nausea and vomiting that affect many pregnant women. It tends to occur in the first three months after conception, but sometimes it continues throughout the pregnancy. Some women find that nausea strikes at any time of the day or night. Others feel worse in the evening, after a long day at work. For some it's triggered by certain smells.

Usually, morning sickness begins at around the sixth week of pregnancy – about the same time as the placenta begins serious production of human chorionic gonadotrophin (HCG), a pregnancy hormone. In most women, symptoms peak during week eight or nine and ease off after week 13. The encouraging news is that morning sickness seems to be a sign that the pregnancy is going well. One large study found that pregnant women who vomited during their first trimester were less likely to miscarry or deliver prematurely.

More good news is that morning sickness seems to be at its worst in first pregnancies. The chances are, you won't be so bad next time around. Armed with those positive thoughts, try the following remedies.

Experiment. What worked for your sister, your best friend or the woman down the road may not work for you. 'There are as many remedies as there are women,' says midwife Deborah Gowen. You may need to try a couple of methods before you find one that suits you.

Although the kitchen may be the last room a nauseous pregnant woman wants to visit, you'll find several helpful drinks there. Obstetrician Gregory Radio recommends drinking small amounts of clear fluids frequently. He suggests clear broth, fruit juice and herbal teas such as ginger or chamomile.

You could also try sports drinks like Lucozade Sport or Isostar: these help to maintain electrolytes – vital substances that regulate your body's electrochemical balance.

Eat the way your baby eats. The child growing inside you nourishes itself by raiding your bloodstream for glucose 24 hours a day. If you don't replenish the supply, your blood sugar levels can drop sharply, making you feel nauseous.

Your best tactic, says midwife Tekoa King, is to change the way you eat to the way the baby eats: a little at a time. Put glucose into your system quickly and easily by eating simple sugars, such as fruit sugars, that are already half broken down. Grapes and orange juice are excellent.

Avoid fried, fatty foods. That bacon sandwich with fried onions may have looked delicious last week, but you might not want to risk it now. Anything fried seems to make pregnant women feel nauseated, says King. And the body takes longer to digest fried foods, she says, so they sit in the stomach longer.

Take a bag of almonds with you. Snacking on the nuts fulfils the need for small, frequent meals. They contain some fat, some protein and are high in calcium and potassium. They're portable, too, and taste better than dry crackers, says Gowen.

Keep nibbles on the bedside table. If nausea strikes first thing in the morning, keep biscuits or crackers by the bed. Getting up on an empty stomach can make you feel worse, says King. So eat something to bring your blood sugar up before you get out of bed in the morning, or in the middle of the night.

Nibble to keep away heartburn, too. You should always have something in your stomach, even if it's just a rich tea biscuit, advises obstetrician Gregory Radio. 'The stomach makes more acids during pregnancy, and those acids need something to work on.'

Sip ginger ale. Ginger has long been used as a remedy for nausea, and ginger ale – commonly used as a mixer with whisky – can work well for pregnancy sickness, too, says obstetrician Yvonne Thornton.

Talk to your doctor about your iron pills. Some brands of iron or vitamin supplements can exacerbate nausea in pregnant women. Your doctor or midwife may be able to recommend a different brand that won't upset your stomach, says Gowen.

Trust your body's wisdom. Eat whatever you fancy, as long as it's not junk, says Gowen. 'Avoid caffeine, artificial sweeteners and all drugs. But if all you crave is pasta, then eat it. It really does work when women listen to their bodies.'

WHEN TO CONSULT A DOCTOR

Consult your doctor about your morning sickness if:

- you notice you've lost a kilo or so. Normally, weight gain continues during pregnancy even if you can't keep all your meals down;
- you feel dehydrated or are not urinating;
- you find that you can't keep anything down – no water, juice, nothing – over a period of four to six hours.

At its most severe, morning sickness can spiral into a condition doctors call hyperemesis gravidarum. Left untreated, it can disturb the electrolyte balance in your body, cause an irregular pulse, and, in its severest form, damage the kidneys and liver. It also endangers your unborn child. The ketones that result when your body breaks down fat already stored in the body can cause neurological damage to the baby.

Women with hyperemesis gravidarum are usually admitted to hospital overnight and treated with an intravenous solution of glucose, water and vitamins, plus certain medicines if necessary.

Doctors usually don't know why some women are more affected than others by morning sickness, but hyperemesis is more common in women who are having twins, and it can also occur in a rare condition called hydatidiform mole, which produces very high HCG levels. Blood tests and scans will establish whether these are responsible.

All medications are best avoided in early pregnancy, but in severe morning sickness that is not quite bad enough for hospital admission, a short course of an antihistamine may be given. There is no evidence that this is harmful to your baby.

Keep calm. If you continue to put on weight, and dehydration isn't a problem for you, you're probably doing fine.

Women don't tend to lose more than their body reserves can cope with, says King. You can be pretty sick with morning sickness, but continue nourishing your baby perfectly well.

Drink ginger tea. Ginger, used to quieten the nausea associated with motion sickness and food poisoning, can also help with morning sickness, says clinical herbalist Douglas Schar. Many women say that their symptoms are greatly reduced with regular doses of ginger tea. 'I am very wary of women taking any herbs while pregnant,' says Schar, 'but this remedy is known to be safe, and unlike many herbal remedies, is actually a pleasure to take!'

MOTION SICKNESS

20 ways to stop it

Even the most seasoned sailors can suffer from seasickness. In the air, it's airsickness. On land, it's carsickness. Or you may be hit with nausea on a seemingly endless roller-coaster ride. Regardless of what you call it, it's all the same thing – a queasy, uneasy feeling known as motion sickness.

Motion sickness occurs when the brain receives wrong information about the environment, explains ear, nose and throat specialist Rafael Tarnopolsky. To keep our bodies in balance, our sensory systems continually collect information about our surroundings and send it to the inner ear, where the information is organized before being sent on to the brain.

When our balance system notes a discrepancy between what our inner ears sense and what our eyes sense, motion sickness can result, says Horst Konrad, an ear, nose and throat specialist. Not everyone gets it, but the signals are pretty clear when it does occur. Dizziness, sweating, pale skin and nausea. If things don't improve, you throw up.

Once you feel the symptoms coming on, motion sickness can be very difficult to stop, especially if you've reached your particular point of no return – usually once nausea sets in. But the following remedies can help to soothe the symptoms, perhaps even cutting them short. Better still, they may keep them from starting in the first place next time you're rolling on a choppy sea.

Don't think about it. 'Motion sickness is partly psychological,' says Dr Konrad. 'If you think you're going to throw up, you probably will.'

Instead, shift your thoughts to something wonderful.

Avoid nasty smells. Smells such as engine fumes, airline food passing you on the flight attendant's trolley or even strong perfume can contribute to nausea, says Dr Konrad. Point your nose elsewhere.

Don't smoke. If you're a smoker, you may think that lighting up will calm you down, deterring motion sickness. You're wrong. Cigarette smoke contributes to impending nausea, says Dr Konrad. Non-smokers should move as fast as possible to a smoke-free area when they feel queasiness coming on.

Leave nursing the sick to someone else. It's a common oc-currence. You're on a boat. Every-thing's fine until someone's sick. You watch sympathetically, maybe even offer a comforting shoulder. Before long, you're the next one down. It's the domino effect in ac-tion. As cruel as it may sound, it's best to ignore others who are being sick, says Dr Konrad. Otherwise, you'll probably end up in the same proverbial boat.

Travel at night. Your chances of feeling sick diminish when you travel at night because you can't see the motion as clearly as you can during daylight, says op-tometrist and motion sickness ex-pert, Roderic Gillilan.

Don't eat the wrong foods. If certain foods don't suit you when you're on solid ground, they'll suit you even less when you're on the move. As tempting as the meals

KITCHEN CURES

These remedies from the kitchen cupboard might be worth a try.

Ginger. A tried and tested remedy, ginger recently passed scientific scrutiny when a trial showed powdered ginger capsules to be more effective than a popular over-the-counter motion sickness pill in preventing motion sickness. Chewing on crystallized root ginger or fresh ginger has the same effect.

Olives and lemons. Motion sickness causes you to produce excess saliva, which can make you nauseated. Olives, on the other hand, produce chemicals called tannins, which make your mouth dry. So, the theory goes, eating a couple of olives at the first hint of nausea can help to diminish it, as can sucking on a lemon.

Cream crackers. They won't stop salivation, but dry crackers may help to absorb the excess fluid when it reaches your stomach.

may be during your travels, don't over-indulge, advises Robert Salada, who runs a travellers' health centre.

Breathe fresh air. Get rid of nausea with a breath of fresh air, recommends Dr Salada. In the car, open a window. On a boat, stand on deck and inhale the breeze. On a plane, turn on the overhead vent.

Think before you drink. 'Too much alcohol can interfere with the way the brain handles information about the environment, setting off motion sickness symptoms,' says Dr Konrad. What's more, alcohol can dissolve into the fluids on your inner ear, which can send your head spinning, he says. Drink in moderation, if at all, when travelling by air or sea.

Get enough sleep. 'Your chance of getting motion sickness increases with fatigue,' says Dr Gillilan. Get enough sleep before setting off. If you're a passenger in a car or plane, having a nap en route can help, too.

Sit still. Your brain is confused enough without your creating extra motion. In particular, try and keep your head especially still.

Get in front and look ahead. In a car, move to the front seat and focus on the road ahead or the horizon, says Dr Tarnopolsky. This brings signals from your body and your eyes into balance.

Better still, drive. When you're behind the wheel, you're sensibly looking straight ahead, says Dr Gillilan, and you have the added advantage of anticipating any quick changes in motion.

Catch up on your reading another time. Don't read while you're travelling by car or on a bumpy flight or boat trip, says Dr Tarnopolsky. The movement of the vehicle you're in makes the printed matter on the page move, which can lead to terrible dizziness.

Find the centre of most resistance. On board a ship, get a cabin midship, where the least amount of rolling and bouncing occurs.

Wear acupressure wristbands. Sold in some pharmacies and health food shops, these lightweight wristbands have a plastic button that is supposed to be worn over what Eastern doctors call the Nei-Kuan acupressure point inside each wrist. Pressing the button for a few minutes protects you against nausea.

Focus on something stationary. It'll help get your sensory system back in balance – though standing in a bobbing boat and watching the horizon may make you sick because the horizon will bob along with you. Instead, fix your sights on a stationary point in the sky or the land in the distance.

Take a preventative. If motion sickness is as inevitable as rain on a summer Bank holiday, consider taking an over-the-counter medication like Kwells or Sea Legs. Taken a few hours in advance, these drugs can prevent symptoms from occurring in the first place, says Dr Salada. One or two tablets last for up to 24 hours. But make sure you take the medication in advance, because it isn't effective once symptoms start.

MOUTH ULCERS
10 ways to ease the sting

No one knows exactly why some people get mouth ulcers and others don't. For most people, a coffee burn heals in two or three days with little or no pain, but for others it can lead to a sore that won't heal for two weeks. Heredity, certain foods, over aggressive toothbrushing, ill-fitting dentures, chewing on the inside of your mouth and emotional stress can all lead to painful, craterlike ulcers.

Viruses such as herpes simplex can be responsible for crops of painful so-called aphthous ulcers: they tend to come up in crops in the mouth or on the tongue and may be triggered when you're unwell for any reason, or run down.

Whatever the cause, treating an ulcer is a difficult task, says Robert Goepp, a surgeon who specializes in oral medicine. Nothing sticks well to the skin in your mouth, and it's one of the most bacteria-laden places in the body. Ulcer remedies aim to minimize pain by protecting the ulcer, and killing infection.

Mouth ulcers occur more often in young people, and become much less frequent with age. Meanwhile, if ulcers are making you miserable, try the following remedies.

Read labels. Look for over-the-counter ulcer treatments that contain benzocaine, lidocaine, menthol, camphor, eucalyptol or alcohol in a liquid or gel, such as Rinstead gel and Anbesol liquid. They often sting at first, and most need repeated application because they don't stick, but they're also effective.

Brush carefully. It is important to keep your mouth and teeth clean while a mouth ulcer heals, but be careful. You don't want to scratch a healing sore with a toothbrush.

Dab on an alternative. Propolis, used by bees to construct their hives, and tea tree oil both have antiseptic properties and can be dabbed on a mouth ulcer with a moist cotton bud, says Andrew Weil, a professor of medicine. Both products are available in health food stores.

Apply a paste coating. Some over-the-counter pastes form a protective 'bandage' over the sore. To get pastes like Orabase to work, dry the sore with one end of a cotton bud, then immediately apply the paste with the other end. It works only on new sores, however.

Disinfect your mouth. Dilute one tablespoon of hydrogen peroxide in a glass of water and swish it around in your mouth to disinfect the sore and speed up healing, says Dr Goepp.

Use milk of magnesia as a mouthwash. Don't swallow your milk of magnesia. Instead, wash it around your mouth and allow it to coat the ulcer before spitting it out. It may also have some antibacterial effect, says Dr Goepp.

Try calendula. Make a strong tea of calendula flowers (available at health food stores) and use it as a mouthwash. Or you can make a paste with a bit of water and apply it directly. 'Calendula has an antiviral and anti-inflammatory effect that can really make a difference,' says clinical herbalist Douglas Schar.

Avoid food irritants. Coffee, spices, citrus fruit, nuts high in the amino acid arginine (especially walnuts), chocolate and strawberries irritate mouth ulcers and can even trigger them in some people, says Dr Goepp.

Rely on vitamins. Craig Zunka, a dentist and homeopath, recommends squeezing vitamin E oil

---

KITCHEN CURES

Eating four tablespoons of natural yoghurt a day may help to prevent mouth ulcers by sending in helpful bacteria to counter the harmful bacteria in your mouth, says dermatologist Jerome Litt. Look for live yoghurt that contains active *Lactobacillus acidophilus*.

Dr Litt also recommends applying a wet tea bag to the ulcer. Tea contains tannin, an astringent that 'may pleasantly surprise you' with its pain-relieving ability.

WHEN TO CONSULT A DOCTOR

A mouth ulcer should heal within two weeks. 'If ulcers last a long time or you are unable to eat, speak or sleep properly, you should see a doctor or dentist, advises mouth specialist Robert Goepp. You will probably be prescribed topical steroids or oral antibiotics.

Sometimes aphthous ulcers are signs of other conditions such as Crohn's disease or coeliac disease, although with these conditions there will usually be other bowel-related symptoms as well.

Oral thrush (candidiasis) can be painful and mistaken for mouth ulcers: it is common in babies and in people with dentures, but can also occur with diabetes, immune deficiency and people taking steroid tablets or using asthma inhalers. It is important to see your doctor if a mouth ulcer fails to heal after three weeks, even if it is painless, as cancer of the mouth or tongue may be the cause.

from a capsule onto an ulcer. Repeat several times a day to keep the tissue well oiled. Also, at the first tingle of an ulcer, take 1000mg vitamin C with bioflavonoids and then take 500mg three times a day for the next three days. It's very important that you use vitamin C with bioflavonoids, he says, because vitamin C by itself doesn't work on mouth ulcers. The homeopathic remedy Borax 12x may also help.

MUSCLE PAIN

31 ways to make it better

Pain can strike any one of the 600 or more muscles in your body, taking the form of a strain, soreness or cramp. In all three cases, overuse is to blame: doing too much, too soon or too often, says Ted Percy, an orthopaedic surgeon who specializes in sports medicine. If you've already overdone it, don't worry. There are plenty of things that you can do to ease muscle pain.

Take it easy. 'Every time you exercise, your muscles are injured,' says Gabe Mirkin, a doctor who specializes in sports medicine. 'It takes 48 hours for muscles to heal from exercise. Soreness means damage, and you should stop exercising when you feel sore.'

You don't have to be running a race or playing a hard tennis match to injure your muscles. Working in the garden, lifting a struggling toddler, sitting in an awkward position – or simply sitting in the same position for a long time – can cause muscle problems.

How much rest you should give your muscles depends on the situation, says sports medicine expert Allan Levy. A cramp may require only minutes, a severe strain may need weeks. But if you're hiking and strain a muscle, at least rest it for a couple of hours, then carefully stretch the muscle before trying to continue.

Use an ice pack. Ice is the first line of defence against swelling and should be used immediately after injury, says Carol Folkerts, a former physiotherapist. She recommends using an ice pack or wrapping ice in a towel or plastic bag and applying it for 20 minutes at a time throughout

---

Stretch to strengthen

Give muscles the attention they need, and they tend to do their jobs quietly. Ignore them, and they'll demand attention by cramping or becoming strained when moved the wrong way.

When that happens, you may be able to soothe them with some simple stretching. But if you want them to remain quiet, you will probably have to make stretching a regular part of your life.

Here are a few suggestions from doctors, physiotherapists and athletics trainers.

Toe the towel. To stretch and strengthen ankle muscles, sit on the floor and loop a towel around the ball of your foot while holding the ends of the towel in your hands. Alternately point your toes up and down while pulling the ends of the towel towards your face and keeping your leg straight. Repeat several times with both feet.

Toe the towel again. Only this time don't move your toes. Lean back with the towel looped around your foot until you feel the stretch in the calf muscle. Hold for 15 seconds and repeat several times.

Use the steps. To stretch your calves, stand on the bottom step of a staircase and hold the rail for balance. Move one foot back so that the ball of the foot is at the edge of the step and your heel hangs off the back. Then, with both knees slightly bent, drop your heel below the step and feel a stretch in the back of your lower leg. Hold for 30 seconds, then switch legs.

Sit on the bed. Actually, sit with one leg stretched out on the bed and hang the other leg over the side. Then lean forwards until you feel the stretch in your hamstring (the back of the thigh) and hold for

the day. But keep the ice off the affected area for at least as long as you keep it on. Ice constricts blood vessels, and it's not good to constrict your blood vessels for too long. You could kill living tissue in the area.

Note: People with heart disease, diabetes and circulatory disorders should use ice with caution, and then only with the consent of a doctor.

Follow with heat. After starting the ice, you can switch to heat for acute soreness or strain, Folkerts says. People usually prefer heat; it's more relaxing. The heat dilates blood vessels and promotes healing. Remember not to switch from ice to heat too soon, or the injured area may swell up.

Wrap it up. An stretchy crepe bandage will keep the swelling down. Just be careful not to wrap too tightly, Dr Levy warns, or you could cause swelling below the injured area.

---

10 to 15 seconds. Repeat several times, then switch positions and stretch the other hamstring.

Stand on one leg. To stretch your quadriceps (the front of the thigh) muscles, stand on one leg and hold your opposite foot so that the ankle is touching your buttocks and your knee points toward the floor. Hold for 10 seconds. Repeat five times with each leg.

Reverse the conventional sit-up. For a safer way to strengthen abdominal muscles, lie back with your arms at your sides or your fingers on your stomach. Then bend your knees and raise them above your chest. Lower your legs slowly while concentrating on your abdominal muscles. Repeat 5 to 10 times.

Reach back. For a good shoulder stretch, place one arm, with elbow bent, behind your

head, and using the opposite hand, gently pull your elbow behind your head.

Reach around. Another good shoulder stretch is to hold one arm, with elbow bent, across your midriff and use the opposite hand to gently pull the arm across the front of your body.

Stretch your wrists. Make a fist, then span or spread your fingers as far as possible. Relax. Repeat three or four times.

Stretch your forearms. Hold your arms straight out in front of your body with your palms facing down. Bend your hands up, so that your palms face away from you. Hold that stretch for 5 seconds. Then bend your hands down, so that your palms are facing towards you. Hold that stretch for 5 seconds. Repeat three or four times.

Put your feet up. If you've injured your foot or lower leg, raise the injured part higher than your heart to prevent blood from pooling and causing swelling, says former football trainer Bob Reese.

Rub in some arnica. This herbal remedy is exceptionally good for muscles that have been overworked or strained, says clinical herbalist Douglas Schar. 'When people overdo it at the gym or get over-enthusiastic about re-arranging the furniture, and find themselves paying for the exertion the next morning, arnica is just what the doctor ordered.' Lotions are available at health food stores and at some pharmacies. Test a small patch of skin before applying, as some people are allergic to arnica.

Take crampbark for stress-related muscle pain. Stress affects different people in different ways, and some find it goes straight to their muscles. Cramps and cricks mysteriously arise when the stress is on. If your muscle pain is stress related, says Schar, try using crampbark (also known as black haw or *Virbunum prunifolium*) to soothe the discomfort. It works best in tincture form: take 5ml tincture 1:5 three times a day.

Use heat-penetrating rubs carefully. Our experts don't all agree on this point. Heat-penetrating rubs are valuable because they keep the temperature of the affected area up, says Dr Levy. But athletics trainers, for the most part, are less enthusiastic: 'they can irritate the skin,' says sports medic Mike McCormick, 'and they give a false sense of security – they warm, but it's only surface warmth. They don't warm the muscles.'

Use an anti-inflammatory. Take aspirin or ibuprofen. These over-the-counter nonsteroidal anti-inflammatory drugs – or NSAIDs – will help to reduce pain and inflammation, says Dr Percy.

Note. Avoid aspirin if you're under 16. If you are over 75, or you have a history of stomach ulcers or frequent indigestion, you should not use any anti-inflammatory without checking with your doctor first. Check too if you are already on other medications.

Incorporate variety. If you're a walker experiencing sore lower leg muscles, add some swimming or cycling (which works the upper legs) so that you can continue to exercise while your lower leg muscles heal, says Dr Mirkin. It's a good idea to swap exercises each day, following a 'hard-easy/hard-easy' routine, because it takes 48 hours for muscles to recover.

Stretch. For cramps and spasms, if you gradually stretch the muscle out, you'll get it to relax. Stretching exercises can take care of any current soreness, as well as prevent pain in the future. Stretching is important

Cure a midnight calf cramp

If you wake from a deep sleep with cramp in your calf muscle, you want to get rid of the pain and, hopefully, stop a recurrence later in the night.

Stretch in bed. If the cramp is mild, you might get away with stretching the calf muscle in bed by contracting the opposing muscles in the front of your lower leg. Do this by drawing your foot up in the direction of your knee, assisting with your hand if necessary. If that doesn't work, there's nothing for it but getting out of bed and walking around the bedroom.

Lean into the wall. Stand a metre or so away from a wall, keeping your heels flat and your legs straight. Lean into the wall in front of you as you support yourself with your hands. Hold for 10 seconds and repeat several times.

Massage the cramp. Massage the calf by rubbing upwards from the ankle towards your heart. If night cramps are a regular problem, try doing this before you go to sleep. If you often get night calf cramps, do this exercise every evening before you go to bed.

Loosen the covers. The weight of heavy blankets on your legs could be partly to blame.

Use an electric blanket. An electric blanket can do more than keep you warm all over on cold winter nights; it can keep your calf muscles warm and pain-free, too

Sleep on your side. Sleeping on your front with your legs straight out can trigger cramping. Instead, sleep on your side with your knees bent and a pillow between them.

Get enough calcium. A calcium deficiency can make muscles contract strongly. The UK recommended daily intake for calcium is 700mg.

See your doctor. If you get persistent night cramps, see your doctor to rule out any underlying problem. She may also be able to prescribe quinine tablets to relieve muscle cramps. If you already have intermittent claudication, (see *Leg Pain*, page 380) and you develop night cramps, see your doctor **urgently**, as this may indicate a significant worsening of your condition.

because muscles injured during exercise shorten during the healing process, Dr Mirkin explains. And unless the muscles are then lengthened, they will remain tight and thus are more likely to be injured or torn (see box, *Stretch to strengthen*, page 402).

WHEN TO CONSULT A DOCTOR

Most of the time, the pain of a sudden muscle cramp, strain, or even extreme soreness is a lot more serious than the injury. But not always.

Cramping could be the result of a nerve injury, says sports medicine expert Allan Levy. Or, in rare cases, it could be the result of thrombophlebitis – inflammation of a vein (see *Phlebitis*, page 443).

A strain may not even be what it seems. 'This is very rare,' says Dr Levy, 'but I once had a patient who thought he had badly strained a thigh muscle on an exercise. It never improved, and when we finally performed surgery we found a large tumour in the muscle.' The point here isn't to scare you, but to make you aware that muscle problems that take on abnormal characteristics and linger *may* be more serious. Consult your doctor.

Muscle pains can occur in other conditions too: infections like flu or Lyme disease; rheumatic disorders like polymyalgia or lupus; autoimmune disorders like dermatomyositis; or electrolyte disturbances causing potassium or calcium deficiencies. Consult your doctor if muscle pains persist or are associated with other symptoms. Certain medications can also cause muscle pains, for example cholesterol-lowering drugs, diuretics and some treatments for hypertension. See your doctor before stopping any prescribed medication, though.

Give muscles a massage. Rub gently and, as with exercise, stop if it hurts, Dr Levy says. You also may want to warm the sore area before massaging it.

Wear warm clothing. If you're exercising in cold weather and feel yourself getting stiff and a little sore, warm up by putting on more layers. You may be able to halt muscle problems before they start.

Loosen your clothing. If you feel a leg cramp coming on, try removing lycra tights or any other snug clothing to give your muscles more room.

Stand up. It's simple, but sometimes standing up is all it takes to stop a cramp in the leg or foot, says Dr Levy.

Change positions. Whether you're bent over a keyboard typing or bent over a bicycle pedalling, your wrists and forearms are vulnerable to cramping and soreness, says chiropractor Scott Donkin. But the difference between cyclists and office workers is that when cyclists buy bikes, there's usually a salesperson there to make sure they choose the bike that best fits them. But office workers, who have hands and fingers of different sizes, use the same office equipment. With the wide choice of ergonomic accessories now available, all it takes is a little research and testing to find a set-up that puts you in a comfortable, ergonomically correct position.

'The wrist and hands should be used in what is known as the neutral position,' says Dr Donkin. 'In this position, the wrist is bent neither forwards, backwards, inwards or outwards.'

If you have long hands and fingers, you can reduce the strain by adjusting the keyboard to a more horizontal position (flat with the work surface) as long as it does not put your arms or shoulders in a strained position. For those who have short hands and fingers, a higher incline on the keyboard or calculator will make the keys easier to reach.

Repeat the activity that made you sore. It sounds counterproductive, but it helps. 'Do the activity again the very next day,' Reese says, 'but with much less intensity. It will help to work out some of the soreness.'

Be realistic. Running is one of the riskiest sports for injuries. If it always makes you sore, then you may have to find another form of exercise.

Slow down instead of stopping suddenly. After hard exercise or physical work, the bloodstream is loaded with lactic acid, which collects in the bloodstream when there is a lack of oxygen, explains Dr Mirkin. When the acid reaches high levels, it disrupts normal chemical reactions of the muscles and can make your muscles hurt.

'The most effective way to clear the bloodstream is to continue exercising at a slow, relaxed pace,' he says. This may lessen immediate soreness, but it won't protect you from soreness the next day. That soreness is caused by torn muscle fibres.

Change your shoes. If you're wearing the wrong kind of shoes or wearing shoes that don't fit well, that could explain the foot, leg and even back pains you feel while exercising, says McCormick.

Be patient. The more serious the injury – a badly pulled hamstring, say – the more patience you will need to ensure a relapse-free recovery.

Lose weight. Chronic sore muscles and muscle strains could be due to having to move extra weight.

Drink up. Dehydration often contributes to cramp, says McCormick. It's vital to drink plenty of fluids, before, during and after physical activity.

Nail Problems

20 strategies for strong, healthy nails

One of the first things many doctors do when examining a patient is look at their nails. 'There is so much you can find out,' says family doctor Stephen Amiel. 'It's the nearest I get to being Sherlock Holmes. Lifestyle, bad habits, mental state, underlying illnesses, nutritional state, occupation – all can be revealed by someone's nails. My biggest coup was working out that a patient was a left-handed guitarist (not much use medically, but it impressed him mightily!).'

Three problems commonly affect our nails – brittleness, discoloration and ridges. The most common causes of brittle nails are ageing, frequent hand washing and exposure to household cleaning products. Nail varnish can also play a role. Brittle nails can be hard or soft. Hard, brittle nails are caused by dehydration – too little moisture in and around nails. Soft, brittle nails result from immersion in water, which leaves nails waterlogged. The water makes nails expand and then shrink, eventually becoming brittle.

Nail discoloration can be caused by a variety of conditions, from a reaction to medicines to nail infection. Smoking can stain nails brown, while some nail varnishes can leave them tinged an unnatural orangy-yellow. But the most common cause of discoloured nails is a fungal infection under the nail; this tends to cause yellowish discoloration and affects toenails more often than fingernails.

Nail ridges can be vertical or horizontal. Vertical ridges are generally perfectly normal and related to ageing or genes. But severe ridging and cracking or the sudden onset of vertical ridges warrants a visit to the doctor, as these could be a sign of poor general health or nutritional deficiency. They may also indicate rheumatoid arthritis or a circulatory or kidney disorder.

Horizontal ridges can occur as a result of hormonal changes, genetics and the way your body uses calcium. They can also result from stress, illness or malnutrition. Some ridges are due to the nervous habit of picking at or chewing the nail and cuticle. Horizontal ridges on the toenails of footballers and tennis players are often the result of sports injury.

Less commonly, the nails can be pitted by psoriasis or alopecia, or distorted by anaemia, liver disease, lung disease or heart problems.

Brittle Nails

Reach for hand cream. Apply a moisturizing cream to your hands and nails after each washing and drying. The cream traps moisture, keeping your hands and nails from drying out, says dermatologist Paul Kechijian.

WHEN TO CONSULT A DOCTOR

Don't ignore a fungal nail infection. If left untreated, it can spread to other nails and eventually make everyday activities, such as walking or writing, painful and difficult. See your doctor if:

• you notice unexplained changes in the colour of your nail;

• your nails look abnormally thick;

• your nails are painful or tender;

• the skin surrounding the nail is swollen;

• the nail appears to have separated from the nail bed.

A fungus is best caught and treated in its early stages. Treating nail fungus can take up to six months, so be patient. If the discoloration is a symptom of something more serious, early detection is even more important. Discoloured nails might indicate heart disease, anaemia or other illness. Sudden nail changes (such as the appearance of nail ridges) or swelling and pain could signal a serious problem and warrant a visit to the doctor. If your nails hurt or affect the everyday function of your hands, then you should also have them looked at.

Choose a sweet smell. Over-the-counter moisturizers come in a range of scents and textures. Find one you really like, says dermatologist Dee Anna Glaser, as you'll be more likely to use it. She also encourages people with brittle nails to keep small tubes of moisturizer wherever they'll need them so that they can apply it after every hand-washing. Stash tubes by any basins or sinks at home as well as in your glove compartment and your desk drawer at work.

Keep nails short and sweet. Longer nails are more vulnerable to cracking or getting caught and tearing. Dr Kechijian also recommends cutting your nails after a bath, when they're softer and less likely to break.

Eat a well-balanced diet. Brittle nails can be the result of something you are – or aren't – eating, says Dr Glaser. Eat a well-balanced diet and take a daily multivitamin/mineral supplement. Avoid fad diets in which only a few foods are eaten, or which exclude certain groups of foods.

Double glove. If washing dishes is a daily job, Dr Kechijian suggests buying several pairs of cotton gloves to wear under your rubber gloves. The vinyl exterior of the dishwashing gloves keeps the water and cleaning

KITCHEN CURES

Rub oil or thick hand cream into your nails while applying your hand moisturizer for better results, says dermatologist Audrey Kunin. You can buy expensive creams or use vegetable oil or margarine.

Dermatologist Dee Anna Glaser recommends this extra-soothing night-time treatment. Before you go to bed, apply vegetable oil to your hands, then put on vinyl gloves or wrap your hands in cling film to keep the oil off the bedding. The gloves or plastic wrap will also force the oil to penetrate and moisturize your skin.

products off your nails, while the cotton gloves absorb sweat so that your nails and hands don't get soggy inside the glove.

Avoid acetone removers. 'Acetone nail polish removers are stronger, but they can take moisture out of your nails and make them brittle,' says dermatologist Ralph Daniel. Instead, try a nail polish remover like Cutex acetone-free nail poish remover.

Add some calcium. A lack of calcium in the diet is another cause of brittle nails, says dermatologist Audrey Kunin. Calcium supplements can work wonders for strengthening nails. If your diet doesn't include three helpings of milk, cheese or yoghurt every day, then take a 500mg calcium supplement every day if you are under 50, or 1000mg if you are over 50.

Give soya a try. Dermatologist Boni Elewski says that just five grams of soya protein a day helps to toughen up brittle nails. Try including tofu or soya milk, available in supermarkets, into your diet. A 250ml glass of soya milk provides six grams of soya protein and is cholesterol-free.

Take biotin. Biotin (vitamin H) can increase the thickness of nails by 25 per cent, according to a Swiss study. 'Biotin doesn't work in every case, but I've found it effective in a third to half of the cases I've seen,' says Dr Daniel. Good dietary sources of biotin include soya flour, rice, barley and nuts. Supplements are available: try taking 300mcg of biotin four to six times a day with food. You should notice an increase in your nail thickness within six months.

Check your medicines. Some common drugs, such as diuretics, can cause dehydration and could worsen a pre-existing case of brittle nails. Check with your doctor if you think your drugs are affecting your nails.

Discoloured Nails

Keep clean. 'Clean, dry feet resist disease,' says Dr Kechijian. 'A strict regime of washing the feet with antibacterial soap and water every night before bedtime, and remembering to dry them thoroughly, is the best way to prevent an infection.' Be sure to check your feet and toes regularly for signs of infection.

Cut nails short. 'Longer nails can get caught on things or rub against tighter shoes, which can cause the nail to lift from its bed,' says dermatologist Coyle Connolly. 'That opening can let fungus in.' Clip toenails straight across so that the nail doesn't extend beyond the nail bed.

Keep them cool. Use a good quality foot powder and wear shoes that fit properly and are made of materials that breathe, says Dr Daniel. 'Sweating makes matters worse, since it creates a warm, moist environment – perfect for spreading nail fungus.'

Wash your hands. Fungal infection can spread from your feet to your hands. So wash your hands after inspecting your feet, says Dr Connolly.

Be wary of nail products. Ordinarily, any moisture that collects underneath the surface of the nail passes through the porous structure of the nail and evaporates. Acrylic nails applied to the top of the nail may impede that, however. Trapped water can become stagnant and unhealthy, ideal conditions for fungi to thrive, says Dr Daniel.

Also, the pigments in some varnishes can turn nails an ugly yellowish orange. Red nail varnish is the most likely to stain, followed by brown shades. One simple remedy is to vary your colour choices – alternating lighter shades of nail polish with your reds and browns from time to time, suggests beautician Barbara Bealer.

Bring on the bleach. Bleaching nails at home is relatively simple. Try using hydrogen peroxide every few days for three weeks to get your nails back to their normal colour. Beautician Rita Johnson suggests mixing one tablespoon of hydrogen peroxide with three

KITCHEN CURES

Superficial staining of the nail responds quite well to wiping clean, dry nails with a half-water, half-fresh-lemon-juice solution. Allow the nails to dry and repeat two or three times, says beautician Joni Keim Loughran. Moisturize afterwards as lemon juice can dry out nails and skin. Skip a day or two and then repeat the process until the discoloration has gone.

tablespoons of baking soda. Apply to nails (underneath and over tops) with a cotton wool ball. Leave on for three to five minutes, then rinse with warm water and apply hand lotion.

Nail Ridges

Buff them. Gently buff your nails with a nail buffer to minimize the ridges, suggests Dr Glaser. But be gentle. Don't completely buff out the nail ridges, since over-zealous buffing can weaken the nail plate.

Eat a well-balanced diet. Ridged nails can be the result of something lacking in your diet, says Dr Glaser. 'When people come into my surgery with severe nail changes, I ask for their dietary history to make sure that they aren't on some faddy diet that's keeping them from getting their recommended daily allowance of vitamins and minerals,' she says. If you're not eating a well-balanced diet, then a proper diet and perhaps a vitamin supplement might benefit your nails.

NAPPY RASH

10 easy solutions

Nappy rash can interrupt the peaceful routine of an otherwise carefree baby, and it won't do much for a parent's quality of life either. Babies have a knack of making their problems their parents' problems, and if your baby has nappy rash, you'll certainly know about it.

During the first year or two of a baby's life, just about every parent shares in the nappy rash experience at least once. It's not surprising, given that the most common rash-triggering irritants come from what is found in baby's nappy – bowel movements and urine. Most nappy rashes go away by themselves within a day or so, but some can last for days.

Breastfed babies have less nappy rash than bottle-fed babies (they tend after the first three months to pass fewer stools than bottle-fed babies, and they are less likely to develop sensitive skin or eczema), and this resistance continues long after a baby is weaned. In some babies, nappy rash may be a harbinger of future skin problems such as eczema or sensitive skin. If your baby has nappy rash, here's how to clear it up.

Give it some air – or water. The oldest advice is sometimes still the best. 'Give that baby's bottom some air,' says childcare expert Anne Price.

Simply take the baby's nappy off and lay her chest down with her face turned to one side, on a towel on top of a waterproof sheet. Leave her

The 'bead bottom' mystery

An article in a medical journal tells of parents reporting a strange nappy rash that looks like 'small shiny beads' covering their babies' bottoms. Doctors investigating the mysterious outbreak of 'bead bottom' noticed that the affected infants all wore super-absorbent disposable nappies. Was there a connection? Yes. The 'beads' are actually the gelling material that makes super-absorbent nappies so absorbent. Small amounts of the material can pass through the top sheet of the nappy and end up on the infant's skin. Doctors say that the material is non-toxic and nothing to worry about.

lying on her chest as long as you're there to keep an eye on her. Try and do this for an hour or so several times a day until her bottom is healed, advises family doctor Stephen Amiel. Another option is to put the baby in a basin or bath of lukewarm water for several minutes every time you change her nappy. This keeps her bottom clean and may comfort her, too.

Wash with herbal tea. Nothing is more pathetic than a baby with a bad case of nappy rash, says clinical herbalist Douglas Schar. Babies express their misery through tears and it's enough to make a grown-up cry too. But herbal medicine can come to the rescue. A strong brew of calendula tea, regularly applied, will quickly clear up the condition. Add two tablespoons of dried calendula flowers to 500ml of water and simmer in a covered pan for 20 minutes. Strain the brew, use it to wash baby's bottom every time you change the nappy, and the inflammation will quickly subside, says Schar. Or buy calendula cream at the health food store and apply several times a day.

Don't give your baby beer and curry. Spicy foods, alcohol and acidic fruits might affect the quality of your breast milk and cause the baby's urine and stool to be more irritant to the skin. Experiment with your diet, suggests Dr Amiel.

Let super nappies come to the rescue. Super-absorbent disposable nappies are a lifesaver in your baby's battle for a dry bottom. 'I think they're the best thing there is for preventing nappy rash,' says paediatrician Morris Green.

Studies confirm this observation. Nappies containing absorbent gelling material significantly reduce skin wetness and leave skin closer to its

WHEN TO CONSULT A DOCTOR

Stubborn nappy rash may be due to thrush (candida). The skin is usually more red than with normal nappy rash, your baby is unhappier when you change him or her, and the rash may extend into the skin folds or have small satellite patches at its margins. The baby may have white thrush spots in the mouth and, if you are breastfeeding, you may have sore nipples. See your doctor for an anti-fungal cream, oral medication or both. A mild steroid may be combined with the anti-fungal cream to reduce inflammation.

Occasionally, a bacterial infection may affect the nappy area. The skin will tend to be particularly warm, red and tender, and the baby will be miserable and possibly feverish. There may be small, pus-filled spots. See your doctor immediately for antibiotics.

---

normal pH than other disposables or cloth nappies. Don't wait too long between changes, though. Some parents wait until disposable nappies are saturated, which actually increases the baby's risk of nappy rash.

Change often. Change your baby as soon as you notice a dirty nappy, says Dr Amiel, and if she already has nappy rash, give her a clean nappy up to 12 times a day. Disposable nappies may have chemicals in the lining that can irritate certain babies. Try a different brand, or change to cotton towelling nappies.

If you do use cotton nappies, make sure you wash them in non-biological detergents, rinse them at least twice and tumble dry rather than use fabric softeners. Eco-friendly detergents are not necessarily skin-friendly ones, notes Dr Amiel.

Give fabric nappies a vinegar rinse. Nappy rash enzymes are most active in a high-pH environment, which often exists in cloth nappies after washing, says Price. To counter this, add four tablespoons of vinegar to four litres of water for the final rinse. Or try a nappy laundering service, suggests Price. 'They go to a lot of trouble to get the pH balance right, and they're not all that expensive. If you're using cloth nappies and your baby has a bad rash, I recommend giving them a try.'

Cleanse gently. Don't use economy baby wipes that contain alcohol because they can burn irritated skin and worsen the condition. Instead, choose thick, soft alcohol-free brands (Huggies, Pampers and Johnson's are all good). The simplest cleanser is cotton wool dipped in warm water.

Or use warm water in a plant sprayer bottle to rinse the baby's bottom before patting dry with a muslin cloth.

Don't throw the baby into the bathwater. Even special babycare bath products can irritate some babies' skin. If your baby's skin seems to be sensitive, use a dermatological cream like aqueous cream as a soap substitute, or just use water alone, says Dr Amiel.

Blow-dry the bottom. Keeping the nappy area clean promotes healing, but drying with a towel can irritate sensitive skin. 'Try a blow-dryer,' says paediatric nurse practitioner Linda Jonides. Dry the nappy area with a hair dryer set on 'low', which saves rubbing wet skin. When the area is dry, apply a zinc oxide ointment like Sudocrem. Petroleum jelly such as Vaseline also provides a protective coating, even on sore, red skin. Don't dust baby's bottom with baby powder as this can trigger breathing problems in little ones.

Make the cranberry connection. When urine and faeces mix in the nappy area, the result is a high pH that irritates the skin and promotes nappy rash. Unorthodox as it may sound, Jonides suggests giving 50ml of cranberry juice to older infants; this leaves an acid residue in the urine, helping to lower pH and reduce irritation.

NAUSEA AND VOMITING

13 stomach-soothing solutions

The world is full of things that make our stomachs turn. Depending on the situation, anything from the smell of hard boiled eggs to giving blood to opening a credit card statement can make you feel like retching. And when that twisting, turning gut becomes too much to bear, you throw up. Below are tips to help you keep nausea in check before you actually vomit. If it's too late, and you've already lost your lunch, there are tips to nurse your stomach – and the rest of you – back to good health.

Sip on syrup. If you're not *that* nauseated, try a spoonful of golden syrup. The cola syrup concentrate used to make fizzy drinks at home seems to work really well, too, says pharmacist Robert Warren.

Choose clear liquids. Even if you crave food, stick to clear liquids like tea and juice, says gastroenterologist Kenneth Koch. Drink the liquids

WHEN TO CONSULT A DOCTOR

There are many diseases that can cause chronic nausea, says gastroenterologist Kenneth Koch. If your nausea doesn't disappear in a day or two, it's a good idea to see your doctor.

Prolonged vomiting could also indicate something serious is going on, and may itself have serious consequences – dehydration and, if very violent, tearing of the lining of the oesophagus (gullet). If you are vomiting a lot, or it's bloody, seek medical advice, says A&E doctor Stephen Bezruchka. You should also see a doctor if you've gone 24 hours without being able to keep any food or fluids down and nothing seems to help, adds Dr Koch. Furthermore, if your thirst is severe and you're not urinating very much – and especially if you feel light-headed when you stand up – see a doctor, as these are all signs of dehydration.

On the other hand, if you know it's flu, or suspect something you've eaten, you might try and last a bit longer. Young and middle-aged adults who are otherwise healthy can easily manage 24 hours or even more of vomiting without harm, even if they're keeping nothing down. On the other hand, vomiting in babies, the frail elderly, and anyone with known chronic heart, lung or kidney disease, cancer or diabetes should be checked by a doctor after a maximum of 12 hours.

Nausea or vomiting associated with crushing or pressing central chest pain may indicate a heart attack. **Call 999**. This is one case of nausea where aspirin is a good idea, as it protects the heart against further damage. Take one 300mg or four 75mg tablets immediately.

You should also seek **immediate** medical attention if the person vomiting is drowsy or unconscious, is complaining of very severe headache, or has a rash that does not fade on pressure (see the glass test for meningitis, *Rashes*, page 464).

warm or at room temperature, not cold, so as to avoid further shock to your stomach. Drink no more than 30 to 60ml at a time. One good choice is peppermint tea: mint has a very relaxing effect on the stomach.

Try a flat fizzy. As our experts advise against both cold and carbonated drinks, do as A&E doctor Stephen Bezruchka suggests. Leave fizzy drinks – such as cola, ginger ale or lemonade – to stand until flat and lukewarm. To speed up the process, stir the drink until it goes flat.

Eat starchy foods first. If you need something to eat, and your nausea isn't too bad, eat light carbohydrates in small amounts – toast or crackers, for instance, Dr Koch says. As your stomach starts to settle, graduate to light protein, like chicken breast or fish. Fatty foods are the last thing to add to your diet. If your problem is not nausea but vomiting, start with jelly. Then follow the progression described above to introduce other foods back into your diet.

Take some medicine. Pepto-Bismol is good for stomach upsets caused by indigestion. It's slightly constipating, so it may help if you have associated diarrhoea. Other antacids may help, too, but avoid aspirin-containing so-called stomach settlers like Alka-Selzer, which can irritate an inflamed stomach further.

Find relief in the meadow. The herb meadowsweet can be quite effective in reducing nausea, says doctor and herbalist Lois Johnson. To make a soothing cup of meadowsweet tea, mix a tablespoon of dried herb per cup of boiling water, and steep for five to 10 minutes before straining. Then sip slowly. Rosemary is another good herb to add to the mixture.

End it all. One of the most effective ways to stop nausea is to let yourself vomit. At the very least, you'll gain a temporary respite from that queasy feeling. We don't recommend *making* yourself vomit, however.

Replace vital fluids and nutrients.
Anyone vomiting a lot needs to avoid becoming dehydrated, says Dr Koch. You lose a lot of fluid vomiting, so the best thing you can do is drink water, tea and weak juices to replace them. Lucozade, Dioralyte or juices like apple and cranberry also help to replace nutrients flushed out through vomiting.

The sugar and electrolytes in non-diet colas and lemonade makes them a suitable (and cheaper) alternative to things like Lucozade and Dioralyte. Children especially may prefer the taste. Remember to stir out the fizz.

Sip – don't gulp. Sipping fluids in tiny swallows lets your irritated stomach adjust, advises Dr Koch.

Do just *one* thing

Try ginger. Herbalist Daniel Mowrey swears by it. Take it in capsule form rather than eating fresh ginger – the flavour is too strong for most people with nausea. Ginger ale or gingernuts may work if your symptoms are very mild.

You could also try taking ginger 30 minutes before you begin an activity that you know will cause nausea (like going on a boat). Take two 500mg capsules of dried ginger or drink an equivalent amount of ginger tea.

Find the pressure point

The Chinese have known for centuries that acupressure is an effective, painless, drugless remedy for nausea. The idea is to use it before you start vomiting, says acupuncturist Joseph Helms. Apply pressure to the webbed area between your thumb and index finger on either hand. Use firm, deep pressure and a rapid massaging movement for several minutes, he says. Using the same kind of motion and pressure, rub with your thumb or thumbnail on the top of your foot between the tendons of the second and third toes. Your nausea should ease off after a few minutes.

Check your urine. If your urine is deep yellow, you're not drinking enough. The paler it gets, the better you're doing to prevent dehydration.

A herbal soak. A herbal foot or hand soak can be very soothing to someone who is vomiting. Mix a tablespoon of fresh grated root ginger or powdered ginger with a litre of hot water, and let it cool. Then soak your hands or feet in the soothing liquid until the vomiting subsides.

NECK PAIN

23 ways to relieve the stiffness

When undue strain isn't placed on your neck, its vertebrae and muscles do a pretty good job of holding up your head. But your head weighs four or five kilos – a pretty heavy load sitting on a relatively small structure. A common cause of neck pain is holding your head in an awkward position for a long time, says former physiotherapist Joanne Griffin.

Some people, because of their occupations, are more at risk than others. Hairdressers, for example, work in a bent-over position all day long, observes neurologist Robert Kunkel. Whatever your job or lifestyle, neck pain can be eased by replacing bad habits with good and giving your neck regular exercise. And most tension headaches arise from the neck and shoulders, says family doctor Stephen Amiel. So look after your neck and your head will thank you, too.

Use ice. Ice helps to reduce swelling, so it's a good choice when stiffness settles in, Griffin says. If your neck has been slightly injured, apply an ice pack, wrapped in a thin cloth to protect your skin, for 15 minutes. Repeat every few hours as needed.

Use heat. After ice has reduced any inflammation, heat is a wonderful soother. Try a heating pad or a hot shower.

Press on the painful spot. Relieve muscle tension by applying moderate pressure to the area for three minutes. Don't press as hard as you can, but use your fingertips to exert steady, constant pressure on the affected point. At the end of three minutes, your pain should have improved dramatically.

Take a painkiller. Over-the-counter anti-inflammatories such as aspirin or ibuprofen will help to reduce pain and inflammation. Simple analgesics like paracetamol aren't as effective, but if you can't take anti-inflammatories, they will certainly help. And if your pain is particularly bad, says Dr Amiel, combine the two sorts, rather than exceeding the recommended daily dose of either.

Take essential fatty acids. Essential fatty acids, found in certain plant oils, makes the body less prone to inflammation and can therefore help to reduce neck pain. Flaxseed (or linseed) is one such oil and contains alpha linolenic acid, a substance similar to the omega-3 fatty acids found in fish. Take two teaspoons a day, recommends Mark Gostine, a specialist in pain management. Refrigerate flaxseed oil, as it spoils quickly.

Other options include evening primrose oil, borage oil, blackcurrant seed oil and hempseed oil. 'Hempseed oil is the best all around essential fatty acid seed oil,' says clinical herbalist Douglas Schar. 'A teaspoon a day is plenty.' But don't expect instant relief, he adds. These oils can take several weeks to work and should be seen as a long-term investment in reducing your symptoms.

If you like it fishy. Oily fish, such as salmon, trout, mackerel, herring and sardines, contain omega-3 fats. Among other health benefits, these fats have natural anti-inflammatory substances that can help to relieve the pain of arthritis and prevent the condition becoming worse, says Dr Amiel. Daily supplements are a suitable alternative if you can't eat oily fish two or three times a week. A recent study in the *British Journal of Nutrition* suggested that 750mg daily is sufficient, as long as each dose contains at least 3mg of vitamin E, although some sources suggest far higher doses are necessary to see an effect.

WHEN TO CONSULT A DOCTOR

If you have severe neck pain, pain that comes on suddenly or lasting neck pain, you need to see your doctor. Seek medical attention immediately if you have severe neck pain following an accident or blow to the head. You may have sustained a whiplash injury or damaged a vertebra.

You should also see a doctor if, in association with neck pain, you develop weakness, numbness or pins and needles in your arms or legs. Damage to the vertebrae or discs between them may be putting pressure on the nerves or spinal cord.

If your neck is painful or stiff and you also have a fever, a rash or vomiting, you should contact a doctor urgently. Swollen glands in the neck can often cause pain and stiffness, but your doctor will want to rule out meningitis.

As a general rule, persistent neck pain warrants professional medical evaluation. It's extremely remote, but it's possible that neck pain could be a sign that there's a tumour on the spine.

Turn to herbs. Neck pain can come from an old or new injury (inflammation) or from a muscle spasm (tension and stress). Herbal medicine offers remedies in both instances, says Schar. For inflammation, try taking white willow bark. Like aspirin, white willow reduces inflammation and makes moving the neck a lot easier. For tension-related neck cramp, try valerian or cramp bark. All of these can be bought at health food stores and should be taken according to label instructions.

Give glucosamine a try. Some evidence suggests that this natural sugar substance may help to relieve pain in osteoarthritic joints, although the evidence of benefit in soft tissue injury is not clear. Dr Gostine recommends taking 1500mg a day to ease neck pain, but be patient; it can take several weeks before you feel an effect. Chondroitin is another supplement which, like glucosamine, is derived from cartilage. It too shows promise in relieving symptoms of neck pain caused by arthritis. You need to take 800mg or more a day to benefit.

Take your vitamins. Antioxidant vitamins such as vitamins C and E, taken on a regular basis, can help to prevent the painful deterioration of joints in your neck and elsewhere in your body. Vegetable oils, wheatgerm oil, nuts and green leafy vegetables are the main dietary sources of vitamin E. Fortified cereals often contain vitamin E too. Fresh fruit and vegetables are the best source of vitamin C. If your diet is deficient in either of these vitamins, supplements are available. Take 1000mg of vitamin C and 250mg of vitamin E per day.

Sit in a firm chair. In the words of the song, the backbone is connected to the neck bone. Sitting in a chair without good back support can make neck problems worse and even cause new ones, says chiropractor Mitchell Price.

Support your lower back. Roll up a towel and place it against the small of your back when sitting. It will align your spine and provide support, says Griffin.

Take a break. Just as the feet need rest from constant standing, the neck needs a rest from constant sitting, says Griffin. Periodically stand up and walk around.

Keep your chin up. Keep your head level but pull your chin in as if you were making a double chin, says Griffin. Also, avoid lowering your head all the time when working at a desk or reading, she advises. This helps to prevent straining the muscles in the back of the neck.

Realign yourself. If you suffer from chronic neck and back problems, invest in some Alexander Technique lessons, says Dr Amiel. Developed over the past century, this technique helps you to rediscover how to move and support yourself, and how to perform daily tasks using your body's natural alignment in relation to gravity. To find a teacher in your area, contact the Society of Teachers of the Alexander Technique (STAT), 1st Floor, Linton House, 39–51 Highgate Road, London NW5 1RS; tel: 0845 230 7828; or visit their website at www.stat.org.uk.

Position your screen. If you look at a computer monitor all day, position it at eye level. If you force yourself to look up or down hour after hour, your neck may spasm, says Dr Price.

Get a telephone headset. Holding the telephone in the crook of your neck and shoulder so that you can talk and write at the same time puts your neck in an awkward position – an invitation to stiffness and pain.

Sleep on a firm mattress. A lot of neck problems begin, and worsen, with poor sleeping habits that put the spine out of alignment. Having a firm mattress is important, Dr Price says.

Get rid of your pillow. 'A lot of people with neck pain feel better sleeping flat – without a pillow,' says Dr Kunkel.

Exercise neck pain away

Here are some exercises to combat stiffness and prevent problems in the future. Do each exercise five times twice a day. Do the first three exercises for two weeks before starting the rest.

- Slowly tilt your head forwards as far as possible. Then tip it backwards as far as possible.

- Tilt your head towards one of your shoulders, while keeping your shoulder still. Straighten, then tilt towards the other shoulder.

- Slowly turn your head from side to side as far as possible.

- Place your hand on one side of your head while you push towards it with your head. Hold for five seconds, then relax. Repeat three times. Then do the same exercise on the other side.

- Do basically the same exercise as above, only provide slight resistance to the front of your head while you push your head forwards. Then provide slight resistance to the back of your head while you push your head backwards.

- Hold light weights – say, 1 to 2 kilos – in your hands while shrugging your shoulders. Keep your arms straight.

Or buy a cervical pillow. These pillows, available from specialist medical supply stores and online, give the neck proper support, says Dr Price.

Don't sleep on your stomach. This is bad not only for your back but also for your neck, says Dr Price. Instead, sleep in the foetal position – on your side with your knees up towards your chest.

Wrap up. When it's cold and damp outside, keep your neck warm. The weather can aggravate neck stiffness and pain, Dr Kunkel says.

Relax. Being tense can tighten the muscles in your neck and put you in pain. If you're under a lot of pressure, meditation or other relaxation techniques can help. CDs and cassettes are also available to teach you how to relax.

NIGHT BLINDNESS
9 ways to deal with the dark

Night blindness is that frightening time of day or night when an extreme change in light drastically reduces visibility. It affects everyone to some degree, because it usually takes a moment for the retina to adjust to changes in light, explains ophthalmologist Alan Laties.

But for some people, night blindness is more than momentary. Short-sighted people can be slower to adapt to the dark, says Dr Laties. Other people simply *can't* see in the dark because of a congenital form of night blindness, or because of eye conditions like glaucoma or cataract.

Unfortunately, doctors cannot prescribe ready cures for night blindness. But if you don't see well at night and your doctor has ruled out an eye disorder, our experts offer the following practical advice for driving safely at night, when night blindness poses the biggest problem.

Drive safely at night. On a clear day from the driver's seat, you can usually see 300 to 400m down a straight road, says research scientist Quinn Brackett. But at night with only your headlights as your guide, you can see only about 100m. So you need to give yourself every advantage.

Get a pair of night glasses. Millions of people wear glasses to improve their vision. Your pupils dilate in low light, making you naturally more nearsighted, so night driving can make a small degree of daytime myopia (nearsightedness) noticeable, or worsen undercorrected myopia. Glasses can also improve night myopia, which is defective night vision, especially of distant objects, says ophthalmologist Creig Hoyt.

Pilots say that they have more trouble seeing runways at night. To combat this problem, they often wear stronger glasses at night. What works for a pilot trying to land a plane on a narrow strip of tarmac should help you to keep you and your car on the road and out of the front garden. Consider wearing stronger glasses at night, or getting glasses for night driving – even if you don't wear glasses during the day.

Keep your headlights, and glasses, clean. Dirty headlights really reduce visibility and will make your problem worse, says safety researcher Charles Zegeer. Keep your glasses clean too. It's amazing how much dirt and grease people carry around on their glasses without noticing the impact it has on their night vision.

Take off the shades. Don't wear sunglasses at night or even at dusk. They will further reduce the light coming into your eyes, says Dr Brackett.

WHEN TO CONSULT A DOCTOR

If you have glaucoma, a condition of raised pressure within the eye, you may be taking drops which constrict the pupil. This will affect your eyes' ability to adapt in low light. Mention this to your doctor if you need to drive at night on a regular basis, in case there are alternative treatments. Don't stop your treatment, even temporarily, without consulting your doctor first, though.

Many older people find driving at night particularly difficult as a result of cataracts. Clouding of the lens of the eye by cataracts causes scattering of light as it enters the eye, so driving at night can be like looking through a windscreen in the rain when the wipers aren't working. Your optometrist or doctor will be able to tell you if you are developing cataracts and, if severe enough, they can easily be treated surgically by an ophthalmologist. Younger people may occasionally also develop cataracts, especially if they have diabetes.

Whatever your age and state of health, consult your doctor or optometrist if you're having problems with night vision that are not easily corrected by glasses. It's the best way to protect your vision.

Plan ahead. Careful route planning can make night driving easier and safer. When possible, choose dual carriageways or roads with little traffic.

Slow down. That will give you more time to react to any unexpected hazards. Increase your stopping distance to allow an extra few precious seconds between you and the car in front. Remember, the roads don't belong just to cars, but to walkers, runners, cyclists and wayward animals as well. It's your responsibility to watch for others sharing the road.

Respect the rain and fog. These two conditions make night driving especially dangerous, Zegeer says. He recommends keeping your dipped headlights on in fog for better visibility. If driving conditions become too bad, says Zegeer, pull off at a service area, garage or lay-by. But don't stop on the hard shoulder.

Look to the left. If you look towards the verge at the edge of the road, this will help you to avoid the glare of oncoming headlights.

Leave driving until tomorrow. If night blindness while driving is really a problem, drive during the day. Even on well-lit roads, such as in a town, night driving can still be hard for someone with night blindness.

NOSEBLEED

15 hints to stop the flow

Whether it's a boxer in the ring, a child hit on the nose by a football or an office worker who's walked into a door, nosebleeds can be alarming and are often painful.

Vast amounts of blood circulate through capillaries in the nose, so bleeding can be copious when blood vessels break. Nosebleeds can also occur when your mucous membranes become irritated by a cold, or by dry indoor heat in winter. People with high blood pressure or atherosclerosis (hardening of the arteries) are especially vulnerable to nosebleeds, as are those taking certain medications, such as anticoagulants, antiinflammatories and aspirin. Nose blowing, nose picking, allergies, excessive sneezing and foreign objects in the nose can also prompt it to bleed. But whatever the cause, there are several ways to stop most nosebleeds.

Blow the clot out. Before you try to stop your nosebleed, give your nose one – and only one – good, vigorous blow, says ear, nose and throat specialist Alvin Katz. That should remove any clots that are keeping the blood vessel open. A clot acts like a wedge in the door, he explains. Blood vessels have elastic fibres. If you can get the clot out, you can get the elastic fibres to contract around that tiny opening.

Then stop. Don't blow your nose again for at least twelve hours after a nosebleed. Give the broken blood vessel time to heal.

Pinch the fleshy part of your nose. As soon as you've blown your nose, use your thumb and forefinger to squeeze shut the soft part of the nose. Apply continuous pressure for five to seven minutes. If the bleeding doesn't stop, pinch again for another five to seven minutes. The bleeding should then stop.

Sit up straight. If you lie down or put your head back, you'll just swallow blood, says Dr Katz. If blood is trickling down the back of your nose into your mouth, lean forward slightly and spit it into a bowl.

Apply ice. An ice pack pack on the bridge of the nose can sometimes help, says general surgeon Christine Haycock, especially following injury. The cold causes blood vessels to narrow and reduces bleeding.

Don't pick. It takes a week to 10 days to completely heal the rupture in the blood vessel that caused your nose to bleed. Bleeding stops after the clot forms, but the clot becomes a scab as healing continues. If you pick your nose during the next week and knock the scab off, you'll trigger another nosebleed, says ear, nose and throat surgeon Jerald Principato.

Take iron? If you're prone to frequent, heavy nosebleeds, you may make yourself anaemic. Get your haemoglobin and iron stores checked by your doctor before taking iron supplements, says family doctor Stephen Amiel. 'A little bit of blood can look like an awful lot: it takes a lot of big nosebleeds to make an otherwise healthy person with a good diet anaemic.'

Watch your aspirin intake. Aspirin can interfere with clotting. If you're prone to nosebleeds, use paracetamol for pain and fever relief rather than over-the-counter aspirin. If you're taking aspirin on medical advice for heart or circulatory problems, consult your doctor.

Watch your salicylate intake, too. John Henderson, an ear, nose and throat surgeon, advises his patients to avoid foods high in salicylate, an aspirin-like substance. It is found in coffee, tea, almonds, apples, apricots, peppers, berry fruits, cherries, cloves, cucumbers, currants, grapes, mint, peaches, pickles, plums, raisins and tomatoes.

Watch your blood pressure. People with high blood pressure are more prone to nosebleeds, even though most nosebleeds are caused by other

WHEN TO CONSULT A DOCTOR

Nosebleeds can be serious. Head for the A&E department if:

- you've applied pressure for 10 to 15 minutes, but your nose is still bleeding;
- your nosebleed results from a head injury. This may indicate other skull or facial injuries. Bleeding that looks thin and watery could indicate the presence of cerebral fluid;
- you have been diagnosed with atherosclerosis or high blood pressure, and your nose has bled for more than 10 minutes;
- you find yourself bleeding from the back of the nose.

In rare instances, continuous bleeding may indicate the presence of a growth. If nosebleeds become more frequent and don't seem to be associated with a cold or irritation of the mucous membranes, see your doctor. See your doctor also if you have signs of bleeding elsewhere: unexplained bruising, blood in your urine or stools, black, tarry stools or bleeding gums.

things, says Dr Amiel. It's a good idea to get your blood pressure checked every few years, anyway, whether you get nosebleeds or not.

If you are already being treated for high blood pressure, follow your doctor's advice on taking medication, controlling your weight, eating a low cholesterol diet and stopping smoking, and get your blood pressure checked at least every six months.

Get plenty of vitamin C. Vitamin C is needed for the formation of collagen, a substance essential to the health of body tissue, says Dr Henderson. The collagen in the tissues of your upper respiratory tract helps mucus to stick where it's supposed to, creating a moist, protective lining for your sinuses and nose. Good sources of vitamin C are fresh fruits and vegetables, especially citrus fruit, kiwi fruit and leafy greens.

Try a humidifier. When you breathe, the moist lining in your nose works to humidify the air that reaches your lungs. It follows that when your surroundings are dry, your nose has to work harder. A humidifier helps to moisturize airways and tissue linings.

Or alternative sources of moisture. Keep nostrils moist by taking a shower and breathing deeply to get moisture into your nose, suggests Dr Amiel. Smear a little petroleum jelly inside your nostrils to keep them moist. A saline solution spray may also help. You can make your own solution by dissolving a teaspoon of table salt in a pint of boiled water.

Ask about your Pill. Anything that changes the oestrogen balance in your body – including menstruation and some oral contraceptives – can make you more prone to nosebleeds. If nosebleeds are a problem, mention it to your doctor when choosing your birth control pill.

Don't smoke. Smoking dries out the nasal cavity, says ear, nose and throat specialist Mark Baldree, making you more prone to nosebleeds.

OSTEOARTHRITIS

25 ways to end the aching

Osteoarthritis (OA) is a condition that affects the joints. Half of us will have x-ray evidence of OA by the time we're 65, and over 10 per cent of over 65s will have significant disability due to it. Many of us don't even realize we have it though, until an x-ray for an unrelated condition reveals it. OA is generally thought of as a degenerative disease, causing progressive loss of the cartilage that lines and lubricates our joints, but some of its symptoms arise from the body's attempts to repair the damage with the formation of irregular knobs of bone called osteophytes. The surface of the joint is damaged and the surrounding bone grows thicker.

Osteoarthritis is also known as degenerative joint disease. It affects about eight million people in the UK, although only one in eight of these asks for treatment. It can affect the fingers, knees, ankles, feet, hips, neck and spine, causing stiffness, swelling and pain. It is usually considered just a natural sign of ageing, the result of normal wear and tear on our joints, but the commonest form of OA, primary OA, usually begins in middle age. Secondary OA may result from a variety of insults to the joints including injury and overwork (that's where the wear and tear comes in), infection and inflammation from other joint diseases. Some of the factors that influence it, like heredity, are out of your control. Others, including numerous lifestyle decisions, can help to prevent and relieve the painful symptoms. Here are the best remedies that our experts have to offer.

Eat for the long term. Rather than focusing on individual nutrients, rheumatologist Justus Fiechtner recommends looking at the big picture as your best dietary approach. 'Keeping your weight under control is the best thing you can do to prevent osteoarthritis,' he says. 'Eating a well-balanced diet is the best way to get there.'

The Arthritis Research Campaign – www.arc.org.uk – has an excellent website with lots of valuable advice. Its three golden rules to help your arthritis are:

• eat a balanced diet that gives you all the vitamins and minerals you need and that also keeps your weight down;

• eat more fruit and vegetables;

• take regular exercise.

It also stresses that your diet should give you all the important basic nutrients, particularly minerals like calcium and iron. If it does not, then your general health will suffer and this will make your arthritis worse.

Focus on fibre. Eating high-fibre foods is important for preventing and minimizing osteoarthritis for two reasons, says nutritionist Neal Barnard. One, fibre fills you up on fewer calories, so you're less likely to overeat and gain weight. Two, fibre is the great waste collector for your internal organs. It picks up inflammatory toxins and hormones that aggravate arthritis and carries them out, reducing your chances of experiencing osteoarthritis pain.

Drink lots of water. 'Hydration helps to prevent arthritis,' says pain management expert Michael Loes. Your joints need to be moist to move smoothly, just like a well-oiled machine. Dr Loes recommends drinking two to three litres of water every day to prevent osteoarthritis pain. If you drink lots of coffee or other caffeinated beverages, which act as diuretics and flush water out of your body, then drink even more water.

Exercise aerobically. Whether it's walking, riding an exercise bike or swimming, daily aerobic exercise can help to reduce stiffness and pain, preserving or improving the health of your bones and joints. If you're just starting, Dr Barnard recommends a half-hour walk three times a week.

Add some weight training. A weight-training programme builds strength in muscles, bones and joints. If muscles aren't strong, joints tend to slip out of alignment, causing more pain. If you have osteoarthritis, talk to a physiotherapist before beginning a weight programme.

Stretch. Stretching is important for maintaining the strength and agility of your joints. Start with gentle range-of-motion exercises. These include simply rotating your arms, legs and trunk, slowly, in as full a range of motion as possible without pain. Dr Loes recommends a TheraBand stretcher (available online), a piece of elastic that offers resistance as you stretch various body parts. Similar products are available in sports shops.

Start slowly and gently. Overexertion can make osteoarthritis pain worse. If exercise causes pain that lasts longer than half-an-hour after you finish, you've probably done too much. Cut back and increase gradually, says Dr Loes. If you're unsure of your limits, talk to your doctor, who can diagnose your physical limitations, and your physiotherapist, who can devise a routine to keep you sufficiently challenged within those limits.

Exercise after a hot shower. The hot water loosens you up, says rheumatologist Ted Fields, so you're less likely to experience pain while exercising.

Buy good shoes. Walking is a great aerobic exercise to reduce your arthritis pain. If you plan on becoming a regular walker, however, Dr Loes recommends investing in a good pair of walking shoes. Try to get comfortable, lightweight shoes that are made of breathable material, are wide enough to accommodate the ball of your foot, and have good arch support and a padded heel.

Exercise on a soft, flat surface. Arthritic joints don't respond well to impact: jogging in particular jars the weight-bearing joints in your knees, hips and spine that are particularly prone to OA. Ideally, walk on grass. If you must jog, grass playing fields or a vulcanized rubber running track are excellent choices.

Get into the water. 'Among retired people, it's not the golfers who are the healthiest,' says Dr Loes, 'it's the swimmers.' Swimming tops all our experts' lists of low-impact, aerobic exercises for arthritis. Backstroke and sidestroke condition the paraspinal muscles – tiny nerve-rich muscles surrounding the spine. Strengthening these muscles will help to ease back pain and improve mobility. Water aerobics also helps to relieve and reduce arthritis pain.

Use Epsom salts. Added to bathwater, these magnesium sulphate crystals provide soothing comfort for arthritis pain because they help to draw carbon – one of your body's waste products – out through your skin.

Stand up straight. Bad posture puts pressure on your joints, causing wear and tear on your bones and cartilage. It also can cause a lot of extra pain for people with arthritis, says rheumatologist Alan Lichtbroun. Standing up straight now could save your knees and hips in the long run.

Apply heat or cold. If you feel arthritis pain flaring, Dr Fields recommends heat or ice to quell the burning. Use ice for sudden flare-ups, chronic pain, or when your joints are inflamed. Keep heat treatment – like a hot bath, heating pad or a hot pack wrapped in a towel – for when you feel sore and achy.

Rely on paracetamol. Safe and effective, taking paracetamol on a daily basis is the standard recommendation for minor arthritis pain. If this is insufficient, adding codeine is probably the best choice, although constipation can be a problem.

The problem with taking aspirin, ibuprofen or other anti-inflammatories every day is that they increase your risk of developing stomach ulcers. In any case, only a relatively small part of the pain from OA results from inflammation of the surrounding soft tissues. 'I particularly try to avoid anti-inflammatories in older people over 75,' says family doctor Stephen Amiel. 'If I feel an anti-inflammatory is essential, I generally prescribe medication to protect the stomach as well.'

Treat your joints to ginger. Some studies suggest that ginger root blocks inflammation as effectively as anti-inflammatory drugs – and without side-effects. Steep a few slivers of fresh ginger in a cup of freshly boiled water for 10 minutes. Allow to cool a little, strain and drink.

WHEN TO CONSULT A DOCTOR

If arthritis pain is persistent or if you have five to ten minutes or more of significant morning stiffness on any given morning, see your doctor. Also see your doctor if you have loss of movement or swelling in a joint or if pain stops you from doing activities that are important to you.

You should also talk to your doctor if paracetamol or other over-the-counter painkillers don't help with the pain. Apart from reviewing your medication, your doctor may be able to refer you to a dietitian for a weight reduction programme, or to physiotherapy for exercise advice, heat treatment, hydrotherapy or perhaps electrical stimulation pain relief with a TENS machine. You may also benefit from occupational therapy advice about aids and adaptations.

If your arthritis is severely disabling, you may need a referral to an orthopaedic surgeon for consideration of joint replacement or resurfacing. Reconstructive surgery for osteoarthritis has come on hugely in recent years. 'You're virtually never too old to benefit,' says family doctor Stephen Amiel. 'In fact it used to be the case that only older people were offered replacement surgery, as the new joints had a limited life expectancy. With new techniques, younger people can be offered effective and longlasting benefit, and older and frailer people can be treated safely and quickly.'

Make friends with SAM. Sometimes used as an alternative treatment for depression, SAM (S-adenosylmethionine) also helps arthritis, says family doctor Sol Grazi. 'SAM gets into the joint and acts as a building block to make the substances a joint needs.' In addition to regenerating cartilage, SAM also reduces inflammation. Take 200 to 800mg a day until your joint pain lessens, advises Dr Grazi.

Try MSM. A sulphur-containing compound found in trace amounts in food, MSM (methylsulphonylmethane) is not as well-researched as other joint remedies. It does seem to relieve arthritis pain and inflammation by increasing the effectiveness of cortisol, the body's own natural inflammation fighter, explains surgeon Stanley Jacob. He recommends taking 1000mg twice a day with food for the first two to three days. Then each week, add an extra 1000mg to your daily intake (up to 8000mg a day) until the pain subsides.

Try glucosamine and chondroitin sulphate. With all the buzz surrounding these two supplements, you might think they're *the* definitive cure for arthritis. But the jury is still out, with some of our experts a bit sceptical over the early study results. There is some reasonable evidence that symptoms of OA may be relieved, but claims that damaged cartilage can be rebuilt have yet to be confirmed. If you decide on taking them, follow package instructions and allow at least three weeks for effects to become noticeable.

Keep up with your vitamins. If you follow the Arthritis Research Campaign's advice for a healthy diet with plenty of fresh fruit and vegetables, you should be getting plenty of vitamin C, which will help to preserve the health of your collagen and connective tissue. The anti-oxidant vitamin E may also help vitamin C, glucosamine and chondroitin to do their work. Vegetable oils, wheatgerm oil, nuts, and green leafy vegetables are the main dietary sources of vitamin E. Fortified cereals often contain vitamin E too. Supplements of both vitamin C and E are available in pharmacies if you are unable to get enough in your diet.

Don't forget vitamin D. Vitamin D may prove to be one of the most important vitamins in preventing OA, says Dr Amiel. Evidence suggests that low levels are associated with more wear and tear of the cartilage in weight-bearing joints and a big study is under way to see if supplements reduce the damage to joints affected by OA. Good dietary sources of vitamin D are fortified cereals, juices and dairy products. Plenty of sun will help your body to synthesize vitamin D, or you can take supplements (250mg per day).

Mix in magnesium. In addition to these other nutrients, Dr Loes recommends 60mg of magnesium a day. As well as helping bones, magnesium helps to ward off cramp and improves sleep.

Oil squeaky joints. Granny may have been right about cod liver oil. 'Many of my patients swear by cod liver oil for arthritis,' says Dr Amiel. 'Some liken it to an oil can

Do just *one* thing

Lose weight. 'Being overweight is like carrying around heavy luggage,' says Neal Barnard, a nutrition expert. 'It hurts the knees, hips, literally every joint in the body.' It's not just the extra weight that causes arthritis problems in obese people, he says. Extra body fat causes hormonal changes and builds up levels of oestrogen, and research suggests that higher levels of oestrogen lead to a higher risk of osteoarthritis. For every extra four kilos of bodyweight, your risk of osteoarthritis in your knees increases by 30 per cent.

for squeaky joints, rather like the tin man in *The Wizard of Oz*.' They may well be right, or almost. The omega-3 fatty acids in fish oils seem to switch off enzymes in the joints that are responsible for breaking down cartilage. Yet another reason maybe to include oily fish (mackerel, salmon, tuna, sardines and pilchards) in your diet. If Granny insists, you can take cod liver oil supplements, though it's slightly more palatable in capsule form than from the dreaded spoon.

Combine your fatty acids. Some limited research suggests that combining omega-3 fatty acids with an omega-6 fat like borage oil, blackcurrant seed oil or evening primrose oil may reduce inflammation in some forms of arthritis, but there is not yet any convincing evidence of benefit in osteoarthritis.

OSTEOPOROSIS

16 ways to preserve bone strength

Osteoporosis is a weakening of the bones that then break easily – hence its popular name, brittle bone disease. Our bones are made up of a thick outer shell with a honeycomb mesh inside. When the gaps in this honeycomb become bigger, osteoporosis occurs, making bones fragile. The wrists, hips and spine are particularly at risk.

The condition affects one in three women and one in 12 men in the UK. It is responsible for a staggering 200,000 breaks per year and 40 deaths a day. The scary thing about osteoporosis is that it's a silent disease. It develops over decades without causing pain or any other symptoms. You don't even suspect there's a problem until it is too late. One day you'll simply fracture a bone doing an everyday job. Weak bones break easily – so easily, in fact, that even the mildest stresses, such as coughing, bending over to tie your shoelaces or lifting a heavy bag of shopping can cause a fracture.

Although brittle bones are associated with old age, recent research suggests that the roots of the disease lie in adolescence. A poor diet during childhood and the teenage years can lay the foundations for osteoporosis later on. On a positive note, bone is constantly regenerated – new cells are created while older cells are taken away. There are various ways to boost this process and restore bone while also slowing down the rate at which bone is removed. Whether you have osteoporosis already or you want to reduce your risk of getting it, here are some strategies to keep your skeleton strong.

Eat a calcium-rich diet. Think of calcium as the cement that makes bones strong. Even though bones are loaded with calcium, cells called osteoclasts constantly break down bone and 'steal' calcium for use in other parts of the body. If you don't get enough calcium in your diet, your bones forfeit the mineral for other functions in your body.

Your peak bone-building years end at the age of 30. After that, bones can get dangerously weak, especially after menopause, when declines in oestrogen levels cause women's bones to lose calcium at an accelerated rate. Men go through a similar process with a decline in their testosterone levels, almost like a menopause, although not as dramatic. Therefore, men are also susceptible to bone loss.

Dietitian Jane Clarke says that young children need about 525mg of calcium per day, adults about 800mg, and breast feeding and pregnant women about 1200mg per day.

Your body only absorbs about 30 per cent of the calcium you take in, says Melba Iris Ovalle, who is medical director of an osteoporosis clinic. So you have to ingest a lot more than your body actually requires.

Luckily, calcium is among the easiest nutrients to get through diet, especially if you eat dairy foods, says Robert Recker, who runs an osteoporosis research centre. Your recommended daily requirement of calcium is found in 660ml (just over a pint) of semi-skimmed milk, 400g of natural yogurt or 100g of Cheddar cheese.

Choose fortified foods. If you don't like or cannot tolerate dairy foods, there are plenty of dairy-free calcium sources to choose from. Many fortified juices and breakfast cereals contain as much calcium as a glass of milk. Some breads and snack bars are also fortified with calcium.

Eat your greens. Salad leaves, broccoli, Brussels sprouts and other vegetables and fruits provide useful amounts of calcium. Baked beans, bony fish and dried fruit are other good sources of the mineral.

Eat soya foods. Some brands of soya foods are calcium-fortified, but that may not be the only reason that soya protects the bones. Soya contains phytoestrogens, chemical compounds that act like a weaker form of the bone-protecting hormone, oestrogen. Although there is some evidence that these substances may help symptoms of the menopause, like hot flushes, there is no strong evidence as yet that they influence osteoporosis. Phytoestrogens are also present in wholegrain cereals, vegetables such as sweet potatoes or yams, fruits and chickpeas.

Supplement your diet. If you have a diet poor in vitamin D, or if you are frail, elderly or housebound, it may be a good idea to take supplements of calcium, preferably combined with vitamin D.

Take supplements with meals. Calcium is absorbed more efficiently in an acidic environment. 'Take supplements with food because that's when stomach acidity rises,' advises Dr Ovalle.

Consider calcium citrate supplements. All calcium supplements are equally effective, but those that contain calcium carbonate may cause bloating. Supplements with calcium citrate are easier on the stomach, says Dr Ovalle. Also, calcium citrate supplements don't require a high-acid environment for good absorption. They are a good option for people with ulcers who may be taking drugs to reduce stomach acid production.

Get enough vitamin D. This nutrient is vital for bone health because it helps to transport calcium from the blood into your bones. Many breakfast cereals are fortified with vitamin D. It's also found in most multivitamins. 'Older people don't absorb vitamin D as well as they did when they were younger, so supplementation makes sense,' says Dr Ovalle.

People on an Asian diet eating unleavened bread are also at more risk of vitamin D deficiency. Your best bet may be to take a combined calcium and vitamin D supplement. These are available over the counter or can be prescribed by your doctor. Aim for 1000mg of extra calcium and 250mg (400iu) of vitamin D daily.

Enjoy the sun. Every time your skin is exposed to sunlight, your body produces bone-protecting vitamin D. If you don't use a sunscreen, 20 minutes of sun exposure gives you about 100mg of vitamin D, says Dr Ovalle. Sunscreen blocks out vitamin D production almost completely. But on balance, protect your skin from too much sun, and let your vitamin D come from your diet, supplements or both.

Make soup. An easy way to get more calcium into your diet is to make stock for soup from bones. Add a little vinegar when making the stock – the vinegar dissolves the calcium out of the bones. Around 500ml of homemade stock provides as much calcium as a litre of milk.

Eat less salt. Salt depletes the body's calcium stores in two ways. It reduces the amount that's absorbed from foods or supplements, and it increases the amount that's excreted. 'The greater your intake of salt, the greater the loss of calcium,' says Dr Recker. It's fine to sprinkle a little salt on your food, but try to avoid processed and packaged foods, which tend to be very high in salt.

Drink alcohol in moderation. For men, that means no more than 21 units a week; for women, 14 units a week is the upper limit. (A unit is a small glass of wine, a single pub measure of spirits, or half a pint of beer.)

Excessive alcohol consumption decreases bone formation and reduces your body's ability to absorb calcium. Furthermore, people who drink heavily often eat a poor diet, which results in lower calcium intake.

Get plenty of exercise. It slows down the rate of bone loss and can lead to an increase in bone density. Virtually any type of exercise is helpful, but the best for bone health is weight-bearing exercise such as walking, in which you move your body against gravity, and resistance exercise such as lifting weights, says Dr Recker.

Exercise has other benefits as well. Because it improves muscle tone, coordination and balance, it can dramatically reduce the risk of falls, the leading cause of fractures in the elderly, says Dr Ovalle.

You don't have to be a body builder to strengthen bones with exercise. You don't even have to join a gym. Any activity that gets you on your feet and moving against gravity for 30 minutes four or five times a week adds significant amounts of bone to your skeleton. Add a 15-minute weight-lifting session, and your bones get even stronger.

'Start with 30 minutes three times a week, then gradually work up to five times a week,' says Dr Ovalle. You don't need to do the exercise all at once. You can spread it out – by doing 15 minutes in the morning, for example, and another 15 minutes later in the day.

Here are some of the best exercises for bones.

- Walking is a weight-bearing exercise that increases stress on bones in the legs and hips. The stress stimulates bone-building cells to create new bone, which is why women who walk regularly have greater bone density and get fewer fractures than those who are sedentary.

- Running, dancing, aerobics and other high-impact activities are even better for bone growth than walking. If you already have osteoporosis, ask your doctor if your bones are strong enough for high-impact exercises.

- Flexing your wrists – by holding a soup can in each hand and bending your wrist towards your forearm, for example – strengthens wrist bones and reduces the risk of fractures or other injuries.

- Household activities can strengthen the bones just as much as formal workouts, as long as you do them vigorously. Gardening is good because it involves a lot of pushing and pulling. Even cleaning the house – sweeping, hoovering and walking up and down stairs – helps to keep bones strong.

Drink fewer soft drinks. Soft drinks, especially colas, contain phosphorus, which can draw calcium out of bones if present in too high a concentration compared with your calcium levels. You need to match your

WHEN TO CONSULT A DOCTOR

Everyone over the age of 65 should have a bone-density test to determine if they're at risk for osteoporosis – or if they already have it. Some people are more at risk of osteoporosis than others. Risk factors for osteoporosis include:

- for women: a lack of oestrogen caused by early menopause, early hysterectomy (before the age of 45), missing periods for six months or more through excessive exercising, low bodyweight or dieting;

- for men: low levels of the male hormone testosterone;

- long-term use of high dose corticosteroid tablets (for conditions such as arthritis and asthma);

- family history of osteoporosis (mother or father), particularly if your mother suffered a hip fracture;

- other medical conditions such as Cushing's syndrome and liver and thyroid problems;

- malabsorption problems such as coeliac disease or Crohn's disease;

- long-term immobility;

- heavy drinking;

- smoking.

See your doctor if you fall into any of these categories. He or she may want to refer you for bone studies. These will calculate your bone density relative to other men or women of your age and indicate a danger of osteoporosis (relative thinning, also called osteopenia) or osteoporosis itself. If the density is lower than it should be, you can discuss various treatment options, including calcium and vitamin D, oestrogen supplements in the form of HRT, or other non-hormonal drugs like bisphosphonates or raloxifene. These treatments may prevent further bone loss and reduce your risk of some osteoporosis-related fractures, but the evidence that they will significantly add to bone mass is slight. Guidelines published in late 2003 suggest that HRT should no longer be considered a first choice for the prevention of osteoporosis; it should rather be reserved for the short-term treatment of menopausal symptoms, with other agents then being used to prevent bone loss in the longer term.

If you have established osteoporosis, speak to your doctor about ways of minimizing your risk of falls and fractures. He or she may refer you for physiotherapy or occupational therapy and you may be recommended to use hip protectors.

phosphorus intake with calcium, so if you drink lots of cola, increase your calcium too. The other downside is that soft drinks often replace calcium-rich milk in the diet.

If you smoke, try to quit. Lifelong smokers are 10 to 20 times more likely to develop osteoporosis than non-smokers, says Dr Recker.

Find out more. Visit the National Osteoporosis Society's website at www.nos.org.uk for the latest research, advice and details of local support groups.

PEPTIC ULCERS
15 tips for quick relief

Every time you eat, your stomach bathes foods in acids to continue the digestion that began in your mouth. The acids that break down proteins and fats are actually strong enough to damage the stomach and the duodenum, the part of the small intestine nearest the stomach. The only reason they don't is that the tissues are coated with a protective, sponge-like mucous lining that resists the acidic onslaught.

Sometimes, however, the tissues break down, causing a peptic ulcer. Most ulcers – small, painful sores that are generally about the size of a shirt button – occur when a corkscrew-shaped bacterium called *Helicobacter pylori* bores through the lining of the duodenum or stomach and allows acids to damage the delicate tissue underneath. Over-the-counter medications such as aspirin and ibuprofen can strip away the stomach's protective lining and cause similar problems.

Some people with ulcers have no symptoms, but others experience abdominal pain. Peptic ulcers are more likely from early middle age onwards. There are two main types: duodenal ulcers, and the less common gastric ulcers. Between them, peptic ulcers will affect about one in 10 men and one in 15 women at some point in their lives.

The pain of a duodenal ulcer is often described as a burning or gnawing hunger pain, usually just below the breastbone or sometimes going through to the middle of the back; it is usually eased by eating, and can often be worse at night. A stomach ulcer can cause a sharp tummy pain when you eat and be worse during the day. Other symptoms may include belching, loss of appetite (more so with gastric ulcer) or, occasionally, increased appetite (more so with duodenal ulcer), nausea and vomiting or waterbrash, when the mouth suddenly fills with saliva.

Ulcers can clear up on their own within one to three weeks once aspirin or other tissue-damaging medications are stopped. But they usually recur if *Helicobacter* is present and not treated. In the meantime the pain can be intense. To stop the pain and prevent recurrences, here's what doctors advise.

Take an antacid. During ulcer flare-ups, taking an antacid is the quickest way to relieve the pain, says gastroenterologist Samuel Meyers.

Antacids contain calcium, aluminium, magnesium or a combination. Aluminium makes some people constipated, while magnesium can lead to diarrhoea. If you tend to be constipated, avoid aluminium-based antacids; likewise, if you are prone to diarrhoea, keep away from magnesium. Ask your pharmacist for advice on the best antacid for you.

Reduce acid production. Over-the-counter medicines called H_2 blockers are among the best ways to treat ulcers, says Dr Meyers. Drugs in this class include Pepcid AC (famotidine), Zantac 75 (ranitidine) and Tagamet 100 (cimetidine). They reduce the output of acid-secreting cells in the stomach, which reduces discomfort and helps ulcers heal more quickly. 'I usually recommend Pepcid or Zantac because these don't interact with other medications that people may be taking,' he adds. (Cimetidine interacts with a lot of other medicines, making the other drug more or less potent.)

One of the best ways to get relief from ulcer pain is to combine antacids with H_2 blockers. Antacids will ease discomfort within 10 to 15 minutes, and H_2 blockers provide longer-term protection.

Note: If you're using H_2 blockers, don't take antacids at exactly the same time, as they'll interfere with absorption. Take the H_2 blocker at the recommended time, then wait an hour or two before taking an antacid.

Give up orange juice for a while. Doctors aren't sure why, but oranges – as well as tomatoes and possibly grapefruit – may trigger the release of pain-causing chemical messengers, or neurotransmitters, in those with ulcers, says gastroenterologist Philip Miner.

Don't believe the milk myth. For a long time, doctors encouraged people with ulcers to drink milk. They thought that milk's smooth texture would coat and soothe painful ulcers. Research has shown, however, that the protein and calcium in milk stimulate acid production and can make ulcers worse, says Dr Meyers.

Soothe with yoghurt. Although milk can aggravate an ulcer, yoghurt can actually soothe one. Researchers from Sweden analysed the diets of 764 people with ulcers and 229 people without. They found that the men

WHEN TO CONSULT A DOCTOR

If you're having ulcer symptoms, especially if they are relieved temporarily by antacids or over-the-counter H$_2$-blockers, ask your doctor to test for the presence of *Helicobacter pylori*. It can be detected with a blood test, a stool sample or a breath test. If the test is positive, your doctor will probably prescribe a combination or two or three medications for one to two weeks. It is vital to take these exactly as instructed. The medication may cause diarrhoea and nausea, and your symptoms may not resolve immediately. But in about 97 per cent of cases, the ulcer never comes back following *Helicobacter* eradication therapy. In fact, about 90 per cent of ulcers clear up with home remedies on their own, but without medical treatment they nearly always recur.

The complications of a peptic ulcer can be very dangerous and warrant seeing a doctor urgently. Bleeding from the ulcer is the most common complication. Symptoms include:

• vomiting blood, which usually looks like brown coffee grounds;

• blood in the faeces;

• black, tarry faeces.

Sometimes the ulcer can perforate the stomach or duodenal lining. This can cause a very dangerous inflammation in the abdomen called peritonitis. Symptoms include:

• sudden severe constant abdominal pain;

• pain spreading to the back.

Doctors sometimes worry that over-the-counter medications for indigestion and ulcer-type pains can be too effective, masking symptoms of more serious disease and delaying people consulting their doctor for further investigation. Avoid this risk by seeing your doctor if:

• you have difficulty swallowing or food seems to stick on its way down;

• you have persistent vomiting;

• you're losing weight;

• you are anaemic;

• you're over 55 and you've developed indigestion or ulcer-type symptoms only in the last year;

• you're over 45 and your symptoms have been more or less continuous since onset;

• more than two close relatives (your parents, siblings or children) have a history of cancer of the stomach, oesophagus or small bowel.

and women who ate the most yoghurt reduced their risk of ulcers by 18 per cent, compared with those who ate the least. The friendly bacteria in yoghurt, such as *Lactobacillus bulgaricus* and *L. acidophilus*, may be the therapeutic substance.

Guard with garlic. Long known as a natural antibiotic, some alternative experts suspect that garlic may also inhibit the growth of *H. pylori*. In one laboratory study, the extract from the equivalent of two cloves of garlic was able to stop the growth of this ulcer-causing bacterium.

Ask your doctor about liquorice. It's a traditional folk remedy for ulcers, and there's some evidence that it's effective. Liquorice contains glycyrrhizic acid, a compound that is thought to strengthen the intestinal lining and help ulcers to heal more quickly, says Dr Miner.

Read the label on the packet – much 'liquorice' is actually made with liquorice flavouring, which won't have the same effect as the real thing. The recommended dose is 1.5 to 3 grams per day.

Note: Liquorice should not be used on a regular basis for more than four to six weeks, because long-term daily use of liquorice can cause high blood pressure. Talk to your doctor before taking it.

Eat more frequently. Even though the stomach's acid production increases during and after meals, the presence of food in the stomach helps to buffer its corrosive effects. Eating also increases bloodflow to the stomach, which helps to protect it from digestive acids. Rather than having two or three large meals a day, eat five or six small meals instead, Dr Miner advises.

Try a different painkiller. Aspirin and ibuprofen are among the most effective over-the-counter painkillers ever discovered, but long-term use of these medications is a common cause of stomach ulcers, says Dr Miner. Along with other nonsteroidal anti-inflammatory drugs (NSAIDs), aspirin and ibuprofen inhibit the body's production of prostaglandins, chemicals that help to maintain the stomach's protective lining. About 20 per cent of people who use these drugs regularly go on to develop ulcers.

If you need long-term pain relief – because of arthritis, for example – your doctor may advise you to switch to paracetamol. It is as effective as aspirin or ibuprofen for easing many types of pain, but is less likely to damage the stomach lining.

Reduce the stress in your life. For a long time, emotional stress was thought to be a leading cause of ulcers. Doctors now believe that stress probably doesn't cause ulcers – but does worsen symptoms if an ulcer is present, possibly because the stomach produces more acid in response to stress. Anxiety, tension and a highly strung approach to life can also increase the brain's perception of pain, says Dr Meyers. If you already have an ulcer – or have had one in the past – it makes sense to include stress reduction in your overall treatment plan.

Everyone controls stress in different ways. Vigorous exercise – walking, running or cycling, for example – is a great way to dispel tension at the end of a hectic day. Others use more formal stress reduction strategies, such as deep breathing or meditation. The idea isn't to completely eliminate stress, but simply to find ways to prevent it from taking over your life – or disrupting your insides.

Quit smoking. People who smoke are much more likely to get ulcers than those who don't, Dr Meyers warns. Smoking slows down the healing time of ulcers, increases the risk of relapses, and may also make the body more susceptible to infection-causing bacteria.

Drink alcohol in moderation. Alcohol can erode the stomach's protective lining, resulting in inflammation and bleeding. It is even more likely to cause problems if you also smoke or take aspirin regularly, says Dr Meyers. For men, the daily alcohol limit is three drinks; for women, the upper limit is two drinks a day. If ulcers continue to cause problems, you may want to give up alcohol altogether.

Cut back on coffee. Both standard and decaffeinated coffee increase levels of stomach acids. Coffee is unlikely to cause ulcers, but it can increase discomfort while an ulcer is healing, Dr Meyers says.

Drink a lot of water. Drink at least two litres of water a day when ulcers are active, and drink a full glass whenever you have pain. Water helps to dilute acid in the stomach, says Dr Meyers. And unlike milk, it won't stimulate the production of more acid.

PHLEBITIS

12 remedies to keep it at bay

Those who have experienced phlebitis know it as a painful, frightening affliction that can claim a victim's life without warning via a blood clot lodged in the veins of the lungs.

Phlebitis just means inflammation of the veins. It is more correctly known as thrombophlebitis – 'thrombo' is the blood clot that constitutes its main danger. Two basic types of phlebitis exist: deep vein thrombophlebitis (or thrombosis), or DVT for short, which is the more dangerous condition by far, and superficial thrombophlebitis, the more common, less serious condition that we deal with here. Superficial thrombophlebitis is very rarely dangerous. Both are caused by long periods of inactivity, perhaps a long car journey, a long flight or an extended period of bed rest – such as after an operation. Your genes might also put you at a greater risk of developing the condition, and you are more at risk if you have varicose veins.

Rather than panicking about the tender, ropy veins you can feel just below the surface of your skin, try these home remedies that may help to complement medical treatment.

Come off the combined Pill. If you have had a history of phlebitis or blood clots, you shouldn't use combined oral contraceptives containing both oestrogen and progestagen, says vascular specialist Jess Young. The incidence of deep vein thrombophlebitis in combined oral contraceptive users is estimated three to four times higher than in non-users.

Studies have shown that in a quarter of cases of superficial thrombophlebitis, some deep vein thrombosis is present too, so even an essentially harmless superficial thrombophlebitis precludes combined pill use. Progestogen-only pills (sometimes called the mini-pill) are safe though and, according to world authority

---

KITCHEN CURES

High-fibre foods are important to vein health for one simple reason – they keep you regular. If you're constipated, you tend to push too much and too frequently when you have a bowel movement, which puts extra pressure on the valves in the veins of your legs. Try to get around 30 grams of fibre a day from foods like bran cereals, oats and beans. And remember to drink extra water. Without plenty of water, adding fibre could make your constipation worse.

Professor John Guillebaud, may even decrease the risk of thrombosis.

You do not need to go off the pill before a long-haul flight, as long as you exercise regularly and drink plenty of non-alcoholic fluids. And if you do discontinue the pill, make sure you have suitable alternative contraception.

Know your risks. Once you've had phlebitis, you're at increased risk of getting it again. Long periods of bed rest make you especially vulnerable. While you might not be able to prevent prolonged bed rest following an injury or serious illness, certain types of risk, such as elective surgery, can be avoided if you're prone to clotting disorders. Talk to your doctor about risk factors, and be aware that getting up and about as quickly as possible can help to reduce the risks of developing phlebitis after surgery.

Give it rest and warmth. Treat superficial phlebitis by putting your leg up and applying warm, moist heat, says cardiovascular expert Michael Dake. You don't need to stay in bed, but resting with the leg raised 15 to 30cm above the heart seems to speed up healing. The inflammation of superficial phlebitis usually disappears in a week to 10 days, though it may take three to six weeks to subside completely.

Get some exercise. Exercise – especially walking – tends to keep the veins emptied, says vascular expert Robert Ginsburg. Keeping your legs moving when they feel fine will help to improve your circulation, so it's a good way to prevent a recurrence of phlebitis. 'The veins are a low-pressure system, and if the valves that keep blood from flowing backwards in the legs aren't working properly, such as in varicose veins, the only way you're going to prevent blood from pooling is by walking.'

Make lots of journey stops. If you've had phlebitis in the past and are going on a long car journey, then be sure to stop frequently and exercise, says Dr Dake. Don't stop just once during the trip for a long walk. Instead, stop four or five times and walk shorter distances. Exercise prevents your circulation from becoming sluggish as a result of sitting still for long periods.

Beware the friendly skies. We have all heard of 'economy class syndrome' following a long flight. It rarely seems to strike passengers in roomy first-class seats, but nobody seems to be quite sure of its cause. Possible culprits are cabin pressure, lack of movement and alcohol intake.

Long flights or car journeys, or any long period of inactivity, can increase the risk of thrombosis, says Dr Young. But on aeroplanes you tend to be confined to your seat more than when travelling by car, when you can make regular stops. So if you're on a long-haul flight, especially if you

WHEN TO CONSULT A DOCTOR

Even the most innocent phlebitis can be the sign of a more serious problem. Swelling or tenderness around a reddened area on your leg is something you should at least show your doctor. If you have a history of superficial phlebitis or varicose veins, you might also be at risk for deep vein thrombophlebitis. And see your doctor if you feel any prolonged pain or swelling in your calf or thigh, and that pain is coming mainly from the back of the calf.

have phlebitis, get out of your seat and walk up and down the aisle every 30 minutes after taking off. Ask for an aisle seat so you don't disturb the passengers sitting next to you, or if you can't get one, move your feet up and down frequently to improve the circulation back from your legs to your heart. Drink plenty of fluids and avoid alcoholic drinks.

Put your feet up when you're bedridden. 'If you've had phlebitis and you're going to be bedridden for any length of time,' says Dr Young, 'raise the foot of the bed several inches to increase bloodflow through the veins.' He also suggests that you exercise your legs as much as you can while in bed. Try this exercise once an hour: flex your feet, lifting your toes while keeping your heels down, as though you're pumping a piano pedal. Repeat for a minute or two.

Wear support tights. These stockings, available in pharmacies and department stores, help to prevent blood from pooling in the small blood vessels closest to the skin. While there's no documented evidence showing that support stockings do any good in preventing phlebitis, they do seem to relieve pain. The advice is to wear support hose if you're prone to swollen legs and ankles or varicose veins.

Give up smoking. If you smoke and experience recurring phlebitis, you should quit, says Dr Young. You could have Buerger's disease, a severe and progressive condition affecting the small arteries, mainly in the legs and feet. It is directly related to smoking, and the only cure is to give up all forms of tobacco. It's possible that Buerger's could be misdiagnosed as phlebitis, in which case continuing to smoke would be very dangerous.

Investigate aspirin. Some studies suggest that the blood-thinning properties of aspirin may help to reduce phlebitis by preventing rapid clot formation in those prone to the disease. These studies advise that you take aspirin before prolonged periods of bed rest, travel or surgery, all of which tend to make circulation sluggish and increase the possibility of clotting. While such simple advice sounds enticing, not all doctors agree on its effectiveness. If you do decide to try aspirin, be aware that this is a medical treatment – and talk to your doctor first.

Add vitamin E. A supplement to try is vitamin E for its mild blood-thinning action. Take doses of 250 to 500mg per day.

PHOBIAS AND FEARS
15 coping measures

A phobia can be defined as 'an irrational, involuntary, inappropriate fear reaction that generally leads to an avoidance of common everyday places, objects or situations,' says phobia expert and psychologist Jerilyn Ross.

In reality, though, a phobia is the fear of fear itself. 'A phobia is a fear of one's own impulses,' says Ross. 'It's a fear of having a panic attack, feeling trapped and losing control.'

Phobias are classified into three types: simple or specific phobias, social phobias and agoraphobia. People with specific phobias experience a dread of certain objects, places or situations. People with social phobias avoid public situations, like parties, addressing a meeting, or even talking on the telephone, because they're afraid they'll do something to embarrass themselves. Agoraphobics are victims of a complex phenomenon based on a fear of being in public places without a familiar person or an escape plan.

The onset of a phobia is generally unprovoked and rapid. 'Usually, people who develop phobias do so in areas in which they had no previous fear,' says Ross. Increasing evidence suggests that phobias are caused by a combination of psychological and biological factors. They tend to run in families, suggesting some genetic basis. So if one of your parents had a phobia, you may be predisposed to one, but not necessarily the same one. More often than not, phobias strike people who have a history of separation anxiety and perfectionism.

People with phobias always recognize that their fear is inappropriate to the situation, says Ross. For example, if you're flying in an aeroplane during a thunderstorm, then feeling afraid is normal. If, however, your boss tells you you'll have to make a business trip in a few weeks and you immediately start worrying about having a panic attack on the plane, that's inappropriate.

Here's some rational advice for irrational behaviour from those who deal with the problem every day.

Reverse your thinking. In a phobic situation, negative thoughts and scary images trigger the physical symptoms of fear, explains Manuel Zane, who runs a phobia clinic. You should allow the fear to come, but try to shift from the negative thoughts – 'that dog will bite me' – to something realistically positive, like 'that dog is on a lead and can't get away'.

Come face-to-face with fear. Avoiding your fear prevents you from overcoming it, says Dr Zane. Instead, desired control can be achieved through a process called exposure treatment, in which, with the guidance of a therapist, you expose yourself to the object of your fears little by little. Gradually, you'll learn that what you imagine and expect to happen does not actually occur. Such graduated exposure also helps you get used to the object of your fear, he says.

For example, say your phobia is spiders. In exposure treatment training, you start to face your fear – usually in the presence of another person – by looking at pictures of spiders. When you learn to handle this, you may move on to looking at a dead spider, then a live spider, and you may even progress to holding one in your hand. Each time you may still feel some fear, but you learn that the awful things you dread don't actually occur.

Researchers are currently evaluating computer-based self-help programmes of exposure training. A national network of group-based support is also available for people wanting to explore this method further. Contact Triumph Over Phobia (see tip *'Find out more'*, page 450) for availability in your area.

Pat yourself on the back. Functioning successfully with a level of fear is a big achievement, says Dr Zane. Dealing with it successfully is much more plausible and realistic than trying to completely erase your fear. Each encounter that you overcome in your exposure treatment training should be considered a personal victory, thus helping build your self-confidence.

Play mind games. 'When you feel your fear taking hold, do manageable things like counting backwards in threes from 1000, reading a book, talking out loud or taking deep breaths,' says Dr Zane. 'When you are involved with doing something manageable in the present, you reduce your involvement with fear-generating thoughts and images. Your body quietens down and you maintain control.'

Measure your fear. Label your fear on a scale of nought to 10, suggests Dr Zane. You'll find that the severity of your fear is not constant, that it

WHEN TO CONSULT A DOCTOR

Phobias can dominate, and ruin, lives. Even a specific phobia may blight a career, or at least your holiday options, if you can't fly or are phobic about snakes, for example. A social phobia may make someone go to extraordinary lengths to avoid speaking to people on the phone, and agoraphobia can literally make people prisoners in their own homes. 'I've had patients who for years on end have been unable to get to the surgery or even telephone me to tell me of their phobia,' says family doctor Stephen Amiel.

If a phobia interferes with your life or someone's close to you, seek professional help. Your doctor can refer you for psychological assessment and treatment: behavioural techniques like cognitive behavioural therapy (CBT) or exposure training have good results.

Medication, usually with drugs similar to those used for depression may also be recommended. If you can't get out to the doctor, a home assessment can usually be arranged.

goes up and down. Write down thoughts or activities that make it increase and decrease. Knowing what triggers, increases and decreases the fear may help you to learn to control it.

Look over the rainbow. Use thoughts, fantasies and activities that make you feel good to shift yourself away from frightening thoughts, suggests Dr Zane. For example, focus on the high probability of a safe flight and the pleasures of lying on that sandy sunny beach instead of reacting to the remote dangers of the flight.

Beware of the effects of caffeine. 'People who have repeated panic attacks may be very sensitive to caffeine,' says David Barlow, an expert in anxiety disorders. 'Caffeine recreates some of the symptoms they have during panic attacks.' When you're offered a drink from the in-flight trolley, remember that caffeine isn't limited to coffee; it's also in tea, colas and chocolate.

Don't resort to alcohol. A calming alcoholic drink – or three – may seem the logical solution for someone with a phobia trying to cope with the prospect of, say, a flight. Don't be fooled, says family doctor Stephen Amiel. 'Alcohol will stop you being able to reason with yourself, will prevent you being able to respond to others reassuring you and, with social phobias, might make you more likely to do the thing that most frightens you – lose control in public,' he says. 'As the alcohol wears off, you are also much more likely to feel increased anxiety, or even go into a full-blown panic attack.'

Calm down with soothing herbs. 'Phobias and fears go hand in hand with adrenaline,' says clinical herbalist Douglas Schar. 'Keeping calm and worry free will help to keep your fight-or-flight reflex to a manageable level.' Displacing terrifying thoughts for soothing, relaxing ones always helps. But herbal remedies may be helpful, too. Chamomile, valerian, passionflower and California poppy are four gentle remedies for anxiety.

Listed in ascending order of strength, try chamomile first and work your way up the ladder until you find the one that works best for you.

How one woman overcame panic attacks

'I felt like I was standing in the middle of a motorway with cars coming at me from all sides.' That's how 26-year-old Tanis describes how it felt whenever she tried to leave her home. Tanis has the most common of all phobias, agoraphobia, a fear of being away from a safe person or place.

Just the thought of venturing outside her house brought on a paralysing panic attack. 'One minute you feel fine, the next, you feel like you're about to die,' she says. 'Physically, my heart started beating faster, I felt sick and shaky and as if I was about to faint.'

But Tanis did manage to leave her house for therapy, and it worked. Now she's out all the time, helping others still stuck indoors. Here are some of the tactics Tanis learnt in therapy that helped to set her free.

Recognize the attack. 'If a panic attack comes on, recognize it for what it is,' she says. 'You've had them before, so you know you're not going to die. You've got through it before and you can do it again. Acceptance is the key.'

Be sensitive to yourself. People with phobias are usually perfectionists and are hard on themselves, but you shouldn't be, says Tanis. When you are going through exposure treatment, be kind to yourself. Give yourself credit because you endured the exposure, even if it brought on an attack.

Go slowly. Start out slowly, but do some exposure treatment every day. Set goals for yourself. Once you start dealing with your phobia over and over again, it really does become conditioned.

'As impossible as it may sound to a phobic, you can do things like a normal person again.'

Buy the remedies in tincture form, and keep them to hand. If you feel the pressure building up, take a dose straight away. Don't wait until you are in the middle of a full-blown attack, says Schar. And if you know you are heading for a situation that will push your fear buttons, use one of these remedies in advance to keep your cool.

The remedies are available in health food stores and should be taken according to label instructions.

Burn that adrenaline. In a panic attack, you have an excess of adrenaline in the body. Moving burns it up, says phobia expert Christopher McCullough, So don't try and relax; you need to burn up that adrenaline, so walk around or exercise during an attack.

Or play muscle games. If you can't move around, the next best thing to do is to tighten and relax various muscles in your body. 'Tighten the large muscles of your thigh, then do a quick release,' suggests Dr McCullough. Then go on to the other muscles in your body. 'This kind of rhythmic tensing and releasing will also burn adrenaline,' he says.

Find out more. Further help and advice is available from various organizations such as: NO PANIC (National Organisation for Phobias, Anxiety, Neuroses, Information & Care) tel: 0808 808 0545 or online at http://nopanic.org.uk; Triumph Over Phobia (TOP UK), tel: 0845 600 9601 or online at www.triumphoverphobia.com; or National Phobics Society, tel: 0870 7700 456 or online at www.phobics-society.org.uk.

PREMENSTRUAL SYNDROME

27 ways to treat the symptoms

Most women undergo some physical or psychological changes in the week or so before a period – tender breasts, headaches and a tendency to tearfulness are common. But for some women, symptoms are bad enough to disrupt their daily lives. Premenstrual Syndrome (PMS) is a recognized medical condition that may affect between a third and half of all women between the ages of 20 and 50. It is caused by fluctuations in the female hormones oestrogen and progesterone. Symptoms include mood swings, aggression, fatigue and depression along with physical effects such as bloating, weight gain, skin problems and painful breasts. Some women

Combat the sugar craving

If you followed supper last night with a bar of chocolate or a tub of ice cream, don't be too hard on yourself, especially if your period is due. Your hormones were probably responsible. You don't overeat at this time of the month because you're a weak character. Research has shown that you're almost driven to it by the effects of progesterone on the brain, says Peter Vash, a specialist in eating disorders. It seems that the high levels of progesterone released by the ovaries at around the middle of the menstrual cycle affect the areas of the brain responsible for carbohydrate cravings.

Try to manage those cravings, says Dr Vash, because giving in to them can make you feel worse. Here's how to steel yourself.

Be prepared. You know that the cravings will last for a week to 10 days each month, so mark those days on your calendar, says Dr Vash. Bear in mind that they will stop, and rise above them.

Put up a fight. Get enough sleep, drink lots of fluids, and eat fresh fruit when your body demands something sweet.

also crave sweet things or drink too much alcohol. The most severe form of PMS, known as premenstrual dysphoric disorder, can have such a marked effect on mood that a doctor may prescribe antidepressants.

There are more than 150 symptoms associated with PMS and the number and type of symptoms varies from person to person. You can feel lousy for days. Then, miraculously, your period begins and you feel instantly better.

Not all women respond to the same treatments. Finding the best way to handle your PMS will require trial and error. These tips come from experts who have worked extensively with women suffering from PMS.

Calm your environment. Women with PMS seem to be particularly sensitive to environmental stress, says Susan Lark, a doctor who runs a help and advice centre for women with PMS.

Surrounding yourself with soothing colours and soft music can contribute to a sense of calm.

Breathe deeply. Shallow breathing, which many of us do unconsciously, decreases energy levels and leaves you feeling tense, making PMS feel even worse, says Dr Lark. Practise inhaling deeply and exhaling slowly.

Make love. The aching muscles and sluggish circulation that often accompany PMS can be relieved by having sex and reaching orgasm, says Dr Lark. The stimulation helps to move blood and other fluids away from congested organs.

Soak in a bath. Indulge yourself in a mineral bath to relax muscles from head to toe, Dr Lark suggests. Add a cupful of sea salt and a cupful of baking soda to warm bathwater. Soak for 20 minutes.

Take chasteberry. Most herbalists recommend chasteberry (*Agnus castus* fruit extract) as the best remedy for PMS symptoms, and there is some good research evidence showing that over half the women who took it daily for three cycles reported a better than 50 per cent improvement in their symptoms. Take it in tea, tincture or capsule form – available from health food stores. Take chasteberry every morning, as you would the birth control pill. You'll need to give it two or three cycles before you notice a change.

Do just *one* thing

Exercise. Experts agree that it may be the best prescription for PMS. Moderate exercise increases your bloodflow, relaxes your muscles and fights fluid retention, says PMS expert Susan Lark.

What's more, says researcher Edward Portman, exercise increases your brain's production of endorphins, natural opiates that make you feel better all over.

Walk briskly in the fresh air, swim, jog, take up dancing or karate – do something you enjoy on a daily basis. For best results, increase your level of activity for the week or two before PMS symptoms begin.

Black cohosh to the rescue. Though many people think of black cohosh as a herb for menopause, this does the remedy a great disservice, says clinical herbalist Douglas Schar. Known as squaw root by Native Americans, the herb has long been used for menstrual problems. Like chasteberry, black cohosh should be used for two or three cycles before its effects can be judged. Buy from a health food store and take according to label instructions.

Get extra sleep. If insomnia is part of your PMS, prepare for it by going to bed a little earlier for a few days before PMS sets in, says Dr Lark. It may help to alleviate the tiredness and irritability that go hand in hand with insomnia.

Stick to a routine. Set reasonable goals for each PMS day to avoid feeling overwhelmed, even if

WHEN TO CONSULT A DOCTOR

The symptoms of premenstrual syndrome rarely call for medical intervention, but drastic circumstances demand drastic measures. If you've tried almost everything here and nothing seems to help, talk to your doctor. In addition, if the symptoms of PMS are seriously affecting your health and other daily activities, see your doctor.

Sometimes, symptoms blamed on PMS may be due to something else: anxiety or depression, or relationship difficulties for example; or to other physical causes of fatigue or breast tenderness. Keep a diary and show your doctor: this will help to clarify if there is a definite monthly pattern, or if your mood problems or physical symptoms are bad throughout the month, and perhaps only a little worse pre-menstrually.

In addition, if the symptoms of PMS are seriously affecting your health, your relationships, your work or your general sense of wellbeing, your doctor may also be able to help. Hormonal strategies using the pill to stop ovulation, or a combination of an oestrogen and a hormonal intra-uterine device may be suggested. Antidepressants like fluoxetine (Prozac), used for depression, may also be suggested, even if you are not clinically depressed. There is good evidence that they help PMS symptoms by increasing serotonin levels in the brain.

Finally, if you feel that PMS is making you irritable or aggressive towards your children, don't be afraid to seek help from your doctor or health visitor.

this means cutting back your normal routine, Dr Lark suggests.

Organize your social life for another time. Don't even attempt to entertain when you know you're likely to be suffering from PMS. It'll only make an already tense situation worse, says Dr Lark.

Eat lots of small meals. Poor nutrition doesn't cause the condition, says Edward Portman, a researcher into PMS, but certain dietary factors can exacerbate it. Try eating small meals, high in starch but low in sugar and fat, several times a day, to help keep your body and mind in better balance.

Avoid empty calories. Avoid low-nutrient foods like soft drinks and sweets, says Guy Abraham, an obstetrician and gynaecologist. Giving in to a sugar craving will only make you feel worse by contributing to anxiety and mood swings. Instead, snack on fresh fruit and raw vegetables.

Help from supplements?

Many claims have been made for various combinations of diets, mineral and vitamin supplements, but the research evidence of benefit to PMS sufferers is generally lacking. Sticking to a healthy diet should usually make supplements unnecessary, but the following information on vitamins and minerals may help.

Vitamin B₆. There is some evidence that vitamin B₆ (pyridoxine) can help alleviate symptoms of PMS such as mood swings, fluid retention, breast tenderness, bloating, sugar cravings and fatigue. Good dietary sources are fortified cereals, beans, meat, poultry, fish, and some fruits and vegetables, or you can use supplements. Do not take more than 100mg a day, as an excess can damage the nervous system.

Vitamins A and D. These two vitamins work in tandem to improve the health of your skin. Because of their importance to the skin, they may play a part in suppressing premenstrual acne and oily skin.

Vitamin C. An antioxidant, vitamin C may help to relieve the stress felt during PMS. Vitamin C is also a natural antihistamine and can help women whose allergies worsen before a period.

Vitamin E. The evidence of benefit from this antioxidant vitamin is slight, but supporters claim it will relieve painful breast symptoms, anxiety and depression.

Calcium and magnesium. These two minerals work together. Calcium helps to prevent premenstrual cramps and pain, while magnesium helps the body to absorb calcium. Magnesium may also help to control premenstrual food cravings and stabilize moods.

Evening primrose oil. Some women have found evening primrose oil capsules helpful for some PMS symptoms, particularly painful breasts. Again, hard evidence for benefit is lacking, and doctors are no longer able to prescribe it for this problem.

Formulated supplements. Various combination supplements for PMS are available in pharmacies and supermarkets. If you are tempted by these, discuss with your doctor first.

Cut down on dairy foods. Eat no more than one or two servings per day of skimmed or semi-skimmed milk, cottage cheese or yoghurt, says Dr Abraham. The lactose in dairy products can block your body's absorption of the mineral magnesium, which helps to regulate oestrogen levels and increases its excretion.

Talk about it. Talking about your PMS problems with your partner, friends or colleagues at work helps. You can also talk to the National Association for Premenstrual Syndrome (NAPS), a medical charity providing information, advice and support to women affected by PMS, their partners and families. They have a Helpline, 0870 777 2177, and an excellent website at www.pms.org.uk.

Restrict salt. Eat a low-salt diet for a week before the onset of your period to combat water retention, suggests women's health expert Penny Wise Budoff. This means no restaurants or takeaways, processed foods, ready made soups or bottled salad dressings.

Fill up with fibre. Fibre helps your body to clear out excess oestrogens, says Dr Abraham. Eat plenty of vegetables, beans and wholemeal bread.

Cut down on caffeine. Consume only small amounts of coffee, tea, chocolate and other caffeine-containing substances, says Dr Abraham. Caffeine has been shown to contribute to painful breast tenderness, anxiety and irritability.

Abstain from alcohol. The depression that often accompanies PMS is exacerbated by alcohol, says Dr Portman. Drinking can also worsen PMS headaches and fatigue and cause sugar cravings, says Dr Lark.

Don't take diuretics. Many women with PMS take diuretics as a temporary measure against water-retention and bloating. But some over-the-counter diuretics draw valuable minerals out of your system along with water, says Dr Lark. A better approach is to avoid substances like salt and alcohol that make you retain water in the first place.

PROSTATE PROBLEMS
21 ways to ease the discomfort

The prostate – the gland responsible for producing most of the fluids in semen – is situated directly beneath the bladder. It fits around the urethra like a collar. (The urethra is the tube through which urine and semen pass out of the body.) Roughly the size of a pea at birth, the prostate begins growing rapidly during puberty, when testosterone levels rise. In adults, it's the size and shape of a conker. When a man hits his mid-40s, his prostate often begins to grow again, probably due to changes in hormone levels. The result is a condition called benign prostatic hyperplasia, or BPH, the technical term for enlarged prostate.

More than 90 per cent of men over 70 have BPH, and by this age, about one in three will be experiencing symptoms from it. The symptoms of BPH include frequency, urgency and discomfort when urinating, weak urinary flow, difficulty starting urination, dribbling at the end of urination, getting up at night to urinate and a feeling that the bladder is not completely empty.

BPH isn't the only ailment that strikes the prostate. At one time or another, roughly 50 per cent of all men develop prostatitis, a condition in which the prostate gland becomes inflamed or, more rarely, infected with bacteria. Prostatitis is not a life-threatening condition. It may come on acutely with flu-like symptoms (high temperature, muscle and joint pains), pain and bleeding on urinating, pain in the rectum, and discharge from the penis; or it may be chronic, with symptoms similar to BPH, plus pain in the genitals or abdomen which is sometimes worse on ejaculation, fluctuating temperature and fatigue.

Prostate cancer is rare before the age of 50. Half of all cases occur in men who are over 75. Overall, a man's average lifetime risk of getting prostate cancer in the UK is about one in 12. Many prostate cancers are slow growing: they are often found by chance, and may have little impact on health or life expectancy. There is little to distinguish the symptoms of early prostate cancer from those of BPH. Increasing attention has been given to a blood test for prostate disease, PSA, as a way of screening for cancer, but experts in many parts of the world, including Britain, doubt its usefulness as a general screening test, even in those with prostate symptoms. If you have prostate symptoms, or you have a family history of prostate cancer, or you are worried about cancer, discuss the pros and cons of the PSA test with your doctor before deciding to have it.

Harvest the power of saw palmetto. The berry extract of this palm tree is widely used to treat an enlarged prostate. In 1998, scientists wondered if its reputation was warranted. They examined 18 clinical studies and concluded that saw palmetto yielded improvements similar to those produced by finasteride – a commonly prescribed testosterone-lowering drug – but with fewer side-effects. Among the benefits reported were stronger urinary flow, fewer night-time trips to the loo, less urine held in the bladder following urination and less urinary frequency.

Two to three 500mg capsules per day of saw palmetto extract should result in an improvement in one to three months.

Note: See your doctor for proper diagnosis and monitoring before self-treating a serious condition like enlarged prostate

Take nettle root. Nettle root extract is becoming increasingly popular as a treatment for BPH, says clinical herbalist Douglas Schar. Scientifically, it is thought to act in similar way to saw palmetto. As no one drug, herbal or otherwise, works for all people, nettle root is worth a try if saw palmetto doesn't work for you, says Schar. But, he adds, be sure that you buy nettle root: nettle leaf is not effective for treating BPH. Buy capsules from health food stores and take according to label instructions.

Try pygeum. Several studies have found this fruit of an African evergreen effective, possibly because of its anti-inflammatory properties. 'The active extract seems to reduce symptoms of frequent night-time urination and difficulty urinating,' says nutrition expert Winston Craig. The standard dose is 100 to 200mg per day in capsule form.

Eat pumpkin seeds. Pumpkin seeds contain high levels of phytosterols and zinc – both important for prostate health. The seeds were first used to treat prostate problems by Native Americans. The key to success is daily intake: anyone with BPH – or trying to prevent it – should eat a teaspoonful or two of pumpkin seeds every day, says Schar. You can buy hulled seeds at any health food store. They are nutty and delicious. Sprinkle them on salads, add to breakfast cereals or munch them straight from the bag.

Add some tomatoes. Lycopene, the compound that makes tomatoes red, can do more than add colour to your salad. Research shows that eating tomatoes is associated with a reduced risk of prostate cancer. Urologist Martin Gelbard prescribes tomatoes for his patients with BPH and prostatitis. 'It helps to relieve symptoms and may prevent the progression of prostate enlargement.' Eat two or three tomatoes or tomato-based products a day, he says.

What not to eat. Some foods and drinks can make matters worse for men with prostatitis. Avoid spicy foods, fizzy drinks, caffeinated drinks and acidic foods such as citrus fruits and juices. These irritate the lining of the prostate, says Dr Gelbard. Spirits do the same, but beer and wine are okay.

Stop smoking. One study in the USA found that BPH symptoms were reduced in cigarette smokers, but before you reach for the packet and light up, other studies have shown an increased risk of aggressive prostate cancer with heavy smoking. Given the 200-plus other reasons to quit smoking, there's still no contest. Give them up!

Keep on your toes. Men whose jobs involve hours of sitting, especially occupations that constantly put pressure on the prostate area, such as

WHEN TO CONSULT A DOCTOR

Problems with urinating are the most common symptoms of prostate disease. The Prostate Research Campaign UK advises you to visit your doctor if you experience any one of the following:

- a weak, sometimes intermittent flow of urine;
- difficulty starting to urinate;
- a need to urinate frequently;
- a need to urinate urgently (that is, you don't feel able to put it off);
- having to go to the toilet several times during the night (for a period of time);
- a feeling that your bladder is not completely empty after you have finished urinating;
- pain or burning when passing urine;
- blood in your urine.

lorry driving, are more prone both to BPH and prostatitis. Take regular, frequent breaks from sitting, recommends holistic practitioner Willard Dean. Getting out of your seat helps to stop circulation being reduced in that area of the body and relieves symptoms.

Get some exercise. 'Men who exercise more are less likely to have symptoms of BPH,' says researcher Elizabeth Platz. By contrast, their inactive counterparts – those who, according to her study, spent 41 or more hours a week watching television – are 42 per cent more likely to develop BPH and exhibit more severe symptoms. According to Dr Platz, walking for just two or more hours per week yields positive results.

Cycle on a split seat. If cycling is your favourite form of exercise, beware – it puts pressure on the prostate. This can lead to prostatitis or exacerbate an existing condition, says Dr Gelbard. 'Get a split bicycle seat,' he recommends. A split seat is cushioned on either side, so your weight rests on the bones of your pelvis, keeping pressure off the prostate.

Consider alcohol. Moderate alcohol consumption may produce a possibly reduced risk for BPH. Dr Platz found that men who drank two to three beers a day (or the equivalent) reported fewer symptoms of BPH. Researchers aren't sure why. It could be that muscle relaxation plays a role. 'Alcohol tends to relax muscles. It might relax muscles important to bladder control,' suggests Dr Platz. This doesn't mean you should start drinking alcohol to reduce symptoms, but don't feel you have to stop moderate drinking. Bear in mind, however, that alcohol can irritate the bladder and may aggravate urinary frequency.

Sit in a warm bath. A warm bath brings heat to the prostate gland and relaxes lower abdominal muscles. 'It reduces inflammation and cuts down on pain and urgency,' says Dr Gelbard. Soak in deep warm water for 15 minutes a day. If you are finding it difficult to pass urine at all, get into a bath as hot as you can bear: the heat will relax your bladder, allowing you to pass urine into the bathwater.

Wear loose cotton underpants. Tight, restrictive underwear restricts bloodflow to the area surrounding the prostate. 'Good bloodflow brings nutrients to the gland and carries away waste products,' says Dr Dean. And synthetic fabrics trap sweat, while cotton absorbs moisture and allows skin to breathe.

Make love more. 'Since the prostate is directly involved in the production of semen, ejaculation can be therapeutic,' says Dr Dean. During ejaculation, muscles surrounding the prostate contract. 'Think of it as exercise for the prostate,' he says. 'It's very good for blood flow.'

Try a foot rub. Reflexology is a natural therapy that can be helpful for prostate ailments, says Dr Dean. The principle behind reflexology is that the hands and feet contain sensors that connect to all other parts of the body. By massaging the reflex points related to the prostate, you send a signal to the gland that stimulates healing. The point for the prostate is located at the base of the heel on either side. (Charts showing actual points are available from some health food stores.)

Once you find the point, rub it with your thumb, a marble or a pencil rubber. 'Rub for 20 to 30 seconds a couple of times a day,' says Dr Dean. The spot may be sore at first, indicating that the gland is in need of balance. With continued rubbing, it will become less sensitive.

Avoid cold cures. Decongestants and antihistamines can cause the muscles that control urine flow to contract, making urination more difficult. If you suffer from allergies, ask your doctor to prescribe cold and allergy medicines that don't contain antihistamines.

Avoid constipation. A full bowel may obstruct your urine flow as it pushes on an already narrowed urethra. Eat plenty of fibre to keep your bowel moving regularly and easily.

Drink plenty of water. If you're tempted to drink less because you're tired of so many trips to the loo, don't give in to the temptation, warns Dr Gelbard. Dehydration will make things worse. Drinking enough water every day is important for proper functioning of the kidneys and can prevent urinary infections. Aim for six to eight 250ml glasses a day.

But not before bed. If you want to cut back on night-time visits to the toilet, don't drink any liquids after 6pm, advises Dr Gelbard. Empty your bladder completely before going to bed but go back to the toilet a few minutes later: you'll usually manage to pass a little more urine by using this 'double voiding' technique, and often save yourself an extra trip to the loo in the middle of the night.

Take a load off. If you're troubled by difficulty in getting started, don't be embarrassed to sit down to urinate – you'll find it much easier, especially if you take your time, and relax.

Do away with the dribble. If dribbling at the end of urination is a problem, hold some toilet tissue to the end of your penis before you do yourself up: the tissue draws out the last few drops of urine from your urethra, saving your trousers from a telltale wet patch.

PSORIASIS
17 skin-soothing remedies

Psoriasis is a disease in which the skin cells multiply very rapidly. Normally, skin renews itself in about 30 days – that's the time it takes for a new skin cell to work its way from the innermost layer of skin to the surface. In psoriasis, that cell reaches the top in just three days, as if the body's brakes have failed. The result is raised areas of skin called plaques, which are red and often itchy – psoriasis is derived from the Greek word 'psora', which means itch.

After the cells reach the surface they die like normal cells, but there are so many of them that the raised patches turn white with dead cells flaking off. Psoriasis usually goes through cycles of flare-ups and remission, with flare-ups most commonly occurring in winter. Sometimes it disappears for months or years. The condition can improve or get worse with age, and can affect the nails and joints as well as the skin.

Around two per cent of people in the UK have psoriasis to a greater or lesser degree. The condition is not contagious.

The cause of psoriasis is unknown, although it does tend to run in families, so a genetic component is likely. If you are susceptible, you might notice new spots coming up soon after the skin is cut, scratched, rubbed, or severely sunburned. Psoriasis can also be activated by infections, such as strep throat, and by certain medicines. Flare-ups sometimes occur during winter months, as a result of a combination of dry skin and lack of sunlight, and can also be precipitated by stress.

There is no known cure for psoriasis, but many things can soothe the itching and reduce the severity of the condition. Here are some strategies to try.

Adopt a new attitude. Accepting that you have psoriasis and focusing your attention on learning how to manage it is the best thing you can do, says dermatologist Philip Anderson. 'Don't waste energy fussing over every bump.'

Feed your skin. Emollients top every dermatologist's list of over-the-counter treatments. Psoriatic skin is dry, and that can mean a worsening of the psoriasis and increased flaking and itching. Emollients help your skin to retain water. The emollient can be your favourite non-irritating body oil or something as mundane as vegetable oil or petroleum jelly. It's most effective applied straight after a bath, when you're still wet. For a natural alternative, try a herbal cream with calendula and beeswax to seal in moisture. An aloe vera-based cream may also be helpful.

Don't scratch. The more you scratch, the more you'll itch. Sit on your hands, keep your nails short, wear gloves at night if you find you're scratching in your sleep. An antihistamine that is slightly sedating, like hydroxyzine (Atarax) can sometimes help at night.

Turn on the lamp. Buy yourself a small ultraviolet A/ultraviolet B sunlamp to treat patches of psoriasis, suggests dermatologist Laurence Miller. Each person's needs vary, and UV light does increase risks of skin cancer, so consult your doctor first. You may prefer the high UVA and low UVB light found in tanning studios, but this light is weaker and needs much more time to work.

Use tar. Over-the-counter coal tar preparations are weaker than prescription versions but can be effective in treating mild psoriasis, says Dr Miller. You can apply the tar directly to the plaques or immerse yourself in tar bath oil and treat your scalp with tar shampoo like T Gel or Polytar. New tar products are available that are more elegant and cosmetically appealing in gel form. They don't smell strongly of tar, they can be used every day and they wash off easily.

Note: If any tar product causes burning or irritation, stop using it. Never use tar on raw, open skin.

Get wet and warm. Baths and heated swimming pools are excellent for psoriasis, Dr Miller says. They flatten plaques or cut down scaling. But don't bath in hot water as this can make itching worse.

Or get wet and cold. A cool-water bath, maybe with a cup or so of cider vinegar added, is great for itching. 'Another thing that really works is ice,' Dr Miller says. 'Just put some ice cubes into a small plastic bag and hold it against the affected skin.'

Try hydrocortisone for small areas. 'Over-the-counter hydrocortisone creams are much weaker than prescription versions, but they're worth trying, and they're safer on the face and genital areas,' Dr Miller says. 'But if you use it all the time in these areas, it will become less effective, and when you give up on it, the psoriasis can rebound. Just use it until you show some improvement, and then gradually wean yourself off.'

Stronger steroid creams and ointments are available on prescription. These are useful for short-term relief, but using them for long periods can cause permanent damage to the skin. Do not use any steroid without an antibiotic on skin that looks infected.

Don't risk injury. New patches of psoriasis often appear where the skin has been injured, says Dr Anderson. Researchers believe damage to the skin sends the body into ungovernable overdrive. 'People with psoriasis shouldn't go blackberry-picking, just as a man with a bad back shouldn't be a piano mover,' he says. You can injure your skin with all sorts of things, from tight shoes or watch-straps to blunt razors and harsh chemicals.

Lose weight if you're over-weight. While there is no scientific proof that obesity worsens

Do just *one* thing

Get some sun. With regular doses of strong sunlight, 95 per cent of people with psoriasis improve. Ultraviolet waves seem to fight psoriasis, and UVB rays work the fastest. But UVBs are also the rays that give you sunburn and increase your risk of skin cancer. They can also cause people with psoriasis to break out in previously unaffected areas.

The answer, says dermatologist Laurence Miller, is to use a good sunscreen on the places where you don't have psoriasis and only expose affected areas to the full force of the sun.

WHEN TO CONSULT A DOCTOR

The impact of psoriasis on people's lives can range from mildly annoying to completely debilitating. If your symptoms are out of control, your doctor can prescribe a number of treatments including emollients, dithranol-based creams, vitamin D derivatives like calcipotriol, and steroid creams or ointments. For more severe psoriasis, you may need referral to a dermatologist, where phototherapy, mixed drug and light therapy (PUVA), or the drug methotrexate may be offered to you.

psoriasis, there is a link, says Dr Anderson. Losing weight helps many people with psoriasis. 'If you lose weight and maintain a normal weight, psoriasis is almost always better.'

Try to relax. Overwhelming evidence shows that stress triggers psoriasis, says dermatologist Eugene Farber. 'If you lie on a beach for a week, you get better. Even going into hospital for surgery can make your psoriasis better. Although it's stressful, you're relaxing and being cared for. Any absence from your daily stresses for any length of time is helpful.'

Avoid alcohol. If you're a heavy drinker, the nutritional problems that accompany binge drinking will make your psoriasis worse.

Try fish oil. Taking fish oil capsules containing a fatty acid known as EPA may help. Although the largest trial showed no benefit from fish oil over corn oil, a small research study found that fish oil supplements benefited 60 per cent of those studied. The area and thickness of the plaques decreased, as did redness and itching.

'But a small number of people will not improve, and a small number will get worse,' says dermatologist Vincent Ziboh. Furthermore, fish oil affects blood clotting, so it can enhance the blood-thinning effects of other

KITCHEN CURES

Try this treatment if psoriasis is affecting your scalp. Warm some olive oil until it reaches body temperature. Massage the oil into your scalp. Put on a shower cap and leave it to 'cook' for 30 minutes – or even overnight. Wash out the oil with a dandruff shampoo. Do this every night until your skin clears up, and then continue the treatment once or twice a week.

drugs you may be taking. Before trying EPA, talk to your doctor.

It's a good idea to eat oily fish such as salmon or mackerel, too. But you'd have to eat up to a kilo a day to get the recommended 5g of EPA.

Oregon grape to the rescue. Oregon grape was first introduced as a psoriasis cure in 1869 – by a company that has since become a pharmaceutical giant. The most effective way to use it is as a tincture, says clinical herbalist Douglas Schar. Take 5ml of tincture (strength 1:5) three times a day. You'll need to take it for at least two months before judging its effects. It may be slow acting, but it makes a huge difference. The tincture is available in health food stores.

Treat infections. A well-documented but unexplained link exists between infections and the initial onset of psoriasis. Existing psoriasis is also known to worsen when an infection strikes. It's important to treat all infections promptly, and to devote extra attention to psoriasis when you have any type of infection.

RASHES
18 soothing solutions for contact dermatitis

Just about everyone can get a rash if their skin is exposed for long enough to everyday materials that are irritant enough. Especially if you've got sensitive skin to start with, contact dermatitis, another name, really, for one form of eczema, can result from exposure to soap, detergents, bleaches and solvents. Red, burning, bubbling, itching, cracking and even bleeding patches of skin are the result. Some people get a much more marked and prolonged dermatitis in response to certain materials which don't bother most of us at all. These people have allergic contact dermatitis, and the triggers that cause it are known as allergens.

Common rash-producing allergens include:

- nickel, a metal often used in glasses frames, cheap jewellery and belt buckles;

- wet cement;

- cosmetics, hair dyes and perfumes;

- rubber and latex found in products such as rubber gloves and condoms;

- plants and flowers such as dahlias, primulas and chrysanthemums.

Almost anything can cause a rash, though, including food and drugs (see *Allergies*, page 28). Children with a family history of allergies and sensitive skin can be very vulnerable to rashes. If you and your doctor are unable to identify and remove the cause of the allergy, then a referral to a paediatrician, dermatologist or allergy clinic for allergy tests might be necessary. Working out what triggered a rash can be very difficult. You need to go to your doctor armed with a complete list of substances you've come into contact with and take it from there. Meanwhile, here are some common causes and cures for rashes.

Nickel Rash

Nickel is often mixed with other metals to make rings, watch cases, necklaces and bracelets. Costume jewellery is by far the most common cause of nickel reactions. But nickel allergy is easy to diagnose because the rash appears wherever nickel touches your skin, says dermatologist Ralph Daniel. For example, you may get a rash on your ears if you wear earrings with nickel in them. Here's what to do.

Change your jewellery. Many women have allergic reactions to costume jewellery with nickel. If you stop wearing that particular jewellery, the rashes will disappear, says Dr Daniel.

Go for gold. 'I've never heard of anyone who's allergic to pure gold,' says dermatologist Larry Millikan. So perhaps it's time to replace the jewellery that's giving you problems with something made of gold.

Don't sweat in it. Perspiration can aggravate dermatitis in nickel-sensitive people. Items containing nickel can cause an itchy, prickly sensation within 20 minutes of touching a sweaty palm. But the same items can be worn for several hours without any problems if you're not sweaty, says Dr Daniel. So take off your jewellery before you go to the gym.

Cement Rash

This is a common cause of contact dermatitis. The culprit is a chemical called chromate found in

Do just *one* thing

Avoid scratching. However maddening the itch, scratching will damage skin that is already suffering, and it will release histamines into the skin that will just make the itch much worse the minute you stop scratching. Break this itch-scratch cycle: keep nails short; wear cotton gloves at night if you scratch in your sleep; wear cool, cotton clothes; keep your room cool at night; and use ice packs to deaden the jangling nerve endings in your skin.

cement, paints and anti-rust products. Builders, decorators and DIY enthusiasts can all be exposed to chromate.

Wear gloves. If you can't avoid the chemical, at least stop it from getting on your hands. Wear a sturdy pair of waterproof work gloves to keep chromate from irritating your skin.

Wash often. Make sure your wash your hands often when working with chromate to ensure that if any of the chemical does get on your skin, it's not there very long. And because frequent washing dries out your skin, follow with a good moisturizer.

Use a lighter. Some matches also contain chromates, so touching unlit matches can contaminate your fingers. Even keeping a book of unlit matches in a pocket will contaminate the pocket lining of those trousers. Put your hands in your pockets, and bingo – a rash. Carry a lighter instead. Better still, give up smoking.

WHEN TO CONSULT A DOCTOR

A rash developing over much of the body could be a symptom of an infectious disease, particularly if it's associated with a fever or feeling unwell. Consult your doctor, especially if it's a child who has the rash. You may need antibiotics if you have a rash that has pus-filled spots or the golden crust typical of impetigo. You may have other skin conditions that might be mistaken for contact dermatitis, such as psoriasis, atopic eczema, or seborrhoeic dermatitis.

See your doctor if you have a rash that:

• doesn't show signs of healing after five to six days;

• develops after you take a medicine;

• is evident on more than one person in your household.

Purpurae: the 'meningitis rash'. Purpurae are small purple marks on the skin – tiny bruises that can appear spontaneously. Occasionally they may indicate septicaemia caused by one of the bacteria (meningococcus) responsible also for meningitis. If you or a child develops spontaneous purpurae or larger bruises, especially in association with fever, drowsiness, vomiting, stiff neck or headache, seek **immediate** medical attention.

The glass test. If you suspect that a rash may be caused by purpurae, press the side of a glass firmly against the skin. *With purpurae, the rash doesn't fade.*

Additive Rash

Exposure to preservatives and fragrances used in hand creams, lotions and other skin-care products causes rashes in many people. Washing-up liquids and household cleaning products, soaps, shampoos and fabric conditioners can all cause contact dermatitis.

Read labels. If you know that a particular additive causes you problems, check the labels of other products and avoid that additive.

Be consistent. Find products that work for you and keep to them, says Dr Daniel. If you're using a particular washing powder and your skin becomes irritated, switch to another one. 'If you find something that works for you and doesn't cause you any problems, stick with it.'

KITCHEN CURES

For a soothing compress, make some runny oatmeal porridge and allow it to cool. Then scoop the mixture into an old sock and strain out the liquid. You can use this sock as a compress to apply to the rash for 10 minutes every two hours. Do this until the symptoms subside.

Rubber Rash

Chemical additives in rubber products, especially latex gloves, can often cause allergic reactions and rashes, including itching, burning and even welts. They're common among people who wear tight-fitting rubber gloves, such as medical personnel. Here are some approaches to try.

Try a different glove. Powderless rubber gloves may be less allergenic, or vinyl (or other synthetic gloves) may be used as a substitute.

Use hypoallergenic condoms. Vaginal irritation and soreness may occur in women who are allergic to the rubber in condoms (the lubricant may also be responsible). Men too may be affected. Ask for hypoallergenic condoms at the pharmacy or your family planning clinic.

Change your underwear. Underclothes are common triggers of rubber rashes – it's the elasticated waists. Visit the lingerie section of a department store and ask for advice on underwear with covered waistbands.

Check your shoes. Many cases of allergic contact dermatitis are caused by ingredients used to make shoes, such as leather, certain dyes, adhesives and rubber. But because so many parts of your shoe could be causing that foot rash, see if your doctor can arrange a patch test to determine what exactly you are allergic to before you buy new shoes.

Plant Rashes

Florists and people who work in garden centres and who notice an outbreak of dermatitis in autumn are probably allergic to chrysanthemums. A rash on the fingertips might be triggered by touching the bulbs of tulips or hyacinths, while primulas can cause a local rash where the plant has been touched, or widespread urticaria (nettle rash). The list of potential allergens in the garden is too large to summarize here, but if you develop a rash after gardening then put plants at the top of your list of suspects.

Rinse well. After touching a plant allergen wash yourself straight away with water. If possible, wipe the area with surgical spirit and follow that with a thorough wash in water, says dermatologist William Epstein.

Use what you have. If you don't happen to have surgical spirit to hand, wet wipes or baby wipes are a good alternative if you have them.

Take a pill. If a maddening itch develops, take an oral antihistamine, suggests dermatologist Robert Rietschel. 'You could even take your hay fever medicine if it happens to be an antihistamine,' he adds.

Cover with a compress. Put a cotton cloth soaked in cool water over an itchy rash and let a fan blow onto it, Dr Rietschel advises. The cooling and evaporating effect works like calamine lotion. It's also a good idea to rub ice on the affected area.

RAYNAUD'S SYNDROME
16 ways to warm up

If you have Raynaud's syndrome, then you know that gloves and mittens are never enough. Not only are your fingers (and sometimes toes) often cold, but the reaction to sudden cold as your blood vessels constrict and blood flow slows can be excruciatingly painful. As blood flow to the affected area slows down, the lack of oxygenated blood causes fingers and toes to turn pale, and maybe even take on a bluish tinge.

The condition affects around one in ten people in the UK. Ninety per cent are women, with young women being particularly susceptible.

Not everyone experiences Raynaud's in the same way. Some feel numbness from the lack of blood, then their fingers turn red again when the blood returns. In advanced stages of Raynaud's, poor blood supply can weaken the fingers and damage the sense of touch.

Cold isn't the only culprit. This odd affliction can also result from injury to the blood vessels caused by vibrations from powerful equipment like chain saws and pneumatic drills, hypersensitivity to drugs that affect the blood vessels, or disorders of the connective tissue or nerves.

Our experts provide some protective suggestions.

Condition yourself to overcome chills. Train your hands to heat up in the cold by adapting this technique devised by US Army researchers in Alaska. Choose a room that's a comfortable temperature and put your hands in a bowl of warm water for three to five minutes. Then go into a cold room and again dip your hands in warm water for 10 minutes.

The cold environment would normally make your peripheral blood vessels constrict, but, instead, the sensation of the warm water makes them open. Repeatedly training the blood vessels to open despite the cold eventually enables you to counter the constriction reflex even without the warm water.

Twirl your arms to generate heat. Force your hands to warm up through a simple exercise devised by dermatologist Donald McIntyre. Swing your arm downwards behind your body and then upwards in front of you at about 80 twirls per minute. (This isn't as fast as it sounds – give it a try.) The windmill effect, which Dr McIntyre modelled after a skier's warm-up exercise, forces blood to the fingers through both gravitational and centrifugal forces. This warm-up works well for chilled hands no matter what the cause.

Eat iron-rich foods. Lack of iron may alter your thyroid metabolism, which regulates body heat. Iron-rich foods include poultry, fish, lean red meat, lentils and leafy green vegetables. Orange juice is good, too, because it increases your body's ability to absorb iron.

Eat a hot meal. The very act of eating causes a rise in core body temperature. This is called thermogenesis. So eat something before you go out to stoke your body's furnace. Something hot will boost that stoking: a bowl of hot porridge before your morning walk, a cup of soup or a hot lunch will help to keep your hands and feet warm even in chilly weather.

Drink up. Dehydration can aggravate chills by reducing your blood volume. Ward off the cold by drinking plenty of warm fluids such as herbal teas or homemade vegetable or chicken stock.

Say no to coffee. Coffee and other foods or drinks containing caffeine constrict blood vessels. The last thing you want when you have Raynaud's syndrome is to interfere with your circulation.

WHEN TO CONSULT A DOCTOR

Raynaud's syndrome may be a symptom of an underlying disorder, such as rheumatoid arthritis, scleroderma or lupus. Cold feet may be a result of arterial circulation problems secondary to diabetes or hardening of the arteries, rather than Raynaud's, so you should always check with a doctor – as a matter of urgency if the problem comes on suddenly.

Some medications, for example beta blockers for high blood pressure or angina, can cause cold hands and feet. Speak to your doctor if you think you are affected, but don't stop the medication beforehand.

Avoid alcohol. Don't be tempted by a hot toddy. Alcohol temporarily warms your hands and feet by increasing blood flow to the skin and making you feel warmer. But that heat is soon lost, reducing your core body temperature. In other words, alcohol actually makes you colder.

Dress warmly. Keep your core body temperature warm by dressing suitably in cold weather. Before you go out, warm your hands before you put your mittens on: mittens keep you warmer than gloves because they trap your whole hand's heat rather than one finger at a time. And wear a hat: you lose most of your body heat through your head.

Try portable heating aids. Some people find that electrically heated gloves are helpful. There are many small portable heating aids available from outdoor shops and catalogues. For more information contact the Raynaud's & Scleroderma Association, 112 Crewe Road, Alsager, Cheshire ST7 2JA; tel: 01270 872776; www.raynauds.demon.co.uk.

Wear loose clothes. None of your garments should pinch. Tight-fitting clothes can cut off circulation and eliminate insulating air pockets.

Dress in layers. If you're going out in the cold, the best warming measure you can take is to dress in layers. This helps to trap heat and allows you to peel off clothes as the temperature changes.

Waterproof your body. Choose a breathable, waterproof jacket or windjammer. Gore-Tex shoes and boots are a good choice for keeping your feet warm and dry. And wear warm socks, too.

Use a foot powder. 'Absorbent foot powders are excellent for helping to keep feet dry,' says foot specialist Marc Brenner.

Note: If you have severe cold feet problems caused by diabetes and peripheral vascular disease, be sure to use a talcum shaker not a foot spray, as the mist from the spray can freeze your feet.

Don't smoke. Cigarette smoke cools you down in two ways. It helps to form plaque in your arteries and, more immediately, it contains nicotine, which causes narrowing of the small blood vessels thus restricting the amount of blood available to keep your hands and feet warm.

Stay out of smoky pubs, too. 'Raynaud's patients are sensitive even to other people's smoke,' says vascular surgeon Frederick Reichle.

Chill out to warm up. Keeping calm may help you to keep warm. Stress has a similar effect on your body as cold. Blood is redirected from the hands and feet to the brain and internal organs to enable you to think and react more quickly.

RESTLESS LEGS
20 calming techniques

Restless legs syndrome (RLS) causes unpleasant burning, prickling, tickling or aching sensations in the muscles of the legs. It is sometimes referred to as Ekbom's syndrome after the doctor who first recognized it. Classic symptoms include fidgety, crawling or jittery feelings in the lower limbs, usually when the sufferer is in bed at night.

The condition affects at least five per cent of the population in the UK, although this may be a conservative estimate: some experts think the true number of people affected may be more like 10 or 15 per cent.

RLS tends to run in families and is most likely to affect middle-aged women, the elderly, pregnant women, people who drink a lot of coffee or other caffeine-containing drinks and people who smoke heavily.

It usually affects both lower legs but it's not always symmetrical; sometimes it occurs in only one limb. Its cause is unknown. Whatever the cause, restless legs syndrome can be very frustrating to those who have it, and it can significantly disrupt your sleep, and that of your partner. Here are a few steps to calm those jumpy legs.

What about iron and folate supplements? Some studies have shown a relationship between RLS and the way certain brain cells fail to utilize iron, and other small trials have shown benefit with high doses of iron supplements. Folate supplements have also been suggested for pregnant women with RLS. 'The truth is,' says family doctor Stephen Amiel, 'the evidence is by no means compelling, and unless you have proven iron or folate deficiency, I would not recommend supplements. Even if blood tests show deficiencies, there is no guarantee that the supplements will make any difference to the part of the brain responsible for RLS.'

Don't eat a big meal late. Eating a lot late at night may get your legs really jumping. The activity of digesting a big meal may trigger something that causes symptoms, suggests neurologist Lawrence Stern.

Avoid sleeping pills. They may provide short-term benefits but many people build up a tolerance to them, and then they have two problems – restless legs syndrome *and* dependence on the drugs, says Dr Stern.

Don't use alcohol as a sedative. Again, you set yourself up for double trouble, Dr Stern says.

Give up coffee. Some studies have shown a link between relief of restless legs syndrome and stopping caffeine, syas neurologist Ronald Pfeiffer.

Avoid cold and sinus remedies. These may increase symptoms.

Give up smoking. Smoking may not cause restless legs syndrome, but smokers are significantly more likely than non-smokers to have RLS.

Come in from the cold. Several studies have found that prolonged exposure to cold may cause restless legs syndrome.

Walk before going to bed. This can noticeably reduce bedtime bouts of RLS, says Dr Stern. 'Exercise changes chemical balances in the brain – endorphins are released, which may promote more restful sleep.'

Massage your legs. Rubbing your legs just before bedtime may be beneficial, says neurologist Richard Olney. Gentle stretching also may help.

Take two aspirins at bedtime. Doctors can't say why aspirin helps, but apparently it does reduce symptoms in some people.

Lower your stress level. 'Stress worsens the problem,' says Dr Stern. Being organized, giving yourself quiet time, taking deep breaths and practising relaxation techniques are good ways to reduce stress.

Get plenty of rest. Symptoms may be more severe if you get overtired.

WHEN TO CONSULT A DOCTOR

If you have restless legs syndrome, you probably don't have anything to worry about – except for the sleep it sometimes makes you miss.

But if you're experiencing symptoms for the first time – pronounced sensations in the legs, usually at night – see your doctor. The symptoms of restless legs syndrome could be warning signs for serious medical problems such as lung disease, kidney disease, diabetes, Parkinson's disease and many neurological disorders. RLS may also be associated with sleep apnoea and narcolepsy, as well as with treatment with some antidepressants or major tranquillizers used for certain mental illnesses.

To be on the safe side, let your doctor make the diagnosis. If jittery legs are keeping you up at night and home remedies aren't helping, your doctor may be able to prescribe something to help.

Get up and walk. Restless legs syndrome tends to strike at night, when you're at rest. When you feel the urge to move, the quickest way to satisfy it is to give in with a walk around the bedroom, says Dr Pfeiffer.

Wiggle your feet. Easy – just move your feet backwards and forwards when symptoms arise.

Change sleeping position. Some people develop symptoms more often sleeping in one position than in another, says Dr Stern. Try different sleeping positions. It's harmless and may prove to be worthwhile.

Make your bed less comfortable. RLS seems to be worse for some people the more comfortable they are, says Dr Amiel. Try a harder bed or sleeping on the floor.

Soak your feet in cool water. 'It works for some,' Dr Pfeiffer says. But don't immerse your feet in iced water; you could cause nerve damage.

Warm up. While cold helps some people, others find using a heating pad more soothing and effective, Dr Pfeiffer says.

Massage your legs with a vibrator. Some people say that this reduces symptoms; in a few people, however, it could make things worse.

ROAD RAGE
16 tips for a happier, safer drive

Drivers in the UK are more likely to lose their tempers than any other European drivers, according to the RAC Foundation. This emerged from a survey of 10,000 drivers in 16 countries. It's probably largely due to the fact that we have the highest number of vehicles per mile of road in Europe, says the RAC. The study found that while the Dutch and Germans go in for tailgating, and the Italians tend to swear and shout, drivers in Britain are likely to resort to more dangerous behaviour like forcing a car off the road or attacking other drivers.

Most people don't participate in serious road rage, says psychologist Leon James, but we all are aggressive drivers. We learn competitive and aggressive attitudes in the car from our parents and from television. By the time we start driving, our attitudes are pretty fixed.

Some of the 'symptoms' of aggressive driving include feeling stressed behind the wheel, swearing, speeding, yelling or honking, making insulting gestures, tailgating, cutting up others, indulging in violent fantasies, or feeling enraged, competitive or compelled to drive dangerously.

Anonymity is a major contributor to the problem, says psychologist Arnold Nerenberg. In cars, we tend to dehumanize each other. 'We don't think, this is a human being just like me, with fears, aspirations, love and vulnerabilities. It's some jerk who's cut me up and I'm going to teach him a lesson.' But there may be a price to pay. An aggressive driver who causes a crash, injury or death is likely to end up in court, or worse.

So here are some tips from the experts on how to relax behind the wheel, as well as some ways to steer clear of aggressive or angry drivers.

Leave more time. Often we're a time bomb waiting to go off before we even get into our car, rushing to get to a meeting, or pick the children up, cutting it fine to catch a plane or get to a show. We've already shouted at the kids, had a row with our partner and missed breakfast. A traffic jam, a wrong turn, red lights against us or roadworks mean we're going to be late – our stress levels boil over and we're ready to kill. Plan ahead instead: work out how long your journey is likely to take, factor in some delays, plan your route and, if necessary, tell your family that the film starts twenty minutes before it actually does.

Lend support. Instead of competing with other drivers, support them, says Dr James. 'If they want to enter the lane ahead of you, make space. If they want to pass, move over and let them,' he says. 'When you're a supportive driver, the stress not only vanishes, you begin to enjoy traffic.'

Drive in the slow lane. 'Try life in the left lane,' Dr James suggests. People often avoid the slower lane because they fear losing time. But if you drive in the slow lane, you'll keep pace with less aggressive drivers and may discover it's not that slow after all.

Control yourself. Don't let other drivers do it for you, says Dr Nerenberg. He asks aggressive drivers: 'do you want to give control to those people you're calling idiots?' Losing your cool is nothing short of giving control away.

Report it. If you or anyone you know is the victim of a road rage incident, report it to the police immediately. And visit www.reportroadrage.co.uk, a website sponsored by the RAC Foundation that aims to reduce road rage.

Listen to your passengers. 'Backseat drivers have a bad reputation,' says Diane Nahl, a researcher into aggressive driving, 'but they may have a point.' So listen to the complaints of your partner, your children and others who drive with you.

Be responsible to your passengers. Drivers often feel they are captain of their ship. They control the temperature, radio station and speed. Try asking your passengers what they'd like. They'll appreciate the consideration, and you'll feel better about yourself and calmer when driving.

Be silly. Feeling tense behind the wheel? Try making animal noises, machine sounds or anything else you find amusing. 'Laughter not only interrupts your negative thinking or anger, but it also disperses stress,' says Dr Nahl.

Entertain yourself. Take your mind off the drive without taking your eyes off the road: listen to music that soothes you, or you can sing along to; play a tape of a favourite book or comedy; get the family to join in a quiz.

Take a break. Driving is tiring and stressful. If your concentration lapses on a long journey, or you're tired, your anticipation of hazards and your reaction time are affected. A near miss, which may be your own fault, can be terrifying. But fear often turns to anger. The adrenaline that is pumped out in response to a shock is part of our survival mechanism: fright, then flight or fight. Don't drive when you're overtired, and of course don't drive when you've taken an appreciable amount of alcohol; stop regularly on long journeys to stretch your legs, get some fresh air and, if necessary, take a short nap.

Forgive and forget. If you are the victim of an aggressive driver, remind yourself that retaliation isn't worth it. Think about the people waiting for you to get home safely. 'You don't want to do anything that would endanger your life or anyone else's,' says Dr James.

Honk with care. 'Even honking has become dangerous,' says Dr Nahl. 'People often take honking as a great insult, as a sign of disrespect.' So be careful about when, where and why you tap or blast that horn.

Don't engage. Avoid confrontations. Never tailgate or make eye contact with an angry driver. Don't get out of the car or attempt to have a conversation. And don't go home or to work if someone is following you. 'You don't want them to know anything about you,' Dr Nerenberg says. If you feel frightened or threatened, go to a safe place, such as a police station or fire station.

Talk about it. Have regular family chats, especially if you have

Do just *one* thing

Acknowledge your aggression. It's a hard thing for people to do, says researcher Dr Diane Nahl. People with road rage are often focused on other people – those on the other side of the windscreen, she says. 'We rarely focus on our own behaviour.'

One way to tune in is to talk behind the wheel. 'The act of speaking your thoughts out loud while you're driving creates awareness,' she says.

Better still, tape-record yourself while driving, and listen later. Research shows people often are surprised by what they've said.

Or keep a notebook in the car. When you arrive at your destination, write down your thoughts and feelings about the drive. Your observations will lend insight that may help you to change aggressive patterns.

teenagers, and talk about safe driving, says Dr Nahl. Ask for feedback on your own driving, allow other family members to openly discuss driving habits or problems, and discuss potential scenarios and courses of action.

Teach your children. Babies and toddlers learn a lot in their car seats. 'We call this the road-rage nursery,' says Dr Nahl. Before they even learn to speak, children absorb the attitudes of adults they drive with. They witness the shouting, the swearing, the gestures.

So learn to turn those actions round. Say something like, 'naughty mummy for shouting at that man. I mustn't do that.' Also ask for your children's help. They might remind you to put on your seat belt, for example. Thank them and encourage them. 'You'll create a completely different culture in your car,' says Dr Nahl. That may pay off in the long run, and your children may be less aggressive when it's *their* turn to drive.

ROSACEA

14 ways to soothe the redness

Rosacea is a relatively common skin complaint, which causes a red rash-like mask around the nose and cheeks. To begin with, rosacea (pronounced 'rose Asia') starts with a simple, and perhaps prolonged, flushing of the face. This may be triggered by eating certain foods such as spicy foods or citrus fruits, drinking alcohol or hot drinks, stress, exercise, the wind, rain, sunshine, too moist an atmosphere, too dry an atmosphere, simply talking to people and thinking that you may be blushing – or nothing you can pinpoint.

After a while, people with the condition may develop permanently enlarged spider veins and acne-like small raised, red lumps, which lead to permanent facial redness and, in men, permanent thickening and mis-shaping of the nose. In some cases, the eyes look watery or bloodshot.

There is no known cause for rosacea, and anyone can get it, although it is more common in people with fair complexions. It is not contagious. The condition is still often called acne rosacea, and is often mistaken for common acne, or an allergy. Because the trigger factors and treatment options for rosacea are very different, though, it's important to get an early diagnosis and make the lifestyle changes necessary in order to keep the condition under control. The main task is to find out what triggers your flare-ups and avoid those things as much as possible.

Trigger Avoidance

As a rule, anything that causes a rosacea sufferer's face to redden or flush may trigger a flare-up. Among the most common trip wires are alcohol, heat, hot drinks, spicy foods, caffeine, stress and exposure to the sun. To avoid a flare-up, make the following lifestyle changes.

Use a sunscreen. Sunscreens are helpful in decreasing rosacea. Use a good quality sunscreen every time you go outdoors for any extended period of time, says dermatologist Ralph Daniel.

Dermatologist Dee Anna Glaser recommends using a broad-spectrum sunscreen with a protection factor (SPF) of at least 15 on your face all year round. This will protect you from both UVA and UVB radiation.

Wear a hat. If you're off to the beach, wear a hat with a 10cm-wide brim, to keep the sun off your face and neck, says Dr Glaser.

Follow the shade. In summer, minimize your sun exposure, says Dr Daniel. Whether on the beach or in the garden, sit under a big umbrella.

Watch your alcohol intake. Alcoholic drinks can trigger flare-ups of rosacea. Use common sense – if alcohol aggravates your condition, reduce your intake or avoid alcohol altogether, says Dr Daniel.

Allow hot drinks to cool. A cup of piping hot coffee may be a problem for some people with rosacea because hot drinks can make your face flush. Decreasing the temperature of your drink, even slightly, may be all that's needed to carry on enjoying coffee and tea.

Watch what you eat. Hot, spicy food is a common rosacea trigger. If spicy foods make your rosacea worse, then cut them down or cut them out, says Dr Daniel. Other foods that may cause problems include aubergines, avocados, cheese, chocolate, citrus fruit, green beans, liver, soya sauce, spinach, vanilla, vinegar, yeast extract and yoghurt.

Food additives can also aggravate rosacea. Monosodium glutamate (MSG), a food flavour enhancer, can sometimes cause so-called 'Chinese Restaurant Syndrome', with palpitations, headaches and flushing that can be particularly noticeable in rosacea sufferers. Food preservatives like nitrates and sulphites, found particularly in cured meats and alcohol respectively may also trigger symptoms.

Keep a diary of what you eat and how it affects your rosacea, suggests Dr Glaser, and adjust your diet accordingly.

Avoid intense exercise. Exercise is a vital part of a healthy lifestyle, but too much exertion can cause rosacea to flare up, says Dr Glaser. It's best to exercise three times a day for 15 minutes rather than 45 minutes in one go. This will stop you from overheating. In summer, exercise in an air-conditioned room or in the evening when the sun isn't so hot.

Keep cool. When exercising, drink cold fluids or suck ice cubes to keep yourself from getting too hot; keep a bottle of cool water nearby when you exercise and take regular sips.

Don't indulge in saunas or hot tubs. The heat of hot tubs and saunas can aggravate your condition, says dermatologist Larry Millikan.

Be gentle when cleansing. Begin each day with a thorough, but gentle cleansing of your face, says Dr Millikan. Think simple. People with

WHEN TO CONSULT A DOCTOR

If you think you may have early symptoms of rosacea, it's wise to see your doctor. He or she will probably prescribe some medication for the condition, usually an antibiotic lotion like metronidazole, or long-term antibiotics like oxytetracycline. Once your rosacea is under control, a tablet two or three times a week may be enough to keep it that way.

Your doctor may also refer you to a dermatologist who may review your treatment, and also cover areas such as how to properly wash your face and care for your skin, how to identify things that trigger flare-ups and how to avoid them, and what sort of make-up is best for concealing the redness. The sooner you have that information, the better.

rosacea get into trouble when they start using expensive scented soaps, or soaps with abrasive textures. Spread a gentle cleanser onto your face softly with your fingertips. Then rinse your face with lukewarm, not hot, water, says Dr Daniel. Let your face air dry for a few minutes before applying any topical medication or skin-care products. Then allow the medication to completely dry for five to ten minutes before applying a moisturizer or make-up. Repeat the same cleansing process at night.

Avoid harsh skin-care products. Steer clear of products that include alcohol or other irritants, which may cause your face to burn or turn red.

Self-esteem Boosters

The redness, blemishes and swelling caused by rosacea can take a psychological toll. It can make you camera-shy and damage your self-esteem and self-confidence. Here are some tips to stop that from happening.

Explain to others. If, during one of your flare-ups, you find yourself subject to stares or comments, turn this awkward situation into an educational one by openly discussing your rosacea.

Wear the right clothes. Avoid red or black-and-white garments, which accentuate your redness. Instead, choose softer shades like blues, yellows, khakis and other neutral colours.

Keep make-up simple and natural. Apply a contrasting concealer, usually a green tone, to offset rosacea's red appearance. Then apply a good foundation in the correct skin tone. Follow with a loose powder to finish, to make blemishes or redness less striking or noticeable.

SAD (SEASONAL AFFECTIVE DISORDER)

15 steps to a brighter outlook

Every winter, as the days grow shorter, an estimated half a million people in the UK get the blues. SAD – short for Seasonal Affective Disorder – is a type of winter depression that can affect people between October and April, but in particular during December, January and February. They may experience mild to severe depression, weight gain, lethargy, a desire to sleep more and an increased appetite or cravings for carbohydrates such as cakes and biscuits.

SAD is caused by a hormone imbalance that can occur in winter due to shorter daylight hours and a lack of sunlight. For some people, SAD is a disabling illness that stops them from leading a normal life without medical treatment. For others it is a milder condition known as the winter blues. When spring arrives, the symptoms of SAD almost magically wane. Sufferers feel energized, sociable and generally happy.

There is no test for SAD. Diagnosis is based on a group of symptoms that usually begin around October and fade around April and appear for two or more consecutive winters. Because other conditions such as poor thyroid function are similar to those of SAD, talk to your doctor before attempting to treat yourself, especially if you are feeling very depressed. But if your symptoms are mild, try any or all of these tips to chase away the winter blues.

Bring in the light. Make your home shine, says Norman Rosenthal, a psychiatrist and expert in SAD. Add more lamps, brighten up rooms with light-coloured paint and carpets, pull up the blinds and open curtains.

Duplicate the sun. Specially designed light fittings, boxes and visors offer full-spectrum lighting that replicates natural light without the harmful ultraviolet rays. Light therapy has been shown to improve symptoms of depression significantly after exposure for as little as half an hour daily, although periods of up to six hours a day are sometimes recommended. Some studies have shown a correlation between length of exposure and melatonin levels, the hormone thought to be involved in SAD. Properly controlled clinical trials of light therapy are difficult to design, however, and use of this therapy is still controversial (see box, *Lighten up with sun lamps*, page 483).

Do just *one* thing

Walk outside. Go outdoors on a bright winter's day and you'll naturally soak up some of that feel-good light, says psychiatrist and SAD specialist Norman Rosenthal. Even on a cloudy day you'll get more light than you would indoors. And it doesn't matter if you are well wrapped up – it's the light that you get through your eyes that helps to lift your mood.

Aim for at least half-an-hour a day for an emotional and physical boost.

Wake up to light. If your symptoms are mild, put a bedroom light on a timer set to come on about an hour before you get up in the morning, says Dr Rosenthal. 'It helps people to wake up in the morning, it helps them to feel better – even though it's just an ordinary bedside lamp – simply because our eyes are so very sensitive at that hour of the morning.'

Even better, buy a specially designed dawn simulator (www.outsidein.co.uk sells a dawn simulator called Bodyclock).

Dawn simulation is a technique in which a light comes on very slowly in the early morning, to mimic a natural sunrise. Research has found that our body clocks respond to this stimulus by speeding up and reinforcing the waking-up process so that we have more or less woken up even before our eyes open.

Take a window seat. Sit by a window at work if you can. Although the glass diminishes the sunlight's potency, you'll still reap some mood-enhancing benefits.

Get fit. Whether you walk, jog or cycle indoors or out, aerobic activity heightens mood-boosting brain chemicals that banish winter blues, says Dr Rosenthal. For two pronged attack against SAD, combine exercise with light. Go for a walk outside or set up a light box in front of your exercise bike.

Brave the weather. 'Winter weather can provide positive stimulation,' says professor of medicine Andrew Weil. 'Find some outdoor chores to do when the sun turns the sky a brilliant blue.' Enjoy the crispness of a frosty morning or the sensation of snowflakes on your cheeks. Dress warmly and keep moving.

Manage stress. People with SAD don't deal with stress that well in winter, says Dr Rosenthal. Don't set yourself deadlines in winter if you can help it. In the same vein, try and avoid long days at work that keep you out of the light.

WHEN TO CONSULT A DOCTOR

Severe seasonal affective disorder can be helped by antidepressants known as selective serotonin re-uptake inhibitors, or SSRIs. See a doctor if your symptoms are interfering with your work or relationships.

Also seek help if you feel despair about the future or are suicidal, or if you have major sleeping problems or a change in eating habits – such as weight loss or weight gain of 5 to 10 kilos.

Don't use light therapy without talking to your doctor first: some medicines make your eyes sensitive to light.

Prepare for winter. Anticipate the months when your energy might flag, says Brenda Byrne, a psychologist who runs a programme for people with SAD. Instead of waiting until the build-up to Christmas to shop for presents or write cards, do those jobs in the brighter months when you feel more energetic.

Pencil in a holiday. Then take one. Even three or four days in a warm, sunny climate may lift you out of the doldrums, especially if your blues are mild. 'Most people notice that within a few days they really do feel better,' says Dr Byrne.

Get warm. Some experts believe that temperature affects seasonal changes in behaviour. 'Lots of people with SAD also hate cold weather and say that they can't get warm in winter, no matter how many layers they put on,' says Dr Byrne. People who dislike the cold may simply avoid going outdoors in winter and get less sunlight, thereby worsening their blues. Some strategies for keeping warmer include tweaking the central heating thermostat up, stopping draughts in your home, using an electric blanket or heating pad or sipping hot drinks. (See *Hypothermia*, page 328.)

Cut down on carbohydrates. 'Many SAD patients claim to be carbohydrate addicts,' says Dr Rosenthal. But overdosing on comfort foods like biscuits, cakes, chips, bread and pasta can lead to lethargy and weight gain. Try eating high protein meals, especially for breakfast and lunch.

Get your B vitamins. Although studies of the impact of B vitamins on mood are inconclusive, a balanced diet with adequate natural B_6, thiamine and folate is recommended. Meat, especially meat juices, dairy products, fish, wholegrain cereals, dark green vegetables, potatoes, beans,

Lighten up with sun lamps

There are now many companies selling full-spectrum lights for the treatment of seasonal affective disorder (SAD) or winter blues. Light boxes are not available on the NHS and have to be bought from specialist retailers; they are free of VAT and start at less than £100. For more information on SAD and treatment options contact the SAD Association, PO Box 989, Steyning, BN44 3HG, or visit their excellent website at www.sada.org.uk.

nuts, yeast extract (Marmite) and bananas should give you plenty. Overdosing on B vitamin supplements can be dangerous.

Try a herbal remedy. St John's wort (hypericum) helps some people with winter depression. Try taking a 300mg capsule three times a day, says Dr Weil. Because St John's wort can take six to eight weeks to work, start this remedy well before the dark days of winter begin.

Note: Do not combine St John's wort with light therapy without consulting your doctor and your optician. The herb may make your eyes very sensitive to light.

Too sensitive to winter

The importance of light's influence on human behaviour makes sense from an evolutionary point of view, says psychiatrist Norman Rosenthal. 'We evolved in a 24-hour day in which part is dark and part is light, and there's a different biology of what we do when it's dark and when it's light,' he says. 'When it's dark, we rest. When it's light, we hunt and are active and explore the world. That is all dependent on our vision, on when it's safe to be out and about. And it's only safe when you can see.' Animals are also tuned in to seasonal changes. Some respond by gaining weight to prepare for winter hibernation, for example. Some change colour to camouflage themselves against the snow. In some extra-sensitive people, too, a set of behavioural changes occurs with the change in seasons. It is this seasonal awareness that can cause SAD in humans.

SCARRING
10 ways to limit the damage

Scar tissue is produced by the body when the skin has been cut or broken open. It is the body's way of replacing damaged tissue with healthy tissue. Scar tissue is tougher and less flexible than normal tissue. It is also usually paler then the surrounding skin, flush with the surface of the skin and, normally, less sensitive to touch or pain. Some skin types scar more easily than others – olive and dark skins, for example. These skin types also tend to be prone to conditions called keloids and hypertrophic scars, in which the body produces an excess of scar tissue. Both cause raised scars that tend to be darker than the surrounding skin and more sensitive to touch.

Scars are permanent, although many can fade until they are almost unnoticeable. How you treat a cut can determine what kind of scar may develop. Then, how you care for that scar can determine how fast and

Stretch marks

During periods of rapid weight gain or growth, like pregnancy or adolescence, the skin has to stretch to accommodate your increased body size. Stretch it too far or too fast and its deepest layer will tear, leaving the skin surface above it looking thin and streaky. These stretch marks may, like scars, look purplish red and ugly to start with. Like scars, they are permanent but, also like scars, they usually fade almost to nothing with time.

Pregnant women spend millions of pounds on creams, oils and ointments and some resort to laser surgery. 'Unfortunately,' says family doctor Stephen Amiel, 'there is precious little evidence that any of them work. Vitamin E compounds are popular, as are creams containing collagen and elastin. Just because these are constituents of normal skin doesn't mean rubbing them onto your skin will have any impact at all. Use an ordinary moisturizer by all means, but don't waste your money on expensive potions.'

Some women are more prone to stretch marks than others, but you can help avoid them by trying to keep your weight gain in pregnancy under control. Eat well, but don't eat for two.

WHEN TO CONSULT A DOCTOR

Generally, you'll be able to tell if a cut or graze is severe enough to warrant medical attention. Here are a few guidelines for those in-between situations, when you're not sure if a trip to the doctor is appropriate or not. See a doctor if:

- blood spurts or continues to flow after several minutes of pressure;
- dirt or debris remains imbedded in the wound even after a thorough cleaning;
- you can't easily close the wound;
- you notice any redness, drainage, heat or swelling – or the wound isn't healing properly;
- the wound is deep and dirty (see *Cuts and Grazes*, page 153).

Keloid scarring may possibly be helped by cryotherapy (freezing), injections with steroids, pressure bandaging, radiotherapy or surgical removal. Talk to your doctor about a referral to a dermatologist or plastic surgeon.

to what extent it will fade over time. These are some suggestions from the experts.

Don't get cut or burned! Every time the skin gets cut, it scars, says plastic surgeon Gerald Imber. And some people are more prone to scarring than others.

Protect your skin by wearing gloves, long trousers and long sleeves when working with or near thorny, sharp or jagged objects. If you cycle, rollerblade or skateboard, wear elbow and knee pads and wrist and shin-guards to prevent accidental cuts and grazes.

Keep boiling kettles and saucepans and irons well out of reach of small children or the frail elderly. Use electric radiators rather than electric bar fires and keep a guard around open fires. Keep matches, lighters and fireworks away from small children, and if you must smoke, make sure you do not hold your cigarette down at child level.

Don't pick scabs. Your mum was right. Picking a scab off a healing wound will increase the chances of a visible scar, says dermatologist John Romano.

Close gaps with a butterfly suture. If you do get cut and the cut is large enough, you should go to a doctor for stitches, particularly if the cut is on the face where a scar would be most visible. But if a cut is small and you are concerned about scarring, consider using adhesive butterfly sutures, such as Steri-Strip skin closures, says Dr Romano. Available from pharmacies, these dressings can help to keep the wound closed for better healing and minimal scarring. Use only after the wound has been thoroughly cleaned.

Moisturize scars. Sweat glands, oil glands and hair glands are all destroyed by a scar, leaving it more at the mercy of the elements than the rest of your skin, says dermatologist Paul Lazar. He advises keeping large scars, such as those from a third-degree burn, lubricated with a good skin cream to protect them from abrasions.

Wash scars gently. You can easily damage tender scar tissue by using a flannel or loofah too roughly. Dr Lazar recommends cleaning scars very gently. If you shave in the shower or bath, lather generously, and shave slowly. Replace your blade frequently to prevent cuts and skin irritation.

Don't be too alarmed. Fresh scars are often quite noticeable, but don't be too concerned. Remember that the colour of a scar usually fades over time by itself, says Dr Lazar.

Eat a balanced diet. Wounds won't heal properly unless your body has what it takes to make them heal properly. Protein and vitamins, provided through eating a good, well-balanced diet, are essential. Of particular importance to wound healing is the mineral zinc. Good sources of zinc include pumpkin and sunflower seeds, Brazil nuts, Swiss and Cheddar

SCIATICA

Do just *one* thing

Thoroughly clean the wound. A wound that heals quickly and neatly is less likely to develop a scar than a wound that festers. Make sure that any cuts and grazes are properly cleaned, and try to keep the wound slightly moist with an antiseptic ointment while it heals, says dermatologist Jeffrey Binstock. If dirt and debris remain in the wound after washing, use tweezers cleaned with surgical spirit to remove any particles.

cheeses, peanuts, the dark meat from turkey and lean beef.

Cover scars with sunblock. Scars have less pigment in them than the rest of your skin. They therefore lack the ability to develop a protective tan and are especially vulnerable to sunburn. Protect scars with a strong sunscreen whenever you go outside on a sunny day, says dermatologist Stephen Kurtin.

SCIATICA

19 strategies to kill nerve pain

Nearly everyone experiences back pain from time to time, but only an unlucky few have to endure the agonizing pain of sciatica.

The sciatic nerve stretches from the lower back region down the back of the legs to the ankles. Anything that puts pressure on the nerve, such as a herniated spinal disc, a bone spur or spinal misalignment can result in sharp, shooting pains in the buttock, leg or both, often with numbness and pins and needles in the same region.

A herniated disc (usually called – rather misleadingly – a slipped disc) is the most common cause of sciatica among young, active adults. It occurs when the outer wall of the disc, which normally functions as a shock absorber between the vertebrae, gets torn, and the inner cushioning material moves into the spinal canal, where it compresses a nerve root.

Sciatica is often short-lived, but sometimes it can come and go for years. Even simple daily activities – bending over, sneezing or having a bowel movement – can trigger attacks. Once the nerve has been irritated or damaged, the pain can persist even when you are lying still.

Because so many things can cause sciatica, and because the nerve can be permanently damaged without prompt treatment, it's essential to see a doctor at the first sign of symptoms. Surgery is occasionally required, but sciatica can usually be controlled with a combination of medicines and home care. Here are a few ways to stop the pain and protect the nerve from further harm.

Try and keep moving. Strict bed rest, sometimes for weeks, used to be recommended for back pain and sciatica. No longer. Recovery is quicker if you keep moving around as normally as you can.

Ice it quickly. At the first sign of pain, apply a cold compress to the lower back for 15 to 20 minutes at a time, every two to three hours. The easiest thing to use is a gel pack, available from sports shops and some pharmacies. The packs remain flexible even after they're chilled in the freezer. Otherwise, a small bag of ice cubes or a packet of frozen peas wrapped in a tea towel will do. The compress can be moulded to the contours of your lower back, putting the cold exactly where you need it. Keep it cold for 24 to 48 hours. Cold reduces inflammation and helps to prevent muscle spasms, which cause much of the pain even when a disc has torn, says back specialist Andrew Cole.

Use a heating pad. After applying cold for a day or two, switch to heat, advises chiropractor John Triano. Apply a hot-water bottle or a heating pad to your lower back for 15 minutes at a time. Repeat the treatment every hour, and keep doing it for as long as it seems to help. Heat relaxes muscles and helps to prevent painful spasms. It also increases circulation and helps to flush pain-causing toxins from around the nerve. But no matter how much better heat makes you feel, don't use it for more than 15 minutes at a time.

Take anti-inflammatories. When you first feel the pain of sciatica, take aspirin or ibuprofen. These are nonsteroidal anti-inflammatory drugs (NSAIDs), which inhibit the body's production of prostaglandins – inflammatory chemicals that increase pain and swelling. Take the recommended dose four times a day, says Dr Cole. If aspirin or ibuprofen upset your stomach, it's fine to take paracetamol – but bear in mind that this works mainly as a pain reliever – it has little effect on inflammation.

Note: Remember aspirin should not be given to anyone under 16. Consult your doctor before taking anything other than paracetamol if you're pregnant.

Go for a swim. Or simply walk in water. The combination of warm water and gentle exercise will often loosen muscles and help to relieve spasms and pain. Also, water supports the body, which may relieve painful pressure on the back.

'Swimming and aquatic exercises are among the best rehabilitation tools available,' says orthopaedic surgeon John Heller. Swimming isn't recommended at the peak of an attack, however, but it's fine once the pain diminishes. It's also a good preventative strategy for anyone who has had sciatica in the past. Avoid butterfly stroke, and if you use breast-stroke, don't arch your back to keep your head out of the water.

Walk if it's comfortable. Walking is one of the best exercises for relieving and preventing sciatica. It keeps muscles flexible and improves circulation throughout the body, including the area of the damaged nerve.

If you're in the acute stage of sciatica and walking causes sharp, stabbing pains, don't do it, says Dr Triano. 'But if you've had the pain for more than a few days and it's mainly a dull ache, it's important to gently push through the discomfort with walking or other forms of gentle exercise.'

Strengthen your trunk muscles. These are the muscles that surround and support the spine. 'The basic curl-up is a good exercise for strengthening the muscles,' says Dr Cole. Curl-ups are easy to do. Lie on your back with your pelvis tilted to flatten your back against the floor, your knees bent at about a 90-degree angle, your feet flat on the floor and your arms at your sides. Using your upper abdominal muscles, raise your head and shoulders off the floor. Your arms should be stretched out in front. Then lower your shoulders to the floor in a slow, controlled motion. You don't want to raise your shoulders more than an inch or two, because that will overwork the muscle that links the lumbar spine to the legs and increase strain on the lower back.

Have a massage. It will make you feel better by reducing muscle spasms and increasing flexibility, says Dr Cole, although it won't reverse underlying nerve or disc damage. The massage needs to be gentle and done by an expert who knows when to leave tissues that are too inflamed alone, and when something more serious might be going on.

Let your legs do the work. Whether you have sciatica now or have had it in the past, the ways in which you move your body every day are crucial. Bending from the waist, for example, is just about the worst thing you can do. Even if you're doing nothing more strenuous than picking up a sock, kneel or squat down and use your leg muscles to get back up.

Hold things close to your body. Whether you're carrying a bag of heavy shopping or a laundry basket, hold it as close to your body as possible, Dr Cole advises. Holding weight close to your body takes some of the pressure off the lower spine.

WHEN TO CONSULT A DOCTOR

The only good thing about sciatica is that the pain is usually temporary. It often begins to ease within four or five days, and most people will be well on the way to recovery within six weeks.

'There's no need to panic if you get sciatica, but it can be extraordinarily painful,' says John Heller, an orthopaedic surgeon.

It's important to see a doctor as soon as possible, he adds. For one thing, you'll probably need medicine to control the pain. You also want to make sure that you aren't risking permanent nerve damage. Your doctor will want to exclude any serious underlying cause for your sciatica such as infection in the bone, a tumour, or collapse of a vertebra, and also make sure that the pain you are getting is not due to something else such as blockage of an artery.

One of the most serious warning signs is a loss of muscle function – your foot is dragging, for example, or you stumble when you walk. Even more serious is a loss of bowel or bladder control, or loss of sensation in the pelvic area around your anus or genitals. If you have any one of these symptoms, contact your doctor immediately, as you may well need urgent hospital admission.

You should see your doctor urgently if your sciatica or acute back pain occurs in any of the following situations:

• you are under 20 or over 55;

• you have suffered recent injury to your back, such as in a road accident;

• the pain is in your upper back;

• you have a history of cancer;

• you have a history of osteoporosis;

• you have been taking long-term oral steroid tablets;

• you have HIV/AIDS;

• you feel generally unwell or have lost weight;

• you have pain, numbness or pins and needles in other limbs.

Support your lower back. Sciatica can take weeks or even months to improve. In the meantime, giving your back extra support – by using a pillow or a rolled-up towel when you're sitting, for example – reduces pain and helps the injured area to heal more quickly, says Dr Triano.

Even better are pillows that inflate automatically with the turn of a valve. Available from camping shops, shops that specialize in back care and online, they allow you to easily change the firmness every 15 to 20 minutes. 'They're a superb way of inexpensively minimizing back pain,' says Dr Triano.

But don't regard back supports as a substitute for exercise or strong supporting muscles in your back, says Dr Heller. Those muscles, built up through regular exercise, become your internal back support.

Avoid slouching in deep, soft armchairs or sofas. Sit comfortably upright on a straight backed chair with a little lumbar support. Use a lumbar support in your car too.

Take frequent breaks. Sitting is surprisingly hard on the lower back, especially when the sciatic nerve is inflamed and irritated. In fact, sitting without a back support can put about twice as much pressure on the spine as standing.

'If you have sciatica, your enemy is any prolonged, static posture,' Dr Triano says. 'The elastic properties of your tissues are used up in about 20 minutes. After that, you will put increased stress on the area.'

If your job involves a lot of sitting, give your back a break by getting up at least every 15 to 20 minutes, or whenever your back starts feeling tense or tired. Walk around for a few minutes. Stretch. Give your muscles a chance to unwind before sitting back down again. 'Bear this in mind during long flights or car journeys, too,' says Dr Heller.

Put a foot up. The back naturally has a slight curve, but when you're standing flat on both feet, the curve is accentuated, which can aggravate a sensitive sciatic nerve. A more 'relaxed' posture gives the nerves slightly more room.

'One of the best things you can do when you're standing is alternately to prop one foot up and then the other,' says Dr Triano. Lifting one foot slightly increases the free space around the sciatic nerve, and shifting from one foot to the other on a regular basis helps to maintain elasticity in the spinal discs and surrounding tissues, he explains.

When standing, rest your foot on a low stool or a step whenever possible. In the supermarket queue, rest one foot on the lower rung of the shopping trolley. On the pavement, use a curb or the base of a lamppost. Many people with sciatica find that lifting one foot even a few inches is enough to temporarily eliminate the pain.

Watch your weight. The lower back supports a hefty amount of your body weight. The heavier you are, the more weight it has to carry – and the more likely you are to experience sciatica or other back problems.

Stay out of the car. Apart from the fact that most car seats are notoriously hard on the lower back, cars vibrate at four to five cycles a second – a frequency that can damage discs, increase muscle inflammation or

Do just *one* thing

Try stretching and flexibility exercises. They are among the best ways to reduce the inflammation and muscle spasms that often accompany sciatica, says chiropractor John Triano. Everyone responds differently to exercises. Some people do best with extension exercises, which include lying face down, arching your back, and rising up on your elbows. Others require flexion movements – for example, lying on your back and bringing your knees to your chest. You'll have to experiment a bit to discover what works best for you.

'Stretching exercises encourage movement of the spine and associated joints, muscles and ligaments, which can prevent adhesions or stiffness due to scar tissue formation after an injury,' says back surgeon John Heller. If exercises make you feel better, keep doing them. But they should never make the pain worse or cause it to radiate down one or both legs. If they do, you know it's the wrong exercise for you and you should get professional advice.

spasms and generally put more strain on the sciatic nerve.

Until your back is better, spend as little time in the car as possible. Even when you're not in pain, it's a good idea to limit driving time to two hours in any one day. And then it's worth getting out of the car every 20 to 30 minutes to stretch and move around.

Find a comfortable position. Everyone with sciatica has at least one posture or position that puts least strain on the nerve. Some people experience less discomfort when their back is pitched slightly forwards. Others do better when they stand militarily upright. Although good posture is important in the long run, don't worry about it when you're in pain. Find whatever position feels most comfortable and hold it until the pain goes.

Get plenty of sleep. It's hard to do when you're in pain, but studies have shown that the body undergoes much of its healing during sleep. If pain is keeping you awake, try raising your knees with a small pillow. It takes some of the pressure off the nerve, says Dr Triano. If you usually sleep on your side, curl up and put a pillow between your knees.

If you smoke, try to give up. Cigarette smoke weakens the spinal discs and slows down recovery time from sciatica. If you need surgery for the condition, smoking increases the risk that the operation won't be successful. And the pain of sciatica will certainly remind you that you're coughing more than you should.

SHIN SPLINTS

10 ways to soothe sore legs

Shin splints are common in those who take lots of vigorous exercise, especially when that exercise is on a hard surface. Shin splints – an injury technically known as medial tibial stress syndrome (MTSS) – affects athletes involved in sports that involve running and jumping, including football, basketball, rugby and sprinting. Marathon runners and ballet dancers are especially susceptible.

There are a number of related overuse injuries of the lower leg. Shin splints occur when repeated running cycles of pounding and push off result in higher forces being applied to the periosteum, the fibrous layer over the lower leg bone (the tibia). The periosteum becomes inflamed and, with further overuse, causes a stress reaction within the bone itself, sometimes leading to an actual stress fracture. A more chronic condition, known as compartment syndrome, can arise when the muscles in the lower leg become too large for the tight fibrous compartment they are contained in, causing compression of the blood vessels and nerves within.

Symptoms of shin splints include tenderness over the inside of the shin, lower leg pain which is worse on bending the toes or foot downwards, and sometimes some swelling or redness over the inside of the shin. Early in the condition, pain tends to come on at the beginning of a run, but disappear as running continues, recurring with subsequent runs, or the following morning. Pain-free intervals get shorter though, as the condition progresses, and if one small area becomes particularly tender to the touch, you may have a stress fracture.

With compartment syndrome, the pain tends to come on during exercise, but continues throughout and goes on for some time after you stop exercising. People who increase muscle bulk over too short a period of intensive training are at particular risk of compartment syndrome.

Rest is the key to treating shin splints. You may need to stop running completely for a period, sometimes weeks, and when you start again, you will have to do less to start with, both in terms of intensity, duration and intervals between runs. These other remedies are designed to help keep shin splints from progressing to the point of stress fracture and to let you continue your active lifestyle without causing irreparable harm. Let pain be your guide. If anything recommended here hurts, don't do it.

Start with the ground. Hard surfaces can cause shin splints. 'If you're walking, running, dancing or whatever on a hard, unyielding surface, then you need to change where you exercise,' advises athletics trainer Marjorie Albohm.

For those who do aerobics, injuries are commonest on carpeted concrete floors, while suspended wooden floors are the least damaging. If you must dance on a solid floor, make sure that you do only low-impact aerobics or that high-quality foam mats are provided. Runners should opt for grass or clay before asphalt, and asphalt before concrete. Concrete is very unyielding and should always be avoided.

Then look at your shoes. If you can't change your surface, or if you find that's not the problem, look at different footwear. Choose a well-fitting shoe with good arch support and shock-absorption in the sole, says Albohm.

If your activity involves a lot of impact on the ball of the foot – such as aerobics – select a shoe for its ability to absorb shock in that area. The best test is to try the shoes on in the shop and jump up and down, both on the toes and flat-footed. The impact with the floor should be firm but not jarring.

For runners, the choice is a bit more difficult. Research has shown that at least half of all runners with shin splints also have what is known as overpronation – which means that their feet roll inwards too much as they run. Good sports shops sell shoes specially designed to combat this problem – rigid, durable, control-orientated running shoes that limit pronation.

Buy new shoes regularly. One way to make sure your shoes retain as much cushioning ability as possible is to replace them frequently. Runners who put in 25 miles a week or more need new shoes every two or three months, says Gary Gordon, a foot surgeon who specializes in sports medicine. Less mileage means new shoes every four to six months. People who do aerobics or play tennis twice a week also need new shoes two or three times a year, while those who participate up to four times a week need them every two months.

Put it on RICE. As soon as you notice shin splint pain, follow the rules of RICE: rest, ice, compression and elevation for 20 to 30 minutes a day. The experts swear by it. Prop your leg up, bind it with a stretchy crepe bandage and put an ice pack on it for 20 to 30 minutes.

Go for contrast. The contrast bath involves alternately bathing the lower legs for one minute in iced water and one minute in hot water. Do this for at least 12 minutes before any activity that might cause shin splint pain.

Master massage. If you have shin splints in the front of the leg, massage the area right near the edge of the shin – not directly on it, advises sports

WHEN TO CONSULT A DOCTOR

Because some experts believe shin splints may actually be stress fractures in an early stage, telling the difference between the two is sometimes tricky. Even so, shin splints can become stress fractures with continued abuse, so seeing your doctor for an early diagnosis is important.

If your doctor suspects compartment syndrome, you may be referred for a pressure check and possible surgery to release the fibrous sheath constricting the muscles.

masseur Rich Phaigh. To massage away shin splint pain, sit on the floor with one knee bent and the foot flat on the ground. Start by lightly stroking both sides of the bone using the palms of your hands, gliding them backwards and forwards from knee to ankle. Repeat this stroking motion several times. Then wrap your hands around the calf and, using the tips of your fingers, stroke deeply on each side of the bone from ankle to knee.

Correct faulty feet. Flat feet or high arches can sometimes cause shin splints, Dr Gordon says. 'If you have flat feet, the muscle on the inside of your calf has to work harder and gets tired more quickly,' he says, 'so the bone takes more of a pounding.' If you're flat-footed, you may need additional shock-absorbing material or arch supports in your shoes. Inserts are available at sports shops, but it might be best to see a podiatrist before adding inserts on your own.

Pain on the outside of the lower leg is sometimes associated with very high arches. 'That requires a lot of stretching exercises, as well as strengthening the muscles and maybe adding orthotics inside your shoes,' says Dr Gordon.

Stretch those calves. Stretching the Achilles tendon and the calf muscles is an excellent preventative measure for shin splints, says Albohm. Stretching helps because shortened calf muscles tend to throw more weight and stress forwards to the shins. Place your hands on a wall, extend one leg behind the other, and press the back heel slowly to the floor. Do this 20 times and repeat with the other leg.

And the tendons. Dr Gordon offers this simple technique for stretching the Achilles tendon: keep both feet flat on the ground about 15cm apart. Then bend your ankles and knees forward while keeping your back straight. Go to the point of tightness and hold for 30 seconds. 'You should feel it really stretching down in the lower part of the calf,' he says. Repeat the exercise 10 times. Or try standing on the bottom stair with the balls of your feet on the stair and your heels hanging over the edge. Holding onto the banister, drop your heels downwards until you feel the stretch in your calves and hold for 30 seconds. Repeat 10 times.

Build muscle, reduce pain. Shin splint pain can sometimes be prevented by strengthening the muscles surrounding the shin. These muscles help to decelerate the foot and reduce shock whenever you walk or run. Help to strengthen them with the following.

- Try cycling with pedal clips. Concentrate on pulling up with the muscles in front of the shin every time you pedal. (Cycling also gives you a good aerobic workout without aggravating shin splints.)

- If you don't have access to a bicycle, walking around on your heels does much the same thing, forcing you to tighten and pull up with the muscles around the shin each time you take a step.

- If you're looking for a conditioning exercise that's a bit more strenuous, try this: sit on the edge of a table that's high enough to keep your feet from touching the ground. Place a sock filled with coins over your foot, or make a 2-kilo weight from an old paint tin by filling it with gravel (hang this over the foot with a shoe on so the handle doesn't hurt). Flex the foot upwards at the ankle, then relax, then flex the foot upwards again. Repeat this as many times as you can, tightening your shin muscles as you pull the foot up.

SHINGLES

13 tips to combat the pain

Shingles, known medically as herpes zoster, is a painful, blistering rash caused when the long-dormant chickenpox virus suddenly reawakens in nerve cells. It affects only a limited area of skin, depending on the area supplied by the affected nerve, but it makes you feel surprisingly tired, run down and miserable.

A few days before the rash appears you may feel slightly unwell and develop a localized area of burning pain and tenderness. This pain can be severe, to the point where, when the affected nerve supplies the chest area, it can occasionally be mistaken for the pain of a heart attack. One or more crops of red spots appears on the chest or back, or, more rarely, on the face, arms, legs and even inside the mouth. The spots quickly turn into tiny blisters called vesicles. They always affect only one side of the body (left or right), and never cross the midline.

Because shingles is caused by a reactivation of a dormant virus in the nerves of people who have previously had chickenpox, it can unfortunately occur more than once.

In some people shingles pain can persist long after the rash disappears. This complication, called post-herpetic neuralgia, results from damaged nerve fibres. It can be very painful and difficult to treat.

Stress, illness and a vulnerable immune system are thought to be contributing factors to an outbreak of shingles. Most sufferers are older adults: up to half of those over the age of 80 may develop this uncomfortable illness. It's important to see your doctor for this complicated condition. Meanwhile, here's what you can do to make yourself as comfortable as possible.

The Early Stages

Here is what the experts recommend for the beginning stages of shingles.

Take painkillers. Aspirin and ibuprofen are anti-inflammatory and will work best.

Take St John's wort. This herbal remedy may help to reduce nerve pain and has antiviral properties as well, says Sota Omoigui, a doctor who specializes in pain management. He recommends taking 200 to 300mg of St John's wort (hypericum) two or three times a day until the pain goes.

Reach for maitake. Maitake is a medicinal mushroom grown in Japan. It acts as a powerful antiviral agent through immune system stimulation. Most people who get shingles are run down, says clinical herbalist Douglas Schar. Maitake jump starts the immune system and helps to get the virus at the root of the shingles outbreak under control. Schar recommends taking six 300mg tablets a day while the condition is active.

Try lysine. Several studies show that the amino acid lysine can help to inhibit the spread of the herpes virus – although not all studies on lysine reach that conclusion. But taking lysine supplements at the onset of shingles certainly can't hurt and might help, says Leon Robb, a pain management specialist.

Amino acids may not be suitable if you have liver or kidney problems, or if you are pregnant or breastfeeding. As with all such supplements, there is no official guarantee of safety, purity or effectiveness. Good dietary sources of lysine include fish, chicken, cheeses, potatoes, milk, brewer's yeast and beans.

For Shingles Blisters

Once the blisters appear, there are several ways to obtain relief.

Do nothing. Leave the blisters alone unless your rash is really bad, says Dr Robb. 'You can slow down healing if you irritate the skin by applying too many creams and ointments.'

Cool with a flannel. Dip a flannel or towel in cold water, squeeze out and apply to the affected area, says dermatologist James Nordlund. 'The cooler it is, the better it feels.'

Keep cool. Avoid anything that will make your blistered skin hotter, says Dr Robb.

Sink into a soothing bath. If you have shingles on your forehead, ignore this tip. But if the rash is below your neck, this may help. Add a handful of cornflour or colloidal oatmeal, such as Aveeno Colloidal Bath additive (available from pharmacies) to your bathwater and have a soak, says Dr Nordlund.

   The relief may not last long, but a soak before bedtime combined with a painkiller may help you to sleep.

Add salt. A cupful of household salt added to the bathwater will help the healing process once your spots have blistered and scabbed.

Zap the infection with hydrogen peroxide. If the blisters become infected, try dabbing them with hydrogen peroxide solution. You can buy 6 per cent (20 vols) and 3 per cent (10 vols) from pharmacies, both of

---

Can you catch shingles?

'The short answer is no,' says family doctor Stephen Amiel. 'Shingles is the reactivation of your own previous chickenpox virus infection. So you can't catch shingles from someone else who has either shingles or chickenpox. But, if you haven't previously had chickenpox, the viruses shed by someone with shingles can give you chickenpox.'

Chickenpox is a trivial illness in children, but very unpleasant in adults, and can be very dangerous to the foetus if you catch it when you're pregnant. So if you have shingles, warn people in close contact with you.

WHEN TO CONSULT A DOCTOR

If you have symptoms of shingles and notice a rash beginning to develop, try and see your doctor as soon as possible, preferably within 72 hours. That's because the prescription antiviral drugs used to treat shingles need to be started early in the course of the illness. Taken straight away, these drugs have been shown to shorten the duration of the virus, help the rash to heal more quickly and reduce the intensity of shingles pain and the time it lasts.

There is also good evidence that antiviral drugs given during the acute stage of shingles can prevent or reduce post-herpetic neuralgia, the nerve pain that lingers after the skin heals. Amitriptyline, an antidepressant increasingly used for various forms of neuralgia, may also prevent neuralgia if given early, and there are several helpful drugs for helping established neuralgia too. If your shingles pain is more than you can stand, see your doctor as soon as possible. This is no time for stoicism. Ignore your discomfort, and you could end up with years of pain.

While most people who develop shingles have no serious underlying condition to trigger it, your doctor may want to test for conditions causing reduced immunity.

which are suitable for cleansing sores. Don't dilute it; straight out of the bottle is fine, says Dr Robb.

Post-blister Care

If you still have some pain after the blisters have gone, here's what to do.

Try eating hot spices. Eating hot spicy foods may bring pain relief. Hot chillis contain capsaicin, a substance thought to block the production of a chemical needed to transmit pain impulses between nerve cells. Sprinkle cayenne pepper on eggs, soups and casseroles, or use it in marinades.

Cool it with ice. If you still have pain after the blisters have healed, put ice in a plastic bag and stroke the skin vigorously, says Dr Robb.

Talk to someone. For some people, long-lasting shingles pain may point to some underlying emotional need that is not being met, says dermatologist Jules Altman. Could the pain be diverting your attention from another problem? Or is the pain diverting much-needed attention to you? This is an issue worth considering, he says, and one which you may like to discuss with your doctor.

SIDE STITCHES

9 ways to avoid the stab of pain

A stitch in the side – a sharp, temporary pain beneath the ribs – is caused by a spasm of the diaphragm. It happens when the diaphragm, a muscle between the chest and abdomen, can't get the oxygen it needs. It often happens to runners.

Whenever you raise your knee, you contract your stomach muscles, which increases the pressure inside your abdomen. The result is a cramping of the diaphragm because the bloodflow is shut off.

You also can get a stitch from walking – and even from laughing. Here's how to handle it.

Stop. When the pain hits you, stop whatever you are doing. You need to relax in order to calm the muscle.

Slow down and walk. If you're running when you get a stitch, sometimes just slowing down to a walk is enough to calm that contracting muscle, says fitness expert Suki Munsell. When the twinge fades, speed up again.

Press where it hurts. Using three fingers, press on the area where the pain is worst until it stops hurting. Or, use those three fingers to gently massage the painful area. This is often enough to release the pain, says sports psychotherapist David Balboa.

Exhale deeply. As you begin to knead the cramp from your diaphragm, take a breath, then purse your lips and blow it out as hard as you can. Take another breath and exhale again. The inhaling followed by a deep exhalation works like yoga, says Balboa, providing an internal massage for your pinched muscle.

Breathe in, breathe out. Continue to massage your aching side and slow your breathing down to a normal rate. Getting your breathing back to a steady rhythm will help to stop the pain.

Practise abdominal breathing. Before you go out walking or running again, you need to know how to breathe to prevent stitches arising. Look down at your chest and watch as you take a deep breath, says Balboa. What is moving? If only your chest moves, you are breathing with your chest cavity – and that's not enough. To fight side stitches, you need your diaphragm to be involved in the breathing exercise.

One way to tell if you're using the right muscles is to get your chest and abdomen to move when you breathe. Keep an eye on your tummy. Inhale. Exhale. It should move in and out.

As you practise abdominal breathing, take deep breaths. Exhale deeply. Be aware of your breathing while you exercise, and within a couple of weeks, you won't even need to think about diaphragm breathing – it will become a habit.

Warm up your diaphragm. Like any muscle, the diaphragm needs to be warmed up before it exercises. So before you stretch your legs, give your diaphragm a breath massage to get it working. Sit on the floor and place one hand on your chest, the other on your stomach. As you breathe, both hands should move up and down, indicating that you're using your full breathing capacity, including your diaphragm. A warmed-up diaphragm is less likely to stitch.

Don't hold your breath. People hold their breath when they are frightened or cold or when they want to avoid pain, says Balboa. If you let yourself feel your emotions rather than trying to avoid them by holding your breath, you're more likely to breathe naturally when exercise demands a constant flow of air.

Stop to go. Even though side stitches are caused by a pinched diaphragm, you can get a similar feeling from trapped wind, says Dr Munsell. Any aerobic activity will slow down or stop the digestive process while the blood rushes to help the muscles, says Balboa. That's why runners are told not to eat for at least two hours before a race. It's also the reason runners sometimes get diarrhoea if they drink a lot of water during a race. So be careful what and when you eat before you exercise, and if you are prone to side stitches, perhaps try to have a bowel movement before you begin.

SINUSITIS
16 infection fighters

Sinuses are air-filled pockets that act as small air-quality-control centres under your cheekbones, above your eyes and nose, and behind your eye sockets. They help to warm, moisten and purify the air you breathe before it reaches your lungs. When they're working properly, airborne bacteria gets trapped and filtered out by mucus and the minute nasal hairs, called cilia, that line your sinuses. This little air-flow system may gum up, however, if something impedes the cilia, if a cold clogs the sinus openings or if an allergen or irritant swells the sinus linings. Then air gets trapped, pressure builds up, the mucus stagnates and bacteria or other organisms can breed. Infection and inflammation of the sinuses can set in, and you have sinusitis.

When you sleep, nasal fluid drips down into your throat, sending you into coughing spasms. You feel pressure and pain around your face, teeth or eyes. The pain is usually worse on one side and increases when you lean forwards. You may have a headache and you'll have a thick green or yellow nasal discharge. You lose your sense of smell, your temperature may rise and you feel pretty rough. Acute sinusitis is usually caused by viruses or bacteria and can last a month or longer. Occasionally the sinuses can become infected following injury to the skull or from spreading tooth or gum infection.

If you get clogged up too often, you may end up with a permanent thickening of the sinus membranes and a chronic stuffy nose. Chronic sinusitis, which usually lasts longer than eight weeks, is often caused by allergies – especially to dust, mould, pollen and certain fungi. Other causes can be nasal obstruction following injury or caused by polyps (grape-like swellings of the membranes lining the nose, usually resulting from chronic allergy).

Doctors generally prescribe antibiotics for bacterial sinus infection. But there are also various steps you can take to feel better. Here are some ways to unblock your sinuses and reduce pain.

Inhale steam. Humidity is vital to keep cilia working, mucus flowing and sinuses drained, says ear, nose and throat specialist Stanley Farb. Twice a day, take a steamy shower or bath, or lean over a bowl of steaming water with a towel draped over your head and the bowl to create a tent, and sniff.

Steam on the go. If you feel stuffiness during the day at work or on the run, get a cup of hot coffee, tea or soup, cup your hands over the top of the mug, and sniff, suggests allergy expert Howard Druce.

Humidify your home. Using a humidifier in your bedroom stops your nasal and sinus passages drying out, says ear, nose and throat specialist Bruce Jafek. Be sure to clean the humidifier every week to prevent a build-up of fungi.

'Get a quick and economical blast of steam,' says family doctor Stephen Amiel, 'by boiling an electric kettle with the lid off to disable the auto switch-off, but make sure it doesn't boil dry and keep it well out of harm's way.'

WHEN TO CONSULT A DOCTOR

If you've tried self-treatment for three or four days and still have sinus pain, pressure and stuffiness, you need to see a doctor to help clear up the infection, especially if the discharge from your nose is offensive-smelling and bloody as well as yellow or green. If your nasal obstruction is one sided only, or you have numbness on one side of your face, you should also seek an early appointment: in rare cases, a tumour in the sinus could be causing your symptoms. In severe and neglected cases, your sinuses could form an abscess affecting your eye or even your brain.

You may also have chronic sinusitis, which can be a recurrent or prolonged disorder lasting for months or even years. Depending on the cause, you may need to take a longer course of antibiotics than for acute sinusitis, or long-term anti-allergic medications.

Your GP may refer you to a specialist who can perform x-rays or other tests to discover what is causing your congestion, be it chronic infection, an obstruction from a deviated nasal septum, polyps or chronic allergy. You may also need to be considered for surgical drainage of a chronically blocked sinus.

Wash out your nostrils. To flush out stale nasal secretions, Dr Jafek suggests using saline nasal sprays or drops, or mixing a teaspoon of salt with 300ml of warm water and a pinch of baking soda. Put this into a squeezy bottle or medicine dropper, tip your head back, close one nostril with your thumb, and squirt the solution into the open nostril while sniffing. Then blow that nostril gently. Repeat on the other side.

Drink up. Drinking extra water or other liquids – both hot and cold – throughout the day, thins down the mucus and keeps it flowing, says Dr Farb. Sipping hot herbal teas made with fenugreek, fennel, anise or sage may help to move mucus even more.

Blow one nostril at a time. This helps to prevent pressure build-up in the ears, which can send bacteria further back into the sinus passages, says Dr Farb.

Go ahead and sniff. Sniffing is also a good way to drain the sinuses and send stale secretions down the throat, says Dr Farb.

Try decongestant tablets. The best over-the-counter medicines to help drain sinuses are single-action tablets that contain only decongestants,

Foods that make your eyes water or your nose run can help to clear blocked sinuses. Here's what allergy expert Howard Druce recommends.

Garlic. This pungent herb contains the same chemical found in a drug that makes mucus less sticky.

Horseradish. This hot root contains a chemical similar to one found in decongestants. The sauce in a jar is fine.

Hot spicy foods. Hot curries and cajun dishes are made with chilli peppers, which contain capsaicin, a substance that appears to act as a natural nasal decongestant. Smaller varieties of chilli are usually hotter and contain more capsaicin than larger ones. Dried chilli works well, too: just sprinkle ground cayenne pepper into your cooking.

such as Sudafed or Actifed tablets, says Dr Farb, although the evidence for benefit from any kind of decongestant is slight. Decongestants constrict the blood vessels, which may reduce the swollen membranes. Air can then pass through the nose, and pressure is alleviated. Avoid products that contain antihistamines if you're stuffed up from an infection, he adds. 'They work by drying out nasal secretions and may block you up even more.'

Use nasal sprays sparingly. Medicated nasal sprays or drops, such as Vicks Sinex nasal spray or Otrivine Sinusitis nasal spray, are fine to use occasionally, but frequent use could prolong the condition or make it worse, warns Terence Davidson, an expert on nasal disorders. It's what specialists call the 'rebound effect'. Initially, the sprays shrink your nasal linings. 'But then the mucosa reacts by swelling even more than before. It can take weeks for the swelling finally to subside after you stop using the sprays.'

Stop smoking. 'If you light twenty little bonfires under your nose every day, it's hardly surprising if your sinuses get inflamed and your cilia get paralysed,' says Dr Amiel. 'Reason number 202 to give up.'

Go for a walk. Exercise, says Dr Farb, may bring relief because it releases adrenaline, which constricts the blood vessels thereby possibly reducing swelling in the sinuses.

Apply pressure. Rubbing your sore sinuses brings a fresh blood supply to the area and soothing relief, suggests Dr Jafek. Press your thumbs firmly on both sides of your nose and hold for 15 to 30 seconds. Repeat.

Use heat. Applying moist heat over tender sinuses is an easy way to wash away sinus pain, says Dr Druce. Put a warm flannel over your eyes and cheekbones and leave it there until you feel the pain subside.

SNORING
12 tips for a silent night

Snoring has long been the subject of jokes, cartoons and sitcoms, but for many people it's no laughing matter. Snoring can be a serious problem, disrupting normal sleeping patterns and disturbing partners as they try to sleep through the noise.

Snoring is extremely common. Around 15 million people in the UK snore (10.4 million men and 4.5 million women), but because snoring often keeps partners awake, its impact is widely felt and can even threaten marriages.

The noise of snoring is caused by air passing through narrowed airways, in the mouth, nose or throat area, causing vibrations. The nasal passages, the tongue, the soft palate, the uvula (the wobbly bit hanging down at the back of the throat, the muscles of the back of the throat and the larynx may all be involved.

The main snoring triggers are being overweight, smoking, drinking too much alcohol, fatty or glandular tissue around the neck and allergies. In a minority of cases the anatomical structure of your airways and the nerve supply to the muscles of the palate and throat may be responsible. 'Some people just snore whatever,' says family doctor Stephen Amiel ruefully. 'I could snore for Britain, even though I don't smoke, hardly drink, don't suffer from allergies and have the body of a Greek god (well, maybe not quite, but I'm certainly not overweight).'

Joking apart, a heavy snorer may have a serious sleeping disorder called obstructive sleep apnoea needing medical attention, but for light or occasional snoring, there are several ways to achieve a quiet night.

Go on a diet. Most snorers tend to be middle-aged overweight men. Most women snorers are past the menopause. Slimming often stops snoring. 'If a moderate snorer loses weight, the snoring becomes less loud, and in some people it disappears,' says professor of medicine Earl Dunn.

Avoid a nightcap. Drinking alcohol before going to bed makes snoring worse, says Dr Dunn. It relaxes all the muscles in the throat that vibrate. And it's dose-related – the more you drink, the louder you'll snore.

Don't take sedatives. Sleeping pills may make *you* sleep, but they will keep your partner awake. 'Anything that relaxes the tissues around the head and neck will tend to make snoring worse. Even antihistamines will do it,' says Dr Dunn.

Quit smoking. Smokers tend to be snorers, says Dr Dunn. This could be because smoking causes swelling and inflammation of the throat tissues, making them more likely to vibrate and produce snoring.

Change your sleep position. Sleep on your side. 'Heavy snorers snore in virtually any position,' says Dr Dunn. 'But moderate snorers only snore when they are on their backs.'

Try the old tennis ball trick. In order to keep you from rolling over onto your back, sew a small pocket onto the back of your pyjama top. Then put a tennis ball inside. When you try and roll onto your back, you'll hit this hard object and unconsciously you'll roll back onto your side.

Get rid of your pillow. Anything that puts a kink in your neck makes you snore more, says Dr Dunn.

Instead, raise the head of your bed. This can lessen snoring. 'Elevate your upper torso, not just your head,' says Philip Westbrook, an expert in sleep disorders. Put a brick under each leg at the head of your bed.

Deal with allergies. Sneezing and snoring go together. 'Snoring can develop because of allergies or colds,' says Dr Westbrook. 'Use a nasal decongestant if your snoring is intermittent, but only for a few days at a time to avoid rebound congestion.

Saline nose drops will relieve mild congestion and can be used long term. Dissolve a teaspoon of salt and a pinch of baking soda (sodium bi-

---

You think you've got problems?

The world's loudest snorer, Melvin Switzer, trumpeted his way into the *Guinness Book of World Records* with a snore registered at 87.4 decibels.

This is equivalent to a large lorry driving through your bedroom. His wife apparently went deaf in one ear as a result of the nightly onslaught.

WHEN TO CONSULT A DOCTOR

The louder your snore, the more likely it is to be related to a medical problem. One of the worst problems associated with snoring is a condition called obstructive sleep apnoea (OSA), a potentially life-threatening disorder, in which breathing actually stops during sleep for at least 10 seconds and up to a minute, or even longer (see box, *Are you at risk of OSA?*, page 508)

This can happen hundreds of times a night, contributing to high blood pressure, cardiovascular disease, memory problems, impotence and headaches. Sleep-deprived apnoea patients often have problems at work and may be unsafe behind the wheel.

Symptoms of OSA include loud snoring, that is, loud enough to be heard outside the room; snoring punctuated by periods of silence, gasping or choking; and extreme tiredness during the day. If this sounds like you, see your doctor.

If you don't have someone sleeping (or trying to sleep) next to you to observe your snoring pattern, but you think you're getting OSA, set a tape recorder next to your bed as you drop off to sleep. If your snoring reaches a crescendo and then stops for short periods before starting again after a choking or spluttering sound, see your doctor. If obvious causes cannot be relieved, you may need a referral to a sleep disorders clinic for an overnight sleep study. Treatment options may include removing nasal polyps or correcting a deviated nasal septum; a mandibular advancement splint worn at night to hold the lower jaw forward; CPAP (a machine delivering a constant stream of air through a nasal cannula, forcing the airways to stay open); or laser surgery to the uvula and soft palate.

If you have a child who snores badly and has obstructive sleep apnoeic attacks, he or she may have enlarged adenoids and tonsils needing fairly urgent removal. Report such symptoms to your doctor.

carbonate) in 300ml of warm water. Put this into a squeezy bottle or medicine dropper, tilt your head back and insert a few drops into each nostril. If you snore during the hay fever season, use a steroid (like Beconase) or cromoglicate (Rynacrom) nasal spray throughout the season.

Try a nasal splint. A spring-loaded adhesive strip across the bridge of the nose, similar to those used by some sportsmen, can hold the nostrils open and relieve night-time nasal obstruction. They can be bought in

Are you at risk of OSA?

You can check your obstructive sleep apnoea (OSA) risk with the 'Epworth Sleepiness Score'. How likely are you to doze off or fall asleep in the following situations? Choose the most appropriate number for each situation from the following scale:

0 – would never doze;
1 – slight chance of dozing;
2 – moderate chance of dozing;
3 – high chance of dozing.

- sitting and reading
- watching television
- sitting inactive in a public place (such as a cinema or a meeting)
- as a passenger in a car for an hour without a break
- lying down to rest in the afternoon when circumstances permit
- sitting and talking to someone
- sitting quietly after lunch without alcohol
- in a car, while stopped for a few minutes in traffic

If your score adds up to more than 9, you may have OSA and should see your doctor.

different sizes at pharmacies, or you can make your own much more cheaply, says Dr Amiel. Cut strips of thick clear plastic, approximately 7cm in length and 1cm wide, from food containers or packaging, rounding off the sharp corners. The plastic needs to be thick enough to spring back into shape when it's flexed. Cover each end with double sided adhesive tape (the strongest and least irritant to the skin is wig tape).

Before you go to bed, clean the sides of your nose just above the curve of the nostrils with an alcohol-based cleanser to remove grease, and stick firmly.

Give your partner earplugs. If all else fails, the one on the receiving end of your snoring can wear earplugs to bed. They're cheap and can be bought at any pharmacy.

Find out more. For further information on the causes and treatments for snoring and sleep apnoea, contact the British Snoring & Sleep Apnoea Association, 2nd Floor Suite, 52 Albert Road North, Reigate, Surrey RH2 9EL; or online at www.britishsnoring.com; or tel: 01737 245638.

SORE THROAT

15 ways to soothe the pain

A burning, irritated throat can disrupt your sleep, interfere with your work and make you feel generally miserable. Your sore throat may be an early symptom of a cold, flu or some other viral or bacterial infection. Pain from the throat may be referred to the ear too and the inflamed small blood vessels may sometimes rupture when you cough, causing alarming streaks of blood to appear in your phlegm.

Sometimes a sore throat is just a minor irritation caused by the low humidity of centrally heated environments in winter, or too much cheering at a football match. Whatever the cause, here are some ways to make it feel better.

Suck lozenges. If your sore throat is caused by a viral infection, antibiotics won't help. Most lozenges are soothing, and pharmacists recommend medicated lozenges containing a local anaesthetic like benzocaine – Dequacaine or Merocaine lozenges, for example. These numb nerve endings so your throat doesn't feel as scratchy. Follow label directions.

Spray away pain. Phenol-containing throat sprays, like Ultra Chloraseptic spray, can also give topical relief. But as pharmacologist Thomas Gossel points out, the duration of contact between the spray and the irritated tissue is relatively brief. Lozenges simply last longer.

Try zinc. Zinc lozenges can help a sore throat associated with a cold, says medical researcher Donald Davis. His studies have shown zinc to lessen both the severity and the duration of a sore throat, although other research has failed to confirm this effect. Suck zinc lozenges, such as Nature's Way Zinc lozenges or Strepsils Zinc Defence lozenges, following label directions, until your symptoms subside.

Note: Don't take more than the recommended dose. Taking more than 40mg of zinc a day can impair your body's ability to absorb copper.

Gargle to bathe and soothe. If it hurts when you swallow, the sore area may be high enough in your throat for gargling to help, says ear, nose and throat specialist Hueston King. So gargle frequently with one of the solutions below.

Salt water: Mix a teaspoon of table salt in 500ml of warm water, says Dr Gossel. That's just enough salt to mimic the body's natural saline content, so you'll find it very soothing. Use every hour or so.

Echinacea tea: According to clinical herbalist Douglas Schar, even severe cases of tonsillitis can be remedied with echinacea tea – you need to ask for the echinacea root. Buy it as a tincture from the health food store and add one teaspoon (5ml) to a cup of warm water. Gargle with the tea and then swallow, three times a day.

Goldenseal tea: Though goldenseal tastes unpleasant, it does wonders for a sore throat, says Schar. It's antimicrobial and anti-inflammatory – so it attacks the infection causing the sore throat, and reduces the tissue inflammation. Buy the tincture at the health food store. Add a teaspoon (5ml) to a cup of hot water and gargle every two hours. In this case, says Schar, do not swallow after gargling.

Whisky. Add a spoonful of whisky to a glass of warm water and gargle, says Dr Gossel. 'It's just enough alcohol to help numb a sore throat.'

Humidify the room. If your throat is sore when you wake up, you may have been sleeping with your mouth open. Ear, nose and throat specialist Jason Surow recommends a bedroom humidifier to keep the environment moist. Humidifiers are available from some pharmacies, department stores and online. For a cheaper alternative, boil an electric kettle (with the lid off to disable the auto switch-off), but make sure it doesn't boil dry and keep it well out of the reach of small children.

Breathe steam. Run very hot water in the bathroom basin to build up steam. Lean over the basin, drape a towel over your head to create a steam tent, and inhale deeply through your mouth and nose for five to ten minutes, topping up the hot water as necessary. Repeat several times a day. A safer and more convenient alternative can be bought at the pharmacy: a device like a baby's feeding mug with an attached mask that fits over your nose and mouth. Half fill with steaming water and inhale.

Clear your nose. If you are breathing through your mouth because your nose is blocked up, says Dr Surow, clear it with an over-the-counter medicated decongestant nasal spray or drops, such as Otrivine or ephedrine. However, they shouldn't be used for longer than seven days. Over-use can have a rebound effect, and make your nose even more blocked than it was before.

Mimic a sea breeze. If you can't actually go to the seaside, get the same sort of salty atmosphere from a saline nasal spray or drops, such as Salex Saline nasal spray, available from pharmacies. Or make your own, using a teaspoon of salt to 300mls of water, and fill an atomizer or plastic

WHEN TO CONSULT A DOCTOR

A strep throat (the commonest form of bacterial tonsillitis) can be particularly unpleasant, although it is impossible to tell by the severity of symptoms alone whether a sore throat is bacterial or not. Complications of a strep throat, like rheumatic fever or kidney disease, are very rare in developed countries, and, left untreated, even a strep throat will get better on its own. 'I usually tell my patients that a strep throat will get better in seven days with antibiotics, and a week without,' says family doctor Stephen Amiel. A throat swab will tell in a few days whether the cause is bacterial but most doctors base their decision on whether to give antibiotics on how generally ill you are otherwise. Antibiotics are also recommended if: you have a one-sided tonsillitis (you may be about to develop a quinsy, a nasty abscess which may require incising in hospital); you have a fine, red, streptococcal rash; and also if you are more at risk with acute infections, for example if you have diabetes or immune deficiency, heart valve disease, or a history of rheumatic fever.

Other important causes of sore throats include mononucleosis, commonly known as glandular fever (a viral infection) and childhood epiglottitis, an acute and sometimes dangerous bacterial infection near the voice box which causes acute swelling that can obstruct the airway.

Sore throats can have many causes, but some symptoms warrant a visit to your doctor. These include:

- severe, prolonged or recurrent sore throats. Ear, nose and throat specialists are more and more reluctant to remove tonsils these days, but if you are getting frequent attacks of bacterial tonsillitis every year for several years running, and missing work or school as a result, they may be persuaded;
- difficulty in breathing, swallowing your saliva or opening the mouth;
- rash or a temperature above 38.3°C (101°F) for more than three days;
- hoarseness lasting three weeks or longer;
- the presence of significant (more than the odd streak) or persistent (more than a few days, however slight) blood in your saliva or phlegm.

garden spray bottle. When you inhale the mist, says Dr Surow, the salt-based spray moistens your nose and drips down the back of your throat to help increase humidity there.

Take a painkiller. It doesn't occur to most people that a sore throat is a pain like any other ache, says Dr Gossel. Paracetamol or ibuprofen will help to ease the pain. Aspirin is a suitable alternative, but has more side-effects and should not be given to anyone under 16. For faster relief, use soluble paracetamol, and gargle with the solution before swallowing it, says family doctor Stephen Amiel.

Increase your fluid intake. Drink as much fluid as you can, says Dr Surow. It doesn't really matter what you drink, he says, although there are a few things to avoid. Thick, milky drinks will coat your throat and may produce mucus, making you cough and further irritating tissues; orange juice may burn an already inflamed throat; and caffeine-containing beverages have a counterproductive diuretic effect.

Suck liquorice for strained vocal chords. Liquorice was used by Greek singers and orators to soothe throats made sore through overuse. This is a very different kind of sore throat from that caused by infection, says Schar, and in this instance, nothing is better than liquorice.

Buy lozenges at the health food store and suck several a day. Make sure that the product contains real liquorice and lots of it!

Use a Russian home remedy. Irwin Ziment, a specialist in respiratory medicine, mixes a tablespoon of grated fresh horseradish, a teaspoon of honey and a teaspoon of ground cloves in a glass of warm water. 'Sip it slowly, and keep stirring – as the horseradish tends to settle – and think happy thoughts,' he says. Or use it as a gargle.

Note: Be sure to peel the horseradish root under a running tap and grate it in the open air, or the pungent fumes will burn your eyes.

What about vitamins? Vitamin C may help to build up your tissues to fight the germs that make your throat sore. A normal healthy diet with plenty of fresh fruit and vegetables should give you plenty of vitamin C.

There is little evidence that vitamin C supplements will reduce the severity or duration of sore throats: the best available evidence shows that taking one gram or more a day reduces the duration of symptoms by only half a day. Claims are also made for vitamin E, but again, firm evidence is hard to find.

Sterilize your toothbrush. Believe it or not, says pathologist Richard Glass, your toothbrush may be perpetuating – or even causing – your sore throat. Bacteria collect on the bristles, and any injury to the gums during brushing injects these germs into your system.

Some dentists recommend replacing your toothbrush after an upper respiratory illness, but sterilizing it in a dilute bleach solution should be fine (you should in any case replace your toothbrush every three months or so).

Raise the bedhead. Another cause of sore throat in the morning – besides sleeping with your mouth open – is a reflux of stomach acids into your throat during the night. These acids are extremely irritating to sensitive throat tissues, says ear, nose and throat specialist Jerome Goldstein. Stop the problem by raising your bedhead by 10 to 15cm – try using bricks or old phone books. But don't simply pile more pillows under your head; they will make you bend in the middle, increasing pressure on your oesophagus and making the problem worse. As an extra precaution, don't eat or drink for an hour or two before going to bed.

SPLINTERS
9 ways to get them out

Splinters are small pieces of wood, glass, metal or other matter that gets caught under your skin. Even though they're often small, they tend to hurt. Whether they are buried deeply or not, you need to remove them as soon as possible so they don't cause infection.

Here are some ideas for relatively painless ways to remove splinters.

Get some help. It's difficult to cause yourself pain, so ask a partner or friend to lend you a gentle, helping hand. First, sterilize a pair of tweezers by cleaning in surgical spirit, says dermatologist Dee Anna Glaser. Use them to grasp the protruding end of the splinter and gently pull it out in the direction it entered. If the splinter is embedded in the skin, your helper will need to use a needle, sterilized with spirit, or over a flame, to make a small hole in the skin over the end of the splinter. Then, lift the skin up to expose the splinter, put the needle under the splinter until it can be grasped with the tweezers, and pull it out.

Make sure that the entire splinter has been removed. If not, repeat the steps above. If the splinter is really small, or if you don't get the entire splinter out on the first try, use a magnifying glass to get a closer look.

Let warm water do the work. If probing with a sterilized needle and tweezers doesn't do the trick, soak the affected area in 300ml warm water with a teaspoon of salt added. A 10 to 15-minute soak will cause the piece of wood to swell, which may help the splinter to pop out on its own, says dermatologist Ralph Daniel.

Try sticky tape. Dr Daniel also suggests using adhesive tape first, if the thought of using tweezers or a needle makes you feel a bit squeamish.

Simply put the tape over the splinter, then pull it off. If the splinter hasn't penetrated too deeply, the adhesive tape will often stick to the splinter. Removing the piece of tape pulls the splinter out painlessly and easily. If that doesn't work, you'll have to resort to tweezers.

Clean it up. After the splinter has been completely removed, clean the wound with surgical spirit or liquid antiseptic and cover with a plaster if necessary, or leave it open to the air.

Take preventative measures. Dr Glaser recommends the following ways to avoid splinters.

• Wear shoes outdoors at all times and whenever you walk on unfinished wooden floors or outdoor wooden decking.

• Clean up all broken glass and metal shavings around the house immediately. Be careful when handling broken glass, and wear hard-soled shoes to protect your feet.

• Wear leather gardening gloves when handling thorny or spiny plants.

• Wear gloves to sandpaper wood or rub down paintwork.

WHEN TO CONSULT A DOCTOR

See a doctor if the splinter is very large or deeply embedded and cannot be easily removed. A deep splinter may necessitate a small incision to remove it. Unless the splinter is removed, it will almost always become infected.

Anyone with diabetes or whose immune system is suppressed for any reason should see a doctor if they have a deeply embedded splinter, because they are at greater risk of infection.

If, after removing a splinter, you see any signs of infection – pain, redness, swelling or red streaks – it may be a sign that the splinter has not been fully removed. Your doctor may prescribe antibiotics, either as an ointment or to be taken internally.

Finally, you may need a tetanus jab. It is now considered unnecessary to have a tetanus booster if you are cut, provided you have had five tetanus injections at any time in your life.

Most children have had four by the time they start school, and a fifth is given in their teens. But as routine immunization only started in 1961, many adults may not have complete immunity. If you have not had five tetanus injections, or you are unsure, get a booster as soon as possible.

SPRAINS
18 self-care strategies

Ligaments are tough bands of tissue that wrap around your ankle and other joints, giving them support and stability. They have a bit of give, but only a little. If stretched beyond their normal limits, they can become damaged or inflamed – in other words, sprained.

You can expect a sprain to heal in about six weeks, provided you treat it properly, says John McShane, an expert in sports medicine. 'But,' he says, 'people tend to ignore sprains, which can result in chronic (long term) problems.' Most sprains can be treated at home without medical attention. This is what to do.

Rest the joint. Sprains don't necessarily hurt a lot at first, and you may assume it's okay to keep doing the activity that caused the sprain in the first place. But pushing an injured joint too hard makes the damage worse.

Minor sprains need a couple of days' rest, advises Dr McShane. You don't have to limit movement completely, but you must avoid vigorous activities that put stress on the injured area.

Ice it immediately. Applying cold to a sprain deadens pain and reduces internal bleeding or the accumulation of fluids in the injured area. It's important to ice sprains immediately because swelling is hard to reverse once it's underway. Put ice cubes or crushed ice in a plastic bag, wrap it in a teatowel and put it over the sprain. Keep applying ice to the area as long as it's sore, especially if there's any swelling.

Or use a bag of frozen peas or coffee beans. This is pliable enough to mould around the joint and apply cold just where it's needed, says Michael Osborne, who specializes in rehabilitation after physical injury.

Buy a gel pack. Available at pharmacies and sports shops, gel packs stay flexible even when frozen and mould themselves to the contours of the joint. 'Gel packs get colder than ice and can cause frostbite if they're put directly onto the skin,' warns Dr McShane. Make sure you put a teatowel between the gel pack and the skin, and don't leave it on for more than 15 minutes at a time.

Bandage the joint. Compressing the area with a stretchy crepe bandage helps to prevent fluid from accumulating, which reduces swelling and pain. Wrapping a joint also restricts movement, which helps the injured ligaments to heal.

WHEN TO CONSULT A DOCTOR

All sprains are painful, and it's difficult even for doctors to tell immediately if the injuries involve torn tissue, fractured bone or other problems.

If there's a lot of swelling or bruising, or if the pain seems unusually severe, it's a good idea to get to an A&E department for x-rays.

All sprains should start feeling better within a few weeks. See your doctor if there isn't a noticeable improvement within two to four weeks.

Note: Don't make the bandage too tight or it will cut off blood circulation. If the area beyond the sprain feels numb or cold, or if the bandage itself is uncomfortably tight, loosen it a bit. 'You should be able to slip a finger snugly under the bandage,' says Dr McShane.

Use a tube. Available at pharmacies, elastic 'tube' bandages come in different sizes for different joints. The problem with the crepe bandages mentioned above is that they can shift when you wear them, which may allow swelling in some areas. Tube bandages work better because they apply even compression all the way around the joint, says Dr Osborne.

Get gravity on your side. For the first day or two after a sprain, raise the injured area for as long as possible. If you've sprained your ankle, for example, put a few pillows underneath your calf. If you've sprained your wrist, keep your hand above chest level – perhaps in a sling. Elevating the joint aids lymphatic drainage from the area and keeps swelling to a minimum, says Dr Osborne.

Take an anti-inflammatory. Aspirin and ibuprofen are nonsteroidal anti-inflammatory drugs (NSAIDs), which means that they inhibit the body's production of prostaglandins – inflammatory chemicals that cause swelling and delay healing time. Paracetamol is effective for pain relief, but it doesn't have any effect on swelling.

Note: If the injury is severe, wait until the bleeding has stopped or the swelling has stabilized before taking NSAIDs, because they also inhibit blood clotting and may delay recovery time. Do not give aspirin to anyone under 16.

Relieve stiffness with heat. Don't treat a sprain with a heating pad or hot-water bottle in the first 48 to 72 hours after injury, because heat increases circulation and may increase swelling. But after a few days, when the swelling has subsided, applying heat – or soaking the area in a hot bath – may help you to feel more comfortable, says Dr Osborne.

Heat also improves the flow of nutrients into the injured area while removing painful metabolic by-products.

Wear a support. If you have a history of ankle sprains, consider wearing an ankle support. Available at sports shops, joint supports protect the joint, which can speed up healing and reduce the risk of further sprains. Some people with ankles prone to sprains wear supports whenever they take part in activities like tennis or netball.

Try not to wear the support at other times though: they're no substitute for exercising and strengthening the muscles that support and stabilize the joint you've sprained.

Wear the right shoes. If you've sprained your ankle once, you may be at greater risk of sprains in future. One way to prevent problems is to buy shoes designed for the activities you do. In other words, wear running shoes for running, but not for playing squash. 'Running shoes don't provide ankle stability, and they may actually create a tendency for the ankle to roll in or out,' says Dr McShane.

Watch the ground. Sprains would be a lot less common if the entire world were as flat as a running track. But hazards – everything from curbs in unexpected places to potholed playing fields – are everywhere. Whether you're walking, hiking or playing sports, always check the ground to see what lies ahead. If you exercise outdoors at night, try to do it in well-lit areas so that you can see where you're treading.

Strengthen the joint. Once the sprain is better, it's worth taking

Do just *one* thing

Start with gentle exercises as soon as possible. It's normal for ligaments to be somewhat tight after a sprain. To prevent stiffness and restore joint mobility, it's helpful to exercise the joint once you're through the initial, painful phase.

Moving the joint may be painful at first, but that's okay. In fact, it's helpful to gently push the joint slightly further than it wants to go, says Dr McShane. 'Ligaments actually heal better when they're slightly stressed.'

If you're recovering from an ankle sprain, use your foot to 'sketch' the entire alphabet once or twice a day. Imagine that your big toe is the tip of a pen. Using the ankle to move the foot, form each letter of the alphabet, from A to Z, in the air. That will help to get the range of motion back, and reduce swelling as well.

the time to strengthen and condition the joint, which reduces stress on the ligaments. Because ankle sprains are so common, this is the area of the body that you may want to focus on – both for relieving stiffness and for preventing future problems. 'The ankle may be weak after a sprain, so you'll want to begin with exercises to increase movement, and then progress to strengthening exercises,' says Dr Osborne. Try these.

- Put a few tins of soup or vegetables into a plastic carrier bag, put your foot through the handles, and lift your toes towards the ceiling. Hold the weight for about three seconds, then lower it back down.

- Put your foot against a wall or another immovable object, and flex and relax the muscles. This type of isometric exercise improves bloodflow and exerts beneficial stress on the ligaments and other tissues.

- While sitting with your legs straight in front of you, flex the top of your foot back towards your body. Hold for a moment, then relax.

- While sitting, loop a towel or an elastic cord around your foot, then flex the muscles in different directions against the resistance.

Stretch away tightness. No one enjoys stretching very much, but it's worth getting in the habit, especially if you're recovering from a sprain and the muscles around the joint are tighter than they should be. At the very least, spend a few minutes a day stretching the muscles around the affected joint.

STRESS

23 ways to beat the tension

We all need a certain amount of stress in order to survive, and at the right level, stress can be healthy – and even enjoyable. But it can get to be too much. The British Health & Safety Executive defines stress as 'the adverse reaction people have to excessive pressure or other types of demand placed on them'. About half-a-million people in Britain experience work-related stress at a level they believe makes them ill, says the HSE. And up to five million of us feel very stressed by our work.

But it isn't only work that makes us stressed. Other common causes of stress include:

- change of social circumstances – this could be the death of your partner, changing your job or getting married;

- pressure to conform to a particular way of behaving, especially where this goes against the grain;
- conflict in relationships, or not feeling valued or being praised by others;
- lack of support, too little free time or time simply to be listened to;
- financial problems, being unemployed or having very limited contact with other people.

Symptoms of stress can include a loss of appetite or binge eating, disrupted sleep patterns, irritability, and the appearance of physical symptoms such as eczema, asthma, psoriasis, irritable bowel syndrome, migraine headaches and stomach ulcers.

But stress isn't all bad. It can be a force you can turn to your advantage. You don't have to run away from it, and you don't have to go on a stress-management course to learn how to handle it. The following tips suggest ways to combat stress – and win.

Change your attitude. 'I think the single most important point you can make about stress is that in most cases it's not what's out there that's the problem, it's how you react to it,' says psychiatrist Paul Rosch. How you react is determined by how you view a particular stress.

'Watch people on a roller-coaster,' says Dr Rosch. 'Some sit at the back, eyes shut, jaws clenched. They can't wait for the ordeal to end and to get back on solid ground. In front are the wide-eyed thrill seekers who relish every steep plunge and can't wait to get onto the next ride. In between are those who appear quite nonchalant, or even bored.

'They're all having exactly the same experience – the roller-coaster ride – but they're reacting to it very differently: bad stress, good stress and no stress.'

Emmett Miller, an expert on stress, uses Chinese wisdom to make this point. 'The Chinese word for crisis is *wuji* – two characters that separately mean "danger" and "opportunity". Every problem we encounter in life can be viewed in that way – as a chance to show that we can handle it.' Changing the way you think – regarding a difficult task at work as a chance to improve your skills, for example – can change a life of stress and discomfort into a life of challenge and excitement.

Think about something else. Anything that will help you to shift your perspective instantly is useful when you're under fire, says Dr Miller. 'You want to distract yourself, to break whatever chain of thought is producing the stress. Thinking about almost anything else will do that.'

Think positive. 'Thinking about a success or a past achievement is excellent when you're feeling uncertain – before giving a presentation, for example, or a meeting with your boss,' Dr Miller says. 'You're instantly reminded that you've achieved before, and there's no reason why you shouldn't achieve this time.'

Take a mental holiday. 'Taking a mini-break in your mind is a very good way to relieve or manage stress,' says Dr Ronald Nathan, author of a book on stress relief. 'Imagine yourself lying in warm sand on a beach, feel the gentle sea breeze and listen to the waves breaking quietly in the background. It's amazing what this can do to relax you.'

Recite an anti-stress litany. Stress can strike anytime, not just at work – in the bathroom before you go to work, in the sandwich bar at lunchtime, in the car on the way home. To help yourself loosen up when unpleasant thoughts knot the muscles in your neck, recite the following litany, suggests Dr Miller.

- 'There's nowhere I have to be right now.'
- 'There's no problem I have to solve right now.'
- 'There's nothing I have to do right now.'
- 'The most important thing I can do right now is to relax.'

You need to think these thoughts consciously, says Dr Miller, because doing so automatically changes the mindset that's causing the stress. If you're reciting the litany, you're not thinking about whatever was bothering you.

Use affirmations. Have some affirmations to hand that you can repeat to yourself when you feel stressed, Dr Miller says. 'They don't have to be complicated. Just chanting "I can handle this" to yourself or "I know more about this than anyone here", will work.' It gets you away from the animal, adrenaline-fuelled 'fright/flight/fight' reflex – rapid breathing, dry mouth, cold or sweaty hands, palpitations, churning gut – and towards the intellectual response to stress, the part of you that really can handle it. And you calm down.

Count to 10. Simply refusing to respond to a stress immediately can help to defuse it, says Dr Nathan. Making a habit of pausing and relaxing just for a few seconds before responding to the routine interruptions of your day can make a big difference to the sense of stress you experience. When the phone rings, for example, breathe in deeply. Then as you breathe out, imagine you are as floppy as a rag doll. 'One of the things pausing like this does is to give you a feeling of control,' Dr Nathan observes. 'Feeling

WHEN TO CONSULT A DOCTOR

Too much stress can directly threaten your health. If your symptoms are new and have no obvious cause, especially if they interfere with your quality of life, see a doctor, says psychiatrist Paul Rosch.

Any of the following stress-related symptoms may suggest that you need medical help:

- frequent headaches, jaw clenching or pain, gritting or grinding teeth;
- stuttering or stammering, tremors, trembling of lips or hands;
- neck ache, back pain or muscle spasms;
- light-headedness or dizziness, ringing, buzzing or popping sounds;
- frequent blushing or sweating, cold or sweaty hands and feet;
- dry mouth or problems swallowing;
- overuse of alcohol or 'recreational' drugs to deal with stress.

in control is generally less stressful than feeling out of control.

Make a habit of using rapid relaxation during the pause before you answer the phone. Deliberately pausing is an instant tranquillizer.'

Look away. 'If you look through a window at a distant view for a moment, and away from the problem that's producing the stress, your eyes relax. And if your eyes relax, the tendency is for you to do the same,' Dr Nathan says.

Get up and leave. 'If you take a saucepan off the hob, it stops boiling,' says Dr Nathan. 'Leaving the scene can also give you a fresh perspective.'

Try 'So Hum' breathing. 'When you're stressed, your pulse races and you start breathing very quickly,' says chiropractor Bradley Frederick. 'Eastern medicine teaches us that we can control our autonomic nervous system and its responses. One example of this is respiration. By making yourself breathe slowly and fully, you can change your body's automatic response to stress. This simple activity can slow down the heart rate and bring oxygen to the brain and muscles, which eases tension and convinces the body that the stress has gone, whether it has or not.'

The right way to breathe is abdominally – feeling your stomach expand as you inhale and collapse as you exhale. While there are many different breathing techniques to calm the mind, a technique described as 'So Hum' breathing is best to begin with. Inhale deeply and mouth 'soooooo', then slowly exhale with 'hummmm'. Pull your stomach in hard. Breathing slowly, fully and calmly at the first sign of stress could change your attitude – and life – forever.

Don't breathe deeply and fast, though, or you risk hyperventilating. During hyperventilation, you blow out too much carbon dioxide. This upsets the acid-base balance in your blood, which makes you dizzy and can cause pins and needles and spasms in your hands, feet and jaw.

Stretch. 'Essentially, every emotion we feel has a physical manifestation,' says Dr Frederick. 'Tightening of jaw and shoulder muscles is a common response to stress. Ideally, we'd prefer to eliminate the causes of stress, rather than treat the symptoms. But because we often cannot do anything about the source of stress, then we need to respond to it. If you stretch your muscles and keep your spine mobile, you'll feel better, be healthier and live longer.'

Massage your target muscles. 'Most of us have particular muscles that knot up under stress,' Dr Miller says. 'It's sort of a vicious circle: stress produces adrenaline, which produces muscle tension, which produces more adrenaline, and so on. A good way to break the cycle is to find out where your target muscles are – the ones that tense under pressure, usually in the back of your neck and upper back – and massage them for a couple of minutes whenever you feel tense.'

Massage your temples. This application of acupressure – the system that uses pressure points to relieve pain and treat a variety of ailments – works indirectly. Massaging nerves in your temples relaxes muscles elsewhere, especially in your neck, says Dr Miller.

Relax your jaw. People under pressure have a tendency to clench their teeth, says Dr Miller. 'Dropping the jaw and rolling it helps the muscles relax, and if you relax the muscles you reduce the sensation of tension.'

Relax your breathing. The tense musculature of a person under stress can make breathing difficult, according to Dr Frederick, and impaired breathing can aggravate the anxiety you already feel. To relax your breathing, roll your shoulders up and back, then relax. The first time, inhale deeply as they go back and exhale as they relax. You could do this while doing 'So Hum' breathing (above). Repeat four or five more times, then inhale deeply again. Repeat the entire sequence four times.

Relax all over. A simple technique called progressive relaxation can produce an immediate and dramatic reduction in your sense of stress by reducing physical tension. Starting at top or bottom, tense one set of muscles in your body at a time, hold for a few seconds, then let them relax. Work your way through all major body parts – feet, legs, chest and arms, head and neck – and then enjoy the sense of release it provides.

Have a hot bath. Hot water works by defeating the stress response, says Dr Frederick. When we're tense and anxious, blood flow to our extremities is reduced. Hot water restores circulation, convincing the body it's safe and that it is okay to relax. Dr Frederick recommends putting warm flannels on your feet, hands and forehead.

At work, try holding your hands under warm running water until you feel the tension starting to drain away.

Exercise. Regular exercise builds up stamina that can help you to fight stress. But even something as casual as a walk around the block can help you get rid of some of the tension that a tough business meeting or a family row leaves behind. Exercise is what your body instinctively wants to do under stress – it's the flight or fight reflex, says Dr Miller. And it works. First, it burns off some of the stress chemicals, and second, tired muscles are relaxed muscles.

Listen to a relaxation tape. Relaxation is the opposite of tension – the antidote for stress, says Dr Miller. And prerecorded relaxation tapes are cheap and effective. You can buy tapes or CDs with voice only, voice with music or just natural sounds – the wind in the trees or waves breaking on the sand. Listen through headphones to block distractions and avoid disturbing other people.

Enjoy music. Relaxation tapes aren't your only option. The right music soothes as perhaps nothing else does. 'Music is an enormously powerful tool for fighting stress,' Dr Miller says. 'You can use it in two basic ways – to relax or to inspire.'

Beat stress with Siberian ginseng. Herbalists call stress-busting herbs adaptogens, because they help us to adapt better to the things that make us stressed. One such herb is Siberian ginseng, says clinical herbalist Douglas Schar. Take it three times a day, following label instructions, during periods of stress.

Note: Make sure you buy Siberian ginseng, as opposed to American ginseng, which can wreak havoc on the menstrual cycle or worsen menopause symptoms.

Avoid stimulants. Piles of empty coffee cups and full ashtrays – the classic television cliché of people coping with stress: a newspaper deadline, a relationship crisis, a difficult business deal. But although small amounts of caffeine may help in performing certain mental and physical tasks, large amounts will increase physical symptoms of anxiety and irritability, and nicotine causes release of adrenaline, increase in heart rate and in blood pressure. So that cup of tea or coffee and a cigarette are just the wrong things to help you deal with stressful situations.

Don't rely on alcohol or cannabis either. Again, a stiff drink, or, increasingly, a joint, is a stock response to a stressful day. But too much alcohol will impair your ability to perform well and increase levels of anxiety as its effects wear off. Cannabis is also often used to relieve stress, but it too can cause anxiety, irritability and paranoia if used to excess, and in susceptible people.

SUNBURN
32 cooling treatments

Most of us like sunny weather. Sunlight is good for our general health and makes us feel great. And because the average British summer so often disappoints, many of us travel abroad specifically in search of a hotter climate. But although sunbathing is enjoyable, it carries risks. A suntan is not a sign of good health, but rather an attempt by your skin at damage limitation. Skin that's exposed excessively to the sun can become permanently damaged and prematurely aged. 'I get to see more bare bottoms than most people,' says family doctor Stephen Amiel. 'The skin there rarely gets to see the sun, and it often looks twenty years younger than the rest of the body.'

Excessive exposure to the sun is also dangerous because of the harmful effects of ultraviolet radiation on the skin, damaging the skin's immune response and increasing the risks of skin cancer. Sunbeds should not be regarded as safe alternatives. Think of sunbathing or using a sunbed as smoking for the skin, and you get the picture, says Dr Amiel.

The sun emits two kinds of ultraviolet rays: UVA, which penetrate deeply into the skin and cause premature ageing and wrinkles; and UVB, which affect the upper layers of the skin and trigger the production of melanin which causes tanning. Too much causes burning, freckling and thickening of the skin. UVB rays can also cause skin cancers, and increasingly it's being suspected that UVA rays can cause cancer too.

UVA and UVB rays can both penetrate cloud. You can also be burnt by sunlight reflected from water, sand or snow. Swimmers are especially at risk of sunburn because the cool water is deceptively comfortable. Furthermore, ultraviolet rays not only penetrate water, but are magnified by it – and in shallow water the rays can reflect off the sand, too. If you are snorkelling, wear a tee-shirt to protect your back.

Sunburn is also a big risk for skiers or climbers. The intensity of sunlight increases with altitude: for every 300 metres you climb, the strength of the sun's rays increases by a frightening four per cent.

If you're reading this, you are probably already sunburnt, in which case here's some helpful advice. And if you aren't burnt, well done – and here are some useful safety tips for staying that way.

Apply soothing compresses. Following a burn, the skin is hot and inflamed. Cool it down with compresses dipped in any one of the following substances. A fan aimed at the sunburned area will enhance cooling.

Cold water. Use cold tap water or add a few ice cubes, says dermatologist Michael Schreiber. Dip a cloth into the liquid and lay it over the burn. Repeat every few minutes as the cloth warms up. Repeat the process several times a day for 10 to 15 minutes at a time.

Witch hazel. Moisten a cloth with witch hazel, says dermatologist Fredric Haberman. This astringent has been shown to provide long-lasting anti-inflammatory relief. Apply often. For smaller areas, dip a cotton wool ball into the liquid and gently stroke it on.

Soak the pain away. An alternative to compresses, especially for larger areas, is a cool bath. Add more warm water as needed to keep the water at a comfortable temperature. Afterwards, gently pat your skin dry with a clean towel. Do not rub your skin, or you'll irritate it. The following substances can reduce pain, itching and inflammation.

Baking soda. Generously sprinkle baking soda into tepid bathwater, suggests Dr Haberman. Instead of towelling dry, let the solution dry on your skin. It is completely non-toxic and will soothe the pain.

Vinegar. Add a cup of cider vinegar to a bath of cool water, suggests dermatologist Carl Korn. A great astringent, it soothes sunburn pain.

Aveeno colloidal bath additive. If the sunburn involves a large area, add ½ cup of Aveeno bath treatment, made from oatmeal, to a tub of cool water, says Dr Schreiber. Soak for 15 to 20 minutes.

Go easy on the soap. Soap can dry and irritate burned skin. If you must use soap, says pharmacologist Thomas Gossel, use a mild brand and rinse it off very well. Do not soak in soapy water and avoid bubble baths.

WHEN TO CONSULT A DOCTOR

Consult a doctor if you experience nausea, chills, fever, faintness, extensive blistering, general weakness, patches of purple discoloration or intense itching. If the burn seems to be spreading, you could have an infection compounding the problem. Your risk of skin cancer is thought to relate not only to total exposure to the sun's UV rays, but also to episodes of sunburn, especially in childhood. Skin cancer itself rarely occurs before adulthood, though. See your doctor if you have:

• new moles;

• a change in existing moles: lumpy texture, pain, itchiness, scabs, crusts, bleeding, change in colour (getting darker or lighter), a halo of lighter pigment around a mole, smaller satellite moles developing around a mole;

• any sores or scabs that are non-healing or reoccurring, especially on the face, ears, lips, nose and hands;

• a scar-like area whose origin is a mystery. Skin cancer can occasionally present in this way;

• any change in skin texture or appearance. Be on the lookout for rough or scaly patches, lumps and bumps and discoloured skin. This will probably turn out to be something entirely innocent, but it's best to be sure.

Moisturize your skin. Soaks and compresses feel good and give temporary relief, says dermatologist Rodney Basler. But they can make your skin feel drier than before if you don't apply moisturizer immediately af-

Are you sensitive to sunlight?

Some drugs increase your sensitivity to the sun (photosensitivity) and can lead to a burn-like dermatitis. Antibiotics, tranquillizers and antifungal medications can all cause reactions. So can some oral contraceptives, diuretics, drugs for diabetes and even PABA-containing sunscreens. Ask your doctor about potential side-effects of any drugs you may be taking.

terwards. Pat yourself dry, then smooth on some bath oil. Let it soak in for a minute, then apply a moisturizing cream or lotion, such as Eucerin.

Chill it. For added relief, try chilling your moisturizer before applying it.

Seek hydrocortisone relief. Soothe skin irritation and inflammation with a topical cream or ointment containing one per cent hydrocortisone, such as HC45 cream and Eurax HC cream.

Use aloe vera juice. Research shows that aloe vera really helps wound healing, says Dr Basler. Although gels and lotions are available, juice straight from the plant, which can easily be grown on a sunny windowsill, is more effective, Simply break a leaf off the plant, cut it lengthwise, and apply the juice.

Note: Test a small area of skin first to make sure you're not allergic to aloe.

Try an ice pack. An ice pack can also provide relief if the burn is mild. Wrap it in a damp cloth and hold it over the sunburn.

Improvise, if necessary, says Dr Haberman. You could use a bag of frozen peas, for instance. But wrap it up first rather than putting the icy package straight onto bare skin.

Drink up. It's a good idea to drink lots of water to help counteract the

KITCHEN CURES

Common foods can be great sunburn soothers. Try any of the following.

Oatmeal. Wrap dry oatmeal in a piece of muslin. Run cool water through it into a bowl. Discard the oatmeal and soak flannels in the liquid. Apply every two to four hours.

Skimmed milk. Mix 250ml skimmed milk with a litre of water and add a few ice cubes. Soak flannels in the liquid and apply for 15 to 20 minutes every two to four hours.

Cornflour. Add enough water to cornflour to make a paste and apply to the sunburn.

Lettuce. Boil lettuce leaves in water. Strain, and cool the liquid for several hours in the refrigerator. Dip cotton wool balls into the liquid and gently pat or stroke irritated skin.

Yoghurt. Apply natural yoghurt to all sunburnt areas. Rinse off in a cool shower and gently pat dry.

Tea bags. If your eyelids are burnt, apply tea bags soaked in cool water to decrease swelling and relieve pain. Tea contains tannic acid, which seems to ease sunburn pain.

Do just *one* thing

Take ibuprofen or another anti-inflammatory. This will help to relieve the pain, itching and swelling of a mild to moderate burn. Take up to 400mg of ibuprofen three times a day.

If you know you've had too much sun, try taking ibuprofen *before* the redness appears.

drying effects of sunburn, says Dr Gossel.

And eat properly. Eat light, nutritious meals. A balanced diet will help to provide the nutrients your skin needs to regenerate itself.

Get a good night's sleep. Sleeping on sunburnt skin can be difficult, but your body needs rest in order to recover from the burn. Try sprinkling talcum powder on the sheets to minimize friction, says Dr Haberman.

Put your feet up. If your legs are burned and your feet are swollen, raise your legs above heart level to help stop the swelling, says Dr Basler.

Be careful with blisters. If blisters develop, you have a pretty bad burn. If they bother you and they cover only a small area, you may carefully drain them, says Dr Basler. But do not peel the top skin off – you'll have less discomfort and danger of infection if sensitive nerve endings are not exposed to air. To drain the fluid, first sterilize a needle by holding it over a flame. Then puncture the edge of the blister and press gently on the top to let the fluid out. Do this three times in the first 24 hours, then leave the blisters alone.

Don't make the same mistake again. After you've been burnt, it takes three to six months for your skin to return to normal, says Dr Schreiber. When you burn and the top layer of skin peels off, the newly exposed skin is more sensitive than ever. That means you'll burn even faster than you did before.

Follow the rules. While the memory of your burn is still painfully fresh, brush up on your sun sense with these tips from dermatologist Norman Levine.

• Apply a sunscreen about 30 minutes before going out, even if it's overcast. (Harmful rays can penetrate cloud cover.) Don't forget to protect your lips, hands, ears and the back of your neck. Reapply often, especially after swimming or if you are sweating.

• Use a sunscreen with a sun protection factor (SPF) between 15 and 30. Sunscreens with SPF 15 protect against 94 per cent of the sun's harmful rays, and those with SPF 30 protect against 97 per cent. Also, look for the ingredients zinc oxide, titanium dioxide or avobenzone in your sunscreen. These block both ultraviolet A and B rays.

- In hotter climates, take extra care between 11am and 4pm when the sun is at its strongest.

- Wear protective clothing when you are not swimming. Broad-brimmed hats, tightly-woven fabrics and long sleeves will help to keep the sun off your skin.

TEETHING

8 ways to help your baby

An infant's teeth start developing months before birth – in fact, tooth buds actually begin appearing by the seventh week of pregnancy. By the time a baby is born, all 20 of the primary teeth that will sprout over the next two-and-a-half years are present in the jawbone.

Usually those first teeth start pushing through from six to eight months after birth, but babies can occasionally be born with visible teeth (in the Middle Ages, it was thought these babies were witches – teeth visible at birth are still sometimes called witches' teeth). At the other end of the scale, some babies don't start teething for a year. The timing is of no significance whatsoever, except sometimes to a mother if she's breastfeeding a baby with teeth (maybe that's where the term 'nippers' comes from?).

Babies react to this new sensation of teething in a variety of different ways. Some babies sail through the teething process with minimal disruption. But for others, the gums become red and sore, and the baby may be much more fretful than normal; one cheek may be more flushed than the other. They often produce a lot of dribble and want to gnaw on anything available – toys, the teats of their bottles, or even your nipples. Dribbling and putting everything in the mouth is normal behaviour for babies from about four months, though, so even this is by no means a cast iron sign that teeth are about to follow.

Be sure to check with your doctor or health visitor if you are worried about your baby – don't dismiss a raised temperature, a bout of diarrhoea or an unusual amount of crying as 'teething'. Teething doesn't make a baby ill. As late as Victorian times, teething was blamed for all sorts of things and was even entered on certificates and church registers as a cause of death. 'Utter nonsense,' says family doctor Stephen Amiel. 'Teething causes teeth, and that's pretty much it.'

If teething is worrying you and your baby, there are ways to ease your anxiety and your baby's discomfort.

Cool baby's gums. 'Chewing on teething rings, particularly those you can put in the refrigerator and keep cold, works very well and feels good on the baby's gums,' says paediatric nurse practitioner Linda Jonides. 'For a baby of six months or older, even a clean, cold flannel to chew on feels good.'

Note: Don't buy a teething ring with anything other than water inside – if it were to crack, the liquid inside might not be safe. And never tie a teething ring around a baby's neck: it could strangle him.

Give lots of love. Give your baby extra cuddles and comfort – anything to help relieve the misery.

Wipe up dribbles. Teething can cause a baby to dribble, a lot. Use a warm flannel often to wipe the dribble off your baby's face to prevent a rash from developing.

Clean the gums. Dentists and paediatricians advise cleaning your baby's mouth before the teeth appear. Use a lightly moistened, small gauze pad or even a soft baby flannel wrapped around your forefinger to massage the gums.

Doing so removes bacteria build-up and gets the baby used to having someone poking around inside her mouth. 'Then, when that first tooth does come in, you can start brushing it right away without any trouble,' says dentist John Bogert. Also, a daily massage makes for much healthier gum tissue.

WHEN TO CONSULT A DOCTOR

Lots of things are blamed on teething – rashes, crying, bad temper, runny noses, more dirty nappies than normal and nappy rash. But none of these signs can be proved to have been caused by teething. And there could be any number of other things happening that might be influencing your baby's behaviour and wellbeing: you may have gone back to work and your baby is exposed to new germs at a nursery, perhaps, or he is beginning to sample an increasingly wide range of foods. It's important not to use teething to explain away what might be the signs of an illness or allergy. If you are at all worried, see your doctor or health visitor.

'We actually recommend you start doing this just days after birth,' Dr Bogert says. 'But you're probably not too late if you begin today. A couple of times a day is good – especially at bedtime.'

When you do start brushing your baby's little teeth, make sure you buy a soft baby toothbrush, and be very gentle.

Give painkillers. 'I recommend using one of the medicines most parents keep handy for baby's pain,' says Dr Bogert. Usually, that's infant paracetamol (like Calpol). The easiest way to give it is using a medicine syringe. Aim the nozzle between the baby's cheek and gums and gently squeeze – don't point it down his throat, or it could make him gag or choke.

Use a teething gel. A number of topical anaesthetics, such as Calgel, are available over the counter at any pharmacy and may do some good in relieving teething pain. Just wipe some on the gums for quick relief.

Avoid gels and other teething medications that contain alcohol, says Dr Amiel. These can sting sore gums and alcohol isn't exactly the ideal sedative to introduce to six-month-old baby.

Keep down sugar intake. As soon as you start your baby on solids, try to encourage a liking for savoury rather than sweet tastes. Limit sugary foods or drinks to mealtimes only. Use her bottle only for water or plain milk – juices should be diluted and offered in a cup. And limit fruit juices as they contain sugar and are acidic, which means that they cause decay and erosion that will, literally, dissolve the teeth. Finally never let your child fall asleep with a bottle in her mouth. The milk will collect around the teeth and begin the process of tooth decay.

KITCHEN CURES

Instead of a standard teething ring, try giving your baby some frozen grapes or bananas in a US-designed product called the Baby Safe Feeder. Designed to stop early eaters from choking on chunks of pear or cucumber, the feeder looks like a dummy but with a small mesh bag (instead of a teat) that can hold a piece of food for your baby to suck or chew. Just a little frozen fruit will give your baby an incentive to bite down and work those teeth through the gums. The replaceable mesh bag needs to be cleaned thoroughly and checked for wear between each use. The feeder is available online from Amazon.com.

TENDINITIS
14 helpful remedies

Like simple muscle soreness from overuse, tendinitisor or tenosynovitis – inflammation in or around a tendon – can be painful. But where simple muscle soreness is temporary, tendinitis is tenacious. It's soreness that doesn't go away with a few hours' rest and an ice pack.

If you continue to use the tendon in the same repetitive motion that triggered the problem in the first place, it's going to be very difficult to heal. That applies to everyone from marathon runners and window cleaners to violinists and keyboard operators.

Work-related upper limb injury (the term now preferred for repetitive strain injury (RSI)) is rightly commanding the attention of occupational health specialists and, in some cases, the courts. In repetitive strain injury, tendinitis commonly affects the hand, wrist, elbows and shoulders, although it may occur in any joint in the body.

With work-related problems, your employer will have certain responsibilities with regard to chair and workstation design, for example, and the provision of frequent short breaks. You may need to take these issues up with your manager, your occupational or HR department, or your trade union. Here are some ways you can lessen the effects of tendinitis and prevent intense flare-ups, but this may mean changing some entrenched habits.

Give it a rest. 'That's a hard thing to get people to do,' says sports physio Bob Mangine. But a runner with Achilles tendinitis, for example, can't realistically expect any improvement if he doesn't take a few days' break.

Of course, resting is easier said than done if the activity triggering your tendinitis is part of your job. If you have occupational tendinitis, it might be a good idea to save a day or two's holiday for times when tendinitis is painfully persistent.

But don't rest for too long. 'Muscles will start to atrophy,' says Mangine. 'For athletes, we never recommend absolute rest,' adds Ted Percy, an orthopaedic surgeon who specializes in sports injuries. The key is to cross-train when possible. Choose an activity that doesn't reproduce the pain, so you can avoid a prolonged rest period and maintain your stamina.

Make a change. If your tendinitis is exercise-induced, a new form of exercise may be just what your inflamed tendon needs. If you're a runner with tendon problems in your lower legs, for example, you can stay on the road if you're willing to hop on a bicycle, which will still give you a good upper-leg workout.

Have a soak. Soaking in warm bathwater is a good way to raise body temperature and increase bloodflow. Warming the tendon before stressful activity decreases the soreness associated with tendinitis, says Mangine.

Use a warm compress. Put a warm, damp towel over the tender tendon, then a plastic bag, then a heating pad, and lastly, a loose elastic bandage to hold everything in place. Keep it on from two to six hours. Keep the heating pad on low so you don't burn yourself, advises athletics trainer Bob Reese. For maximum effect, keep the injured part at a level higher than your heart.

Warm with stretching. The heat treatments above are only the first part of a warm-up. You should always stretch before exercising at full speed, says physiotherapist Terry Malone. Stretching prevents the shortening of muscles and tendons that comes with exercise.

Also, some studies suggest that people who are less flexible are more prone to develop tendinitis, says Mangine. So stretching should be a regular part of your routine. As you get older, your tendons and muscles gradually lose their elasticity, so going into strenuous exercise without warming up and stretching can cause inflammation, pain and even rupture of tendons.

Get braced for action. Even a little extra support and warmth from a flexible support can help during exercise and afterwards, Mangine says. 'There is no truth to the old wives' tale that wearing a support will weaken the tendons and muscles, provided you continue exercising.'

Use ice. After exercising, ice is great for keeping down both swelling and pain, says Mangine (for more information on applying ice, see *Sprains*, page 515).

Note: People with heart disease, diabetes or impaired circulation should be careful about using ice because cold constricts blood vessels and could cause serious problems.

Wrap it up. Another way to reduce swelling is to wrap your pain in a stretchy crepe bandage, says Dr Percy. Just be careful not to wrap the inflamed area too tightly or to leave the area wrapped for so long that it becomes uncomfortable or interferes with circulation. (For more information on bandaging, see *Sprains*, page 515).

WHEN TO CONSULT A DOCTOR

If you only feel the pain of tendinitis during or after exercise, and if it isn't too bad, you may think that you can play through your pain. But this is not a good idea. If pain is severe and you continue to abuse the tendon, it may rupture. That could mean a long lay-off, surgery or even permanent disability.

So exercising through tendon pain today could mean standing on the touchline for the rest of your life. To be on the safe side, stop doing whatever is causing the pain, and see a doctor if the pain is persistent.

Your doctor may be able to prescribe anti-inflammatories, rule out any underlying illness, and arrange for you to have further treatment if necessary. This may include physiotherapy, a cortisone injection into an inflamed tendon sheath or, occasionally, surgery if a tendon is torn or calcified.

Put it up. Raising the painful area above heart level is good for controlling swelling.

Wear a higher heel. For Achilles tendinitis, wearing boots or shoes with a heel some of the time is a good idea, according to Dr Percy. 'It lifts the heel off the ground,' he says, 'and the muscles and tendons don't have to work as hard.'

Take an anti-inflammatory. Aspirin and ibuprofen are effective temporary painkillers for tendinitis, Dr Percy says. They also reduce inflammation and swelling. Do not use aspirin if you're under 16.

Strengthen your body. We're not suggesting you become Mr Universe, says Mangine, just to get better defined muscles by working out at home with light weights. All tissues develop simultaneously, so working out will train muscles, tendons and ligaments. You don't even need a set of weights – just fill a sock with pennies to work your arm muscles.

Take breaks. This is a simple way to at least temporarily relieve physical stress at work, says chiropractor Scott Donkin. 'If you work in an awkward position, tendinitis can develop quite easily, especially in the arms or wrists if you're working at a keyboard or typewriter all day.'

TINNITUS
21 ways to cope with the noise

The noise of the modern world is bad enough, but people with tinnitus have the added burden of hearing sounds in their own heads. This irritating condition causes people to hear clicking, roaring, ringing or buzzing sounds when no external sounds actually exist.

Doctors and audiologists think that tinnitus is caused by damage to the microscopic hairs on auditory cells in the inner ear. Persistent exposure to earsplitting music or other loud sounds is the main cause of tinnitus. It has also been linked to hearing loss, circulatory problems and middle-ear problems. Tinnitus is often accompanied by an intense sensitivity to sounds called hyperacusis.

There is a wide misconception that tinnitus is confined to elderly people, but studies have shown that it can occur at any age, even in young children. Mild tinnitus is common – about 10 per cent of the UK population has it all the time and, according to the British Tinnitus Association, the condition has a detrimental effect on the quality of life of one adult in every hundred. The main treatment approach is to help people to cope with the persistent noise – and to prevent it from getting any worse. Here's what doctors advise.

Avoid loud noises. Chain saws, power motors and the ear-pounding volume of club dance music and rock are just a few of the things that can damage auditory cells and make tinnitus worse.

'If you're two metres away from someone and have to raise your voice to make yourself heard, the environmental noise is probably too loud,' says ear, nose and throat surgeon Douglas Mattox.

Turn down the volume. Millions of young people now seem to club wherever they go – the explosion of personal stereo systems and huge in-car speaker systems is risking a generational epidemic of premature deafness and tinnitus, says family doctor Stephen Amiel. 'I've been at traffic lights, and my car actually shakes with the noise coming from the car behind me. I shudder – sometimes literally – at the thought of what that kind of noise is doing to their ears.' Personal stereos, with in-ear headphones, can do just as much damage. 'Turning down the volume will save your ears, as well as the sanity of all the middle-aged fuddy-duddies (like me!) around you.'

Buy some earplugs. When you know you're going to be exposed to ear-splitting sounds – from a building site next door, for example – buy some earplugs. Pharmacy earplugs work fine, but you'll do better with the type sold in music stores: they let you hear music or voices clearly, but at a greatly reduced volume, says auditory researcher Marshall Chasin.

'The earplugs you buy over the counter never fit very well,' adds Chasin. 'Custom-made earplugs, which are fitted to your ear, are a lot better. They fit like a good pair of shoes – you probably won't even be aware of them.' Different types are available, according to your needs: musicians, gun enthusiasts, pilots, and snorers' partners may all need slightly different types. Customized earplugs are available at some hearing aid shops, or look online for suppliers.

Or wear ear defenders. If you don't like the sensation of earplugs, go to a builder's merchants or DIY store and buy some foam-filled safety muffs, which look like headphones and form a tight seal over the ears. 'They can make you feel hot and sweaty, but they're very effective,' says Dr Mattox. You probably wouldn't wear these in public – to a Robbie Williams concert, say – but they may come in handy when using your hammer drill to put up shelves. If your occupation involves regular use of power tools or heavy machinery, your employer should provide you with ear defenders, but it's up to you to wear them.

Hum away noise. One of the first lessons drummers learn is that humming for a few seconds during the loudest part of the song helps to drown out the crashing sounds of cymbals. You can use the same technique whenever you're anticipating a loud noise – when you're walking past an idling bus, for example, or when you're using power tools at home.

Humming activates a muscle in the inner ear, which pulls tiny bones together and prevents some sound waves from getting through, says Chasin. 'In evolutionary terms, the muscle may prevent our own voices from sounding too loud,' he explains. This protects you from tinnitus, because prolonged exposure to loud noises can cause tinnitus.

Let your hair grow. 'If your hair is reasonably thick, wearing it over the ears will provide three or four decibels of protection,' Chasin says. 'That may not sound like much, but reducing sound by three decibels essentially means that you can be exposed to a sound for twice as long before any damage occurs.' This could help stop your tinnitus from getting worse, and may have saved many a rock musician from even worse problems.

Give your ears a rest. A single loud noise could potentially result in tinnitus, but persistent loud noises are more likely to be a problem. It's important to let the ears 'rest' for about 16 hours after exposure to loud sounds. If you've spent the morning hoovering, for example, don't fire up the strimmer that afternoon, says Chasin.

Use a hearing aid if necessary. About 90 per cent of people with severe tinnitus also have hearing loss. Using a hearing aid often helps both problems at the same time.

'As long as the auditory pathway is occupied by outside sounds, you'll be less likely to hear the tinnitus,' explains Dhyan Cassie, a doctor of audiology. Speak to your doctor about a referral.

Sleep with white noise. The sounds of tinnitus aren't really louder at night, but they often seem as though they are because of the relative silence of the surroundings. Creating a little background noise – the static of a radio set between stations or the whirr of a small fan, for example – helps to mask the sounds of tinnitus and makes it easier to rest, says Dr Cassie.

Wear a sound generator. Available from audiologists, sound generators are hearing-aid-like devices that fill the ears with a soft white noise. 'As long as the auditory pathways are occupied, your brain can't concentrate on the sound of tinnitus, and it will eventually learn to ignore it,' explains Dr Cassie.

Try 'tinnitus retraining'. Studies have shown that when people subject themselves to a quiet sound – static or white noise from a sound generator that's just loud enough to mask the tinnitus sounds – the internal noise may diminish or even disappear. 'Over a period of months, you'll find that the volume of sound needed to mask the tinnitus keeps getting lower,' Chasin says.

Watch what you eat. Red wine, chocolate, pickled and other processed foods that contain chemicals called sulphides may increase tinnitus in some people, says Chasin.

Eat less salt. Tinnitus is sometimes caused by Ménière's disease, a condition that results in excessive amounts of fluid in the ear, and also causes deafness and vertigo. People with Ménière's should limit their use of salt and buy packaged products labelled 'low-salt'. A diagnosis of Ménière's disease should be made by your doctor or specialist.

Cut back on caffeine. If you drink a lot of coffee, tea or cola, you might experience higher levels of tinnitus. That's because caffeine constricts blood vessels and temporarily raises blood pressure, which can make the sounds of tinnitus louder. Giving up caffeine isn't likely to eliminate the problem, but it might make a small difference, says Dr Mattox.

Don't smoke. The nicotine in cigarettes and cigars has the same effect

Do just *one* thing

Distract yourself. It can be hard to ignore the sounds of tinnitus but it's worth making the effort. The more you focus on the sounds, the more likely it is your brain will build additional neural pathways to make your listening more efficient. In other words, you may wind up hearing the annoying sounds even more, says ear, nose and throat surgeon Douglas Mattox.

'The most important thing is to keep the auditory system busy doing other things,' Dr Mattox advises. 'When you're working or doing other quiet activities, create a little ambient noise, like the sound of a small water fountain or an inexpensive noise generator.' An even easier solution is to turn on the radio. Just keep the volume down. You don't necessarily want sounds that you'll pay attention to or find distracting.

as caffeine: it constricts blood vessels and may make tinnitus sounds more noticeable.

Check your medication. Certain drugs can cause tinnitus, including aspirin, some diuretics, and antibiotics like gentamicin. Don't stop prescription drugs without consulting your doctor first.

See your dentist. Tinnitus may sometimes be caused by problems with your temporo-mandibular joints (TMJs) (see *Jaw Pain and TMJ Problems*, page 364). See your dentist or doctor if you think your TMJs are responsible and you've tried our home remedies for TMJ problems without success.

Reduce the noise with baby oil. Build-ups of earwax can impair hearing and potentially make the sounds of tinnitus louder. One solution is to apply a few drops of baby oil with an eyedropper once or twice a day for several days. Once the wax softens, gently flush the ear canal with warm water, using a bulb syringe. Repeating this several times removes excessive wax from the ear canal (see *Earwax*, page 413). Sodium bicarbonate ear drops, available from your pharmacist, are a good alternative.

Note: Check with your doctor before attempting to flush your ear canal. There could be a ruptured eardrum behind the wax.

Practise stress control. 'When people are under stress, they feel it in the weakest part of the body,' says Dr Cassie. 'If you already have tinnitus, high levels of stress are likely to make the sounds seem even louder.'

There are several ways to control stress (see *Stress*, page 518). Some people exercise; others meditate, do yoga or spend an afternoon at the cinema.

WHEN TO CONSULT A DOCTOR

Tinnitus is rarely an indication of a serious disorder, but it is a good idea to see your doctor if you think you might have it. You may have wax in your ears, anaemia, high blood pressure, impacted wisdom teeth, Ménière's disease or (very occasionally) a treatable tumour of the auditory nerve. Persistent tinnitus following a head injury or noise injury should also be checked out. Even if there is no obvious cause for your tinnitus, a referral to a tinnitus specialist may give you access to hearing therapy, where you can be given advice and support, cognitive behavioural therapy (CBT) to help you deal with your tinnitus, or masking aids. Medication may sometimes help if you have Ménière's disease, although on the whole drugs are disappointing in the treatment of tinnitus.

Learn more. You will probably feel better when you find out more about the condition – that it's very common and you're not alone, says the British Tinnitus Association. If you would like to talk to someone about any problems you have, the association can put you in touch with a support group near you. Many of the groups are run by people who have tinnitus and who can share their experiences with you. Contact the British Tinnitus Association, Ground Floor, Unit 5, Acorn Business Park, Woodseats Close, Sheffield S8 0TB; or tel: Freephone 0800 018 0527; or visit the charity's website at www.tinnitus.org.uk.

TOOTH STAINS
10 brightening ideas

Coffee, tea, colas, smoke, acidic juices, certain medicines and highly pigmented foods can take their dingy toll on tooth enamel. Not that teeth were ever meant to be totally white. The natural colour of teeth is actually pale yellow to pale yellowy red, says dentist Roger Levin. But as you age, your teeth tend to darken.

Over time, surface enamel cracks and erodes, exposing dentine. This is the less dense interior of the tooth, which absorbs colour from food. Stains also latch onto plaque and tartar that build up on and between our teeth. Many things can stain teeth, says cosmetic dentist Ronald Maitland, including antibiotics, quirks in individual metabolism and even a high fever. The yellower your tooth stains, the easier it will be to remove them. Deep brown stains, such as those brought on by long-term use of the antibiotic tetracycline, can be very difficult to erase.

But many common stains – the coffee and cigarette variety – can often be washed away between visits to the dental hygienist.

Brush after every meal. If you clean your teeth regularly and conscientiously, stains are less likely to remain on your teeth, says Dr Levin.

Scrub gently. Just as abrasive products can scrub away enamel work surfaces, over-aggressive brushing can rub off tooth enamel, exposing the deeper-coloured dentine, which could make your teeth look even duller.

Polish with baking soda. Mix baking soda with just enough hydrogen peroxide mouthwash (available from pharmacies) to make a mixture the consistency of toothpaste, says Dr Levin, then brush stains away. Follow with a rinse using hydrogen peroxide mouthwash, which you should dilute according to instructions on the label.

Use a discloser. Rinse your mouth out with a disclosing solution from your dentist. The coloured areas show where plaque still clings to your teeth after brushing. These spots are where your teeth will stain if you don't improve your brushing technique, says John Featherstone, an expert in preventative dentistry.

Rinse often. After every meal, rinse the food from your teeth, says Dr Maitland. If you can't get to a bathroom, take a swig from your water glass, rinse and swallow at the table.

Switch to an electric toothbrush. They seem to be better at motivating reluctant brushers to clean their teeth more often than manual toothbrushes. But when it comes to plaque removal, this depends more on the quality of your brushing than the type of toothbrush you use.

Choose an antibacterial mouthwash. All mouthwashes are fine for rinsing, but mouthwashes that have an antibacterial action, such as Corsodyl or Chlorohex, will reduce stain-catching plaque, says Dr Featherstone.

Use a whitening toothpaste or tooth polish. Dentists used to warn patients away from over-the-counter whitening products because they contained gritty abrasives that could erode the tooth enamel. But manufacturers have got better at using peroxide instead of abrasives to give you a slightly brighter after-brushing effect, says dentist Dean Lodding. But don't expect miracles. The peroxides in toothpastes or polishes only stay on the tooth surface for a brief period, so you'll only get a bit of lightening.

Try a whitening system. Pharmacies sell a product called Brilliant Tooth Whitening system, in which a gel is applied to the teeth using a gum shield left in place for five to ten minutes. This keeps the bleaching agent on the teeth a bit longer than a tooth polish, so may get them a bit whiter. Regular use could lighten your teeth by two to three shades, compared to the eight to ten shades of lightening you can get from a cosmetic dental lightening treatment.

Do it all in one visit. If you're impatient, your dentist can bleach your teeth at the surgery by using a concentrated carbamide peroxide solution and a special light that 'powers the material into the dentine,' says Dr Lodding. This treatment is not available on the NHS.

TOOTHACHE
13 tips to relieve the pain

Toothache can be excruciatingly painful, so it's hardly surprising that dentistry was one of the earliest medical disciplines practised. The Ancient Egyptians used some bizarre methods to ward off tooth pain, such as placing a live mouse on the gums of a person with toothache. They believed that, because mice have such strong teeth, some of the effect might rub off on the sufferer. In Ancient Rome, things were little better. One historian noted that a frog tied to the jaws made teeth firmer, and that toothache responded to ear drops made by boiling earthworms in olive oil. We have excluded all mention of rodents, amphibians or worms in the following tips; instead, we've taken some sound advice on toothache from modern dentists.

Rinse. Take a mouthful of tepid water and rinse vigorously, says dentist Jerry Taintor. If the toothache is caused by trapped food, a thorough rinse may dislodge the problem.

Floss gently. If swishing doesn't work, try to prise a small bit of food like a blackberry seed or corn husk from between your teeth by flossing, says Dr Taintor. Be gentle, as your gums are likely to be sore.

Numb it with alcohol. Hold a swig of whisky over the painful tooth, says dentist Philip Corn. Your gums will absorb some of the alcohol, and that will numb the pain.

Rinse with salty water. After each meal and at bedtime, stir a teaspoon of salt into a 250ml glass of tepid water, says Dr Corn. Hold it in your mouth, rinse it around and spit.

Try an ice massage. Wrap a teatowel or handkerchief around an ice cube and rub it into the V-shaped area where the bones of the thumb and forefinger meet. Gently hold the ice on the area for five to seven minutes. Amazingly, this technique can ease toothache pain.

Use oil of cloves. People have been using this remedy for centuries, says dentist Richard Shepard. Drop a little oil directly onto the tooth, or put a little on a cotton wool ball and pack it next to the problem tooth.

Don't bite. If the toothache is caused by an injury to the tooth, try not to use that area when you eat, says Dr Corn. If nothing is damaged, resting the tooth may ease the ache.

Ice it. Treat your tooth as you would treat a bruise with ice, says Dr Corn. Put some ice in a small plastic bag, wrap it in a thin cloth and put it on the adjacent cheek for 15 minutes at a time, three or four times a day.

Be kind to sensitive teeth

If you can't even touch your tooth, you have toothache. But if the tooth is merely reacting to heat or cold, then it's a problem with sensitivity.

Tooth sensitivity affects around 20 per cent of the UK population and is due to the exposure of dentine on the root surface of the tooth below the gum line. Age, receding gums and overzealous brushing can expose dentine. Sometimes, plaque attacks the tooth enamel and exposes the dentine.

Choose a toothpaste designed for people with sensitive teeth, and apply it with soft toothbrush.

If you are aware of sensitivity for the first time, it's a good idea to see your dentist to make sure you have no other problem.

WHEN TO CONSULT A DOCTOR

Toothache can be a symptom of a wide range of problems. The pulpy core of your tooth, or the gum around it, could be infected. A tooth may be cracked or decaying.

An injury, a piece of food caught between two teeth or even a sinus problem may be at the root of your pain. Whatever the cause, if you have toothache, it's important to find out why. See a dentist whenever you have tooth pain, even if the pain subsides.

Soothe and heal with echinacea. It's hard to concentrate on anything when a tooth is throbbing, says clinical herbalist Douglas Schar. But help is at hand: echinacea is one of the best remedies for toothache. It stimulates the immune system to clear the infection at the root of the toothache, and it has a deadening effect on the pain.

Buy echinacea root tincture (1:5) from a health food store. Put a teaspoonful into your mouth and rinse it around the problem tooth. Then swallow. Repeat this procedure four times a day. The effect is often described as miraculous – though it will take a day to begin working.

Keep your mouth shut. If cold air moving across the tooth hurts, just shut off the flow, says dentist Roger Levin. But don't clench your teeth. Some toothaches arise when the bite isn't quite right. If that is the case, try and avoid shutting your mouth as much as possible until the dentist can take a look.

Swallow painkillers. Don't believe the old-fashioned remedy that advises putting an aspirin directly on the aching gum. This can cause an aspirin burn, says Dr Taintor. For pain relief, take paracetamol or ibuprofen every four hours as needed.

Note: Don't give aspirin to children under 16.

Avoid heat. Keep heat away from your aching cheek even if it makes the toothache feel better, warns Dr Corn. 'If it's an infection, the heat will draw the infection to the outside of the jaw and make the infection worse.'

Urinary Tract Infections (Cystitis)

21 germ-fighting strategies

Urinary tract infections (UTIs) are easy to treat, but that's no comfort when you're running to the loo every 15 minutes to pee – and experiencing burning, excruciating pain.

Most urinary tract infections, commonly known as cystitis, occur when bacteria from the bowel enter the urethra, the tube that carries urine from the bladder out of the body. Sex is a common cause of infection because intercourse can 'massage' external bacteria into the urethra. Cystitis is also more common after menopause, when falling oestrogen levels make tissues in the vagina and urethra drier and, therefore, more vulnerable to bacteria.

Pregnancy is another risky time for cystitis – the enlarged uterus can partially obstruct urine outflow and pregnancy hormones relax the smooth muscle of the urinary tract, making backflow and stagnation of urine more likely.

One in five women will get a urinary tract infection – in the urethra, bladder or kidneys – at some point in her life. Some women get them over and over again. Men are much less likely to suffer because their extra inches of anatomy make it harder for bacteria to get inside. UTIs in men often indicate some blockage in the urinary tract, such as an enlarged prostate or a stone, allowing urine to stagnate and become infected. Children can also get UTIs, sometimes as a result of structural problems in their urinary tract allowing reflux of urine back up towards the kidneys when the bladder contracts.

The symptoms of classic cystitis are: pain in the lower abdomen, worse on urinating; frequency; stinging or pain on urination (sometimes likened to passing ground glass); difficulty in starting to urinate; urgency or incontinence; and cloudy, offensive-smelling or bloody urine. If the infection involves the kidneys more, you may have pain in the loins (the area on either side of your back just below your ribs); high fever; shivering attacks (rigors); nausea and vomiting. Sometimes though, particularly in older people and babies, there may be no specific symptoms. Babies may go off their feeds, have vomiting or diarrhoea, or fail to gain weight. Older people may just feel off-colour or perhaps become confused.

Antibiotics are usually recommended to clear up urinary tract infections, and usually relieve the discomfort within a day or two. In the meantime, here are a few steps that will reduce pain and help to prevent the infection from coming back.

Drink lots of water. This is the traditional advice most doctors give, although it has to be said that there is no evidence to prove it makes a difference when you have cystitis. The theory goes that the more you drink, the more you urinate – and frequent urination helps to flush harmful bacteria from the bladder. 'If you keep filling your bladder and flushing it out, you will reduce the numbers of bacteria,' says family planning doctor Diana Koster. Water also dilutes the concentrated salts in urine, which can reduce discomfort when you have an infection.

Drinking lots will mean more uncomfortable trips to the toilet perhaps, but otherwise it can do no harm and, unless and until the evidence becomes conclusive, it's probably still worth a try. Aim for at least eight to twelve 250ml glasses of water a day.

Don't hold back. Drinking lots doesn't give you much choice, but people with cystitis will sometimes delay going to the loo for as long as they can to avoid the pain. This will only make things worse when you do finally go and may even stop you being able to pee at all. You should drink lots and pee often to prevent cystitis too. Young girls in particular need to be encouraged to overcome their reluctance to use school toilets – a common contributory cause of UTIs in school-age girls.

Fight bacteria with baking soda. At the first sign of cystitis, drink a solution made from ¼ teaspoon of baking soda mixed in 250ml of water. Do this once a day until you can get to your doctor for antibiotics. Baking soda makes the bladder environment more alkaline, which inhibits the ability of bacteria to multiply, says urologist Larrian Gillespie.

Drink Evian water. It contains the same bicarbonate as baking soda but without the extra sodium, says Dr Gillespie. It neutralizes acid in the bladder and helps to reduce painful nerve irritation.

Dilute the burning. The concentrated salts in urine can cause stinging pain when you have cystitis. You can reduce discomfort by pouring warm water over yourself as you pee, says Dr Koster. Or try sitting in a warm bath and allowing yourself to urinate in the water.

Relax with a heating pad. Applying heat to the abdomen is a great way to reduce cramps or painful pressure that sometimes accompanies urinary tract infections, says Dr Gillespie. If you don't have a heating pad, a hot-water bottle or flannel soaked in hot water works just as well.

Avoid orange juice. Along with strawberries, grapefruit and pineapple, orange juice has a high acid content. When you have cystitis, it will increase the burning when you pass water, says Dr Gillespie.

WHEN TO CONSULT A DOCTOR

Urinary tract infections respond very quickly to antibiotics, so see your doctor at the first sign of symptoms. For most adult women, a three-day course or even a single dose will be sufficient, although longer courses are usually given to older people, men and children. It's especially important to get a prescription if you're experiencing a fever, loin pains, chills or nausea, along with the usual sensations of burning or urgency. These symptoms may mean you have pyelonephritis, where the kidneys are more seriously affected.

If you have frequent bouts of cystitis, you're male or you have a baby or small child with a UTI, further investigation by a specialist will be required. Sometimes, you might be given a low dose of antibiotics to take continuously or after every time you have sex.

If you pass blood in your urine, especially if there is no pain when you urinate, see your doctor as soon as possible: painless haematuria as it's called may be a sign of a tumour somewhere in the urinary tract.

Don't drink coffee or alcohol. When you have cystitis, coffee and alcohol can make it painful to pee, says Dr Gillespie. Caffeine and alcohol also stimulate the muscular walls of the bladder, which may increase urinary urges and cause further pain.

Take vitamin C for prevention. If you already have a urinary tract infection, don't start taking vitamin C. That would be like trying to put out a fire with petrol, says Dr Gillespie. But to prevent infection, you want urine to be more acidic, which will stop bacteria from adhering to the bladder wall. As a preventative measure, Dr Gillespie suggests taking 1000 to 2000mg of vitamin C a day. 'But if you get a urinary tract infection, stop taking the vitamin.'

Drink cranberry juice. Once you've had cystitis, you'll never want it again. Get a taste for cranberry juice, says Beverly Kloeppel, who runs a student health centre. It's a traditional remedy for preventing urinary tract infections, and scientific research suggests it works. Cranberry juice seems to help prevent the culprit bacterium *E. coli* from sticking to the walls of the urinary tract. If you get frequent urinary tract infections, drink one glass of cranberry juice a day for a few months to see if it makes a difference.

Note: Avoid cranberry juice if you have an overactive bladder, because it can irritate the bladder and make it more sensitive.

Eat blueberries. Cranberry juice is well known for its ability to control the bacteria at the root of a urinary tract infection. What is less well known is that the cranberry's tasty relation, the blueberry, has the same effect, says clinical herbalist Douglas Schar. The berries were traditionally used by Native Americans as a treatment for urinary tract infections, and recent research has proven blueberry to be effective at limiting these infections. Treat yourself to bowl of blueberries a day if you have cystitis or you want to prevent it.

Take immune stimulant herbs. 'In my experience, working women seem to be particularly prone to cystitis,' says Schar. 'This seems to be because they become run-down and overtired. Then a urinary tract infection develops, which makes them even more tired, and by the time they've cleared up one infection, another one is setting in.' The solution, says Schar, is to use a herbal immune stimulant like echinacea, maitake or astragalus, to boost resistance to infection. Take any one of these at the first sign of cystitis to wipe it out before it wipes you out.

Eat more yoghurt. The research isn't conclusive, but there's some evidence that the organisms in live yoghurt, *Lactobacillus acidophilus*, may help to prevent unwanted bacteria from multiplying in the urinary tract and prevent urinary tract infections, says gynaecologist Mary Jane Minkin.

Yoghurt is especially helpful if you're taking antibiotics. While these drugs are very effective at killing harmful bacteria, they also kill 'good' germs, which can lead to urinary tract infections. Eating a cup of live yoghurt daily helps replenish beneficial bacteria while keeping the 'bad' bugs away.

Wash before sex. It's impossible to eliminate infection-causing bacteria from around the anus, but you can prevent them from entering the urinary tract by both partners washing the genital area before having sex, suggests Dr Minkin. This helps to prevent the bacteria from being moved into the vaginal area and urethra.

Urinate before and after sex. It washes out any bacteria that may have entered the urethra during intercourse, says Dr Kloeppel. Ideally, go as soon as you can after sex, and then once more ten minutes or so later: this way, you expel any residual urine in the bladder.

Use a lubricant. If you're experiencing vaginal dryness, it's important to use a water-based lubricant during sex. By decreasing friction, the extra lubrication lessens the possibility of inflammation in the external urethral area, which in turn makes it more difficult for bacteria to cause infection. Menopausal women who get frequent cystitis may be offered an oestrogen cream instead to restore the tissues of the vaginal wall near to which the urethra runs. This cream need only be used two or three times a week.

Change your contraception. Studies have shown that women who use diaphragms and spermicides for birth control have a higher risk of urinary tract infections, probably because using these products can irritate the urethral lining. If you get infections frequently, you may want to talk to your doctor about other forms of birth control.

Use regular tampons. Women tend to get more infections during their periods. This is partly because the warmth and moisture of the blood provides a hospitable environment for germs. Also, super-size tampons can obstruct the bladder and prevent it from emptying completely. It's easier for bacteria to multiply when urine stays in the bladder for a long time, explains Dr Gillespie.

Use pads or regular tampons, and change tampons every time you urinate.

Always wipe backwards. After going to the toilet, wipe from front to back to ensure that anal bacteria don't get pushed forward towards the urethra, says Dr Kloeppel. It's important to teach this to little girls, too, as soon as they begin using the loo on their own.

Don't use 'feminine' products. The chemicals in vaginal deodorant sprays may irritate the tender tissues in the urethra and vagina, making it easier for bacteria to thrive, says Dr Koster.

Similarly, avoid biological detergents for washing your pants, bubble bath, bath salts or Radox, Dettol in the bath and even perfumed soaps if your vaginal area is particularly sensitive.

Take a medicine. Pharmacies sell various preparations that can relieve cystitis symptoms, though they won't kill bacteria. They include Cystopurin or Effercitrate, which contain potassium citrate, or Cymalon, Cystemme or Canesten Oasis, which contain sodium citrate.

VAGINAL AND YEAST INFECTIONS (THRUSH)

13 comforting steps

When we think of yeast, we think of its magical multiplying qualities that turn flour and water dough into bread. Unfortunately, those same qualities can wreak havoc in women when a vaginal yeast called *Candida albicans* (a type of fungus) gets out of control. Usually, *Candida* is kept in check by our immune system and by 'friendly' bacteria that live with it. But the fungus can grow and get out of control when the hormonal and/or bacterial balance of the body is disturbed by taking the contraceptive pill, antibiotics or corticosteroids, during pregnancy, or in certain illnesses like diabetes or immune deficiency (HIV/AIDS for example). It can also be passed between sexual partners.

Candida, like the yeast in bread-making, likes warm, moist, dark places, especially when (as in diabetes and babies' mouths) there's some sugar thrown in. In babies, the mouth, the folds of the neck and the nappy area can be affected; in people who are overweight, the skin in the folds of the groin or under the breasts; in people with their hands in water a lot, the nail folds; in men, the penis; and in women, the nipples if they're breast feeding, and, most commonly of all, the vaginal area.

When *Candida* multiplies in the vagina, it causes itching and irritation and a whitish cottage-cheese-like, usually odourless discharge, commonly known as thrush. Intercourse and urination can be painful, and the outside of the vaginal area can look red and inflamed. About 75 per cent of women will get thrush at least once, and more than 45 per cent will have it twice or more during their lives. Here are some ways to reduce the discomfort of thrush and prevent the infection from returning.

Visit the pharmacy. Women who have had several yeast infections in the past recognize the symptoms, says family planning doctor Diana Koster, but you may want to see your doctor first to be sure it really is a yeast infection. While some strains of yeast require treatment with prescription drugs, others can be controlled with the active ingredients in over-the-counter creams, suppositories or tablets.

Over-the-counter creams and vaginal tablets or pessaries for controlling yeast (such as Canesten) usually contain clotrimazole. Don't skimp on cream, especially if the outer vaginal tissues are irritated. Apply to external areas as well as inside the vagina.

You can also buy over-the-counter oral medications for thrush: Diflucan One (fluconazole) and Canesten Fluconazole oral capsule. These can also be obtained on prescription from your doctor.

Ease irritation with an oatmeal bath. Available in pharmacies, colloidal oatmeal (such as Aveeno) is ground to a fine powder, which enables it to stay suspended in water. Added to a warm bath, it's very soothing for itchy, irritated tissues. 'It's not a cure, but it might relieve some of the discomfort,' says Dr Koster.

Apply a cool compress. When you're feeling unusually itchy or sore, apply a cool, damp flannel to the outer part of the vagina. Both the moisture and the cool temperature will temporarily ease the discomfort.

Pat yourself dry. After showers or baths, rubbing yourself dry with a towel can be irritating. Gently pat yourself dry or allow the area to air-dry.

Wear cotton undies. Unlike nylon and other synthetic fabrics, cotton knickers breathe. In other words, they allow air to get in and moisture to get out, which will reduce your risk of infection, says urologist Larrian Gillespie.

Avoid scented bath products. Harsh chemical scents near tender parts of our bodies can cause irritation, says Dr Koster. Scented bath additives contain chemicals that make you even more uncomfortable. You'll be less vulnerable to yeast or other infections if you wash with water and a mild soap, with a dermatological cream like aqueous cream or E45 or with water alone. Bubble bath (even baby product types), bath salts, Radox and particularly Dettol, should be avoided.

Don't douche. The vagina is self-cleaning, so douching as part of normal vaginal hygiene is unnecessary, at best. It can also be harmful because it disrupts the natural balance of organisms in the vagina and increases the risk of infections, says Dr Gillespie.

Front to back. Vaginal infections often occur when bacteria and yeasts that normally inhabit the anal area move – or are pushed – into the vagina. This can also result in uncomfortable and potentially dangerous infections of the bladder, kidneys or urethra (see *Urinary Tract Infections*, page 544).

One way to keep anal bacteria where they belong is to wipe from front to back after urinating or having a bowel movement. It's important to teach little girls this rule, too, as soon as they begin using the loo on their own.

It's also a good idea for both partners to wash their genital areas with

Do just *one* thing

Wear loose clothes. The yeast fungus thrives in a warm, moist environment. Women who get frequent infections should do everything possible to make the vagina less hospitable by keeping it cool and dry, advises Dr Diana Koster. Wear loose clothes instead of skin-tight jeans. If you swim or work out, change into dry clothes as soon as you've finished.

It's also helpful to wear nothing on your bottom half in bed – wear a long baggy tee-shirt instead of pyjamas – and go without knickers under your skirt or dress when you're at home. Anything that increases air circulation keeps the vaginal area drier. This can reduce discomfort if you have a vaginal infection, and will help prevent future problems.

soap and water before sex to stop bacteria from being pushed into the vagina.

Identify changes in your life. It's not uncommon for women who have never had vaginal infections in the past to suddenly start getting them. Try to work out if you're doing anything different, Dr Koster advises. 'If you get irritated by using a new type of condom or even a different lubricant, change to another product.'

Eat live yoghurt. It won't help if you already have a yeast infection, but researchers believe that the live bacteria in yoghurt reduce the risk of infection. Yoghurt contains *Lactobacillus acidophilus*, which helps the vagina to maintain a healthy acid/alkaline balance. To prevent outbreaks of thrush, eat a tub or two of live yoghurt every day.

Try yoghurt the other end. Some authorties recommend douching with live yoghurt to help the symptoms of thrush. Cold yoghurt may soothe inflamed tissues and the *lactobacillus* may help to colonize the vagina with healthy bacteria. A yoghurt douche can be made by placing six tablespoons (90ml) plain nonpasteurized yoghurt containing live *lactobacillus* culture in a small douche bag with warm water. Douching can be repeated twice a day for three to four days. Check with your doctor before douching.

Practise good glucose control. Women with diabetes can be prone to vaginal infections because they may have abnormally high levels of glucose (sugar) in their blood. Higher-than-normal glucose levels can reduce the vagina's natural protective abilities.

Whether or not you need medication for your diabetes, you can help to keep your glucose levels under control by eating lots of fruits and whole grains, by exercising and maintaining a healthy weight (see

WHEN TO CONSULT A DOCTOR

Women often assume that every vaginal infection is caused by yeast – and then proceed to use over-the-counter medications. But women often misdiagnose their own infections.

If you have never had a vaginal infection, see your doctor at the first sign of symptoms. The infection could turn out to be yeast – or it could be caused by trichomoniasis, a sexually transmitted parasite, or by bacteria that requires treatment with antibiotics.

You should also talk to your doctor if you have four or more yeast infections in one year. You may have a resistant strain of yeast that won't get better without the use of prescription drugs. You may also need checking for underlying illnesses like diabetes or immune deficiency.

Diabetes, page 172). Even if you haven't been diagnosed with diabetes, you may want to have yourself checked if you've been getting frequent vaginal infections. Diabetes can reduce the ability of the immune system to combat yeast and other infections, says Beverly Kloeppel, who runs a student health centre. Men who develop thrush on their penis should also be checked for diabetes, particularly if they don't have a sexual partner who's affected.

VARICOSE VEINS

15 ways to improve the blood flow

Most people don't regard varicose veins as a disease – they think of them only as a cosmetic nuisance. Actually, this is far from the case. 'People with varicose veins have a disease – a disease with cosmetic impact,' says vein specialist Brian McDonagh.

Blue, swollen, lumpy-looking veins – and their cousins, the little fan-shaped purplish thread veins – are just the visible signs of varicose vein disease. People with the condition know only too well that these visible veins often come with aching, tired legs. But the condition is not life-threatening, so there's no need to panic or rush to your doctor.

Varicose veins are very common – up to 20 per cent of people in the UK will probably suffer from the condition at some time. They occur when superficial veins become swollen by blood leaking back from deep veins through valves which no longer work. This can be because of gravity or obstruction higher up increasing venous pressure, or because of a blockage (usually by thrombosis) in the deep veins. They can develop at almost any age, although they are more common as you get older. Pregnant women often get varicose veins, partly due to hormonal changes and partly because, in later pregnancy, the uterus squashes the veins in the pelvis and restricts blood flow back from the legs.

The condition is probably inherited – if your mother or father had varicose veins, you may develop them, too. Your job can also contribute to the risk – people whose jobs involve standing up all day have an increased chance of developing varicose veins, which can cause their legs to ache at the end of the day. People with a sedentary lifestyle are also more prone to varicose veins than active adults. If you have varicose veins, for whatever reason, here are some suggestions from the experts.

Enlist the help of gravity. Veins in the legs are the most susceptible to varicose change, for they are furthest – and straight downhill – from the heart. You can make their job much easier by getting gravity on your side. It's easy. Use a sofa, pillows or a footstool to raise your legs above hip level whenever they ache, and the discomfort should ease, says family doctor Dudley Phillips.

Wear support tights. These look like ordinary tights but extra elastication helps to provide relief. Support tights are sold in chemists and department stores. They resist the blood's tendency to pool in the small blood vessels closest to the skin, explains Dr Phillips. Instead, the blood is pushed into the larger, deeper veins, where it is more easily pumped back to the heart.

Or buy elastic stockings. These special stockings don't look like ordinary tights. They are made from a much thicker, stronger fabric. Support stockings, sold in most pharmacies or medical supply stores, help your leg muscles to push blood upwards by

KITCHEN CURES

Strangely enough, a high-fibre diet may be the kitchen's key to preventing varicose veins. Straining to have a bowel movement puts pressure on the veins in your lower legs. Over time, this pressure promotes the development of varicose veins.

A high-fibre diet can stop this gradual decline before it's too late. Fibre keeps waste moving freely, preventing straining and thus preventing varicose veins in the long run. Try to eat around 25g a day from sources like bran cereals, beans and whole grains.

concentrating pressure near the ankles. Your pharmacist will be able to measure your legs and advise you on the correct size of stocking. Put them on before you get out of bed in the morning. Raise your legs in the air and pull the stockings on evenly; they should not feel tight on your calves or in the groin. Wear them all day.

Put your legs in the air. Dr Phillips suggests that people with varicose veins combine the powers of gravity and support hose in the following exercise. Put on your support tights. Then lie flat on your back and raise your legs straight up in the air, resting them against a wall. Hold this position for two minutes. This allows the blood to flow out of the swollen leg veins and back towards your heart. Repeat throughout the day, if possible, as often as you need to.

Tilt your bed. Make gravity work for you throughout the night by raising the foot of your bed several inches, says dermatologist Paul Lazar.
    Note: If you have a history of heart trouble or if you have any difficulty breathing at night, consult a doctor before adjusting your bed.

Do just *one* thing

Try yoga, says cardiologist John Clarke. This yoga breathing exercise can be done without instruction, without danger and with a good chance that it will relieve the discomfort of varicose veins, he claims.

Lie flat on your back and prop your feet up on a chair. Breathe slowly and evenly from your diaphragm, through your nose. That's all there is to it. While gravity is pulling excess blood out of your raised legs, your full, steady inhalations pull air into the chest cavity, as well as blood from all over the body, including your blood-gorged legs.

Wear sensible shoes. Varicose veins are uncomfortable enough. Don't add to your leg pain by wearing high heels.

Watch your weight. Added body weight means more pressure on your legs. Keep your weight down, and the chances are you'll have fewer problems with bulging veins, says dermatologist Lenise Banse.

Avoid tight-fitting clothes. Tight garments, particularly a too-tight panty-girdle or tights that pinch in the groin area, can act like tourniquets and keep blood pooled in your legs, says Dr Banse.

Try some herbs. Horse chestnut is one of the best herbs available for varicose vein relief, says clinical herbalist Douglas Schar. Take horse chestnut extract, according to label instructions, whenever you

WHEN TO CONSULT A DOCTOR

If you have varicose veins, there are occasions when medical care is warranted. It's important to see a doctor if:

- you have a clot – this is very sore and tender and may be visible as a red lump in the vein that doesn't decrease in size even when you put your legs up (see *Phlebitis*, page 443);

- you cut a varicose vein. Control the resulting flow of blood and dial 999. Varicose veins around the ankle are more inclined to rupture and bleed. Bleeding is more dangerous than clotting because you can lose blood very fast;

- you have red varicose veins;

- swelling becomes incapacitating;

- the skin over your varicose veins becomes flaky, ulcerated, discoloured or prone to bleeding.

put your legs in a stressful situation, such as walking all day or sitting through a long flight. If varicose veins run in your family, think about taking horse chestnut regularly to reduce your risk of getting them too.

Go for a walk. Prolonged sitting or standing can cause problems in your legs because the blood tends to pool. A little exercise taken throughout the day, particularly walking, can often prevent this, says surgeon Eugene Strandness.

Witch hazel to the rescue. This plant has been used for centuries to improve varicose veins, whether in the legs or when they appear as haemorrhoids, says Schar. Apply witch hazel tincture, sold in health food stores, morning and night whenever the condition is troublesome.

Find relief with water. When showering, alternate between spraying hot and cold water on your legs, advises alternative practitioner Mindy Green. Change temperatures at one to three-minute intervals, and repeat the switch three times. The changing temperature gets blood moving by expanding and contracting the blood vessels.

Don't hide from your problem. Much of the discomfort and pain of varicose veins can be masked with painkillers. Varicose veins are a problem that should not be dealt with by hiding the pain. If you've gone through this list of tips and nothing helps, see your doctor.

WARTS AND VERRUCAS
21 healing secrets

After acne, warts are the most common dermatological complaint. At any one time, about 10 per cent of people have a wart, says immunologist Robert Garry. About 25 per cent will get one sometime in their lives.

Warts and verrucas are small thickened growths on the skin, which are caused by a virus. They have a somewhat rough surface, and can look quite ugly. They do not usually hurt but they may itch.

Warts can appear anywhere on the body, but are most commonly seen on the hands. Warts on the feet are known as verrucas. They are flatter as a result of the pressure from body weight, and they grow into the skin more. Verrucas can be painful, a bit like having a small stone in your shoe.

Sometimes people have many warts or verrucas; others have only one or two. They can be picked up from direct contact or in swimming pools or changing rooms. However, because warts and verrucas don't spread rapidly through a family, doctors think that some people are just more susceptible to the virus.

Standard treatments for warts tend to involve burning, scraping, cutting, freezing or zapping with a laser. Some treatments are uncomfortable and may leave scars. These techniques are not always effective, and warts often reappear, no matter what treatment is used. So you may want to try some home remedies before seeing your doctor. Unless stated otherwise, the following can be used for both warts and verrucas.

Leave them alone. According to one estimate, 40 to 50 per cent of all warts eventually disappear on their own – usually within two

---

KITCHEN CURES

The remedy that so neatly dispatched one little growth might leave another completely unscathed. Here are some folk cures – treatments that have never undergone formal scientific scrutiny but have worked for many.

- Apply clove oil or the milky juice of unripe figs directly to the wart.

- Soak lemon slices in cider and a little salt. Leave to stand for two weeks. Then rub the slices onto the wart.

- Rub the wart with a piece of chalk or a raw potato.

- Tape the inner side of a banana skin to a verruca and change daily.

WHEN TO CONSULT A DOCTOR

If you have the slightest doubt about what you're dealing with, see a doctor. It could be a corn, callus, mole or cancerous lesion.

In general, warts are pale, skin-coloured growths with a rough surface, even borders and blackened surface capillaries. Normal skin lines such as fingerprints do not cross a wart's surface. And contrary to popular opinion, warts are very shallow growths – they don't have 'roots' or 'runners' that go down to the bone.

Genital warts can affect both men and women and can be transmitted sexually. Certain sub-types of the genital wart virus have been associated with the development of cancer of the cervix. Use condoms if either partner is affected and see your doctor for regular cervical smear checks.

years. Children, in particular, often lose warts spontaneously.

Warts constantly shed the infectious virus, though, warns dermatologist and foot expert Marc Brenner. If left untreated, they may get larger or spread to other areas. So if your warts start multiplying, take action.

Apply vitamin A. Dr Garry recommends applying vitamin A directly to warts. Break open a cod-liver oil capsule, squeeze some of the liquid onto the wart and rub it in once a day. Different warts respond differently to this treatment. Juvenile warts can disappear in a month, others in two to four months, but verrucas might take two to five months longer.

And another vitamin. Apply a paste of crushed vitamin C tablets and water to the wart and then cover with a plaster so that the paste doesn't rub off. Although no formal research has been done in this area, there is some evidence that the high acidity of vitamin C can kill the wart-producing virus, according to Dr Jeffrey Bland, who spent many years studying the effects of vitamin C. Vitamin C could irritate your skin, so apply the paste only to the wart.

Keep your feet dry. Warts thrive on moisture, so keeping your feet very dry may help to eliminate verrucas. Change your socks at least three times a day, says Dr Brenner, and apply a medicated foot powder frequently.

Buy a wart treatment. The most popular commercial wart remedies are the over-the-counter salicylic acid preparations. Salicylic acid softens

How to avoid a wart

Warts are caused by a virus. It's in the air, and you pick it up in the same way as you do any viral infection. If you're susceptible to the virus and you have a suitable cut or crack in the skin for it to take hold, you'll get a wart. But there are a few things that you can do to lessen your chances of sprouting a wart.

Keep your shoes on. The wart virus thrives in a very moist environment, so always wear flip flops around swimming pools, health clubs and changing rooms to avoid foot contact with it.

Change shoes frequently. Since the wart virus breeds in moist places, change your shoes often and let them dry out properly between each wearing.

Clean up. At a health club or gym, clean the shower out first. Simple household bleach will kill viruses and bacteria.

Look but don't touch. Warts spread easily, so try not to touch them. If you have even a small cut on your finger, you risk getting a wart there.

Care for cuticles. If the wart virus enters a cut around your cuticle, it can cause a nasty type of wart called a periungual wart. This is difficult to treat, so if you get a cut in your cuticle, apply an antiseptic cream and cover it with a plaster until it heals.

Relax. People seem to be more susceptible to warts when they're under stress and eating badly.

and dissolves warts. Liquid, gel, pad and ointment forms are available.

Follow these rules when using salicylic acid, says foot specialist Glenn Gastwirth. First, make sure that it is a wart you're treating (see 'When to consult a doctor' on page 557). Secondly, follow label instructions to the letter. Thirdly, be patient.

You may need to treat a wart, particularly a verruca, for a number of weeks before it finally gives up the ghost.

Liquids and gels, which usually contain only about 17 per cent salicylic acid, may not be strong enough to work on verrucas, which have thick calluses covering them. They will work better if you rub down the area regularly with a pumice stone or an emery board.

Note: Don't use these products if you have diabetes or impaired circulation.

Try an ointment. There are several ointments available from pharmacies, including Verrugon ointment (50 per cent salicylic acid), Salactol paint (16.7 per cent) or Cuplex gel (11 per cent). For best results, soak the wart area in lukewarm water for about 10 minutes to allow greater penetration, advises podiatrist Suzanne Levine. Dry well, then apply a drop of the ointment to the wart. Cover with a plaster. If you're dealing with a verruca, do this at bedtime so that you won't have to walk around on it and rub off the ointment. In the morning, soak the area again and lightly pumice off any softened skin.

Use a pad. Dermatologist Christopher McEwen recommends treating warts with pads impregnated with 40 per cent salicylic acid (such as Scholl Verruca Removal System). These work fairly well for verrucas and can also be effective on hand warts, although it's harder to keep the patch

Believe it's going – and it goes

Go into a trance. Psychiatrist Owen Surman says hypnosis works for treating warts. In one study, he hypnotized 17 people who had warts for a series of five sessions and told them that their warts would disappear. Another seven people were not hypnotized and were told to abstain from using any wart remedies. Three months later, more than half of the hypnotized group had lost at least 75 per cent of their warts. Those who hadn't been hypnotized still had their warts.

Imagine your warts gone. The power of suggestion alone – without hypnosis – may be just as effective at getting rid of warts. Psychologist Nicholas Spanos tells patients to imagine that their warts are shrinking, that they can feel the tingling as their warts dissolve and their skin becomes clear. Initially, he gives them about two minutes of this type of imagery, then he asks them to practise on their own at home for five minutes a day. He can predict who will achieve good results based on the first session. People who report vivid imagery on that first day are more likely to lose warts than those whose visualization was weak.

Be a believer. Other doctors have had success with the power of suggestion. Dermatologist Christopher McEwen treated two children, who could not tolerate freezing, like this. He gave them a harmless lotion to use and stressed that it was a very strong medicine that would knock out their warts. It worked. Belief in a cure may also explain the popularity of folk remedies such as rubbing the wart with a penny and then burying the penny under the porch.

in place on the hand. The main drawback to pads, says Dr Levine, is that people use too large a piece, which irritates the surrounding skin. This can cause an ulcer around the wart that's worse than the wart you had in the first place. Follow directions on the label.

To ensure a good fit, cut out a cardboard template in exactly the shape and dimensions of your wart. Then use the template to cut a supply of patches from the adhesive wart plaster.

Lightly coat the skin around the wart with petroleum jelly to prevent medication from touching your skin.

Take an immune stimulant. Warts are a viral condition and they tend to worsen when someone is under stress, says clinical herbalist Douglas Schar. This is because stress suppresses your immune system, allowing the virus to proliferate.

If you have warts and you know you're heading for a stressful patch, plan ahead, advises Schar. Take a herbal immune stimulant to kick-start your immune system. Maitake and astragalus are both excellent options. Buy either from a health food store and take throughout the stressful period.

WEIGHT PROBLEMS

24 ways to achieve and maintain a healthy weight

More than half of us are overweight in Britain, according to the British Nutrition Foundation, and the numbers are going up. Whilst millions of children across the world face daily starvation, our children face an epidemic of a different, and ultimately perhaps just as deadly form of malnutrition – obesity.

People who are very overweight run a much greater risk of developing diseases like diabetes mellitus and coronary heart disease. But dieting, as most of us know, is hard and boring, and usually fails. You are much more likely to succeed if you set your sights on a sensible weight loss of about 0.5kg a week rather than going for a dramatic fall.

It took some time to get fat – and it's going to take time to get slimmer, too. 'A pound a week doesn't sound much to someone in a hurry,' says family doctor Stephen Amiel. 'But if you keep that up for a year, you'll have lost almost four stones (nearly 24kg). And you're much less likely to put it straight back on.'

There's no mystery to putting on weight – or taking it off again. It's a matter of simple arithmetic. Take in more calories than you burn up –

you put on weight; burn more than you take in – you lose it again. This then is why we are getting fatter – we eat more food than we need for the amount of exercise we take.

Our society makes it very easy to get large. Food is plentiful, and because so much of it is higher in calories than our bodies were designed to cope with, it's easy to eat more than our bodies need. And we have grown very sedentary.

While our ancestors ploughed fields and churned butter as part of their working day, nowadays many of us tap keyboards for a living, and go home at the end of the day to watch television – and eat. Even fifty years ago, children actually consumed more calories than they do today. But they walked to school, and they played outside, instead of sitting with their fast-food dinners in front of the telly or their computers.

Labour-saving devices spare us effort and exercise. Escalators whisk us from floor to floor at stations or shopping precincts; washer-dryers take care of the laundry; remote controls let us change channels from our armchairs.

Eating too many calories is no problem, as long as we have ways to burn them off. Here, we look at ways to use your mind, mouth and muscles to control your weight.

Use Your Mind

Many weight-loss efforts fail as a result of our mental attitude, says Gary Foster, a psychologist who runs a clinic for people with eating disorders. Here's how to use your mind to reduce your waistline.

Resist the hard sell. Regardless of all the rapid weight loss plans you see advertised, the best way to lose weight and keep it off is to make permanent changes to your eating and exercise habits, says Marsha Marcus, a psychiatrist who specializes in eating disorders.

Easy answers to a difficult task like losing weight may be appealing. But if a weight-loss promise sounds too good to be true – then it is.

Aim for 10 per cent. Despite the inspiring advertisements of skinny people holding up the huge clothes they used to wear, the best goal for weight loss is to lose 10 per cent of your body weight, says Dr Foster.

People who aim too high, like losing 20 kilos, do one of two things. They either feel so daunted that they give up from the word go. Or they eat less and less, and exercise more and more – and then give up because no one can go on like that forever.

Instead, says Dr Foster, work out what 10 per cent of your body weight is and aim for that. So if you weigh 80 kilos, try and lose eight kilos. Most people take about six months to achieve this initial goal.

Don't slow down your metabolism. Once you've worked out how much weight to lose to begin with, plan to lose up to 0.5kg (1lb) a week, advises nutrition expert Joanne Larsen. If you go on a very low calorie diet or take far too much exercise and lose more than a kilo per week, your body goes into starvation mode. A body in starvation mode burns fewer calories and resists your efforts to lose more weight.

Enjoy your success. Once they've shed 10kg or so, many clients tell Dr Foster that they sleep better, can climb stairs more easily and have more energy to play with their children or grandchildren. Celebrate your success; treat yourself – perhaps to some new clothes.

Think about the future. An irritating fact of weight loss is that the smaller you get, the fewer calories you can consume and still maintain that new weight, Dr Foster says. After you've lost 10 per cent of your weight, you'll have to eat roughly 10 per cent fewer calories each day than you do now to stay at that weight.

But most people don't think about how they're going to maintain their new weight. They diet, lose the weight and then go back to their old eating habits. The weight goes straight back on. The idea is not to get to your goal and then go back to the way you used to eat.

Take a break. Once you've reached your goal of losing 10 per cent of your body weight, your next goal should be simply to maintain that loss for a while.

'Try to stay at that weight for at least another six to eight months, or longer than it took to lose that initial amount. Really get a feel for what it is to live in your body at that weight,' says Dr Foster. When the time is right and you're ready and willing for even more weight-loss effort, Dr Foster suggests you now try losing five per cent of your body weight. Everyone will lose at a different rate, so it's impossible to predict how long it will take.

Make changes you can live with. Even if you can totally cut out fast food, chocolate and other forbidden foods while you're losing weight, you need to remember that you can enjoy all foods, including these, in moderation for the rest of your life.

'I think that for people with weight problems, it's a question of a lifetime of self-management. That's not to say that one has to *diet* for life,' says Dr Marcus. 'We have to say yes to ourselves and enjoy our food, but we also have to learn to say no.'

Become more aware of your eating behaviour. In order to change your eating behaviour, you first have to *learn* what that behaviour is. It's

WHEN TO CONSULT A DOCTOR

It's a good idea to talk with your doctor if you think you need to lose weight. This is especially important if you have reached or are near menopause or if you have other risk factors for developing a chronic disease associated with overweight and obesity, such as a smoking habit, a sedentary lifestyle, high blood sugar, high blood pressure or high cholesterol levels.

Weight loss during menopause may increase the rate at which bone density is lost, so your doctor should be aware of your efforts to lose weight – you may need calcium supplements.

Weight gain is almost never due to a 'glandular' or metabolic cause, and only uncommonly is it due to fluid retention. A visit to a doctor will reassure you on this, and give you an opportunity to get your blood sugar and blood pressure checked, have your height and starting weight recorded, agree a target weight, and get some dietary advice.

If your BMI (see box page 564) is over 30, or over 28 and you're diabetic or have heart disease, you may be considered for appetite-reducing medication.

a two-step process, explains Dr Marcus. First, start paying attention to what, when, where and with whom you're eating, how you feel and what kind of activities you're doing throughout the day. Next, think about what triggers the eating – the smell of baking bread, the sight of a certain food, boredom or anger.

It's easy to go through our days without paying attention to such details, Dr Marcus says. A lot of us eat all the time without thinking about it. Keep a food diary to record the information, so you can read it later.

Use Your Mouth

It's easy to say that the secret to weight loss is to eat fewer calories than you burn. But because of our fast-paced, sedentary lifestyle, eating well every day isn't that simple.

Ask for help. Individual needs may vary, depending in part on body composition and activity. Gender and genetics have an impact on how your body uses and stores food. For example, women's hormones tend to encourage fat deposition.

A dietitian can help you tailor a weight-loss plan, suggests Larsen. Ask your GP for a referral.

Calculate your body mass index

Most health professionals use a tool called the body mass index (BMI) to determine if someone falls into either the 'overweight' or 'obese' category. The BMI measures body weight relative to height, which usually correlates to the amount of body fat you have. People who have a BMI of 30 or higher are classified as obese. People with a BMI of 25 to 30 are considered overweight, because they weigh more than average for their height.

The excess weight can come from muscle, bone or body water as well as fat. This means that some people, such as bodybuilders, could be overweight but not overfat. BMI values below 25 and down to 18.5 are considered healthy.

You can calculate your own BMI by dividing your weight in kilos by your height in metres, squared (eg 70kg/1.71m x 1.71m = BMI 24).

Or go to the British Nutrition Foundation website at www.nutrition.org.uk and use their automatic BMI calculator (under the section entitled 'What is a healthy weight? What is a healthy shape?').

Eat a balanced diet. High-protein/low-carbohydrate diets, which cut out the bread, pasta and fruit and bump up the meat, have enjoyed a wave of popularity. You might lose weight while enjoying steak and eggs, but it's partly due to fluid loss from the unusual way the body has to turn food into energy, and partly due to eating fewer calories.

Using so much protein as fuel can leave you tired and constipated and puts great demand on your kidneys as they filter excess protein. This is especially risky for diabetics, says nutritionist Mary Friesz.

A diet that's ultra-low in fat isn't good for you, either. In reasonable amounts, the fat in your food makes you feel full, so you want to stop eating. The balanced diet that experts recommend for weight loss or weight maintenance is simple. Every day, try to get about half of your calories from carbohydrates. Good sources of carbohydrates include fruits, vegetables, whole grain breads, pasta, rice and milk.

About a quarter of your calories should come from protein. Good sources include lean cuts of beef, chicken breast, fish and beans. If you're a vegetarian, eat rice on the same day as beans to ensure that you get complete proteins. The remainder of your calories should come from fats and oils, especially olive oil. This is the healthiest for your heart, but it's still high in calories.

Eat frequently. Instead of eating all your food for the day in two or three sittings, eat four to six smaller meals throughout the day, suggests Dr Friesz. When you eat smaller, more frequent meals each day as opposed to a couple of large ones, your body is more likely to use the calories instead of packing them away as fat, she says. You'll also ensure that you aren't starving when you sit down at the table, so you won't wolf down more than you need.

Drink less alcohol. Alcoholic drinks are often very high in calories and have virtually no nutritional value, says Dr Amiel. Dilute wine with sparkling water, drink low sugar beers (they're usually lower in alcohol too) and limit your total intake to three standard drinks daily for men, and two for women.

Don't smoke instead. The increase in smoking amongst women, and now sadly the increase in smoking-related deaths amongst women, has a lot to do with weight. 'So many young women tell me they've started smoking as a way of controlling their weight, and fear of putting weight on is a major reason for not trying to quit,' says Dr Amiel.

Whatever you do, resist the temptation to turn, or turn back, to cigarettes: smoking is an infinitely greater health risk than being moderately overweight.

Eat slowly. Your brain's satiety centre (the part that tells you you're full) is in that part of your brain linked to our emotions, the hypothalamus. Feel good while you're eating and you eat less. You can also fool your satiety centre by chewing your food more (Granny was right – again), taking smaller mouthfuls and having little breaks during a meal.

Well presented food, eaten in pleasant surroundings, in good company will make mealtimes a sensual and pleasurable social experience, leaving you feeling contented and pleasantly full although you've taken in fewer calories.

Beware when eating out. 'If you're full when you leave the table, you've eaten too much,' says Dr Friesz. You need to stop eating before you feel full – when you still have room for food but no longer feel hungry.

Drink plenty of water. Drink eight 250ml glasses of water each day. Keeping some water in your stomach most of the time can help to fool it into thinking it's full, Larsen says.

Strive for 25. Eating at least 25 grams of fibre each day is very helpful if you're trying to lose weight. Foods rich in fibre tend to be nutritious, filling and lower in calories, Larsen says. You can accumulate a total of 25 grams of fibre in a day by eating a bowl of bran flakes for breakfast, a wholemeal muffin with your morning coffee, adding a tablespoon of chickpeas to your salad at lunchtime, snacking on a large apple and stir-frying a serving of broccoli to accompany your evening meal.

Use Your Muscles

The last key component of any weight-loss programme is exercise. Activity burns calories, allowing you to eat more and weigh the same, or eat the same amount and weigh less. Exercise combined with diet is the most effective approach to weight loss and is an integral part of long-term weight maintenance.

Go for a blend. The best exercise programme combines aerobic exercise, strength training and stretching, says physical education professor Joseph Chromiak. Aerobic exercise that is continuous, such as cycling, walking and swimming, strengthens your heart and is best for reducing your risk of many chronic diseases. 'Stop-start' activities like squash are not as good for you.

Strength training, such as weight-lifting, makes muscles stronger and helps to maintain muscle mass. This becomes more important as we get older, because muscle mass starts diminishing in our early twenties. If you don't use your muscles, they get smaller. Because muscle tissue significantly contributes to a person's daily calorie expenditure, the more muscle mass you have, the more calories you use. The daily difference may not be large, but it's huge over time.

Stretching helps to prepare your muscles for a work-out and increases flexibility. But the best time to stretch for long-term results is after exercise, when your muscles are warmed up, advises Dr Chromiak. Try to stretch for 10 to 15 minutes at least three times a week.

Aim for three days a week. Initially, plan to exercise for 20 minutes for a minimum of three days a week, says Dr Chromiak. Build up to 30 to 40 minutes at a time. The more days you exercise, the better, but three days is a good starting point if you haven't been exercising at all.

If your size or fitness level prevents you from working out for 20 minutes a day, start with just 15 minutes and gradually work your way up. Don't put off exercising if you are short of time – even exercising for 10 minutes intermittently during the day helps to strengthen your heart.

Find exercises you enjoy. Think of all the activities you might enjoy, then alternate between them. Variety may make it easier to stick with your programme.

WRINKLES **567**

Ask for help. It's a good idea to talk to a qualified trainer to ensure that you're choosing the right exercises to safely work all the major muscles in your body. If you don't belong to a gym, hire a personal trainer for a few sessions to get you started. Ask at your local sports centre or fitness club.

Put exercise in your diary. If you're not used to exercising regularly, book it as an appointment in your diary, Dr Friesz suggests. Otherwise, you'll forget or find an excuse not to do it. After three months, it should become a habit.

Get help if you need to. If you suspect that your eating or dieting, or someone's you care about, is out of control, professional help is available and should be sought urgently. For more information on eating disorders, contact: Eating Disorders Association, 1st Floor, Wensum House, 103 Prince of Wales Road, Norwich NR1 1DW; tel: 0845 634 1414 (adults) or 0845 634 7650 (young people); or online at www.edauk.com.

WRINKLES
14 ways to lessen their impact

Unlike a fine wine or a single malt, the quality of human skin does not improve with age. Instead, it loses moisture, elasticity and resilience, making it wrinkle.

Skin undergoes two types of ageing, says dermatologist Coyle Connolly. The first, intrinsic ageing, is genetically programmed. You can't do much about that without the help of a dermatologist or plastic surgeon. The second – photoageing – is the result of damage caused mainly by the sun. You can delay photoageing by making certain lifestyle choices. Here's what the experts advise to keep wrinkles from taking too much of a toll on your skin.

Sleep on your back. Sleeping on your side or front with your face squashed into the pillow causes wrinkles, says dermatologist Anne Kleinsmith. Sleeping on your back may eliminate this problem.

Wear sunglasses. A major area for wrinkles is around the eyes, partly caused by screwing up your eyes in bright sunlight. One way to lessen the formation of crow's feet is to wear sunglasses in bright weather, says Dr Kleinsmith.

Keep a straight face. Lots of frowning or smiling, or any other much-repeated facial expression, aggravates wrinkles, says Dr Kleinsmith. 'I'm not saying that you should not smile or frown, but try to be aware of how often you're doing it – especially frowning.'

Avoid smokers' face. 'I can often tell that a person is a long-term heavy smoker just by looking at their face,' says family doctor Stephen Amiel. Smoking robs the complexion of oxygen, by causing constriction in the capillaries and decreasing blood circulation to facial skin.

Smokers' wrinkles have a number of distinctive features: they come on earlier, they are more extensive, especially around the lips and they're deeper and often leathery-looking. In addition, the smoker's face often has a yellow grey tinge.

Use a sunscreen. Whether it's achieved indoors or out, today's tan leads to tomorrow's wrinkles. 'Obviously, excessive exposure to sunlight is going to increase your chances of developing wrinkles,' says dermatologist Audrey Kunin. Choose a sunscreen, preferably with a sun protection factor (SPF) of 30 and with both ultraviolet (UV) A and B protection (also known as broad-spectrum).

Avoid tanning beds. Twenty minutes on a tanning-bed is equivalent to a whole day on the beach without sunscreen. Avoid them for the sake of your skin, says Dr Kunin. 'If you want to look brown, use self-tanning lotion and a bronzing foundation.'

Wear a hat. Whether you're off to the beach or spending time outdoors in the midday sun, put on a hat with a 10cm-wide brim to keep the sun off your face and neck, says Dr Kunin. But don't rely on unlined, loosely woven straw hats. They let the sun's rays through. And baseball caps don't protect your ears, the back of your neck or even most of your face from full sun. A sunhat needs a wide brim and a sun-protective cloth lining.

Stay out of the midday sun. That's 11am to 4pm in summer, and midday to 2pm the rest of the year. This is when the ultraviolet radiation is strongest, says skin-care expert Joni Keim Loughran.

Sit in the shade. Because wrinkles are caused by excessive sun exposure, retreat to a shady spot on sunny days from time to time, says Loughran. At the beach or in the garden, sit under a large umbrella. If you're out walking or boating, wear tightly woven clothing if it's not too hot. This helps to stop UV rays from penetrating your skin.

Keep your weight steady. If your weight fluctuates greatly, your skin will expand to accommodate it, but it might not contract all the way if you lose it again. And as you age, you may need a little more weight on you to keep the wrinkles at bay. Was it Zsa Zsa Gabor who said, 'Darling, after 40, to keep your face you have to sacrifice your body a little'?

Use a moisturizer. If you have dry skin, daily use of a moisturizing lotion can plump up your skin and temporarily hide smaller wrinkles that form on the skin's surface, says Dr Connolly. This is not a long-term solution, but it makes your skin look healthier.

Exfoliate. Alpha hydroxy acids (AHAs), found in plants and fruits, are used in some skin products. They act by removing dead skin cells on the surface to expose the younger cells underneath. And by plumping up the skin, they smooth the areas that cause wrinkles. If your skin is too sensitive for AHAs, you might try beta hydroxy acids (BHAs) such as salicylic acid. It's available in moisturizers and cleansers, and exfoliates the skin like an AHA but with less irritation.

Top up on omega-3s. Two dietary changes can help to maintain skin moisture. Eat oily fish such as salmon, trout, mackerel and fresh tuna (not tinned, as the canning process removes most of the beneficial oils), which are rich in omega-3 fatty acids, at least twice a week to help restore moisture to dry skin. Flaxseed (or linseed) oil, also high in omega-3s, can be stirred into fruit juice or added to salad dressings. Keep the oil in the fridge or it will go rancid.

KITCHEN CURES

Eat your greens. 'Some years ago,' says clinical herbalist Douglas Schar, 'I was talking with a group of unwrinkled women in San Juan, Puerto Rico. I asked them how they managed to stay wrinkle-free, despite the harsh sunny environment. They told me that they ate watercress every day.' Vegetables like watercress are incredibly rich in antioxidants, which are thought to reduce the free-radical damage that causes wrinkling. So add dark green leafy vegetables to your daily diet to slow down the ageing process, says Schar.

SAFETY GUIDELINES
Using herbs, vitamins and supplements

Although most herbs, vitamins and supplements are generally safe and cause few, if any, side-effects, doctors advise that you should use them responsibly. After all, every product has the potential to cause an adverse reaction. When taken to treat or prevent disease, herbs, vitamins and supplements should be regarded as drugs, and treated as carefully. Just because they are organic or 'natural' does not make them intrinsically safe for everyone on every occasion. Remember, too, that many of them are classed as food substances, rather than drugs. The manufacture of these products, clinical trials for their effectiveness and safety, and the advertising claims made for them, are therefore not subject to the same regulations and controls that apply to over-the-counter or prescribed drugs.

If you are under medical supervision for any health condition or are taking any medication, it's a good idea to talk with your doctor before using herbs and supplements. Some natural substances change the way your body absorbs and processes medicines. Furthermore, if you are pregnant, breastfeeding or trying to conceive, do not treat yourself with any natural remedy without the consent of your doctor or midwife.

Herbs

Some herbs are more likely than others to cause adverse reactions in certain people. Though such occurrences are rare, you should be aware of what they are and stop using a herb if you experience an unusual reaction. And never exceed the recommended dose – more is not better.

Aloe *Aloe barbadensis* May delay wound healing; do not use gel externally on any surgical incision. Do not take the dried leaf gel internally, as it is a habit-forming laxative.
American ginseng *Panax quinquefolius* May cause irritability. Do not take if you have high blood pressure.
Arnica *Arnica montana* Do not use on broken skin.
Black cohosh *Actea racemosa* Do not use if taking the Pill or HRT.
Chamomile *Matricaria recutita* Rarely, can cause an allergic reaction when taken by people allergic to related plants (chrysanthemums, asters).
Chasteberry *Vitex agnus-castus* Do not use if taking the Pill or HRT.
Echinacea *Echinacea angustifolia, E. purpurea, E. pallida* Use products with echinacea flowers with caution if allergic to related plants (asters, chrysanthemums). If you have an auto-immune condition like lupus, discuss with your doctor before taking.

Feverfew *Tanacetum parthenium* Chewing fresh leaves can cause mouth sores.

Flaxseed *Linum usitatissimum* Always take flaxseeds with at least 250ml of water. Do not take seeds if you have a bowel obstruction. These notes apply to seeds only. The oil is safe.

Garlic *Allium sativum* Do not take supplements if you are on anticoagulants or before undergoing surgery: garlic thins the blood and may increase bleeding.

Ginkgo *Ginkgo biloba* Do not take with MAOI (mono amine oxidase inhibitor) antidepressants such as phenelzine (Nardil); or with aspirin or other nonsteroidal anti-inflammatory medications; or with blood-thinning medications such as warfarin. Can cause dermatitis, diarrhoea and vomiting in doses higher than 240mg of concentrated extract.

Goldenseal *Hydrastis canadensis* Avoid if you have hypertension.

Hawthorn *Crataegus oxycantha, C. laevigata, C. monogyna* If you have a cardiovascular condition, do not take hawthorn without medical supervision. You may require lower doses of other medications such as high blood pressure drugs. If you have low blood pressure caused by heart valve problems, do not take without medical supervision.

Horse chestnut *Aesculus hippocastanum* May interfere with the action of other drugs, especially blood thinners such as warfarin. May irritate the gastrointestinal tract.

Liquorice *Glycyrrhiza glabra* Do not take if you have high blood pressure, kidney disorders or low potassium levels. Do not take daily for more than 4 to 6 weeks, because overuse can lead to water retention and high blood pressure.

Meadowsweet *Filipendula ulmaria* Do not take if you need to avoid aspirin, because its active ingredient, salicin, is related to aspirin.

Myrrh *Commiphora myrrha* Do not take internally.

Nettle *Urtica dioica* If you have allergies, your symptoms may worsen, so take only one dose a day for the first few days.

Oats *Avena sativa* Do not take if you have coeliac disease.

Parsley *Petroselinum crispum* Do not take if you have kidney disease, because parsley taken in therapeutic amounts increases urine flow. Safe as a garnish or in food.

Psyllium (ispaghula) *Plantago ovata* Take with at least 250ml water and one hour after other drugs. Avoid if you have a bowel obstruction.

Sage *Salvia officinalis* Taken in therapeutic amounts, sage can increase sedative side-effects of drugs. Do not take if you are hypoglycaemic or undergoing anticonvulsant therapy.

St John's wort *Hypericum perforatum* Do not take with antidepressants or other prescription medicine without your doctor's consent. May cause photosensitivity: avoid overexposure to direct sunlight.

Turmeric *Curcuma domestica* Do not take if you have high stomach acid or ulcers, gallstones or bile duct obstruction.

Valerian *Valeriana officinalis* Do not take with sleep-enhancing or mood-regulating medications, because it may intensify their effects. Discontinue use if taking valerian causes heart palpitations or nervousness.

White willow *Salix alba* Can cause stomach irritation, especially when taken with alcohol. Do not take at the same time as aspirin.

Vitamin and Mineral Supplements

Although serious side-effects from vitamin and mineral supplements are not common, they can happen. These guidelines are designed to help you use supplements safely and wisely. The vitamin and mineral doses listed *in italics* below are the UK recommended daily amounts for healthy adults. Some supplements can be harmful if taken in large doses.

Biotin *100–200mcg* Dietary sources are usually sufficient.

Calcium *700mg* Taking more than 1500mg a day can cause serious side-effects such as kidney damage. For best absorption, avoid taking more than 500mg at one time. If you are over 50, look for a formula that contains vitamin D as well as calcium, as you may need more vitamin D than is supplied by a multivitamin alone.

Copper *1.2mg* Dietary sources are usually sufficient. Do not exceed 1mg copper daily in supplements. For best absorption, take supplements containing copper sulphate or cupric sulphate.

Magnesium *300mg for men, 270mg for women* Dietary sources are usually sufficient. Check with your doctor before beginning supplementation in any amount if you have heart or kidney problems. Taking more than 400mg a day can cause diarrhoea.

Niacin (vitamin B$_3$) *17mg for men, 13mg for women* High doses of niacin (17mg in nicotinic acid supplement form; 500mg in nicotinamide supplement form) can cause liver damage and should be taken only under your doctor's supervision.

Vitamin A *700mcg for men, 600mcg for women* Dietary sources are usually sufficient. Taking more than 1500mcg a day can cause headache, double vision, drowsiness or fatigue, nausea or vomiting. Do not take vitamin A while pregnant or trying to conceive as it can damage the foetus.

Vitamin B$_6$ *1.4mg for men, 1.2mg for women* Taking more than 200mg a day over a long period can cause (reversible) nerve damage.

Vitamin B$_{12}$ *1.5mcg* Do not exceed 2mg daily. Take with folic acid to aid absorption.

Vitamin C *40mg (80mg smokers)* Taking more than 2000mg a day can cause diarrhoea. Split up high doses (1000mg should be sufficient) over the course of the day.

Vitamin E *4mg for men, 3mg for women* Do not take more than 540mg daily. Because it acts like a blood thinner, consult your doctor before taking vitamin E if you are already taking aspirin or a blood-thinning medication, such as warfarin. Choose the natural form (d-alpha-tocopherol) over the synthetic form (dl-alpha-tocopherol).

Zinc *5.5–9.5mg for men, 4–7 mg for women* Do not take more than 25mg daily unless advised by your doctor. Long-term use of more than 25mg a day can impair immunity, reduce levels of HDL (good) cholesterol and cause nausea, vomiting, diarrhoea or anaemia.

Other Supplements

Reports of adverse effects from supplements are rare, especially compared to prescription drugs, and supplement manufacturers are required by law to provide information on labels about safe dosages for healthy individuals. Be aware that strength and dosage can vary significantly between products. Note, too, that little scientific research exists as to the safety or long-term effects of many newer supplements, and some supplements can complicate existing conditions or cause allergic reactions. Take supplements with food for best absorption and to avoid stomach irritation, unless otherwise directed. Never take as a substitute for a healthy diet: supplements do not offer the nutritional benefits of food.

Activated charcoal May interfere with the absorption of oral medications or other supplements if doses not taken at least 2 hours apart. Do not take more than 4000mg a day: may cause stomach upset, diarrhoea, constipation or vomiting. May turn teeth black and cause painful stools.

Bromelain Avoid if taking aspirin or anticoagulants (blood thinners). Do not take if you are allergic to pineapple.

Coenzyme Q$_{10}$ Avoid if pregnant or breastfeeding. Talk to your doctor if taking the blood thinner warfarin. Side-effects – heartburn, nausea or stomach ache – are rare and can be prevented by taking with food.

Curcumin May cause heartburn.

Fish oil Do not take if any of the following apply: you have a bleeding disorder, uncontrolled high blood pressure, an allergy to any kind of fish, or you take anticoagulants (blood thinners) or aspirin regularly. Increases bleeding time, possibly resulting in nosebleeds and easy bruising, and may cause upset stomach, belching and flatulence. Diabetics should not take fish oil because large doses increase blood sugar levels. Cod liver oil supplements are best avoided altogether: they contain very high doses of vitamin A, which can cause headache, skin irritation and liver damage. Pregnant women should avoid all vitamin A-containing supplements.

Glucosamine In very rare cases, may cause upset stomach, heartburn or diarrhoea. Take with food to prevent this.

Lysine Avoid if pregnant or breastfeeding. Don't take with arginine (sometimes used for angina), as lysine counteracts arginine's effects.

Quercetin Doses above 100mg may dilate blood vessels and cause blood thinning. Avoid if you are at risk for low blood pressure or problems with blood clotting.

SAM May increase blood levels of homocysteine, a risk factor for cardiovascular disease. People with bipolar disorder should not take SAM.

COMBINATIONS TO AVOID

The following guide can help you to avoid mixing common drugs with herbs, supplements and foods that might cause problems. Please note that this list is not comprehensive. If you are taking a different drug for any of these conditions, consult your doctor or pharmacist about possible interactions. To be on the safe side, tell your doctor about all the medicines you are taking and any medicinal herbs or foods you use therapeutically.

Allergies If you are taking antihistamines such as diphenhydramine (Benadryl) or hydroxyzine (Atarax) then **avoid** sedative herbs such as passionflower and valerian: they may increase the drug's sedative effects.

Angina If you are taking beta-blockers such as propranolol (Inderal) then **avoid** broom and fumitory: they increase the drug's effects.

Anxiety If you are taking hypnotic and mild sedative drugs such as lorazepam (Ativan), diazepam (Valium), temazepam, zopiclone (Zimovane) then **avoid** cowslip, mistletoe and yohimbe: they increase the drug's effects. **Also avoid** sedative herbs such as passionflower, skullcap and valerian: they may increase the drug's sedative effects.

Asthma If you are taking theophylline then **avoid** charcoal and guarana: they decrease the drug's effects; **avoid** St John's wort: it may lower blood levels of the drug; **avoid** ephedra: it intensifies the drug's effects.

Auto-immune disorder, *or inflammatory disease such as tendinitis, or allergies or asthma* If you are taking aspirin or other nonsteroidal anti-inflammatory drugs then **avoid** ginkgo: it may increase the blood-thinning effects of these medications.

Congestive heart failure *or atrial fibrillation* If you are taking cardiac glycosides such as digitoxin or digoxin (Lanoxin) then **avoid** most herbal medicines because these conditions are not suitable for self-medication: you should not take anything without professional consultation.

Constipation If you are taking laxative drugs such as docusate (Dioctyl) or macrogol (Movicol) then **avoid** aloe, cascara sagrada, plantain, rhubarb, senna and yellow dock: they also have a laxative effect.

Cough If you are taking codeine, **avoid** tannic herbs like uva-ursi, black or green tea and raspberry leaf tea: they may inhibit drug absorption.

Depression If you are taking SSRI (selective serotonin reuptake inhibitor) antidepressants such as fluoxetine (Prozac), sertraline (Lustral) or paroxetine (Seroxat), **avoid** herbs that affect nervous system or mood: they may increase the drug's effects and cause excess sedation, lethargy or confusion. If you are taking MAOI (mono amine oxidase inhibitor) antidepressants such as phenelzine (Nardil), **avoid** butcher's broom, capsicum, galanthamine, ginkgo, ginseng and tonka: they may increase the drug's effects or cause toxic reactions.

Epilepsy If you are taking carbamazepine (Tegretol), or phenytoin (Epanutin) then **avoid** St John's wort: it lowers blood levels of the drugs.

Headache or fatigue If you are taking drugs containing caffeine such as Pro-Plus or Do-Do, **avoid** creatine: it decreases the drug's effects. Also **avoid** Asian ginseng, ephedra, guarana, yerba maté and yohimbe: they exacerbate anxiety, insomnia, high blood pressure and rapid heart rate.

Heart attack, *atrial fibrillation, venous thrombosis, pulmonary embolism or stroke* If you are taking anticoagulants then **avoid** most herbal medicines. If you have any of these conditions you should not take anything – even supplements – without talking to your doctor first.

Heartburn *caused by gastro-oesophageal reflux disease* Avoid menthol-containing herbs such as peppermint: they may make the reflux worse.

High blood pressure If you are taking diuretics such as furosemide (Lasix) or indapamide (Natrilix) then **avoid** buchu, cornsilk, dandelion, uva-ursi and yarrow: they are diuretic and will increase the drug's effects.

High blood pressure *or congestive heart failure* If you are taking calcium channel blockers such as amlodipine (Istin), diltiazem (Tildiem) and nifedipine (Adalat); or felodipine (Plendil), then **avoid** grapefruit juice: it boosts absorption of these drugs. If you are taking any of the above, or ACE inhibitors like captopril (Capoten) or enalapril (Innovace), **avoid** most herbal medicines: they may alter the drug's effects.

High cholesterol If you are taking HMG-CoA reductase inhibitors or statins such as atorvastatin (Lipitor), simvastatin (Zocor) or pravastatin (Lipostat) then **avoid** grapefruit juice: it can inhibit intestinal enzymes that help your body to absorb the drug.

Menopausal symptoms If you are taking ethinylestrodiol, conjugated oestrogens (Premarin) or estradiol (Climagest, Cyclo-Progynova) then **avoid** grapefruit juice: it boosts absorption of the drug. If you are taking conjugated oestrogens (Premarin) also **avoid** isoflavone-containing herbs such as red clover: they may cause hormone overload.

Neuralgia If you are taking carbamazepine (Tegretol) then **avoid** St John's wort: it lowers blood levels of the drug.

Nicotine addiction If you are taking drugs containing nicotine then **avoid** blue cohosh: it increases the drug's effects.

Oral contraception If you use oestrogen-containing pills or patches then **avoid** St John's wort: it may reduce contraceptive effectiveness.

Pain If you are taking aspirin then **avoid** ginkgo, horse chestnut, poplar and wintergreen: they may over-thin the blood.

PANEL OF ADVISORS

ACNE **James E. Fulton Jr., M.D., Ph.D.,** is a dermatologist and founder of the Acne Research Institute in Newport Beach, California. He is also c-oauthor of *Dr Fulton's Step-by-Step Programme for Clearing Acne* and co-discoverer of Retin-A (synthetic vitamin A), a prescription drug used to treat a variety of skin problems. **Thomas Gossel, Ph.D., R.Ph.,** is a professor of pharmacology and toxicology at Ohio Northern University in Ada. He is an expert on over-the-counter products. **Peter E. Pochi, M.D.,** is a former professor of dermatology at Boston University School of Medicine. **Douglas Schar, M.C.P.P., M.N.I.M.H.,** is a clinical herbalist practising in London and Washington, DC. He is herbal advisor to *Prevention* magazine and author of *Thirty Plants That Could Save Your Life* and *Backyard Medicine Chest*. An expert in herbs for disease prevention, he is finishing his Ph.D. in herbal medicine at Exeter University. **Maurice Stein** is a cosmetologist and Hollywood makeup artist. He is the owner of Cinema Secrets, a full-service beauty supplier for the public and a theatrical beauty supplier for the entertainment industry in Burbank, California.

ADDICTION **Stephen Amiel, M.A., M.R.C.G.P., D.R.C.O.G.,** is a GP in London working as a family doctor in a large practice of 12,500 patients. In addition to teaching medical students and GPs-in-training, he is co-editor of a textbook on family violence and has broadcast extensively on health matters. **Peter A. DeMaria Jr., M.D.,** is an associate professor of psychiatry and human behaviour in the division of substance abuse programmes at Jefferson Medical College of Thomas Jefferson University in Philadelphia. **Tom Horvath, Ph.D.,** is president of Practical Recovery Services, an addiction treatment centre in La Jolla, California, and president of SMART Recovery, an abstinence-oriented support group for those with addictive behaviours.

AGE SPOTS **C. Ralph Daniel III, M.D.,** is a clinical professor of dermatology at the University of Mississippi Medical Center in Jackson. **Mitchel Goldman, M.D.,** is an associate clinical professor in the division of dermatology at the University of California, San Diego, School of Medicine. **Audrey Kunin, M.D.,** is a cosmetic dermatologist from Kansas City, Missouri, and the founder of the dermatology educational website DERMAdoctor.com. **Nelson Lee Novick, M.D.,** is an associate clinical professor of dermatology at the Mount Sinai-New York University Medical Center in New York City.

ALLERGIES **Stephen Amiel**, see Addiction. **David Lang, M.D.,** is the section chief of allergy and immunology at Thomas Jefferson University, Philadelphia. **Thomas Platts-Mills, M.D.,** is a professor of medicine and head of the allergy and immunology division at the University of Virginia Medical Center in Charlottesville. **Richard Podell, M.D.,** is associate clinical professor in the dept. of family medicine at the University of Medicine and Dentistry of New Jersey-Robert Wood Johnson Medical School in Piscataway.

ALOPECIA **Stephen Amiel,** see Addiction. **Sue Livingston B.Pharm., M.R.PharmS., Ph.D.,** is a pharmacist and medical writer based in London. **Douglas Schar,** see Acne.

ANAL FISSURES **Stephen Amiel,** see Addiction. **John A. Flatley, M.D.,** is a colorectal surgeon in Kansas City, Missouri, where he also served as a clinical instructor of surgery at the University of Missouri-Kansas City School of Medicine. **J. Byron Gathright Jr., M.D.,** is chairman emeritus of the department of colon and rectal surgery at the Ochsner Clinic Foundation and clinical professor of surgery at Tulane University, both in New Orleans. He is also past president of the American Society of Colon and Rectal Surgeons, and Secretary General of the International Society of University Colon and Rectal Surgeons. **John O. Lawder, M.D.,** is a family practitioner specializing in nutrition and preventive medicine in Torrance, California. **Edmund Leff, M.D.,** is a colon and rectal surgeon in Phoenix and Scottsdale, Arizona. **Marvin Schuster, M.D.,** is director emeritus of the Marvin M. Schuster Center for Digestive and Motility Disorders at the Hopkins Bayview Medical Center, and professor emeritus of medicine and psychiatry at Johns Hopkins University School of Medicine, both in Baltimore. **Lewis R. Townsend, M.D.,** is a clinical instructor of obstetrics and gynaecology at Georgetown University Hospital and former director of the physicians' group at Columbia Hospital for Women Medical Center, both in Washington, DC.

ANGINA **Stephen Amiel,** see Addiction. **David M. Capuzzi, M.D., Ph.D.,** is a professor of medicine, biochemistry, and molecular pharmacology and director of the Cardiovascular Disease Prevention Center at Thomas Jefferson University Hospital in Philadelphia. **Kristine Napier, R.D.,** is nutrition director of Nutrio.com, author of *Eat to Heal*, and co-author of *Eat Away Diabetes*. **Howard Weitz, M.D.,** is co-director of the Jefferson Heart Institute of Thomas Jefferson University Hospital and deputy chairman of the department of medicine at Jefferson Medical College, both in Philadelphia.

ANXIETY **Edward M. Hallowell, M.D.,** is a psychiatrist and founder of the Hallowell Center for Cognitive and Emotional Health in Sudbury, Massachusetts. He is the author of *Worry: Hope and Help for a Common Condition* and *Connect: 12 Vital Ties That Open Your Heart, Lengthen Your Life, and Deepen Your Soul*. **Douglas Schar,** see Acne. **Bernard Vittone, M.D.,** is a psychiatrist and founder of the National Center for the Treatment of Phobias, Anxiety, and Depression in Washington, DC. **Andrew Weil, M.D.,** is a clinical professor of medicine and director of the programme in integrative medicine at the University of Arizona in Tucson. He is the author of several books, including *8 Weeks to Optimum Health*.

ASTHMA **Stephen Amiel,** see Addiction. **Kendall Gerdes, M.D.,** is director of Environmental Medicine Associates in Denver. **Elson Haas, M.D.,** is director of the Preventive Medical Center of Marin, an integrated healthcare facility in San Rafael, California, and author of seven books on health and nutrition, including *The False Fat Diet* and *Staying Healthy with Nutrition*. **Thomas F. Plaut, M.D.,** is consultant to *Asthma Update* newsletter and author of *Dr Tom Plaut's Asthma Guide for People of All Ages* and *One-Minute Asthma*.

ATHLETE'S FOOT
Diana Bihova, M.D., is a dermatologist affiliated with the dermatology department at the Columbia University College of Physicians and Surgeons in New York City. **Glenn Copeland, D.P.M.,** is a podiatrist at the Women's College Hospital in Toronto. He is also consulting podiatrist for the Canadian Back Institute and a podiatrist for the Toronto Blue Jays baseball team. **Thomas Goodman Jr., M.D.,** is a dermatologist and former assistant professor of dermatology at the University of Tennessee Health Science Center in Memphis. He is the author of *Smart Face*. **Frederick Hass, M.D.,** is a GP in San Rafael, California. He is on the staff of Marin General Hospital in Greenbrae. **Neal Kramer, D.P.M.,** is a podiatrist in Bethlehem, Pennsylvania. **Suzanne M. Levine, D.P.M., P.C.,** is a podiatrist and a podiatric attending physician at New York-Presbyterian Hospital. She is the author of *Your Feet Don't Have to Hurt*. **Sue Livingston,** see Alopecia. **Dean S. Stern, D.P.M.,** is a podiatrist at Rush-Presbyterian-St Luke's Medical Center in Chicago.

BACKACHE
Edward Abraham, M.D., is an assistant clinical professor of orthopaedics at the University of California, Irvine, College of Medicine, and has a practice in Santa Ana. He originated the concept for outpatient back therapy in the United States. **Stephen Amiel,** see Addiction. **Richard A. Deyo, M.D.,** is a professor of medicine and health services and director of the Center for Cost and Outcomes Research at the University of Washington in Seattle. **Milton Fried, M.D.,** is the founder and director of the Milton Fried Medical Clinic in Atlanta. He also holds degrees in chiropractic and physical therapy. **David Lehrman, M.D.,** is an orthopaedic surgeon affiliated with Mount Sinai Hospital and the Miami Heart Institute in Miami Beach, Florida. **Ronald Melzack, Ph.D.,** is a professor emeritus of psychology at McGill University in Montreal. **Roger Minkow, M.D.,** is a back specialist and founder and director of Backworks, a rehabilitation facility for people with back injuries, in Petaluma, California. **Dennis Turk, Ph.D.,** is the John and Emma Bonica professor of anaesthesiology and pain research at the University of Washington in Seattle.

BAD BREATH
Stephen Amiel, see Addiction. **Roger P. Levin, D.D.S.,** is the chief executive officer of the Levin Group, a dental practice in Baltimore. **Douglas Schar,** see Acne. **Eric Shapira, D.D.S.,** is an assistant clinical professor and lecturer at the University of the Pacific School of Dentistry in San Francisco and a dentist in Half Moon Bay, California. **Jerry F. Taintor, D.D.S.,** is chairman of endodontics at the University of Tennessee College of Dentistry in Memphis. He is the author of *The Complete Guide to Better Dental Care*.

BED-WETTING
Stephen Amiel, see Addiction. **Linda Jonides** is a paediatric nurse practitioner in Ann Arbor, Michigan. **Anne Price** is a former educational coordinator for the National Academy of Nannies, Inc. (NANI) in Denver. **Bryan Shumaker, M.D.,** is a urologist at Michigan Institute of Urology in St Claire Shores, Michigan.

BELCHING
André Dubois, M.D., is a gastroenterologist in Bethesda, Maryland. **Samuel Klein, M.D.,** is a William H. Danforth professor of medicine and nutritional science and director of the Center for Human Nutrition at Washington University School of Medicine in St. Louis. **Richard McCallum, M.D.,** is a professor of medicine and chief of the gastroenterology and hepatology division at the University of Kansas Medical Center and the Kansas City Veterans Administration Medical Center in Kansas City, Kansas. **Douglas Schar,** see Acne. **Marvin Schuster, M.D.,** see Anal Fissures.

BITES, SCRATCHES AND STINGS
Stephen Amiel, see Addiction. **Joseph Benforado, M.D.,** is a professor emeritus of medicine at the University of Wisconsin-Madison and past vice president of the US Pharmacopoeia, which sets American drug standards. **Claude Frazier, M.D.,** is an allergist in Asheville, North Carolina. **David Golden, M.D.,** is an associate professor of medicine at Johns Hopkins University in Baltimore. **Richard Hansen, M.D.,** is past medical director of the Poland Spring Health Institute in Poland Spring, Maine. He is author of *Get Well at Home*. **Herbert Luscombe, M.D.,** is a professor emeritus of dermatology at Jefferson Medical College of Thomas Jefferson University, Philadelphia. He is also formerly senior attending dermatologist at Thomas Jefferson University Hospital, Philadelphia. **Edgar Raffensperger, Ph.D.,** is a professor emeritus of entomology in the department of entomology at Cornell University in Ithaca, New York. **Stephen Rosenberg, M.D.,** is an associate professor of clinical public health at Columbia University School of Public Health in New York City. He is the author of *The Johnson & Johnson First-Aid Book*. **Douglas Schar,** see Acne.

BLACK EYE
Jack Jeffers, M.D., is an ophthalmologist and director of emergency services at the Sports Center for Vision at Wills Eye Hospital, Philadelphia. **Douglas Schar,** see Acne. **Keith Sivertson, M.D.,** is director of the department of emergency medicine at Johns Hopkins Hospital, Baltimore. **David J. Smith, M.D.,** is an ophthalmologist in Ventnor City, New Jersey, and a member of the Medical Advisory Council of the State Athletic Control Board of the State of New Jersey. He is also on the medical team at the Sports Center for Vision at Wills Eye Hospital, Philadelphia. He has examined more than 300 boxers for eye injuries. **Anne Sumers, M.D.,** is team ophthalmologist for the New York Giants and the New Jersey Nets in addition to operating an ophthalmology practice in Ridgewood, New Jersey. She serves as spokesperson for the American Academy of Ophthalmology.

BLISTERS
Nancy Lu Conrad, D.P.M., is a private practitioner in Circleville, Ohio. She specializes in

footwear for children as well as in sports medicine and orthopaedics. **Richard M. Cowin, D.P.M.,** is a private practitioner and director of Advanced Foot Surgery in Lady Lake, Florida, where he specializes in the practice of minimal incision and laser foot and ankle surgery. He is a diplomate of the American Board of Podiatric Surgery and the American Board of Ambulatory Foot Surgery. **Joseph Ellis, D.P.M.,** is a private practitioner in La Jolla, California. He is a consultant for the University of California, San Diego, and is the sports medicine consultant for the Asics-Tiger running shoe company. **Douglas Richie Jr., D.P.M.,** is a sports podiatrist in Seal Beach, California, where he studies the function of socks and their effect on sporting activities. He also is a director of the American Academy of Podiatric Sports Medicine. **Clare Starrett, D.P.M.,** is a professor at the Temple University School of Podiatric Medicine in Philadelphia. **Suzanne Tanner, M.D.,** is a private practitioner in Denver, who specializes in sports medicine.

BODY ODOUR

Lenise Banse, M.D., is a dermatologist in Clinton Township, Michigan, where she is director of the Northeast Family Dermatology Center. She has special expertise in cutaneous oncology as well as cosmetic dermatology. **Hridaya Bhargava, Ph.D.,** is a professor of industrial pharmacy at the Massachusetts College of Pharmacy in Boston. He is a consultant to groups such as the World Health Organization and UNICEF. **Nathan Howe, M.D., Ph.D.,** is formerly a physician in the department of dermatology at the Medical University of South Carolina College of Medicine in Charleston. He was also a zoologist with a special interest in how animals communicate using chemical smells. **Randall Hrabko, M.D.,** is a dermatologist in Los Angeles. **Kenzo Sato, M.D.,** is a professor emeritus of dermatology at the University of Iowa in Iowa City. **Douglas Schar,** see Acne.

BOILS

Rodney Basler, M.D., is a dermatologist and assistant professor of internal medicine at the University of Nebraska College of Medicine in Lincoln. **Michael Blate** is founder and executive director of the G-Jo Institute of Columbus, North Carolina, a natural health organization that promotes acupressure and oriental traditional medicine. **Adrian Connolly, M.D.,** is a dermatologist/Mohs surgeon in private practice in West Orange, New Jersey, and a member of the American Academy of Dermatology.

BREAST PAIN

Stephen Amiel, see Addiction. **Ellen Kamhi, R.N., Ph.D.,** of Oyster Bay, New York, is the author of *The Natural Medicine Chest, Arthritis: An Alternative Medicine Definitive Guide,* and *Cycles of Life.* She hosts radio and TV shows nationally. **Kerry McGinn, R.N., N.P.,** is a staff nurse at Kaiser Permanente South San Francisco; the author of *The Informed Woman's Guide to Breast Health*; and co-author of *Women's Cancers.* **Christiane Northrup, M.D.,** is an assistant clinical professor of obstetrics and gynaecology at the University of Vermont College of Medicine in Burlington and a former president of the American Holistic Medical Association. She practises medicine at Women to Women, a health care centre in Yarmouth, Maine. **Gregory Radio, M.D.,** is a practising obstetrician-gynaecologist and chairman of

primary care and the department of obstetrics and gynaecology at Lehigh Valley Hospital in Allentown, Pennsylvania. **Thomas J. Smith, M.D.,** is a chief of surgical oncology and director of the Breast Health Center at New England Medical Center in Boston. He is also associate professor of surgery at Tufts University School of Medicine, also in Boston. **Sandra Swain, M.D.,** is a former assistant professor of medicine at Georgetown University and former director of the Comprehensive Breast Service of the Vincent Lombardi Cancer Center at Georgetown University School of Medicine in Washington, D.C. **Yvonne S. Thornton, M.D.,** is a maternal foetal medicine specialist and associate clinical professor of obstetrics and gynaecology at Columbia University College of Physicians and Surgeons in New York City. She is also director of the Perinatal Center at St. Luke's Hospital, also in New York City.

BREASTFEEDING

Stephen Amiel, see Addiction. **Kittie Frantz, R.N., C.P.N.P.,** is director of the Breast-Feeding Infant Clinic at the University of Southern California Medical Center in Los Angeles and a paediatric nurse practitioner. She has been working with nursing mothers since 1963. She also spent 20 years as a leader for La Leche League International. **Carolyn Rawlins, M.D.,** is an obstetrician in Munster, Indiana, and a former member of La Leche League International board of directors. **Julie Stock** is medical information liaison for La Leche League International, a support group for breastfeeding mothers.

BRONCHITIS

Stephen Amiel, see Addiction. **Barbara Phillips, M.D.,** is a pulmonologist and associate professor of pulmonary medicine at the University of Kentucky College of Medicine in Lexington. **Douglas Schar,** see Acne. **Daniel Simmons, M.D.,** is a pulmonologist and professor of medicine in the division of pulmonary disease at the UCLA School of Medicine in Los Angeles. **Gordon L. Snider, M.D.,** is a professor of medicine at Boston University School of Medicine and Tufts University School of Medicine in Boston. He is also a pulmonologist and chief of medicinal service at the Boston Veterans Administration Medical Center.

BRUISES

Stephen Amiel, see Addiction. **Sharleen Andrews-Miller** is a herbalist and a faculty member at the National College of Naturopathic Medicine in Portland, Oregon, and medicinary botanical educator at the college's public clinic. **Hugh Macaulay, M.D.,** is an emergency room physician at Aspen Valley Hospital in Aspen. **Sheldon V. Pollack, M.D.,** is a dermatologist and former associate professor of medicine in the division of dermatology at Duke University School of Medicine in Durham, North Carolina.

BURNOUT

Karen Bierman, Ph.D., is a psychologist in Beverly Hills, California. **Peter S. Moskowitz, M.D.,** is the director of the Center for Professional and Personal Renewal in Palo Alto, California. He conducts workshops and lectures and provides career/life coaching for physicians and other professionals on stress management and related life-balance issues. **Jack N. Singer, Ph.D.,** is an industrial/organizational and consulting psychologist and a professional speaker who specializes in burnout. He is author of *Conquering Your Internal Critic So You Can Sing Your Own Song*. He lives in California. **Melissa Stöppler, M.D.**, writes the stress-management column for the website About.com. A consultant on stress and health issues, she is a pathologist at the University of Marburg in Germany.

BURNS Stephen Amiel, see Addiction. **William P. Burdick, M.D.**, is a professor of emergency medicine at MCP Hahnemann University School of Medicine in Philadelphia. **John J. Caimi, D.M.D.**, is a dentist in Ridgway, Pennsylvania. He has been in practice for more than 23 years. **John Gillies, E.M.T.**, is a former emergency medical technician and programme director for health services at the Colorado Outward Bound School in Denver. **Kimberly Harms, D.D.S.**, is a dentist in Farmington, Minnesota, and a consumer advisor for the American Dental Association. **Van B. Haywood, D.M.D.**, is a professor at the Medical College of the Georgia School of Dentistry in Augusta.

BURSITIS Stephen Amiel, see Addiction. **Alan Bensman, M.D.**, is a physiotherapist at Rehabilitative Health Services, P.A., in Golden Valley, Minnesota. **Alison Lee, M.D.**, is medical director of the Barefoot Doctors in Ann Arbor, Michigan, and a specialist in acupuncture and pain management. **Edward Resnick, M.D.**, is an orthopaedic surgeon and director of the Pain Control Center at Temple University Hospital in Philadelphia. **Allan Tomson, D.C.**, is a chiropractor with the Natural Horizons Wellness Center in Fairfax, Virginia.

CALLUSES AND CORNS Nancy Lu Conrad, see Blisters. **Richard M. Cowin, D.P.M.**, see Blisters. **Frederick Hass, M.D.**, see Athlete's Foot. **Neal Kramer, D.P.M.**, is a podiatrist in Bethlehem, Pennsylvania. **Suzanne M. Levine, D.P.M., P.C.**, see Athlete's Foot. **Elizabeth H. Roberts, D.P.M.**, has spent more than 30 years as a prominent podiatrist in New York City, where she is professor emeritus at the New York College of Podiatric Medicine. **Marvin Sandler, D.P.M.**, is a podiatrist in Allentown, Pennsylvania. He was formerly chief of podiatric surgery at Sacred Heart Hospital in Allentown. **Terry L. Spilken, D.P.M.**, is a podiatrist in New York City and Edison, New Jersey. He is on the adjunct faculty of the New York College of Podiatric Medicine in New York City. **Mark D. Sussman, D.P.M.**, is a retired podiatrist who formerly practised in Wheaton, Maryland.

CARPAL TUNNEL SYNDROME Stephen Cash, M.D., is an assistant clinical professor of orthopaedic surgery in the division of hand surgery at Jefferson Medical College of Thomas Jefferson University in Philadelphia and a staff member of the Hand Rehabilitation Center there. **Colin Hall, M.D.**, is a professor of neurology and medicine and director of the neuromuscular unit in the department of neurology at the University of North Carolina at Chapel Hill School of Medicine. **Susan Isernhagen** is a physical therapist and president of Isernhagen Work Systems in Duluth, Minnesota. She acts as a consultant to industries to help reduce work injuries and rehabilitate injured workers.

CHAFING Tom Barringer, M.D., is a family physician in Charlotte, North Carolina. **Robert Boyce, Ph.D.**, is an expert in exercise physiology and owner of Robert Boyce Health Promotion, Charlotte, North Carolina. **Richard H. Strauss, M.D.**, is formerly a sports medicine doctor at Ohio State University College of Medicine and Public Health, Columbus.

CHAPPED HANDS Joseph Bark, M.D., is a dermatologist in Lexington, Kentucky, and the author of *Your Skin...An Owner's Guide*, see Boils. **Diana Bihova, M.D.**, see Athlete's Foot. **Howard Donsky, M.D.**, is a clinical instructor of dermatology at the University of Rochester and a dermatologist at the Dermatology and Cosmetic Center of Rochester in New York. **Thomas Goodman Jr., M.D.**, see Athlete's Foot. **Nelson Lee Novick, M.D.**, see Age Spots. **Stephen Schleicher, M.D.**, is medical director of DERM DX Centers for Dermatology, Inc. in Hazleton, Pennsylvania, with offices throughout eastern Pennsylvania. He is also an advisor for dermatological training to physician assistant students at Arcadia University in Glenside and at King's College in Wilkes-Barre. **Lia Schorr** is a skin-care specialist and director of Lia Schorr Institute of Cosmetics Skin-Care Training in New York City. **Trisha Webster** is a top New York City hand model formerly with the Wilhelmina, Inc. modeling agency. She has almost 20 years of experience in the business.

CHAPPED LIPS Stephen Amiel, see Addiction. **Joseph Bark**, see Chapped Hands. **Rodney Basler**, see Boils. **Diana Bihova**, see Athlete's Foot. **Thomas Goodman Jr.**, see Athlete's Foot. **Nelson Lee Novick, M.D.**, is associate clinical professor of dermatology at the Mount Sinai-New York University Medical Center, New York City. **Glenn Roberts** is director of creative beauty at Elizabeth Arden, New York City.

COLD SORES Stephen Amiel, see Addiction. **Milos Chvapil, M.D., Ph.D.**, is a professor emeritus of surgery in the surgical biology section of the University of Arizona College of Medicine in Tucson. **David H. Emmert, M.D.**, is a family physician in Millersville, Pennsylvania, who, in 2000, summarized cold sore treatments for the medical journal *American Family Physician*. **Richard T. Glass, D.D.S., Ph.D.**, is director of the forensic graduate programme and professor of oral pathology at Oklahoma State University, College of Osteopathic Medicine in Tulsa, Oklahoma. He is professor emeritus from the University of Oklahoma, Colleges of Dentistry, Graduate, and Medicine where he was professor and chairman of the department of oral and maxillofacial pathology and professor of pathology. **Mark A. McCune, M.D.**, is a dermatologist in Overland Park, Kansas. He is chief of dermatology at Humana Hospital in Overland Park. **James F. Rooney, M.D.**, is a clinical virologist and formerly a special expert in the Laboratory of Oral Medicine at the National Institutes of Health in Bethesda, Maryland. **Cal Vanderplate, Ph.D.**, is a clinical faculty member at Emory University School of Medicine in Atlanta and a clinical psychologist specializing in stress-related disorders.

COLDS Stephen Amiel, see Addiction. **Diane Casdorph, R.Ph.,** is an assistant clinical professor and assistant director of the Drug Information Center of the West Virginia University School of Pharmacy in Morgantown. **Samuel Caughron, M.D.,** is an assistant clinical professor in family medicine at the University of Virginia in Charlottesville and a member of the Albemarle Medical Association. **Elliot Dick, Ph.D.,** is a retired virologist and professor of preventive medicine at the University of Wisconsin-Madison. He has conducted research on the common cold for more than 30 years. **Elson Haas, M.D.,** see Asthma. **Sue Livingston,** see Alopecia. **Kenneth Peters, M.D.,** is medical director of the Northern California Headache Clinic in Mountain View. He also practises general internal medicine at El Camino Hospital, also in Mountain View. He has published numerous articles on effective headache management and has done extensive clinical research in the area of new headache medications. **Martin Rossman, M.D.,** is a general practitioner in Mill Valley, California, and author of *Guided Imagery for Self-Healing*. **Douglas Schar,** see Acne. **Keith W. Sehnert, M.D.,** was a physician with Trinity Health Care in Minneapolis and author of several books, including *The Garden Within* and *How to Be Your Own Doctor (Sometimes)*. **Timothy Van Ert, M.D.,** is a staff physician at Western Oregon University in Monmouth, Oregon, where he specializes in self-care and preventive medicine.

CONJUNCTIVITIS Stephen Amiel, see Addiction. **Peter Hersh, M.D.,** is an ophthalmologist and former assistant surgeon in the department of ophthalmology at Massachusetts Eye and Ear Infirmary in Boston. He is also former instructor of ophthalmology at Harvard Medical School. **J. Daniel Nelson, M.D.,** is an ophthalmologist at Regions Medical Center, St Paul, Minnesota. **Robert Petersen, M.D.,** is assistant professor of ophthalmology at Harvard Medical School. He is also a paediatric ophthalmologist and director of the Eye Clinic at Boston Children's Hospital.

CONSTIPATION Alison Crane, R.N., is the founder of the American Association for Therapeutic Humour. **Edward R. Eichner, M.D.,** is an expert in the effects of exercise on the human body, a professor of medicine, and team internist at the University of Oklahoma Health Sciences Center in Oklahoma City. **Patricia H. Harper, M.S., R.D.,** is a research nutritionist at the University of Pittsburgh School of Medicine. She also coordinates diabetes and weight-loss programmes there. **John O. Lawder, M.D.,** is a family practitioner specializing in nutrition and preventive medicine in Torrance, California. **Paul Rousseau, M.D.,** is associate chief of the department of geriatrics and extended care at the Phoenix Veterans Affairs Medical Center in Phoenix. **Douglas Schar,** see Acne. **Marvin Schuster,** see Anal Fissures. **Lewis R. Townsend, M.D.,** is a clinical instructor of obstetrics and gynaecology at Georgetown University Hospital and former director of the physicians' group at the Columbia Hospital for Women Medical Center, both in Washington, DC.

COUGHS Stephen Amiel, see Addiction. **Anne Davis, M.D.,** is an associate professor of clinical medicine at New York University School of Medicine and attending physician at the Chest Service at Bellevue Hospital Center, both in New York City. **Stuart Ditchek, M.D.,** is a paediatrician and assistant professor of paediatrics at New York University School of Medicine in New York City and co-author of *Healthy Child, Whole Child*.

CUTS AND GRAZES Stephen Amiel, see Addiction. **John Gillies, E.M.T.,** is a former emergency medical technician and programme director for health services at the Colorado Outward Bound School in Denver. **Hugh Macaulay, M.D.,** is an emergency room physician at Aspen Valley Hospital in Aspen. **Patricia Mertz** is a former research associate professor in the department of dermatology and cutaneous surgery at the University of Miami School of Medicine in Florida. **Douglas Schar,** see Acne.

DANDRUFF Diana Bihova, M.D., see Athlete's Foot. **Howard Donsky, M.D.,** see Chapped Hands. **Patricia Farris, M.D.,** is an assistant clinical professor of dermatology at Tulane University School of Medicine in New Orleans and a dermatologist in Metairie, Louisiana. **Joseph F. Fowler Jr., M.D.,** is an assistant professor of dermatology at the University of Louisville and a dermatologist in Louisville. In addition, he is a member of the North American Contact Dermatitis Group, an elite skin-allergy research group. **Louis Gignac** is a hairstylist and the owner of the Stella Salons in New York City and Miami. **R. Jeffrey Herten, M.D.,** is an assistant clinical professor of dermatology at the University of California, Irvine, College of Medicine. **Maria Hordinsky, M.D.,** is an assistant professor of dermatology at the University of Minnesota Medical School-Minneapolis and a dermatologist in Minneapolis. **Philip Kingsley** is a trained trichologist who maintains salons in New York City and London. He's also the hair columnist for the style section of *The Times*, London and the author of *Hair: An Owner's Handbook* **Douglas Schar,** see Acne.

DENTURE PROBLEMS George A. Murrell, D.D.S., is a retired prosthodontist in Manhattan Beach, California. He also has taught at the University of Southern California School of Dentistry, Los Angeles. **Eric Shapira,** see Bad Breath. **Richard Shepard, D.D.S.,** is a retired dentist in Durango, Colorado. He is also executive director of the Holistic Dental Association. **Jerry F. Taintor,** see Bad Breath.

DEPRESSION Edward M. Hallowell, see Anxiety. **Douglas Schar,** see Acne. **Bernard Vittone,** see Anxiety. **Andrew Weil,** see Anxiety.

DERMATITIS AND ECZEMA Howard Donsky, see Chapped Hands. **Sue Livingston,** see Alopecia. **Hillard H. Pearlstein, M.D.,** is an assistant clinical professor of dermatology at the Mount Sinai School of Medicine of New York University in New York City. **John F. Romano, M.D.,** is a dermatologist and an assistant clinical professor of dermatology at New York Hospital-Cornell University Medical Center in New York City.

DIABETES Stephen Amiel, see Addiction. **Marc A. Brenner, D.P.M.,** is director of the Institute of Diabetic Foot Research in Glendale, New York; past president of the American Society of Podiatric Dermatology and author and editor of various books. **Marion Franz, M.S., R.D.,** is a nutrition consultant in Minneapolis and co-chairman of the American Diabetes Association's task force to revise nutrition principle recommendations. **Robert Hanisch** is the senior medical exercise physiologist and certified diabetes educator with the Diabetes Treatment Center at Columbia-St Mary's Hospital in Milwaukee. **Angele McGrady, Ph.D.,** is a professor in the department of psychiatry and the director of the Complementary Medicine Center at the Medical College of Ohio in Toledo. **Carla Miller, Ph.D., R.D.,** is an assistant professor in the department of nutrition and co-director of the Diet Assessment Center, both at Pennsylvania State University in University Park. **Harry G. Preuss, M.D.,** is a diabetes researcher and professor of physiology, medicine, and pathology at Georgetown University Medical Center in Washington, DC. **Christopher D. Saudek, M.D.,** is president of the American Diabetes Association and director of Johns Hopkins Diabetes Center in Baltimore. **Aaron I. Vinik, M.D., Ph.D.,** is a professor of internal medicine, pathology, and neurobiology at the Eastern Virginia Medical School and director of the Strelitz Diabetes Research Institute, both in Norfolk.

DIARRHOEA Stephen Bezruchka, M.D., is an emergency physician at Virginia Mason Hospital and Group Health Hospital in Seattle and an affiliate associate professor in the School of Public Health and Community Medicine at the University of Washington in Seattle. **William Y. Chey, M.D.,** is director of the Rochester Institute for Digestive Diseases and Sciences and a physician in Rochester. He is a former professor of medicine at the University of Rochester School of Medicine and Dentistry in New York. **Harris Clearfield, M.D.,** is a professor of medicine and section chief of the division of gastroenterology at Hahnemann University Hospital in Philadelphia. **Thomas Gossel,** see Acne. **David A. Lieberman, M.D.,** is a gastroenterologist and associate professor of medicine at Oregon Health Sciences University School of Medicine in Portland. **Sue Livingston,** see Alopecia. **Lynn V. McFarland, Ph.D.,** is a former research associate with the department of medicinal chemistry at the University of Washington in Seattle and director of scientific affairs of Biocodex, Inc.

DIVERTICULOSIS Samuel Klein, see Belching. **Albert J. Lauro, M.D.,** is director of emergency medical services at Charity Hospital in New Orleans. **Craig Rubin, M.D.,** is a professor of internal medicine and chief of the geriatric section at the University of Texas Southwestern Medical Center at Dallas. **Marvin Schuster,** see Anal Fissures. **Paul Williamson, M.D.,** is an associate clinical professor of surgery at the University of Florida in Gainesville and a colon and rectal surgeon in Orlando.

DIZZINESS Terry D. Fife, M.D., is an associate professor of clinical neurology at the University of Arizona in Tucson and director of the Balance Center at Barrow Neurological Institute in Phoenix. **Joshua Hoffman, M.D.,** is an internist and medical director of Sutter Medical Group hospitalist programme in Sacramento, California.

DRY EYES Phillip J. Calenda, M.D., is an ophthalmologist in Scarsdale, New York. **Stephen C. Pflugfelder, M.D.,** is an ophthalmologist in Houston and a spokesman for the American Academy of Ophthalmology. **Anne Sumers,** see Black Eye.

DRY MOUTH Stephen Amiel, see Addiction. **Anne Bosy** is a dental hygienist and co-founder and clinical director at the Fresh Breath Clinic in Toronto. She is also a professor in the faculty of community services and health sciences at the George Brown College of Applied Arts and Technology in Toronto and a member of the International Society of Breath Odour Research. She has treated thousands of patients with dry mouth associated with bad breath. **John J. Caimi, D.M.D.,** is a dentist from Ridgway, Pennsylvania. He has been in practice for more than 23 years. **Dan Peterson, D.D.S.,** is a dentist from Gering, Nebraska. He has been in practice for more than 25 years and has treated numerous patients with dry mouth syndrome.

DRY SKIN AND WINTER ITCHING **Howard Donsky,** see Chapped Hands. **Kenneth Neldner, M.D.,** is a professor emeritus in the department of dermatology at the Texas Tech University School of Medicine in Lubbock. **Hillard H. Pearlstein,** see Dermatitis and Eczema.

EARACHE AND EAR INFECTION Stephen Amiel, see Addiction. **Gary D. Becker, M.D.,** is a staff physician at Kaiser Permanente Medical Center in Panorama City, California. **Dan Drew, M.D.,** is a physician in Indianapolis. He is also an avid swimmer. **Brian W. Hands, M.D.,** is an ear, nose, and throat specialist in Toronto. **John House, M.D.,** is a clinical professor of otolaryngology at the University of Southern California School of Medicine in Los Angeles. He serves as a national team physician for United States Swimming, the national governing association for competitive amateur swimming that selects the Olympic team. **Donald B. Kamerer, M.D.,** is a professor in the department of otolaryngology at the University of Pittsburgh School of Medicine. **Douglas Schar,** see Acne. **Dudley J. Weider, M.D.,** is an otolaryngologist at Dartmouth-Hitchcock Medical Center in Lebanon, New Hampshire.

EARWAX Stephen Amiel, see Addiction. **David Edelstein, M.D.,** is a clinical professor of otolaryngology at the Joan and Sanford I. Weill Medical College of Cornell University in New York City. **George W. Facer, M.D.,** is an otolaryngologist at the Mayo Clinic in Scottsdale, Arizona.

EMPHYSEMA Henry Gong, M.D., is a professor of medicine and preventive medicine at the University of Southern California in Los Angeles and chairman of the department of medicine at Rancho Los Amigos National Rehabilitation Center in Downey. **Francisco Perez, Ph.D.,** is an associate clinical professor of neurology and physical medicine at Baylor College of

Medicine in Houston. **Robert Sandhaus, M.D., Ph.D.,** is a pulmonary specialist, a clinical professor at the University of Colorado Health Sciences Center, director of Alpha-1 Clinic at the National Jewish Medical and Research Center, and executive vice president and medical director of the Alpha-1 Foundation and AlphaNet, all in Denver. **Robert B. Teague, M.D.,** is an associate professor of medicine at Baylor College of Medicine in Houston.

EYESTRAIN Samuel L. Guillory, M.D., is an ophthalmologist and associate clinical professor of ophthalmology at Mount Sinai School of Medicine of New York University in New York City. **David Guyton, M.D.,** is the Krieger professor of paediatric ophthalmology and director of the Krieger Children's Eye Center at the Wilmer Institute at the Johns Hopkins University School of Medicine in Baltimore. **Meir Schneider, Ph.D.,** is founder of the School for Self Healing in San Francisco. He is the author of *Self Healing: My Life and Vision* and co-author of *The Handbook of Self-Healing*.

FATIGUE Stephen Amiel, see Addiction. **William Fink** was formerly an exercise physiologist and assistant to the director of the Human Performance Laboratory at Ball State University in Muncie, Indiana. **M. F. Graham, M.D.,** is a paediatrician in Dallas and a former consultant to the American Running Association. **E. Drummond King** is a triathlete and a lawyer in Allentown, Pennsylvania. **Rick Ricer, M.D.,** is the vice chairman for educational affairs and a professor of family medicine at the University of Cincinnati in Ohio. **Douglas Schar,** see Acne. **David Sheridan, M.D.,** is the medical director at Palmetto Government Benefits Administrators in Columbia, South Carolina. **Mary Trafton** is a hiker, marathoner, and skier and a former information specialist for the Appalachian Mountain Club in Boston. **Vicky Young, M.D.,** is an occupational health doctor at the TriCity Medical Center Work Partners in Vista, California.

FEVER Eleonore Blaurock-Busch, Ph.D., is associate laboratory director of King James Medical Laboratory and Trace Minerals International, both in Cleveland. She is also the director of Micro Trace Minerals in Hersbruck, Germany; co-chairman of the International Association of Trace Elements and Cancer; and the author of several books. **Thomas Gossel,** see Acne. **Mary Ann Pane, R.N.,** is a nurse clinician in Philadelphia. She was formerly affiliated with Community Home Health Services, an agency catering to people who require skilled health care in their homes. **Stephen Rosenberg,** see Bites, Scratches and Stings.

FLATULENCE Stephen Amiel, see Addiction. **Samuel Klein,** see Belching. **Richard McCallum,** see Belching. **Dennis Savaiano, Ph.D.,** is a professor of foods and nutrition and dean of the School of Consumer and Family Sciences at Purdue University in West Lafayette, Indiana. **Douglas Schar,** see Acne. **Andrew Weil,** see Anxiety.

FLU Stephen Amiel, see Addiction. **Eleonore Blaurock-Busch,** see Fever. **Suzanne Gaventa** is an epidemiologist formerly in the division of viral diseases at the Centers for Disease Control and Prevention in Atlanta. **Thomas Gossel,** see Acne. **Mary Ann Pane,** see Fever. **Jay Swedberg, M.D.,** is a family practitioner at the Family Health Care, P.C., in Casper, Wyoming. **Calvin Thrash, M.D.,** was the founder of Uchee Pines Institute, a non-profit health education facility in Seale, Alabama. He is also co-author of *Breast Cancer: Causes, Prevention, and Treatment.* **Donald Vickery, M.D.,** is president of the Center for Corporate Health Promotion in Reston, Virginia. He is also assistant clinical professor of family medicine and community medicine at Georgetown University School of Medicine in Washington, DC., and associate clinical professor of family medicine at Virginia Commonwealth University School of Medicine in Richmond. He is the co-author of *Take Care of Yourself.*

FOOD POISONING Vincent F. Garagusi, M.D., is professor emeritus of medicine and microbiology and former director of the Infectious Disease Service at Georgetown University Hospital in Washington, DC. **Daniel C. Rodrigue, M.D.,** is an infectious disease specialist at Lexington Infectious Disease Consultants in Lexington, Kentucky.

FOOT ACHES Judith Jackson is a health and beauty consultant in Greenwich, Connecticut. She is also a certified aromatherapist with a degree in massage and aromatherapy. **Neal Kramer,** see Athlete's Foot. **Mark D. Sussman, D.P.M.,** is a retired podiatrist who formerly practised in Wheaton, Maryland. **John F. Waller Jr., M.D.,** is an orthopaedic surgeon specializing in the foot and ankle. He is attending surgeon in orthopaedic surgery at Lenox Hill Hospital, New York City. **Gilbert Wright, M.D.,** was an orthopaedic surgeon in Sacramento, California, and spokesman for the American Orthopaedic Foot and Ankle Society. He was also director of the Sacramento Orthopaedic Foot Clinic.

FOOT ODOUR Diana Bihova, see Athlete's Foot. **Glenn Copeland,** see Athlete's Foot. **Richard L. Dobson, M.D.,** is a professor emeritus of the department of dermatology at the Medical University of South Carolina College of Medicine in Charleston. **Frederick Hass,** see Athlete's Foot. **Neal Kramer,** see Athlete's Foot. **Suzanne M. Levine,** see Athlete's Foot. **Mark D. Sussman,** see Foot Aches. **Stephen Weinberg, D.P.M.,** is director of the running clinic at the Weil Foot and Ankle Institute in Des Plaines, Illinois, and director of podiatric services for the Chicago Marathon.

FROSTBITE Bruce Paton, M.D., is a former clinical professor of surgery at the University of Colorado in Denver. **Tod Schimelpfenig** is director of the Rocky Mountain division of the National Outdoor Leadership School in Lander, Wyoming. He also is a volunteer emergency medical technician. **James Sturm, M.D.,** is a former staff physician in the emergency medicine department at St Paul-Ramsey Medical Center in Minnesota. **Ruth Uphold, M.D.,** is medical director of the emergency department at Fletcher Allan Health Care in Burlington, Vermont

GENITAL HERPES

Stephen Amiel, see Addiction. **Mitch Herndon** is programme manager at the Herpes Resource Center and the National Herpes Hotline at the American Social Health Association (ASHA) in Research Triangle Park, North Carolina. **Judith M. Hurst, R.N.,** is medical advisor to Toledo HELP, a support group for people with herpes in Toledo, Ohio. She is also a retired obstetric nurse. **Stephen L. Sacks, M.D.,** is a professor of medicine at the University of British Columbia and the founder and president of the Viridae Clinic, both in Vancouver. He is also the founder and former director of the UBC Herpes Clinic. A renowned expert on the management of genital herpes, he is the author of *The Truth about Herpes*. **Douglas Schar,** see Acne. **C. Norman Shealy, M.D., Ph.D.,** heads the Shealy Wellness Center in Springfield, Missouri. He is also a professor of energy medicine at Holos University Graduate Seminary, the founding president of the American Holistic Medical Association, and the author of such books as *Sacred Healing* and *Holy Water, Sacred Oil*. **Christopher W. Stout, Ph.D.,** has a private practice near Denver and is a clinical psychologist specializing in psychoneuroimmunology (the study of the connection between the immune system and human emotions). He is also an industrial consultant. **Will Whittington, M.D.,** was a research investigator with the division of sexually transmitted diseases at the Centers for Disease Control and Prevention in Atlanta.

GINGIVITIS

Vincent Cali, D.D.S., is a New York City dentist and author of *The New, Lower-Cost Way to End Gum Trouble without Surgery*. He also has a postgraduate degree in clinical nutrition from the Fordham Page Institute at the University of Pennsylvania in Philadelphia. **Roger P. Levin,** see Bad Breath. **Robert Schallhorn, D.D.S.,** is a dentist in Aurora, Colorado, and past president of the American Academy of Periodontology. **Richard Shepard,** see Denture Problems.

GOUT

John Abruzzo, M.D., is director of the division of rheumatology and a professor of medicine at Thomas Jefferson University in Philadelphia. **Eleonore Blaurock-Busch,** see Fever. **Robert H. Davis, Ph.D.,** was a professor of physiology at the Pennsylvania College of Podiatric Medicine in Philadelphia. He is now retired. **Felix O. Kolb, M.D.,** is a clinical professor emeritus of medicine at the University of California, San Francisco, School of Medicine. **Branton Lachman, Pharm.D., J.D.,** is a practising attorney and consultant pharmacist in Corona, California. He has also taught at the University of Southern California School of Pharmacy, Western State College of Law, Southern California Law School, and within the California public school system. **Jeffrey R. Lisse, M.D.,** is a professor of medicine, head of clinical osteoporosis research, and associate chief of the Arthritis Center at the University of Arizona, Tucson. **Douglas Schar,** see Acne. **Gary Stoehr, Pharm.D.,** is an associate professor of pharmacy and associate dean for student and academic affairs at the University of Pittsburgh School of Pharmacy. **Agatha Thrash, M.D.,** is a pathologist who lectures worldwide. She is also co-founder of Uchee Pines Institute, a nonprofit health-training centre in Seale, Alabama, and author of many books.

Robert Wortmann, M.D., is a professor of medicine and chairman of the dept of internal medicine at the University of Oklahoma College of Medicine, Tulsa.

GREASY SKIN

Howard Donsky, see Chapped Hands. **Kenneth Neldner, M.D.,** see Dry Skin and Winter Itching. **Hillard H. Pearlstein,** see Dermatitis and Eczema.

HAEMORRHOIDS

Stephen Amiel, see Addiction. **J. Byron Gathright Jr.,** see Anal Fissures. **John O. Lawder,** see Anal Fissures. **Edmund Leff,** see Anal Fissures. **Douglas Schar,** see Acne. **Lewis R. Townsend,** see Constipation.

HAIR PROBLEMS

David Daines is a professional hairstylist at Salon in New York City. **Steven Docherty** is the former senior art director of New York City's Vidal Sassoon Salon. He has cared for the hair of some of New York's top magazine and television models. **Lowell Goldsmith, M.D.,** is a professor of dermatology and chairman of the department of dermatology at the University of Rochester School of Medicine and Dentistry in New York. He specializes in hair disorders. **Thomas Goodman Jr.,** see Athlete's Foot. **Joanne Harris** has created character hairstyles for some of Hollywood's top actors and actresses, including Richard Gere (in *Sommersby*) and Gwyneth Paltrow (in *Seven*). She operates the Joanne Harris Salon in Los Angeles. **Lenore S. Kakita, M.D.,** is an assistant clinical professor of dermatology at UCLA School of Medicine in Los Angeles and a dermatologist in Glendale, California. **Philip Kingsley,** see Dandruff. **Jack Myers,** a professional cosmetologist for more than 40 years, is a member of Hair America, the educational body of the National Cosmetology Association. He is also the owner and operator of Jack Myers Hair Styles in Owensboro, Kentucky. **Victor Newcomer, M.D.,** is a professor of dermatology at the UCLA School of Medicine in Los Angeles. **Anja Vaisanen** is a hairstylist at New York City. Trained in Finland, she's been a stylist for more than 10 years.

HANGOVERS

Stephen Amiel, see Addiction. **Kenneth Blum, Ph.D.,** is an adjunct research professor in the department of biological sciences at the University of North Texas in Denton and a retired professor of pharmacology at the University of Texas Health Sciences Center at San Antonio. He is also the president and chief executive officer of NutriGenomics Inc. in San Antonio. **John Brick, Ph.D.,** is the former chief of research in the division of education and training at the Center of Alcohol Studies at Rutgers, the State University of New Jersey, in Piscataway. He is now the executive director of Intoxikon International in Yardley, Pennsylvania. **Seymour Diamond, M.D.,** is director and founder of the Diamond Headache Clinic and the Inpatient Headache Unit at St. Joseph Hospital in Chicago. He also is executive chairman of the National Headache Foundation. He has written several books on headaches. **Von Lierer, Ph.D.,** is a former cognitive psychologist at Stanford University. **Mack Mitchell, M.D.,** is president of the Alcoholic Beverage Medical Research Foundation in Baltimore and chairman of medicine at the Carolinas Medical Center in Charlotte, North Carolina.

HEADACHE AND MIGRAINE Seymour Diamond, see Hangovers. **Harry C. Ehrmantraut, Ph.D.,** is author of *Headaches: The Drugless Way to Lasting Relief.* **Jerome Goldstein, M.D.,** is a private practitioner and director of the San Francisco Headache Clinic and the San Francisco Clinical Research Center. **Robert Kunkel, M.D.,** is a consultant in the department of neurology at the Cleveland Clinic Headache Center in Ohio. He also is president of the National Headache Foundation. **Ninan T. Mathew, M.D.,** is director of the Houston Headache Clinic in Texas. He also is president of the International Headache Society. **Joel Saper, M.D.,** is director of the Michigan Head Pain and Neurological Institute in Ann Arbor. He also is the author of the *Handbook of Headache Management.* **Douglas Schar,** see Acne. **Fred Sheftell, M.D.,** is director of the New England Center for Headache in Stamford, Connecticut. **Patricia Solbach, Ph.D.,** is a neuroscience scientific liaison for Ortho-McNeil Pharmaceutical, a division of Johnson & Johnson in Lawrence, Kansas, and former director of the Headache and Internal Medicine Research Center at the Menninger Clinic in Topeka. **Seymour Solomon, M.D.,** is a professor of neurology at Albert Einstein College of Medicine at Yeshiva University and director of the Headache Unit at Montefiore Medical Center, both in Bronx.

HEART PALPITATIONS James Frackelton, **M.D.,** has a practice in Cleveland and does research on vascular disease and immunology. He is past president of the American College of Advancement in Medicine and president of the American Institute of Medical Preventics. **John O. Lawder,** see Anal Fissures. **Dennis S. Miura, M.D., Ph.D.,** is an assistant clinical professor of medicine at the Albert Einstein College of Medicine at Yeshiva University and director of cardiology at the Bronx/Westchester Medical Group, both in the Bronx. **Douglas Schar,** see Acne.

HEARTBURN Stephen Amiel, see Addiction. **Larry I. Good, M.D.,** is a former member of the Long Island Gastrointestinal Disease Group in Merrick, New York. He also was an assistant professor of medicine at the State University of New York at Stony Brook. **Francis S. Kleckner, M.D.,** is a gastroenterologist in Allentown, Pennsylvania. **Samuel Klein,** see Belching. **Daniel B. Mowrey, Ph.D.,** of Lehi, Utah, is a psychologist who specializes in psychopharmacology and who has been researching herbs in medicine for 15 years. He also is president of American Phytotherapy Research Laboratory in Provo, Utah, and the author of *Herbal Tonic Therapies.* **Betty Shaver** is a herbalist and a lecturer on herbal and other home remedies is based in Grahamsville, New York.

HEAT EXHAUSTION Richard Keller, M.D., is an emergency room physician at St. Therese Hospital in Waukegan, Illinois. **Larry Kenney, Ph.D.,** is a professor of physiology and kinesiology in the Noll Physiological Research Center at Pennsylvania State University in University Park. **Lanny Nalder, Ph.D.,** is a professor in the department of health, physical education, and recreation and director of the Human Performance Research Center and the Wellness Center at Utah State University in Logan. **David**

Tanner is safety director and project manager for Tip Top Roofers in Atlanta.

HICCUPS Stephen Amiel, see Addiction. **André Dubois,** see Belching. **Ronnie Fern** is director of the ACJC Day-Care Center in Easton, Pennsylvania. **Richard McCallum,** see Belching. **Betty Shaver,** see Heartburn. **Douglas Schar,** see Acne.

HIGH BLOOD PRESSURE Stephen Amiel, see Addiction. **David M. Capuzzi, M.D., Ph.D.,** is a professor of medicine, biochemistry, and molecular pharmacology and director of the Cardiovascular Disease Prevention Center at Thomas Jefferson University Hospital in Philadelphia. **Nilo Cater, M.D.,** is an assistant professor of internal medicine and a nutrition scholar at the Center for Human Nutrition at the University of Texas Southwestern Medical Center at Dallas. **Kristine Napier, R.D.,** is nutrition director of Nutrio.com, author of *Eat to Heal,* and co-author of *Eat Away Diabetes.* **Howard Weitz,** see Angina.

HIGH CHOLESTEROL Stephen Amiel, see Addiction. **David M. Capuzzi,** see High Blood Pressure. **Nilo Cater,** see High Blood Pressure. **Kristine Napier,** see High Blood Pressure. **Douglas Schar,** see Acne.

HIVES Stephen Amiel, see Addiction. **Michael Blate,** see Boils. **Leonard Grayson, M.D.,** is a skin allergy specialist and former clinical associate allergist and dermatologist at Southern Illinois University School of Medicine in Springfield. **Jerome Z. Litt, M.D.,** is a dermatologist and assistant clinical professor of dermatology at Case Western Reserve University School of Medicine in Cleveland. He is the author of *Your Skin: From Acne to Zits.* **Thomas Squier** is a retired former US Army Special Forces instructor. He is a Cherokee herbologist, grandson of a medicine man, and writes a newspaper column, *Living off the Land.*

HOSTILITY Stephen Amiel, see Addiction. **Karyn Buxman, R.N.,** is a public speaker who specializes in therapeutic humour and is the president of HUMORx, a company that helps people manage their stress and organizations improve their bottom line through humour, based in Hannibal, Missouri. **Paul A. Hauck, Ph.D.,** is a psychologist in Moline, Illinois. **Aaron R. Kipnis, Ph.D.,** is a psychotherapist in Santa Barbara, California, and the author of *Angry Young Men.* **John Lee, M.A.,** is the founder and director of several mental health programmes related to anger management and the author of *Facing the Fire.* **Lynne McClure, Ph.D.,** is president and consultant of McClure Associates in Mesa, Arizona, and the author of *Anger and Conflict in the Workplace* and *Risky Business: Managing Employee Violence in the Workplace.* **Marilyn J. Sorensen, Ph.D.,** is a clinical psychologist and author of *Breaking the Chain of Low Self-Esteem* and *Low Self-Esteem: Misunderstood and Misdiagnosed.*

HOT FLUSHES Larrian Gillespie, M.D., is a retired assistant clinical professor of urology and urogynaecology and president of Healthy Life Publications. She is the author of *The Menopause Diet* and *The Goddess Diet.* **Mary Jane Minkin, M.D.,** is a clinical professor at Yale University School of Medicine and an obstetrician-gynaecologist in New Haven, Connecticut. She is the co-author of *What Every Woman Needs to Know about Menopause.*

HYPOTHERMIA Stephen Amiel, see Addiction. **Tod Schimelpfenig,** see Frostbite. **James Sturm,** see Frostbite.

IMPOTENCE Neil Baum, M.D., is associate clinical professor of urology at Tulane University School of Medicine and a staff urologist with Touro Infirmary, both in New Orleans. **Richard E. Berger, M.D.,** is a urologist and a professor at the University of Washington in Seattle and director of the Reproductive and Sexual Medicine Clinic at the university. **James Goldberg, Ph.D.,** is research director of the Bari/Goldberg Clinic at Chula Vista, California. **Irwin Goldstein, M.D.,** is a professor of urology at Boston University School of Medicine. **Douglas Schar,** see Acne.

INCONTINENCE Cheryle Gartley is president of the Simon Foundation for Continence in Wilmette, Illinois. **Katherine Jeter, Ed.D.,** is founder of the National Association for Continence in Spartanburg, South Carolina. **Joseph Montella, M.D.,** is director of urogynecology at Jefferson Medical College of Thomas Jefferson University in Philadelphia. **Abraham N. Morse, M.D.,** is an assistant professor of urogynecology at the University of Massachusetts Medical School in Worcester. **Neil Resnick, M.D.,** is a professor of medicine and chief of the division of geriatric medicine at the University of Pittsburgh Medical Center. **Robert Schlesinger, M.D.,** is a urologist at Faulkner Hospital in Jamaica Plain, Massachusetts.

INFANT COLIC Stephen Amiel, see Addiction. **Morris Green, M.D.,** is chairman of the department of paediatrics at Indiana University School of Medicine in Indianapolis. **Linda Jonides,** see Bed-wetting. **Helen Neville, R.N.,** is director of the Inborn Temperament Project at Kaiser Permanente Hospital in Oakland, California, and the author of *Temperament Tools.* **Anne Price,** see Bed-wetting. **Douglas Schar,** see Acne.

INFERTILITY Stephen Amiel, see Addiction. **Serafina Corsello, M.D.,** is medical director of the Corsello Center for Complementary-Alternative Medicine in New York City. She is the author of *The Ageless Woman.* **Linda C. Giudice, M.D., Ph.D.,** is director of the division of reproductive endocrinology and fertility at Stanford University. **John Jarrett, M.D.,** is a reproductive endocrinologist in Indianapolis. **Douglas Schar,** see Acne. **Robert Stillman, M.D.,** is a clinical professor in the department of obstetrics and gynaecology at Georgetown University School of Medicine in Washington, DC, and medical director at the Shady Grove Fertility Reproductive Science Center in Rockville, Maryland.

INGROWING HAIRS Rodney Basler, M.D., see Boils. **Jerome Z. Litt,** see Hives.

INGROWING TOENAILS Glenn Copeland, see Athlete's Foot. **Frederick Hass,** see Athlete's

Foot. **Suzanne M. Levine,** see Athlete's Foot.

INSOMNIA Sonia Ancoli-Israel, Ph.D., is a psychologist and a professor in the department of psychiatry at the University of California, San Diego, School of Medicine and the director of the Sleep Disorders Clinic at the VA Medical Center in San Diego. **Jean R. Joseph-Vanderpool, M.D.,** is an associate programme director for the Sleep Disorder Center at Del Sol Medical Center in El Paso, Texas. **Mortimer Mamelak, M.D.,** is director of the Sleep Disorders Clinic at Baycrest Hospital at the University of Toronto. **Merrill M. Mitler, Ph.D.,** is a professor of neuropharmacology at the Scripps Research Institute in La Jolla, California, and a clinical professor of psychiatry at the University of California, San Diego. He is also associated with Pacific Sleep Medicine Services in La Jolla. **David Neubauer, M.D.,** is an associate director at the Johns Hopkins Sleep Disorders Center in Baltimore. He is also a general psychiatrist in the department of psychiatry at the Johns Hopkins University, also in Baltimore. **Douglas Schar,** see Acne. **Magdi Soliman, Ph.D.,** is a professor of neuropharmacology at Florida A&M University College of Pharmacy in Tallahassee, Florida. **Edward Stepanski, Ph.D.,** is director of the Sleep Disorder Service and Research Center at the Rush-Presbyterian-St Luke's Medical Center in Chicago. **Michael Stevenson, Ph.D.,** is a psychologist and clinical director of the North Valley Sleep Disorders Center in Mission Hills, California. **James K. Walsh, Ph.D.,** is a clinical professor at the St. Louis University School of Medicine and executive director and senior scientist at the Sleep Medicine and Research Center of St. Luke's Hospital in Chesterfield, Missouri.

IRRITABLE BOWEL SYNDROME Donna Copeland, Ph.D., is a professor of paediatrics (psychology) and chief of the behavioural medicine section at the University of Texas M. D. Anderson Cancer Center in Houston. She is also a clinical psychologist and past president of the American Psychological Association's Division of Psychological Hypnosis. **Douglas A. Drossman, M.D.,** is a professor of medicine and psychiatry with the division of digestive diseases and co-director of the UNC Center for Functional Gastrointestinal and Motility Disorders at the University of North Carolina at Chapel Hill School of Medicine. He is a gastroenterologist with psychiatric training. **Nancy Norton** is founder of the International Foundation for Functional Gastrointestinal Disorders in Milwaukee. **Mark Pimentel, M.D.,** is assistant director of the gastrointestinal motility programme at Cedars-Sinai Medical Center in Los Angeles, and lead author of a 2000 study in the *American Journal of Gastroenterology* on bacterial overgrowth and irritable bowel syndrome. **James B. Rhodes, M.D.,** was a professor of medicine with the division of gastroenterology at the University of Kansas Medical Center in Kansas City. **Douglas Schar,** see Acne. **William J. Snape Jr., M.D.,** is a clinical professor of medicine at University of California, Irvine; medical director of clinical motility laboratory at California Pacific Medical Center in San Francisco; and director at the Bowel Disease and Motility Center at Long Beach Memorial Medical Center in Long Beach.

JAW PAIN AND TMJ PROBLEMS Stephen Amiel, see Addiction. **Albert Forgione, Ph.D.,** is a pain specialist and director of research at the Gelb Craniomandibular Orofacial Pain Center at Tufts University School of Dental Medicine, Boston. **Sheldon Gross, D.D.S.,** is a dentist in Bloomfield, Connecticut. He is a lecturer in Tufts University School of Dental Medicine's postgraduate orofacial pain programme, Boston and the University of Medicine and Dentistry of New Jersey/New Jersey Dental School, Newark. He is also on the board of directors of the American Academy of Orofacial Pain, past president of the American Academy of Craniomandibular Disorders, and a member of both the American Pain Association and the American Headache Association. **Andrew S. Kaplan, D.M.D.,** is an associate clinical professor of dentistry at the Mount Sinai School of Medicine of New York University and director of the TMJ and Facial Pain Clinic and attending dentist at Mount Sinai Hospital, New York City. **Harold T. Perry, D.D.S., Ph.D.,** is a lecturer of orthodontics in the School of Dentistry at Marquette University, Milwaukee. He was a professor of orthodontics at the former Northwestern University Dental School, Chicago. He was also the editor of *The Journal of Craniomandibular Disorders* and a past president of the American Academy of Craniomandibular Disorders. **Owen J. Rogal, D.D.S.,** is the director of the Pain Center, Philadelphia, which specializes in many types of pain, including TMJ. He is a past executive director of the former American Academy of Head, Neck, and Facial Neck Pain, now called the American Academy of Craniofacial Pain.

JET LAG Stephen Amiel, see Addiction. **Charles Ehret, Ph.D.,** is a pioneer in the field of chronobiology, the study of time's effect on plants, animals, and people. He is a retired senior scientist from the Argonne National Laboratory, a unit of the US Department of Energy. **Al Lewy, M.D., Ph.D.,** is a psychiatrist at Oregon Health Sciences University School of Medicine in Portland. He has done studies on the effects of sunlight on the human body clock. **Timothy Monk, Ph.D.,** is a professor of psychiatry and director of the human chronobiology research programme at the University of Pittsburgh School of Medicine. **Marijo Readey, Ph.D.,** was formerly a researcher at the Argonne National Laboratory, a unit of the US Department of Energy.

KNEE PAIN Marjorie Albohm is a certified athletic trainer at Ortho Indy in Indianapolis. She served on the medical staffs for the 1980 Winter and 1996 Summer Olympics and the 1987 Pan American Games. **Stephen Amiel,** see Addiction. **Lisa Dobloug** is a fitness and spa consultant in Washington, DC. She is president of Saga Fitness. Many of her clients are older people who wish to remain active and who appreciate her sound advice about warming up, stretching, and cooling down. **James M. Fox, M.D.,** specializes in arthroscopic and reconstructive knee surgery at the Southern California Orthopaedic Institute in Van Nuys, California. He is the author of *Save Your Knees* and was a member of the medical staff for the 1984 Summer Olympics. **Gary M. Gordon, D.P.M.,** has a sports medicine practice in Glenside, Pennsylvania, where he specializes in podiatric medicine and foot surgery.

Rich Phaigh is co-director of the American Institute of Sports Massage in New York City and the owner of a therapeutic massage clinic in Eugene, Oregon. He has taught more than 250 classes in advanced therapeutic technique in the United States and abroad. Phaigh has worked on the likes of running stars Alberto Salazar and Joan Samuelson. **Douglas Schar,** see Acne.

LACTOSE INTOLERANCE Theodore Bayless, M.D., is the clinical director of the Meyerhoff Digestive Disease Center at the Johns Hopkins University Hospital, Baltimore. **Jeffrey Biller, M.D.,** is a gastroenterologist at the Center for Paediatric Gastroenterology and Nutrition, Boston. **Naresh Jain, M.D.,** is a gastroenterologist in Niagara Falls, New York. **Seymour Sabesin, M.D.,** is a gastroenterologist and director of the section of digestive diseases at Rush-Presbyterian-St Luke's Medical Center, Chicago.

LARYNGITIS Robert Feder, M.D., is an otolaryngologist in the Los Angeles area. He is the physician on-call for the Music Center, the Performing Arts Center of Los Angeles County. He is also a former professor of drama and a former professor of otolaryngology at UCLA. **Scott Kessler, M.D.,** is a New York City otolaryngologist specializing in performing-arts medicine. He is the physician for many of the performers at the Metropolitan Opera and the City Opera, as well as for cast members of Broadway plays and cabarets. He is also on the staffs of Mount Sinai and Beth Israel Hospitals in New York City. **Laurence Levine, M.D., D.D.S.,** is an associate clinical professor of otolaryngology at Washington University School of Medicine in St. Louis and an otolaryngologist in Creve Coeur and St. Charles, Missouri. **Douglas Schar,** see Acne. **George T. Simpson II, M.D.,** was chairman of the department of otolaryngology at Boston University School of Medicine, University Hospital, and Boston City Hospital. He was also an attending physician at Children's Hospital Medical Center and the Veterans Administration Hospital and a member of the scientific advisory committee for the Voice Foundation.

LEG PAIN Robert Ginsburg, M.D., is the former director of the Center for Interventional Vascular Therapy at Stanford University Hospital. **Jess R. Young, M.D.,** is the former chairman of the department of vascular medicine at the Cleveland Clinic Foundation in Ohio.

MEMORY PROBLEMS Stephen Amiel, see Addiction. **Gunnar Gouras, M.D.,** is an assistant professor of neurology and neuroscience at the Joan and Sanford I. Weill Medical College of Cornell University and an Alzheimer's researcher at Fisher Center for Alzheimer's Research at Rockefeller University, both in New York City. **Cynthia R. Green, Ph.D.,** is an assistant clinical professor of psychiatry at Mount Sinai School of Medicine of New York University in New York City. She is also president of Memory Arts, a consulting firm that provides memory fitness training to corporate executives, and the author of *Total Memory Workout.* **Allan Hobson, M.D.,** is a professor of psychiatry at Harvard Medical School and director of the Neurophysiology and Sleep Laboratory at Massachusetts Mental Health Center in Boston. **Brigitte Mars**

is a herbalist and teacher at the Rocky Mountain Center for Botanical Studies in Boulder, Colorado. She is also a professional member of the American Herbalists Guild. **Douglas Schar,** see Acne.

MENOPAUSE **Stephen Amiel,** see Addiction. **Connie Catellani, M.D.,** is a physician in Skokie, Illinois. **Larrian Gillespie,** see Hot Flushes. **Mary Jane Minkin,** see Hot Flushes. **Douglas Schar,** see Acne.

MORNING SICKNESS **Deborah Gowen,** a certified nurse-midwife, works for Women-Care in Arlington, Massachusetts. **Tekoa King,** a nurse-midwife, has been delivering babies for more than a decade and has taught nurse practitioners at the University of California, San Francisco. She is affiliated with the Bay Area Midwifery Service. **Wataru Ohashi** is an internationally known teacher of ohashiatsu and founder of the Ohashi Institute, a nonprofit organization in New York City. **Gregory Radio,** see Breast Pain. **Douglas Schar,** see Acne. **Yvonne S.Thornton,** see Breast Pain.

MOTION SICKNESS **Patricia Cowings, Ph.D.,** is director of the Psychophysiological Research Laboratory at NASA's Ames Research Center in Moffett Field, California. **Roderic W. Gillilan, O.D.,** is a retired optometrist in Eugene, Oregon, where he still specializes in the treatment of motion sickness. **Horst Konrad, M.D.,** is former chairman of the Committee on Equilibrium of the American Academy of Otolaryngology/Head and Neck Surgery, and professor and chairman of the division of otolaryngology at Southern Illinois University School of Medicine in Springfield. **Robert Salada, M.D.,** is an assistant professor of medicine at Case Western Reserve University School of Medicine in Cleveland. He is also director of the Travelers Health Care Center of the University Hospitals of Cleveland, a first-of-its-kind service that provides health information and immunizations to travelers and immigrants. **Rafael Tarnopolsky, M.D.,** is a former professor of otolaryngology at the University of Osteopathic Medicine and Health Sciences in Des Moines, Iowa, who now lives in Pittsburgh.

MOUTH ULCERS **Robert Goepp, D.D.S., Ph.D.,** is a professor emeritus in the departments of surgery and pathology, specializing in oral pathology at the University of Chicago Medical Center and hospital in Illinois. **Jerome Z. Litt,** see Hives. **Douglas Schar,** see Acne. **Harold R. Stanley, D.D.S.,** is a professor emeritus of dentistry at the University of Florida College of Dentistry in Gainesville. **Varro E. Tyler, Ph.D.,** was a professor of pharmacognosy at Purdue University in West Lafayette, Indiana, and author of The Honest Herbal. He also served as a Prevention magazine advisor. **Andrew Weil,** see Anxiety. **Craig Zunka, D.D.S.,** is a dentist in Front Royal, Virginia, and is past president and advisor to the Board of the Holistic Dental Association. He also is a diplomate of the Board of Dental Homeopathy.

MUSCLE PAIN **Scott Donkin, D.C.,** is a partner in the Chiropractic Associates, Lincoln, Nebraska. He is also an industrial consultant and author of Sitting on the Job. **Carol Folkerts** is formerly an orthopaedic

co-ordinator of physical therapy at the University of Maryland Hospital, Baltimore. **Allan Levy, M.D.,** has a private practice in sports medicine in Woodcliff Lake and is a team physician for the New York Giants football team. **Mike McCormick** is a partner with AthletiCo Sports Medicine and Physical Therapy Center in LaGrange Park, Illinois. **Gabe Mirkin, M.D.,** is an associate clinical professor of paediatrics at Georgetown University School of Medicine in Washington, DC, and in practice at Mirkin Medical Consultants in Kensington, Maryland. He is author of several sports medicine books, including Women and Exercise, and a syndicated newspaper columnist and broadcaster. **Ted Percy, M.D.,** is associate professor emeritus of orthopaedic surgery and sports medicine and head of the sports medicine section at the Arizona Health Sciences Center at the University of Arizona College of Medicine, Tucson. **Bob Reese** is former head trainer for the New York Jets and past president of the Professional Football Athletic Trainers Society. He is now an associate professor at the College of Health Sciences in Roanoke, Virginia. **Douglas Schar,** see Acne.

NAIL PROBLEMS **Stephen Amiel,** see Addiction. **Barbara Bealer** is the assistant director of the Allentown School of Cosmetology in Pennsylvania. **Coyle S. Connolly, D.O.,** is an assistant clinical professor at the Philadelphia College of Osteopathic Medicine and a dermatologist practising in Linwood, New Jersey. **C. Ralph Daniel III, M.D.,** see Age Spots. **Boni Elewski, M.D.,** is a professor of dermatology at the University of Alabama at Birmingham. **Dee Anna Glaser, M.D.,** is an associate professor of dermatology at St. Louis University School of Medicine. **Rita Johnson** is the director of the Allentown School of Cosmetology in Pennsylvania. **Paul Kechijian, M.D.,** is an associate clinical professor of dermatology and chief of the nail section at the New York University Medical Center in Great Neck. **Joni Keim Loughran,** is the author of Joni Loughran's Natural Skin Care. **Audrey Kunin, M.D.,** see Age Spots.

NAPPY RASH **Stephen Amiel,** see Addiction. **Morris Green, M.D.,** see Infant Colic. **Linda Jonides,** see Bed-wetting. **Anne Price,** see Bed-wetting. **Douglas Schar,** see Acne.

NAUSEA AND VOMITING **Stephen Bezruchka, M.D.,** is an emergency physician at Virginia Mason Hospital and Group Health Hospital in Seattle and an affiliate associate professor in the School of Public Health and Community Medicine at the University of Washington in Seattle. **Joseph M. Helms, M.D.,** is a medical acupuncturist in Berkeley, California, and a clinical instructor at the UCLA School of Medicine in Los Angeles. He is the author of Acupuncture Energetics. **Lois Johnson, M.D.,** is a physician in Sebastopol, California and a professional member of the American Herbalists Guild. **Samuel Klein,** see Belching. **Kenneth Koch, M.D.,** is a gastroenterologist at the Milton S. Hershey Medical Center of the Pennsylvania State University in Hershey. **Daniel B. Mowrey,** see Heartburn. **Robert Warren, Pharm.D.,** is a pharmacist at United Pharmacy in Dinuba, California.

NECK PAIN Stephen Amiel, see Addiction.
Mark Gostine, M.D., is president of Michigan Pain
Consultants, based in Grand Rapids. **Joanne Griffin**
was formerly a senior physical therapist and inpatient
headache treatment therapist in the New England
Center for Headache at Greenwich Hospital in Con-
necticut. **Robert Kunkel,** see Headache and Migraine.
Mitchell A. Price, D.C., is a chiropractor in Reading,
Pennsylvania. **Douglas Schar,** see Acne.

NIGHT BLINDNESS Quinn Brackett, Ph.D.,
is a retired research scientist at the Texas Transporta-
tion Institute of Texas A&M University in College Station. **Jill C. Hennessey, M.S.,** is formerly assistant to
the director of science at the Foundation Fighting
Blindness in Baltimore. **Creig Hoyt, M.D.,** is vice
chairman of the department of ophthalmology at the
University of California, San Francisco, Medical Center.
Alan Laties, M.D., is a professor of ophthalmology at
the Scheie Eye Institute of the University of Pennsylvania School of Medicine in Philadelphia. **Charles
Zegeer** is associate director of the Highway Safety
Research Center at the University of North Carolina
at Chapel Hill.

NOSEBLEED Stephen Amiel, see Addiction.
Mark Baldree, M.D., is an otolaryngologist in
Phoenix. He is a staff member in the division of otolaryngology in the department of surgery at Good
Samaritan Hospital in Phoenix. **Christine Haycock,
M.D.,** is a professor of clinical surgery at the Univer-
sity of Medicine and Dentistry of New Jersey/New
Jersey Medical School in Newark. She maintains a private practice in Newark. **John A. Henderson, M.D.,**
is an assistant clinical professor of surgery at the University of California, San Diego, School of Medicine and
an otolaryngologist and allergist in San Diego. **Alvin
Katz, M.D.,** is an otolaryngologist and surgeon director of the Manhattan Eye, Ear, Nose, and Throat
Hospital in New York City. He is past president of the
American Rhinologic Society. **Gilbert Levitt, M.D.,** is
a retired otolaryngologist and former clinical instructor of otolaryngology at the University of Washington School of Medicine in Seattle. **Jerold
Principato, M.D.,** is an associate clinical professor of
otolaryngology in the department of surgery at
George Washington University School of Medicine and
Health Sciences in Washington, DC. He is also an instructor at the American Academy of Otolaryngology
and an otolaryngologist in Bethesda, Maryland.

OSTEOARTHRITIS Stephen Amiel, see Addiction. **Neal Barnard, M.D.,** is the president of the
Physician's Committee for Responsible Medicine in
Washington, DC, and the author of *Foods That Fight
Pain.* **Justus Fiechtner, M.D.,** is head of rheumatology
at Michigan State University College of Human Medicine in East Lansing. **Ted Fields, M.D.,** is a rheumatologist at the Hospital for Special Surgery in New York
City. **Sol Grazi, M.D.,** is an assistant professor of
family medicine at the University of Colorado School
of Medicine in Denver. **Stanley Jacob, M.D.,** is a professor of surgery at the Oregon Health Sciences University in Portland. **Alan Lichtbroun, M.D.,** is an
assistant professor of rheumatology and the internal
medicine director of the alternative medicine

department at the Robert Wood School in New
Brunswick, New Jersey. **Michael Loes, M.D.,** is
director of the Arizona Pain Institute in Phoenix and
author of *The Healing Response.*

OSTEOPOROSIS Melba Iris Ovalle, M.D., is
medical director of the Osteoporosis Center of
Evanston Northwestern Healthcare in Highland Park,
Illinois. **Robert R. Recker, M.D.,** is director of the
Osteoporosis Research Center at Creighton Univer-
sity School of Medicine in Omaha, Nebraska.

PEPTIC ULCERS Samuel Meyers, M.D., is a
gastroenterologist and clinical professor of medicine at
the Mount Sinai School of Medicine of New York University in New York City. **Philip Miner, M.D.,** is a
gastroenterologist and the president and medical
director of Oklahoma Foundation for Digestive
Research in Oklahoma City.

PHLEBITIS Michael D. Dake, M.D., is an associate professor of radiology and chief of the division of
cardiovascular and interventional radiology at Stanford
University Medical Center. **Robert Ginsburg,** see Leg
Pain. **Jess R. Young,** see Leg Pain.

PHOBIAS AND FEARS Stephen Amiel, see
Addiction. **David H. Barlow, Ph.D.,** is a professor
and director of the Center for Anxiety and Related
Disorders at Boston University. **Christopher
McCullough, Ph.D.,** has a practice in San Francisco.
He is the founder and former director of the San Fran-
cisco Anxiety and Phobia Recovery Center. He is co-
author of *Managing Your Anxiety* and author of *Always at
Ease* and *Nobody's Victim.* **Jerilyn Ross, M.A.,
L.I.C.S.W.,** is president and chief executive officer of
the Anxiety Disorder Association of America, director
of the Ross Center for Anxiety and Related Disorders
in Washington, DC, and co-author of *Triumph over Fear.*
Douglas Schar, see Acne. **Manuel D. Zane, M.D.,** is
founder and former director of the Phobia Clinic at
White Plains Hospital Medical Center in New York.

PREMENSTRUAL SYNDROME
Guy Abraham, M.D., is a former professor of ob-
stetrics and gynecologic endocrinology at the UCLA
School of Medicine in Los Angeles and has conducted
extensive research on PMS. **Penny Wise Budoff,
M.D.,** founded the Women's Medical Center in Beth-
page, New York, and is author of *No More Hot Flashes
and Even More Good News* and other related books.
Susan Lark, M.D., is director of the PMS Self-Help
Center in Los Altos, California, and author of *Dr Susan
Lark's Premenstrual Syndrome Self-Help Book.* **Edward
Portman, M.D.,** is a PMS consultant and researcher
and was formerly the director of the Portman Clinic in
Madison, Wisconsin. **Douglas Schar,** see Acne. **Peter
Vash, M.D.,** is executive director of the Lindora Medical Clinic in Costa Mesa, California. He is also an
endocrinologist and internist on the clinical faculty of
the UCLA Medical Center in Los Angeles and a
specialist in eating disorders.

PROSTATE PROBLEMS Winston Craig,
R.D., Ph.D., is a professor of nutrition at Andrews
University in Berrien Springs, Michigan. **Willard**

Dean, M.D., is a holistic physician in Glorieta, New Mexico. **Martin K. Gelbard, M.D.,** is assistant clinical professor of urology at the University of California, Los Angeles, School of Medicine and the author of *Solving Prostate Problems.* **Elizabeth Platz, Sc.D.,** is an assistant professor in the department of epidemiology at Johns Hopkins University Bloomberg School of Public Health in Baltimore. **Douglas Schar,** see Acne.

PSORIASIS **Philip Anderson, M.D.,** was a professor and chairman of the department of dermatology at the University of Missouri-Columbia School of Medicine. **Eugene Farber, M.D.,** was president of the Psoriasis Research Institute and former professor and chairman of the department of dermatology at Stanford University School of Medicine. **Laurence Miller, M.D.,** is a dermatologist in Chevy Chase, Maryland, and a member of the medical advisory board of the National Psoriasis Foundation and a special advisor to the director of the National Institute of Arthritis and Musculoskeletal and Skin Diseases of the National Institutes of Health. **Douglas Schar,** see Acne. **Vincent Ziboh, Ph.D.,** is a professor of dermatology and biochemistry at the University of California, Davis, School of Medicine.

RASHES **C. Ralph Daniel,** see Age Spots. **Dee Anna Glaser,** see Nail Problems. **Larry Millikan, M.D.,** is chairman of the department of dermatology at Tulane University Medical Center in New Orleans. **William L. Epstein, M.D.,** is a professor emeritus of dermatology at the University of California, San Francisco, School of Medicine. **Robert Rietschel, M.D.,** is a staff dermatologist at the Ochsner Clinic in New Orleans and clinical professor of dermatology at the Louisiana State University School of Medicine and Tulane University Medical Center in New Orleans.

RAYNAUD'S SYNDROME **John Abruzzo, M.D.,** is director of the division of rheumatology and a professor of medicine at Thomas Jefferson University in Philadelphia. **Marc A. Brenner,** see Diabetes. **Murray Hamlet, D.V.M.,** is the former director of cold research at the U.S. Army Research Institute of Environmental Medicine in Natick, Massachusetts. He is now retired and is a consultant and lecturer on environmental medicine. **Donald McIntyre, M.D.,** is a retired dermatologist in Rutland, Vermont. **Frederick A. Reichle, M.D.,** has a practice affiliated with Mercy Suburban Hospital in Norristown, Pennsylvania. He was previously the chief of vascular surgery at Presbyterian University of Pennsylvania Medical Center in Philadelphia.

RESTLESS LEGS **Stephen Amiel,** see Addiction. **Richard K. Olney, M.D.,** is a professor of clinical neurology at the University of California, San Francisco. **Ronald F. Pfeiffer, M.D.,** is professor, vice chairman, and director in the department of neurology at the University of Tennessee Health Science Center in Memphis. **Lawrence Z. Stern, M.D.,** is a professor of neurology at the University of Arizona College of Medicine in Tucson.

ROAD RAGE **Leon James, Ph.D.,** is a professor of psychology at the University of Hawai'i, Honolulu.

He has researched aggressive driving for more than 20 years and is coauthor, with his wife Diane Nahl, Ph.D., of *Road Rage and Aggressive Driving.* Dr James and Dr Nahl run a Website DrDriving.org and are creators of an anti-aggressive driving video series called *RoadRageous.* **Diane Nahl, Ph.D.,** is professor and information scientist at the University of Hawai'i, Honolulu. She has studied aggressive driving for over 20 years. **Arnold P. Nerenberg, Ph.D.,** is a psychologist in Whittier, California, and a road-rage researcher. He is co-author of the American Institute for Public Safety's Road Rage Programme and author of *A 10-Step Compassion Programme,* for overcoming angry driving.

ROSACEA **C. Ralph Daniel,** see Age Spots. **Dee Anna Glaser,** see Nail Problems. **Larry Millikan,** see Rashes.

SAD (SEASONAL AFFECTIVE DISORDER) **Brenda Byrne, Ph.D.,** is a psychologist and director of the seasonal affective disorder programme of the light research programme at Jefferson Medical College of Thomas Jefferson University in Philadelphia. **Norman E. Rosenthal, M.D.,** is a clinical professor of psychiatry at Georgetown University in Washington, DC, and a former senior researcher at the National Institute of Mental Health. He is author of *Winter Blues: Seasonal Affective Disorder* and *The Emotional Revolution.* **Andrew Weil,** see Anxiety.

SCARRING **Jeffrey H. Binstock, M.D.,** is associate clinical professor of dermatologic surgery at the University of California, San Francisco, School of Medicine and a dermatologist in San Francisco and Mill Valley, California. **Gerald Imber, M.D.,** is an attending plastic surgeon at New York-Presbyterian Hospital, New York City. **Stephen Kurtin, M.D.,** is a practising dermatologist and an assistant professor of dermatology at the Mount Sinai Hospital, New York City. **Paul Lazar, M.D.,** is a professor emeritus of clinical dermatology at Northwestern University Medical School, Chicago. He is a former board member of the American Academy of Dermatology. **John F. Romano,** see Dermatitis and Eczema.

SCIATICA **Andrew J. Cole, M.D.,** is the medical director of the Spine Center at Overlake Hospital Medical Center and has a private practice with Northwest Spine and Sports Physicians in Bellevue, Washington. He was the director of Spine Rehabilitation Services at Baylor University Medical Center in Houston from 1993 to 1996, and co-author of *Low Back Pain.* **John G. Heller, M.D.,** is a professor of orthopaedic surgery and director of the spine fellowship programme at the Emory Spine Center at Emory University School of Medicine in Atlanta. **John J. Triano, D.C., Ph.D.,** is director of the chiropractic division of the Texas Back Institute, Plano, Texas. His doctorate is in spine biomechanics. He specializes in prevention, treatment, and rehabilitation of spine disorders.

SHIN SPLINTS **Marjorie Albohm,** see Knee Pain. **Gary M. Gordon, D.P.M.,** has a sports medicine practice in Glenside, Pennsylvania, where he specializes in podiatric medicine and foot surgery. **Rich Phaigh,** see Knee Pain,

SHINGLES
Jules Altman, M.D., is a clinical professor of dermatology at Wayne State University in Detroit and a practitioner in Warren, Michigan. **James J. Nordlund, M.D.,** is a professor in the department of dermatology at the University of Cincinnati College of Medicine in Ohio. **Sota Omoigui, M.D.,** is medical director of the LA Pain Clinic in Hawthorne, California. **Leon Robb, M.D.,** is a pain-management specialist, anaesthesiologist, and director of the Robb Pain Management Group in Los Angeles, where he treats patients with shingles and conducts research. **Douglas Schar,** see Acne.

SIDE STITCHES
David Balboa, M.S.W., is a co-director of the Walking Project in New York City. He is an expert on walking and mind-body relationships. **Suki Munsell, Ph.D.,** a registered movement therapist, is president of the Dynamic Health and Fitness Institute in Corte Madera, California. A fitness consultant, her doctorate is in movement education and body transformations.

SINUSITIS
Stephen Amiel, see Addiction. **Terence M. Davidson, M.D.,** is a professor of head and neck surgery and director of the Nasal Dysfunction Clinic at the University of California, San Diego, Medical Center. **Howard M. Druce, M.D.,** is an associate clinical professor of medicine in the division of allergy and immunology at the University of Medicine and Dentistry of New Jersey/New Jersey Medical School in Newark. **Stanley N. Farb, M.D.,** is a retired chief of otolaryngology at Montgomery and Suburban Mercy Hospitals in Norristown, Pennsylvania. **Bruce W. Jafek, M.D.,** is a professor in the department of otolaryngology at the University of Colorado School of Medicine in Denver. He served as chairman of the department for 22 years before returning to clinical practise and teaching. Dr Jafek practises at University Hospital, Rose Medical Center, the Children's Hospital, and the Denver VA Medical Center.

SNORING
Stephen Amiel, see Addiction. **Earl V. Dunn, M.D.,** is a professor in the department of family medicine, faculty of medicine and health sciences, at the United Arab Emirates University in Al-Ain and a professor emeritus at the University of Toronto. **Philip Smith, M.D.,** is a professor of medicine and a physician in the division of pulmonary and critical care, who specializes in sleep disorders, at the Johns Hopkins University School of Medicine in Baltimore. **Philip Westbrook, M.D.,** is chairman of the board and medical director of Advanced Brain Monitoring, California. He was founder and former director of the Sleep Disorders Centers at the Mayo Clinic in Rochester, Minnesota, and Cedars-Sinai Medical Center in Los Angeles, president of the American Academy of Sleep Medicine, and editor of the journal *Sleep.*

SORE THROAT
Stephen Amiel, see Addiction. **Donald Davis, Ph.D.,** is a research associate at the Biochemical Institute at the University of Texas at Austin. **Richard T. Glass,** see Cold Sores. **Jerome C. Goldstein, M.D.,** is a visiting professor of otolaryngology/head and neck surgery at Georgetown University School of Medicine in Washington, DC, and Albany Medical College in New York. He is also past executive vice president of the American Academy of Otolaryngology in Washington, DC. **Thomas Gossel,** see Acne. **Hueston King, M.D.,** is an associate clinical professor of otolaryngology at the University of Texas Southwest Medical Center in Dallas and the University of Florida in Gainesville. He is also an ear, nose, and throat specialist in Venice, Florida. **Robert Rountree, M.D.,** is a holistic physician in Boulder, Colorado, and coauthor of *Immunotics.* **Douglas Schar,** see Acne. **Jason Surow, M.D.,** is an ear, nose and throat specialist in Teaneck and Midland Park, New Jersey. He's an attending otolaryngologist at Valley Hospital in Ridgewood, New Jersey and Holy Name Hospital in Teaneck. **Irwin Ziment, M.D.,** is a professor of medicine in the department of pulmonary and critical care medicine at UCLA School of Medicine in Los Angeles.

SPLINTERS
C. Ralph Daniel, see Age Spots. **Dee Anna Glaser,** see Nail Problems.

SPRAINS
John M. McShane, M.D., is an associate clinical professor of family medicine at Jefferson Medical College of Thomas Jefferson University and director of sports medicine at Thomas Jefferson University Hospital, both in Philadelphia. **Michael Osborne, M.D.,** is senior associate consultant in the department of physical medicine and rehabilitation at Mayo Clinic Jacksonville, and an instructor at the Mayo Medical School in Jacksonville, Florida.

STRESS
Bradley W. Frederick, D.C., is a chiropractor and director of the International Institute of Sports Medicine in Los Angeles. **Emmett Miller, M.D.,** is medical director for the Center for Healing and Wellness in Menlo Park, California. He is a nationally recognized expert on stress and mind-body medicine. **Ronald Nathan, Ph.D.,** is a clinical professor at Albany Medical College in New York and co-author of *The Doctors' Guide to Instant Stress Relief.* **Paul J. Rosch, M.D.,** is a clinical professor of medicine and psychiatry at New York Medical College in Valhalla. He's also an adjunct clinical professor of medicine in psychiatry at the University of Maryland School of Medicine in Baltimore and president of the American Institute of Stress. **Douglas Schar,** see Acne.

SUNBURN
Stephen Amiel, see Addiction. **Rodney Basler,** see Boils. **Thomas Gossel,** see Acne. **Fredric Haberman, M.D.,** is an assistant clinical professor of medicine at the Albert Einstein College of Medicine of Yeshiva University in Bronx, New York, and director of the Haberman Dermatology Institute in Saddle Brook and Ridgewood, New Jersey, and New York City. **Carl Korn, M.D.,** is an assistant clinical professor of dermatology at the University of Southern California in Los Angeles. **Audrey Kunin,** see Age Spots. **Norman Levine, M.D.,** is a professor of medicine in the department of dermatology at the University of Arizona College of Medicine in Tucson. **Lia Schorr** is a skin-care specialist and director of Lia Schorr Institute of Cosmetics Skin-Care Training in New York City. She is the author of *Salonovations' Advanced Skin Care Handbook.* **Michael Schreiber, M.D.,** is senior clinical lecturer in the department of internal medicine at the University of Arizona College of Medicine in Tucson and a dermatologist in Tucson.

TEETHING Stephen Amiel, see Addiction. John A. Bogert, D.D.S., is a retired dentist in Chicago. Linda Jonides, see Bed-wetting.

TENDINITIS Scott Donkin, see Muscle Pain. Terry Malone, Ed.D., is the director of physical therapy at the University of Kentucky in Lexington. Bob Mangine is chairman of the American Physical Therapy Association's sports physical therapy section. He also is administrative director of rehabilitation at the Novacare Physical Rehabilitation in Florence, Kentucky, and author of *Physical Therapy of the Knee*. Ted Percy, see Muscle Pain. Bob Reese, see Muscle Pain.

TINNITUS Stephen Amiel, see Addiction. Dhyan Cassie, Au.D., is a doctor of audiology and co-ordinator of the Tinnitus/Hyperacusis Management Clinic for Speech and Hearing Associates at the College of New Jersey in Ewing. Marshall Chasin is an audiologist and director of auditory research at the Musicians' Clinics of Canada in Toronto and the author of *Musicians and the Prevention of Hearing Loss*. Douglas Mattox, M.D., is chairman of the department of otolaryngology-head and neck surgery at Emory University School of Medicine in Atlanta.

TOOTHACHE Philip D. Corn, D.D.S., has a practice in Philadelphia. He is a former director of the Pennsylvania Academy of General Dentistry. Roger P. Levin, see Bad Breath. Douglas Schar, see Acne. Richard Shepard, see Denture Problems. Jerry F. Taintor, see Bad Breath.

TOOTH STAINS John D. B. Featherstone, Ph.D., is a professor and chairman of the department of preventive and restorative dental sciences in the School of Dentistry at the University of California, San Francisco. Roger P. Levin, see Bad Breath. Dean Lodding, D.D.S., is a dentist in Elgin, Illinois, and past president of the American Academy of Cosmetic Dentistry. Ronald I. Maitland, D.M.D., is a New York City dentist who specializes in cosmetic dentistry. He is chairman of the Greater New York Dental Meeting and an expert on dental stains.

URINARY TRACT INFECTIONS Larrian Gillespie, see Hot Flushes. Beverly Kloeppel, M.D., is associate director of the Student Health Center at the University of New Mexico in Albuquerque. Diana Koster, M.D., is vice president of medical affairs and medical director of Planned Parenthood of New Mexico. Mary Jane Minkin, see Hot Flushes. Douglas Schar, see Acne.

VAGINAL AND YEAST INFECTIONS Larrian Gillespie, see Hot Flushes. Beverly Kloeppel, see Urinary Tract Infections. Diana Koster, see Urinary Tract Infections. Mary Jane Minkin, see Hot Flushes.

VARICOSE VEINS Lenise Banse, see Body Odour. John Clarke, M.D., is presently a consultant in Milton, Massachusetts, and was formerly a cardiologist with the Himalayan International Institute in Honesdale, Pennsylvania. Mindy Green is director of education at the Herbal Research Foundation in Boulder, Colorado. Paul Lazar, see Scarring. Brian McDonagh, M.D., is a phlebologist based in Chicago. He is the founder and medical director of Vein Clinics of America, the largest medical group in the country dedicated solely to the treatment of vein disorders. Dudley Phillips, M.D., of Darlington, Maryland, has practised family medicine for more than 40 years. He is now retired. Douglas Schar, see Acne. Eugene Strandness Jr., M.D., was a professor of surgery at the University of Washington School of Medicine in Seattle.

WARTS AND VERRUCAS Jeffrey S. Bland, Ph.D., is president and chief science officer of Metagenics, a leading health sciences company in Gig Harbor, Washington. Marc A. Brenner, see Diabetes. Robert Garry, Ph.D., is a professor of microbiology and immunology at Tulane University School of Medicine in New Orleans. Glenn Gastwirth, D.P.M., is executive director of the American Podiatric Medical Association. Thomas Goodman, see Athlete's Foot. Suzanne M. Levine, see Athlete's Foot. Christopher McEwen, M.D., is a dermatologist in Baton Rouge, Louisiana. Douglas Schar, see Acne. Nicholas Spanos, Ph.D., is a former professor of psychology at Carleton University in Ottawa, Canada. Owen Surman, M.D., is an assistant professor of psychiatry at Harvard Medical School and a psychiatrist at Massachusetts General Hospital in Boston.

WEIGHT PROBLEMS Stephen Amiel, see Addiction. Joseph Chromiak, Ph.D., is an assistant professor in the department of health, physical education, recreation, and sport at Mississippi State University in Starkville and a certified strength and conditioning specialist. Gary Foster, Ph.D., is clinical director of the weight and eating disorders programme at the University of Pennsylvania in Philadelphia. Mary Friesz, R.D., Ph.D., is a nutrition and wellness consultant and a certified diabetes educator in Boca Raton, Florida. Joanne Larsen, R.D., designs nutrition software and food and ingredient databases for software companies. She also has a nutrition information website at www.dietitian.com. Marsha D. Marcus, Ph.D., is an associate professor of psychiatry and psychology and chief of the behavioural medicine and eating disorders programme in the department of psychiatry at the University of Pittsburgh School of Medicine.

WRINKLES Stephen Amiel, see Addiction. Coyle S. Connolly, see Nail Problems. D'Anne Kleinsmith, M.D., is a cosmetic dermatologist at William Beaumont Hospital in Royal Oak, Michigan, and is an expert on wrinkles. Audrey Kunin, see Age Spots. Joni Keim Loughran is a skin-care expert in Petaluma, California. Douglas Schar, see Acne.

INDEX

Bold numbers refer to main entries

OTHER RODALE BOOKS
AVAILABLE FROM PAN MACMILLAN

1-4050-3337-1	The Acne Cure	*Dr Terry J. Dubrow and Brenda D. Adderly*	£10.99
1-4050-4099-8	Before the Heart Attacks	*Dr H. Robert Superko*	£12.99
1-4050-0667-6	The Green Pharmacy	*Dr James A. Duke*	£14.99
1-4050-0674-9	The Hormone Connection	*Gale Maleskey & Mary Kittel*	£15.99
1-4050-3339-8	The Immune Advantage	*Ellen Mazo*	£14.99
1-4050-3335-5	Picture Perfect Weight Loss	*Dr Howard Shapiro*	£14.99
1-4050-3286-3	Stay Fertile Longer	*Mary Kittel with Dr Deborah Metzger*	£12.99
1-4050-3340-1	When Your Body Gets The Blues	*Marie-Annette Brown and Jo Robinson*	£10.99

All Pan Macmillan titles can be ordered from our website, *www.panmacmillan.com,* or from your local bookshop and are also available by post from:

Bookpost, PO Box 29, Douglas, Isle of Man IM99 1BQ
Credit cards accepted. For details:
Telephone: 01624 836000
Fax: 01624 670923
E-mail: bookshop@enterprise.net
www.bookpost.co.uk

Free postage and packing in the United Kingdom.

Prices shown above were correct at time of going to press.
Pan Macmillan reserve the right to show new retail prices on covers which may differ from those previously advertised in the text or elsewhere.

For information about buying *Rodale* titles in **Australia**, contact Pan Macmillan Australia.
Tel: 1300 135 113; fax: 1300 135 103; e-mail: *customer.service@macmillan.com.au*;
or visit: *www.panmacmillan.com.au*

For information about buying *Rodale* titles in **New Zealand**, contact Macmillan Publishers New Zealand Limited. Tel: (09) 414 0356; fax: (09) 414 0352; e-mail: *lyn@macmillan.co.nz*;
or visit: *www.macmillan.co.nz*